Imaging and Metabolism

Jason S. Lewis • Kayvan R. Keshari
Editors

Imaging and Metabolism

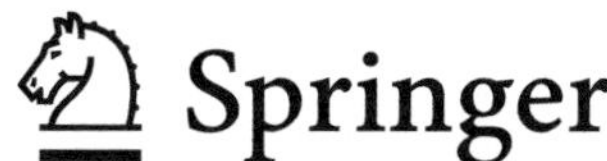

Editors
Jason S. Lewis
Department of Radiology and the Molecular Pharmacology Program
Memorial Sloan Kettering Cancer Center
New York, NY
USA

Kayvan R. Keshari
Department of Radiology and the Molecular Pharmacology Program
Memorial Sloan Kettering Cancer Center
New York, NY
USA

ISBN 978-3-319-61399-4 ISBN 978-3-319-61401-4 (eBook)
DOI 10.1007/978-3-319-61401-4

Library of Congress Control Number: 2017955382

Printed on acid-free paper

This Springer imprint is published by Springer Nature
The registered company is Springer International Publishing AG
The registered company address is: Gewerbestrasse 11, 6330 Cham, Switzerland

Foreword for Imaging and Metabolism

The editors have assembled an impressive and timely synthesis of two of the most dynamic fields in medicine: molecular imaging and metabolism. Recent advances in positron emission tomography, magnetic resonance imaging, and optical imaging not only allow us to image the human body but also to interrogate its physiology. These advances are timely because the worldwide obesity epidemic has forced scientists and physicians to rethink basic concepts of cellular and organismal metabolism. The in vivo metabolic insights being provided by molecular imaging techniques have the potential to revolutionize the understanding of diabetes and obesity, as well as to provide new insight into cardiac disease and other metabolic syndromes. Molecular imaging techniques are also shedding new light on how cellular metabolism is altered during the pathogenesis of proliferative disorders (including cancer and autoimmunity) and degenerative disorders (including Alzheimer's disease and Parkinson's syndrome).

The authors of each of the chapters are leading investigators in the evolving field of metabolic imaging and how it can be applied to the study of disease. For the introductory reader, the early chapters introduce the principles underlining molecular imaging and their application to the disease-related studies of organismal and cellular metabolism. For more advanced readers, the book provides an excellent synthesis of how recent advances in PET, MRI, and optical imaging have combined to advance the field of molecular imaging in pursuit of a greater understanding of human physiology. The later chapters describe the in vivo uses of metabolic imaging in studying the pathogenesis of a wide variety of human diseases.

Collectively, the chapters of this comprehensibly prepared book make a compelling case that molecular imaging of metabolic processes will transform our ability to diagnose and treat traditional and nontraditional metabolic diseases. It is a must-read for investigators interested in imaging and/or metabolism.

Craig B. Thompson
Memorial Sloan Kettering Cancer Center

Preface: Imaging and Metabolism

Both Metabolism and Molecular Imaging have recently received an increased interest across many scientific communities—especially with the emergence of the personalized medicine paradigm and the desire to better understand disease processes in a nondestructive and noninvasive manner.

Molecular imaging, as its name implies, is a field that lies squarely at the nidus of molecular biology and traditional medical imaging and is situated at the intersection of various disciplines—biology, medicine, chemistry, physics, genomics, pharmacology, and engineering. Over the past two decades, two factors have acted in concert to fuel the ascent of molecular imaging in both the laboratory and the clinic: an increased understanding of the molecular mechanisms of disease and the continued development of in vivo imaging technologies, ranging from improved detectors to novel labeling methodologies. Taking cancer as an example, both the cellular expression of disease biomarkers and fluctuations in tissue metabolism and microenvironment have emerged as extremely promising targets for imaging. Indeed, the field has produced effective molecularly targeted agents applied with a wide variety of imaging modalities, from fluorescence and luminescence to nuclear imaging and magnetic resonance.

With molecular imaging as a means to probe the inner workings of a cell, metabolism represents the fundamental biochemical processes that facilitate life. In the past century, an immense literature has been established elucidating the interconnected reactions, which transform nutrients into building blocks and functional cellular components and generate energy. Interestingly, metabolic reactions can establish a steady state that provides differential cell function and when derailed, in response to genomic or environmental changes, can result in a wide range of disease phenotypes. Moreover, dynamic aberrations in metabolism can lead to epigenetic regulation of gene expression, further manipulating cell function and even potentially cell fate decisions. With a reemergence of metabolism to the forefront of biochemical research, novel molecular imaging tools allow for the ability to further connect disease states with their fundamental causes, *in vivo*.

In this book, we sought for the first time to combine the latest insights into metabolism with state-of-the-art imaging technologies. In the first part of the book, we introduce the reader to advanced molecular imaging techniques as well as to the metabolism field. We then focus in Part II on approaches available for imaging metabolism. We complete the book with the specifics of imaging diseases, which have a metabolic component, e.g., cancer, neurodegeneration, diabetes, and fatty liver disease. The aim is to provide the reader with a multi-modality imaging compendium targeted at understanding metabolism from multiple viewpoints. Our overarching goal is for the first edition of this book to become a reference textbook for researchers interested in metabolism and the noninvasive tools that are available to interrogate aberrant metabolism in both the preclinical and clinical settings.

No work of this size can be achieved without significant help from some very special people. We would first like to thank all the contributors to this book—their efforts and work is very much appreciated. We would like to thank our postdocs and students for their insight and help reviewing and editing the chapters as well as Janet Folin and Karthik Periyasamy at Springer for their support and help. Finally, we would like to thank our better halves, Mikel and Parastou, for their patience and understanding while sitting through many evenings when we discussed planning this book over dinner.

New York, NY Jason S. Lewis
New York, NY Kayvan R. Keshari

Contents

Contributors

Erik H.J.G. Aarntzen Department of Radiology, Radboud University Medical Centre, Nijmegen, The Netherlands

Scott C. Beeman Mallinckrodt Institute of Radiology, Washington University, St. Louis, MO, USA

Ronald G. Blasberg Memorial Sloan Kettering Cancer Center, New York, NY, USA

Lewis C. Cantley Department of Medicine, Meyer Cancer Center, Weill Cornell Medicine, New York City, NY, USA

Woo June Choi Department of Bioengineering, University of Washington, Seattle, WA, USA

Derk Draper Department of Tumor Immunology, Radboud University Medical Centre, Nijmegen, The Netherlands

Joel R. Garbow Mallinckrodt Institute of Radiology, Washington University, St. Louis, MO, USA

The Alvin J. Siteman Cancer Center, Washington University, St. Louis, MO, USA

Jan Grimm Molecular Pharmacology Program, Memorial Sloan Kettering Cancer Center, New York, NY, USA

Department of Radiology, Memorial Sloan Kettering Cancer Center, New York, NY, USA

Robert J. Gropler Division of Radiological Sciences, Mallinckrodt Institute of Radiology, Washington University School of Medicine, St. Louis, MO, USA

Andrea L. Gropman The George Washington University School of Medicine, Washington, DC, USA

Katja Haedicke Molecular Pharmacology Program, Memorial Sloan Kettering Cancer Center, New York, NY, USA

Christopher J. Halbrook Department of Molecular and Integrative Physiology, University of Michigan, Ann Arbor, MI, USA

Tiffany M. Heaster Department of Biomedical Engineering, University of Wisconsin-Madison, Madison, WI, USA

Susanne Kossatz Department of Radiology, Memorial Sloan Kettering Cancer Center, New York, NY, USA

Ho-Joon Lee Department of Molecular and Integrative Physiology, University of Michigan, Ann Arbor, MI, USA

Jonathan T.C. Liu Department of Mechanical Engineering, University of Washington, Seattle, WA, USA

Costas A. Lyssiotis Department of Molecular and Integrative Physiology, University of Michigan, Ann Arbor, MI, USA

Division of Gastroenterology, Department of Internal Medicine, University of Michigan, Ann Arbor, MI, USA

Craig R. Malloy Departments of Radiology and Internal Medicine, Advanced Imaging Research Center, University of Texas Southwestern Medical Center, Dallas, TX, USA

VA North Texas Health Care System, Dallas, TX, USA

Jonathan McConathy Department of Radiology, University of Alabama at Birmingham School of Medicine, Birmingham, AL, USA

Division of Molecular Imaging and Therapeutics, University of Alabama at Birmingham, Birmingham, AL, USA

Vesselin Z. Miloushev Memorial Sloan Kettering Cancer Center, New York, NY, USA

Ephraim Parent Department of Radiology, Emory University School of Medicine, Atlanta, GA, USA

Carmen Paus Department of Tumor Immunology, Radboud University Medical Centre, Nijmegen, The Netherlands

Thomas Reiner Department of Radiology, Memorial Sloan Kettering Cancer Center, New York, NY, USA

Darren Roblyer Department of Biomedical Engineering, Boston University, Boston, MA, USA

Melissa Skala Department of Biomedical Engineering, University of Wisconsin-Madison, Madison, WI, USA

Mangala Srinivas Department of Tumor Immunology, Radboud University Medical Centre, Nijmegen, The Netherlands

Greg M. Thurber Department of Chemical Engineering, University of Michigan, Ann Arbor, MI, USA

Department of Biomedical Engineering, University of Michigan, Ann Arbor, MI, USA

Karissa Tilbury Department of Chemical and Biological Engineering, University of Maine, Orono, ME, USA

Sriram Venneti Department of Pathology, University of Michigan Medical School, Ann Arbor, MI, USA

Daniel R. Wahl Department of Radiation Oncology, University of Michigan Medical School, Ann Arbor, MI, USA

Matthew A. Wall Institute for Systems Biology, Seattle, WA, USA

Ruikang Wang Department of Bioengineering, University of Washington, Seattle, WA, USA

Matthew T. Whitehead Children's National Health System, Washington, DC, USA

David Wilson Department of Radiology, University of California San Francisco, San Francisco, CA, USA

Liang Zhang Department of Chemical Engineering, University of Michigan, Ann Arbor, MI, USA

Part I

Basic Principles

1 Molecular Imaging and Molecular Imaging Technologies

Katja Haedicke, Susanne Kossatz, Thomas Reiner, and Jan Grimm

1.1 Definition of the Field

Molecular imaging has become an integral component of modern medicine. Defined by the molecular imaging center of excellence as "the visualization, characterization, and measurement of biological processes at the cellular and molecular level in humans and other living systems", molecular imaging includes two- or three-dimensional noninvasive imaging as well as the quantification of acquired data over time [1]. Clinically, the importance of molecular imaging is paramount in the study and noninvasive diagnosis of diseases—based on molecular signatures rather than anatomic alterations—which in turn enables early detection of abnormalities and evaluation of new treatment approaches for improved survival rates. James and Gambhir summarized the main advantages of molecular imaging approaches: the possibility of studying cells in their natural environment without any disturbance from outside, the analysis of complex biological processes in real time, the investigation of signaling pathways in vivo, the gaining of information about drug delivery and pharmacokinetics, and the obtaining of multiple data sets in adequate resolution from the same patient over time [2].

Molecular imaging probes are an essential component in imaging molecular processes in vivo, in particular, for visualization of a target of interest [3]. The hallmarks of a highly sensitive and selective imaging probe include the ability to bind to the molecular target with high affinity [4]. A molecularly targeted probe must also possess suitable pharmacokinetic properties to avoid undesirable biodistribution, to allow for excretion or biodegradation, and to enable sufficient delivery into the target tissue. In the absence of these traits, false-positive results may occur without specific detection of the targeted biological process of interest, or unwanted accumulation in nontarget tissue may result. An ideal probe is biocompatible, i.e., the compound does not induce side effects, is not toxic, and does not induce an immune reaction or significant biological response within the body. Finally, intracellular targets require additional considerations; biological barriers such as cell membranes must be overcome for effective targeting. Cell membrane barriers may be surmounted either via active (receptor-mediated) or inactive transport, allowing the agent to pass through the barriers. Anatomical barriers present similar challenges,

K. Haedicke
Molecular Pharmacology Program, Memorial Sloan Kettering Cancer Center, New York, NY, USA

S. Kossatz • T. Reiner
Department of Radiology, Memorial Sloan Kettering Cancer Center, New York, NY, USA

J. Grimm (✉)
Molecular Pharmacology Program, Memorial Sloan Kettering Cancer Center, New York, NY, USA

Department of Radiology, Memorial Sloan Kettering Cancer Center, New York, NY, USA
e-mail: grimmj@mskcc.org

J.S. Lewis, K.R. Keshari (eds.), *Imaging and Metabolism*, DOI 10.1007/978-3-319-61401-4_1

most prominently the blood-brain barrier for targets in the central nervous system.

Imaging agent selection and optimization toward the intended use are, however, only two of the hurdles to be considered for targeted probe design. Equally important for successful imaging is the selection of an appropriate readout technology tailored to the biological problem. It should provide high-sensitivity images of sufficiently high resolution to detect early pathological changes on a molecular level. The last several decades have witnessed the development, validation, and evolution of a large array of imaging technologies [2, 5], including ultrasound [6], computed tomography (CT) [7], magnetic resonance imaging (MRI) [8], positron-emission tomography (PET) [9], single photon emission computed tomography (SPECT) [10], and optical imaging using fluorescence imaging (FLI) [11], bioluminescence imaging (BLI) [12], optoacoustic imaging [13], and Cerenkov imaging [14]. Depending on the application, the processes to be visualized, the frequency and time period of image acquisition, the imaging area, and required resolution, one or more imaging modalities can be chosen to detect the structure or process of interest. Figure 1.1 summarizes the sensitivity, penetration depth, and spatial resolution of the most common imaging modalities. CT and ultrasound are typically used to obtain structural and anatomical information. Nuclear imaging modalities like PET and SPECT enable the detection of molecular or metabolic processes but require the application of radioisotopes (e.g., ^{18}F in [^{18}F]-fluorodeoxyglucose (FDG)), to assess the metabolic activity of tumors and metastases [15]. Despite the outstanding sensitivity of nuclear imaging technologies, they lack in resolution and anatomical detail. In contrast, MRI can provide exquisite anatomic and physiologic information but is hampered by inherently low sensitivity. Optical imaging is used sparingly for anatomical or physiological inquiry alone but routinely for the detection of molecular and metabolic alterations [3]. Acoustic imaging can also inform anatomical structures together with physiologic parameters using intrinsic contrast generators to facilitate visualization of molecular entities.

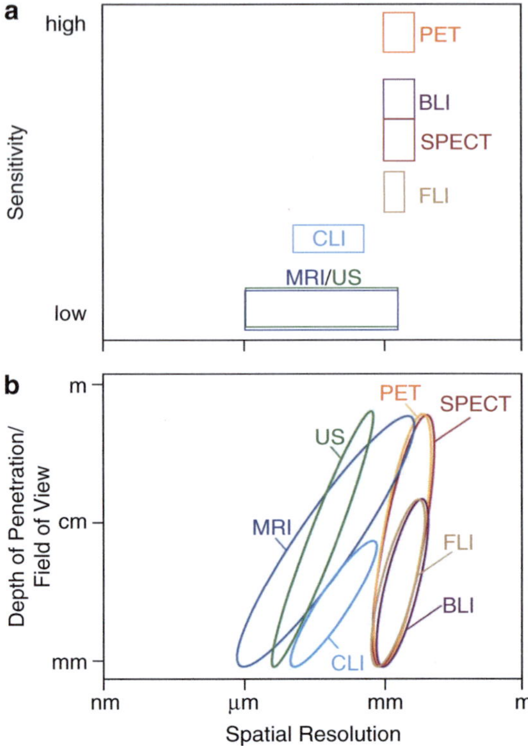

Fig. 1.1 Sensitivity (**a**), penetration depth (**b**), and spatial resolution of the most common molecular imaging technologies: positron-emission tomography (PET), single photon emission computed tomography (SPECT), magnetic resonance imaging (MRI), ultrasound (US), fluorescence imaging (FLI), bioluminescence imaging (BLI), and Cerenkov luminescence imaging (CLI). Adapted from [19]

Superior imaging techniques are required given the emerging emphasis on molecular imaging of disease-related, altered metabolism. Many genomic alterations encountered, e.g., in cancerogenesis, lead to downstream changes in cellular glucose or amino acid metabolism and thus enable the detection of abnormalities and diseases [16]. While the last decades have seen marked improvement in all of the aforementioned technologies and preclinical imaging agents [5], for many applications clinical imaging lags behind other diagnostic tools, e.g., ex vivo methodologies including deep genome sequencing. Therefore, substantial effort is directed toward improving screening methods as well as pre- and intraoperative diagnostics for increased sensitivity and specificity. For intraoperative diagnostics, the visualization of tumor margins as well as remaining tumor deposits play an important role [17], while preoperative diagnostics focus on the overall tumor burden, genomic signatures, and spatial location. Indeed, the field is currently experiencing a paradigm shift, moving into tumor characterization on a molecular level through radiomics or radiogenomics [18]. Similarly, monitoring of modern biological and immunological therapies has attracted intense interest in the molecular imaging community, whereby especially molecular metabolic imaging enables the detection of response to drugs based on alterations of metabolism much faster than conventional anatomical imaging modalities.

1.2 Molecular Imaging Technologies

1.2.1 History

Molecular imaging was pioneered in the field of nuclear medicine in the 1920s when Hermann Blumgart injected bismuth-214 (radium-C) intravenously into patients to study blood flow [20]. In the 1930s, another milestone was reached with the advent of particle accelerators, e.g., the cyclotron enabled production of artificial isotopes [21]. Accelerators allowed scientists to produce a variety of radioisotopes and to select a specific radioisotope geared toward the biochemical process to be studied—indeed, the foundation of modern precision nuclear medicine. Initially, the Geiger counter was used in patients to detect radioactivity from injected radioiodine (^{131}I) to study abnormalities in goiter and hyperthyroidism [22]. The evolution of instrumentation allowed for the development of scintillation detectors, and the development of fast electronics for the detection of annihilation photons by means of coincidence counting. In 1962, David Kuhl introduced emission reconstruction tomography, with which single photon emission computed tomography (SPECT), positron-emission tomography (PET), and transmission X-ray scanning (CT) became the primary tools for nuclear medicine. Medical scanning using ^{99m}Tc was reported first in 1963 by using a gamma camera [23]. In 1983, Henry Wagner generated the first successful PET image of a neuroreceptor using himself as the experimental subject [24]. The now ubiquitous ^{18}F-FDG was first introduced in 1980s to study brain tumors where it was shown that FDG uptake correlates with the degree of malignancy [25]. In 1998, ^{18}F-FDG was used to determine the efficacy of chemotherapy in selected cancers and to predict response [26]. Today, ^{18}F-FDG is the workhorse radiotracer for PET in oncology and beyond, outstanding as the most widely clinically used metabolic marker.

Since its inception in the 1940s, nuclear magnetic resonance (NMR) has been an indispensable tool in the physical sciences for characterization of molecules. However, not until 1971 did NMR begin to revolutionize radiology when it was used to detect tumors. The use of different gradients allowed for image acquisition in 1973 [27, 28]. By 1977, the first whole-body magnetic resonance imaging (MRI) scanner was built to produce images of living human subjects [29]. In essence and in practice, MRI refers to spatially decoded NMR spectroscopy of physiological water protons; intrinsic contrast is generated by the water proton content and their immediate environment in different tissues. This environment may be altered artificially via introduction of paramagnetic cations to enhance contrast. Various cations including manganese (Mn^{2+}), iron (Fe^{3+}), copper (Cu^{2+}), chromium (Cr^{3+}), and the rare earth gadolinium (Gd^{3+}) have been explored with Gd^{3+} being most effective in terms of contrast enhancement due to its seven unpaired f-shell electrons. The first human trial using gadopentetate dimeglumine was performed in 1983 [30], which was approved 5 years later under the name Magnevist® as the first contrast agent for clinical use [31]. Since then, six other contrast agents have been approved with four being Gd^{3+} based and two Mn^{2+} based. In 2003, Paul C. Lauterbur and Sir Peter Mansfield were awarded with the Nobel Prize in physiology or medicine for their discoveries in the field of MRI, making this a routine modality in contemporary medical imaging [32].

The discovery of the piezoelectric effect in 1880 allowed for the development of ultrasound [33]. The piezoelectric effect describes the generation of electrical charges in certain materials as a response to mechanical stress, or vice versa (the inverse piezoelectric effect). This effect is applied using transducers to generate high frequency sound signals (ultrasound). Ultrasound was later used for development of sound navigation and ranging (SONAR) technology in 1912 [34]. In 1942, Karl Dussik became the first physician to use ultrasound in clinical applications, where he demonstrated detection of brain tumors in human subjects [35]. Later in 1948, it was used to diagnose gallbladder stones and made its way into obstetric-gynecology in 1958 [36]. In the late 1960s, it was discovered that small air bubbles could enhance the ultrasound echo signal, although it was not until 1990 when the first microbubble-based contrast agent Albunex™ was clinically approved [37].

The phenomenon of fluorescence was coined in 1852 by a publication of George Gabriel Stokes [38]. By 1887, 660 fluorescent dyes were known. The development of the fluorescence microscope in the early 1900s allowed investigators to study autofluorescence, and subsequently, fluorescent dyes bound to living cells [38]. The first medical applications using fluorescence of endogenous porphyrins in tumors after illumination with UV light date back to 1924 [39]. With the first labeling of antibodies with fluorescein isothiocyanate (FITC) in 1941, the field of immunofluorescence was born [40]. In 1942 the first administration of porphyrins followed by the detection of exogenous red fluorescence took place [39]. The first fluorescent dyes to be synthetically produced were quinine and fluorescein, the latter being used for the first time clinically in 1948 to detect brain tumors [41]. The isolation of green fluorescent protein (GFP) from jellyfish in 1962 followed by its expression in cells allowed fluorescence imaging of intact cell and organisms [42].

Bioluminescence was first documented by Aristotle around 300 BC, and the first book on bioluminescence and chemiluminescence was published in 1555 by Conrad Gesner on self-illumination over marine water as well as in fireflies and glowworms [43]. The oxygen requirement for the bioluminescence process was observed in 1667. In 1873, the two key components of the bioluminescence reaction, luciferin and luciferase, were identified and used to generate light, while luciferin could first be isolated in 1956 [44]. Since then it has been widely used in research for in vivo imaging using the luciferase enzyme as reporter gene [45]. Of the many variants, the luciferase gene of the North American firefly, *Photinus pyralis*, is the most commonly used for research purposes [46].

Cerenkov light was first described by Madame Curie (probably together with radioluminescence), though the phenomenon was first formally examined experimentally in 1934 by Pavel Cerenkov while studying luminescence under irradiation. Ilya Frank and Igor Tamm subsequently described the theoretical basis for the phenomenon from a special relativistic perspective in 1937 [47]. The first Cerenkov images in life science were generated in 2009 using ^{18}F-FDG in tumor-bearing mice [48]. Two years later, Cerenkov emission from ^{89}Zr was used for preclinical image-guided, intraoperative surgical resection of tumors [49]. Clinical Cerenkov luminescence imaging of ^{18}F-FDG was performed in 2014 by visualizing tumor in axillary lymph nodes [50]. Figure 1.2 summarizes the main findings in the field of molecular imaging and its technologies.

1.2.2 Nuclear Imaging

Nuclear imaging is based on the introduction of radionuclides into the patient that emit detectable radiation (gamma or positrons) that can be visualized with single photon emission computed tomography (SPECT) or positron-emission tomography (PET). PET and SPECT (radio) tracers are typically administered in sub-pharmacological doses for noninvasive imaging of biochemical processes. With nuclear imaging, it is possible to observe molecular signatures, e.g., tumor-specific receptors or glycolysis, noninvasively in vivo. With increasing knowledge of relevant targets in pathophysiological processes,

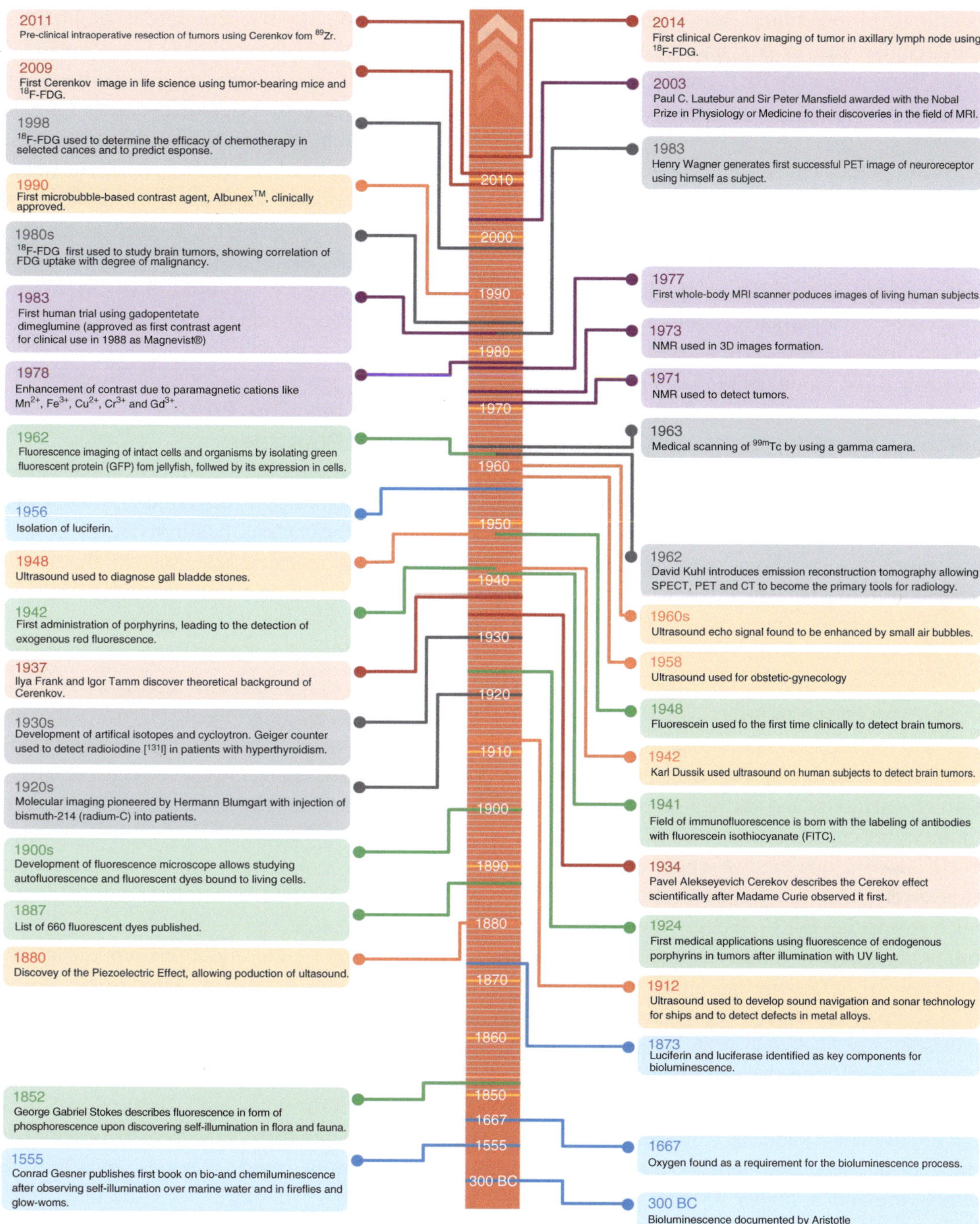

Fig. 1.2 Timeline of the history of molecular imaging and its technologies

e.g., for tumor development, it becomes possible to monitor molecular events in the course of a disease, as well as during treatments such as chemo- or radiation therapy. In addition, molecular markers that reveal prognostic information can be imaged, and disease recurrence can be monitored. Hence, nuclear imaging approaches can be widely applied to answer biological and medical questions in preclinical and clinical settings. Importantly, due to the nature of radioactive decay, predominantly PET, but with newer scanners also SPECT imaging, are quantitative methods.

In the past, a wide array of biologically active molecules has been successfully labeled and translated to the clinic, including sugars, amino acids, nucleic acids, water, molecular oxygen, receptor-binding peptides, antibodies, biomacromolecules, nanoparticles, compounds targeting pH, and hypoxia or cells (e.g., stem cells or heat-inactivated red blood cells). Examples of probes which are on the verge of clinical translation are discussed in the respective PET and SPECT imaging probe chapter below. Based on which type of molecule is radiolabeled, nuclear imaging can measure pharmacokinetic processes (e.g., transport rates, metabolic rates, binding properties) and molecular expression patterns (cell surface receptors, transporters, shed antigens, enzymes). To create nuclear imaging probes, a large number of radioisotopes and labeling techniques have been established, all of which can be tailored to the respective imaging problem at hand. Major advantages of nuclear imaging are its high sensitivity and ability to detect even picomolar tracer concentrations throughout the entire body, allowing quantitative whole-body imaging. Conversely, the most significant shortfall of nuclear imaging is its relatively low spatial resolution, limited to 4–8 mm (clinical) and 1–2 mm (preclinical), impairing the ability to accurately resolve small structures [51]. This is based on the physical characteristics of the detector system, the radiotracer, and the reconstruction methods. Both PET and SPECT have been developed for the use in human subjects, followed by the introduction of dedicated small animal scanners, which provide a higher spatial resolution for basic and translational research [52–54]. Combination of functional imaging with high-resolution morphological/anatomical information via computed tomography (PET/CT and SPECT/CT) has been proven to be superior to single modality imaging and has dramatically improved diagnostic accuracy and spatial localization of many lesions [55, 56]. More recently, hybrid systems combining magnetic resonance imaging with PET have been developed [57], adapted for use in humans, and introduced to the clinic [58]. Currently, the use of PET/MRI scanners is still heavily research based, but more scanners with a clinical focus are being installed. PET/MR imaging presumably will have the most pronounced additional value over PET/CT when investigating diseases in anatomical regions where high soft tissue contrast is required or it is desirable to avoid additional ionizing radiation from CT [59, 60].

1.2.2.1 PET Imaging: Probes and Principles

Radioisotopes suitable for PET imaging decay via the emission of positrons (β^+-emission). Once ejected from the nucleus, positrons travel through space, gradually loosing velocity, until they eventually annihilate through collision with a negatron (electron), producing two high-energy γ-rays (511 keV), released in almost opposite directions. Surrounding PET detectors recognize coincidence photons, i.e., photons detected at the same time on opposite sides of the detector ring (Fig. 1.3, PET imaging) [61]. The point of origin can be reconstructed using the spatial and temporal information. From millions of decay events, three-dimensional images can be reconstructed showing the quantitative distribution of the tracer of interest [62, 63].

For efficient leveraging of this process in biological systems, radiotracers have to be chosen whose half-life matches the desired biological imaging window as well as the biological half-life of the labeled biomolecule in the body. Typically, radioisotopes with physical half-lives of a few minutes to several days are used. The most commonly used isotopes include ^{14}O (~2 min), ^{13}N (~10 min), ^{11}C (~20 min), ^{68}Ga (~67 min), ^{18}F (~110 min), ^{64}Cu (~12.7 h), and ^{89}Zr (~78.4 h). Logistically, the use of isotopes with half-lives of less than 2 h are produced on-site or within close proximity of a cyclotron, while isotopes with a longer half-life can be produced off-site and be shipped to the imaging facility. Some radioisotopes can be produced by a generator (^{68}Ga, ^{82}Rb). Especially for the use of

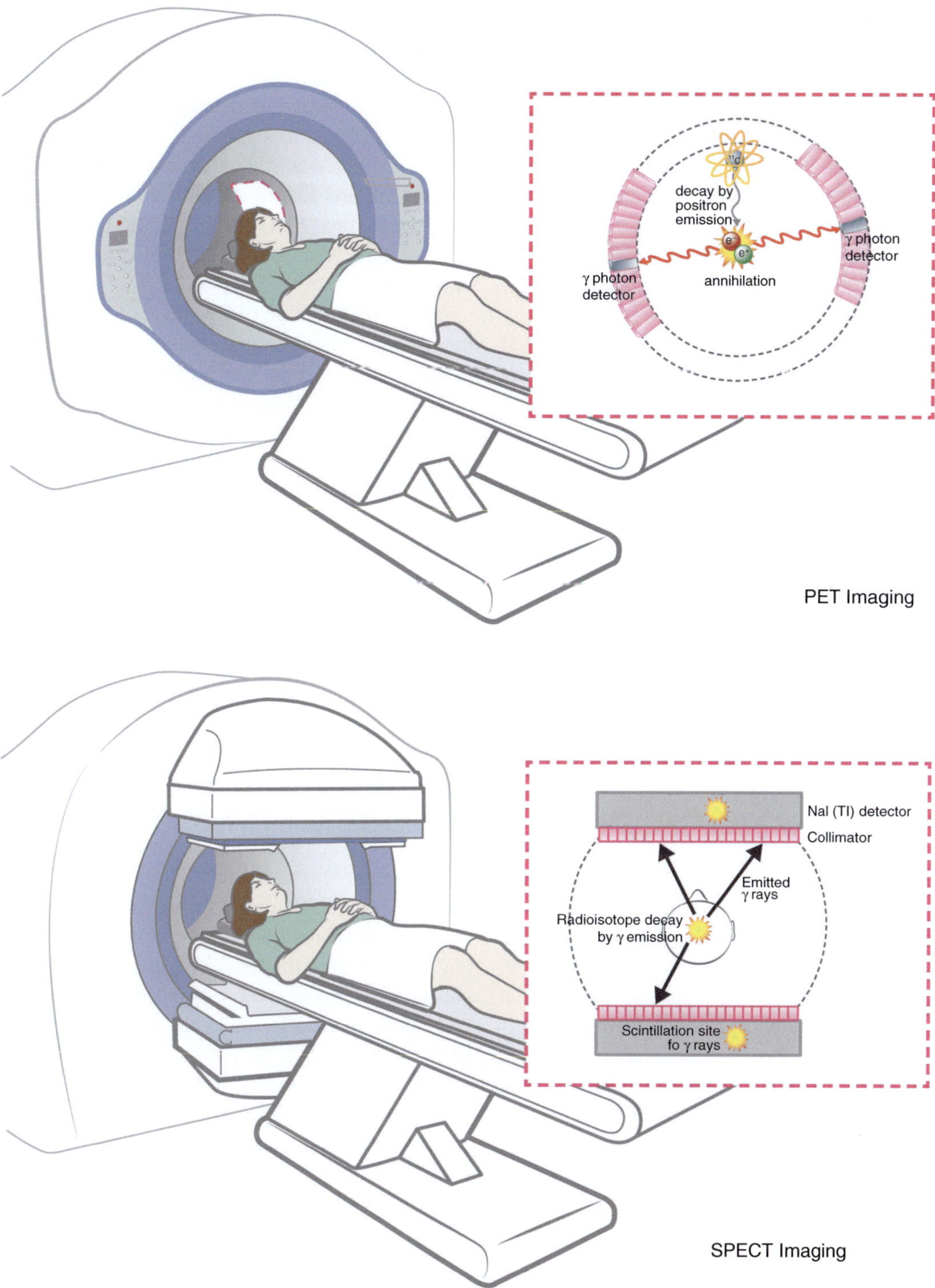

Fig. 1.3 Principle of PET and SPECT imaging

very short-lived isotopes (less than 100 min), the chemistry to incorporate the isotope into the biomolecule and the time to administer the tracer to a patient become a significant logistical consideration and sometimes limiting factor for the routine use of PET/CT to facilities without a cyclotron and the associated chemical production infrastructure.

PET imaging is inextricably linked with ^{18}F-FDG (2-[^{18}F]fluoro-2-deoxy-D-glucose) imaging; in many hospitals, the terms are used synonymously. The metabolically active radiolabeled glucose analog is used to image glucose transport and glycolytic activity of cells. After initial uptake into the cell through glucose transporters, ^{18}F-FDG becomes phosphorylated by hexokinase and is subsequently trapped in the cell due to the newly gained negative charge from the phosphorylation—and with it the radiolabel. Quantification of the ^{18}F-content therefore allows physicians to identify tissues with elevated metabolic rates, a hallmark of malignant growth (Warburg effect) [64–66]. ^{18}F-FDG was developed in 1976 in collaboration between the National Institutes of Health, the University of Pennsylvania, and Brookhaven National Laboratory with the purpose to observe cerebral glucose metabolism [67]. The first images were obtained with a Mark IV radionuclide computed tomography system [68], whose detection mechanism is based on single photon counting (without coincidence) and showed a high concentration of the tracer in the brain of healthy volunteers [69, 70]. In parallel, the first scanners with two opposing scintillation cameras to capture both emitted photons (coincidence) were developed, which led to a major improvement in image sensitivity and resolution [61, 71]. The increased glucose consumption of tumor cells was known since the 1930s [66], and the potential of ^{18}F-FDG to image malignant cells in the brain was established soon after its discovery [72, 73]. During the 1980s whole-body imaging with PET was evaluated, and by the 1990s, PET imaging became an established method for diagnosis, staging, monitoring treatment, and detecting recurrence in a large variety of tumors, making ^{18}F-FDG the single most important tracer in clinical practice today. Similar to most tumor cells, some inflammatory cells also show an increased glucose consumption, which enables the use of ^{18}F-FDG for imaging of inflammatory processes, such as granulomatous diseases [74–76], arthritis [77–79], or atherosclerosis [80–82]. At the same time, this complicates imaging in tumor types that are linked to strong inflammatory processes, since FDG-PET imaging cannot differentiate between malignant and inflammatory masses [83].

Undoubtedly, FDG-PET and FDG-PET/CT has added immeasurable diagnostic value for many diseases, first and foremost for tumor detection, delineation, staging, monitoring, and imaging of recurrence (see [83–97] for reviews and meta-analyses). Irrespective, ^{18}F-FDG it is not a one-size-fits-all imaging agent, as some tumors show low FDG uptake, while some benign processes lead to increased glucose consumption [98–100]. The most common malignancy where FDG-PET is of limited value is (recurrent) prostate cancer [101, 102], but, among others, imaging of hepatocellular carcinoma and primary brain lesions is also challenging using ^{18}F-FDG [103, 104]. To close this gap, the development of other more specialized PET imaging tracers has been pursued. Preclinically, hundreds of different PET tracers were developed, investigating a host of targets and tracer combinations. However, only in the last decade, the FDA approved new PET tracers for use in oncology. A range of additional tracers have now entered clinical use but are still far from being standard. A subset of the novel radiotracers image metabolic processes, in parallel to FDG. Choline radiolabeled with ^{11}C or ^{18}F is a promising tracer of cell metabolism, its retention indicating elevated membrane synthesis. Choline intake in tumor cells is upregulated due to their higher demand for cell membranes building blocks and subsequently elevated phospholipid synthesis rates [105]. Radiolabeled choline has been shown to be most useful in restaging patients with biochemical failure after local treatment for prostate cancer, but studies for other patient subgroups and tumor types are warranted [106–111]. ^{11}C-Acetate is a marker for overexpression of fatty acid synthase, which occurs frequently in prostate cancer. Sensitivity and specificity for primary lesion detection were rather low, but ^{11}C-Acetate imaging can be useful for patients with biochemical recurrence [112–114]. ^{18}F-Fluoro-ethyl-tyrosine (^{18}F-FET) and ^{11}C-Methionine are two amino acid-based radiotracers. They are especially useful for imaging of brain lesions, where FDG-PET is of limited value due to the high glucose consumption of normal brain and consequently high baseline uptake [115–118]. Amino acid-based radiotracers get into cells via the membranous amino acid transporter system and have been shown to be useful for lesion detection with good contrast in low grade and high grade brain tumors, at lower effective doses than ^{18}F-FDG [119, 120]. Both tracers have been established as valuable tools in brain tumor imaging, but ^{11}C-Methionine requires an on-site cyclotron due to the short half-life of the ^{11}C, while that is not necessary for ^{18}F-FET [121–123]. Very recently, a synthetic analog of L-leucine, ^{18}F-fluciclovine (^{18}F-FACBC), was FDA approved for the use in prostate cancer. It has an improved biodistribution, less renal clearance, superior sensitivity, and longer half-life compared to ^{11}C-Choline [124]. Another class of agents, the nucleoside analogs, is represented by ^{18}F-fluoro-deoxythimidine (^{18}F-FLT). This pyrimidine analog is trapped in cells after phosphorylation by thymidine kinase 1 and reflects cell proliferation [125–127]. ^{18}F-FLT was suggested to be superior to FDG for glioma imaging, due to its low background uptake in brain [125], but is also evaluated as imaging agent and prognostic predictor for other tumor types [128–130]. Other types of tracers, which are, e.g., selective for hypoxic tissue, can give insights into prognosis and potential treatment responses/resistance. ^{18}F-FMISO, ^{18}F-FAZA, and $^{62/64}Cu$-ATSM are examples for tracers that can selectively map oxygen deficiency. Their eventual clinical value, distinct characteristics, and which hypoxia tracer is most beneficial under which circumstances are currently being investigated [131–137].

Apart from metabolism tracers, novel radiolabeled peptide and antibody PET probes for receptor imaging are entering the clinical arena. Neuroendocrine tumors, e.g., are known to have a slow metabolism but frequently overexpress somatostatin receptors [138–140]. Hence, radiolabeled somatostatin analogs for diagnosis and therapy have been developed, leading to FDA approval of ^{68}Ga-DOTATATE in June 2016. Other somatostatin imaging agents are under investigation (^{68}Ga-DOTATOC, ^{68}Ga-DOTANOC) [141–143]. More recently, prostate-specific membrane antigen (PSMA) agents for detection of prostate cancer relapses and metastasis have been developed. Small molecule inhibitors have been labeled and have entered the clinical research space (e.g., ^{68}Ga-PSMA-DKFZ-11) [144, 145]. In parallel, the development of gastrin-releasing peptide receptor (GRPr) targeting agents (e.g., ^{68}Ga-RM2, ^{68}Ga-NeoBOMB1), which is also highly overexpressed in primary prostate cancer, is under clinical evaluation [146, 147].

Radiolabeled monoclonal antibodies (mAb) can be summarized under the term immuno-PET. Immuno-PET is an exciting option for imaging of tumor-specific targets but also for guidance and monitoring of mAb-based therapies, e.g., by predicting their biodistribution and assess treatment responses. Here, mostly longer-lived PET isotopes such as ^{64}Cu, ^{124}I, and ^{89}Zr feature a long enough half-life to be able to image the slow accumulation of full-sized antibodies in tumors [148]. The use of shorter-lived isotopes has become available by the application of antibody fragments with faster pharmacokinetics or the development of novel pretargeting approaches [149]. The field of immuno-PET is now rapidly growing, since genomic and proteomic approaches are revealing numerous relevant targets in, e.g., tumor development, progression, and metastasis and therapeutic antibodies are increasingly investigated. A selection of antibodies that have been radiolabeled and preclinically and partially clinically investigated as diagnostic agents is cetuximab, rituximab, bevacizumab and trastuzumab, huA33 and girentuximab [149–152]. Rapid progression toward clinical use will likely lead to the introduction of immuno-PET to the clinical landscape and improve current procedures in diagnosis and therapy monitoring.

Due to the nature for the positron detection with coincidence imaging, for a long time only one isotope could be injected simultaneously, since all positrons annihilate with the same energy—irrespective of the nuclide of origin. However, recent developments are moving PET imaging into multitracer capabilities, e.g., triple coincidence imaging. Positron-gamma emitters generate a significant number of triple coincidences through additional gamma decays [153] that can be extracted from the acquired list-mode data which allows them to be differentiated from the standard PET radionuclides [154]. This new approach allows imaging two PET tracers at the same time and therefore a deeper insight into metabolism.

1.2.2.2 SPECT Imaging: Probes and Principles

Gamma-emitting isotopes can also be used for noninvasive imaging of living subjects using SPECT. In SPECT, usually two gamma cameras are rotated around the subject to collect the γ-rays (Fig. 1.3, SPECT imaging). SPECT probes and instrumentation precede PET imaging and have been developed since the 1960s. Preclinical SPECT can reach submillimeter resolution (0.5–2.5 mm), while clinical SPECT/CT has a lower resolution (7–15 mm). However, recent clinical advances in instrumentation show major improvement in resolution and image acquisition speed without sacrificing sensitivity [155, 156].

Due to the nature of the technique to collect single gammas, as well as scatter and attenuation effects, quantification of the technique is challenging, but more recent developments offer promising solutions [157]. On the other hand, it is possible to detect different isotopes simultaneously, because probes can be labeled with isotopes that emit gamma rays at different energies [158, 159]. Typically, SPECT isotopes have a longer half-life than PET isotopes, ranging from several hours to days. Therefore, SPECT is often used to measure relatively slow kinetic processes. The most commonly used isotopes in SPECT are ^{99m}Tc (~6 h), ^{123}I (~13.2 h), ^{111}In (2.8 days), and ^{131}I (~8.0 days). The generator-produced ^{99m}Tc is the most commonly used medical radioisotope for detection in conventional gamma (scintillation counters) and SPECT cameras [160]. It is used clinically in more than 30 radiopharmaceuticals. A host of SPECT imaging probes have been developed, including monoclonal antibodies, antibody fragments, peptides, and small molecules [161, 162]. ^{111}In- or ^{99m}Tc-labeled monoclonal antibodies have thus far been approved by the FDA for diagnostic imaging [163]. Furthermore, an established clinical application of SPECT is imaging of neuroendocrine tumors (NET) by targeting the frequently overexpressed somatostatin receptor family. The indium-111-labeled peptide ^{111}In-pentetreotide (Octreoscan®) was the first approved radiopeptide for diagnostic use and remains the most successful one [164–167]. The radiolabeled guanethidine analog meta-iodobenzylguanidine (^{123}I-MIBG or ^{131}I-MIBG) has also been suggested for NET imaging, among others for pheochromocytoma and neuroblastoma [168]. Several studies have shown the utility of sentinel lymph node imaging with SPECT/CT using ^{99m}Tc-labeled sulfur colloids by increasing localization, sensitivity, and specificity of imaging compared to planar lymphoscintigraphy [169–171]. Detection of bone metastasis, which occurs in approximately 30% of cancer patients, can be achieved with bone scintigraphy. SPECT/CT imaging with ^{99m}Tc-methylene diphosphonate (^{99m}Tc-MDP) provides whole-body visualization of bone lesions with sensitivity of 62–100% but rather limited specificity of 25% [172, 173].

SPECT has been suggested to be used for imaging of metabolism in various ways. The high cost and limited availability of PET led to efforts to realize SPECT imaging of glucose metabolism. ^{99m}Tc- or ^{123}I-labeled sugar derivatives have been evaluated but did not emerge as effective alternatives to ^{18}F-FDG PET [174]. ^{18}F-FDG has also been directly used for SPECT imaging, indicating sufficient sensitivity and resolution to detect myocardial viability and diagnose malignant tumors, if the pathological structure is >2 cm [175]. ^{123}I-methyltyrosine (^{123}I-IMT) is an example of an amino acid analog for SPECT imaging, which reflects the rate of amino acid synthesis and is especially useful for imaging of brain tumors, because it can cross the blood-brain barrier [176–178].

Other SPECT tracers in preclinical and clinical development are targeting, e.g., prostate cancer, lung cancer, and brain tumors showing the broad range of clinical applications of SPECT/CT in oncology. Especially if used as hybrid technology with CT, the technique is likely to expand due to the combination of availability of hybrid gamma cameras and increasing availability of tracers.

1.2.3 Magnetic Resonance Imaging

Magnetic resonance imaging (MRI) stands out as the imaging technology with a much higher spatial resolution (typically voxel size 100 μm^3–1 mm^3) than nuclear and optical imaging, paired with an extraordinary soft tissue contrast compared to computed tomography but plagued with lower sensitivity than nuclear modalities. MRI is based on measuring energy released by hydrogen nuclei when they relax back into their original spin state (parallel or antiparallel) in a magnetic field after being excited by a radiofrequency pulse (nuclear magnetic resonance, NMR). The endogenous soft tissue contrast depends on basic parameters: proton density, longitudinal (T1) relaxation time, and transverse (T2) relaxation time. By varying the pulse sequence parameters (e.g., repetition time, echo times) and increasing the magnetic field strength, signal intensity and contrast can be enhanced. The technique is free of ionizing radiation and is not limited by depth penetration but is also considerably more costly and time consuming than other methodologies. Therefore, evaluation of cost-effectiveness is an important factor in the decision if MRI or CT is performed. MRI is routinely used for diagnostics of the central nervous system, abdominal organs, pelvis, breast, heart, and vessels [179]. Regarding clinical oncology, MRI is established in lesion detection in soft tissues (e.g., sarcomas), additional lesion characterization, evaluation of physiologic parameters (diffusion, dynamic contrast enhancement), and therapy monitoring. Recently, hardware innovations have made high-resolution whole-body MRI clinically feasible [180, 181], enabling imaging of metastatic spread and bone marrow diseases [182].

Conventionally, MRI is classified as an anatomical-morphological technique, but the use of contrast agents, the development of novel applications, and the identification biomarkers for MRI are bridging the gap to true molecular imaging, supplementing, and enhancing anatomic information. Quantitative MR imaging applications can report on various aspects of tumor biology, including perfusion, cellularity, protein deposition, and metabolism [183].

The low sensitivity of conventional MRI (10^{-3} to 10^{-5} M) can be explained by the low polarization (and therefore NMR signal) of proton nuclei at thermal equilibrium. At body temperate, e.g., only about one of one million nuclei contributes to the measured NMR signal in a standard clinical scanner [184]. The most prominent ways to increase MRI sensitivity are increasing magnetic field strengths (3.0 Tesla (T) compared to the standard 1.5 T leads to a proportional increase in NMR signal [185]) and alternative applications such as whole-body diffusion MRI, MR spectroscopy, and hyperpolarization, which will be discussed below.

Alternatively, visualization of pathologies with MRI can be enhanced by the introduction of external contrast agents, which shorten the relaxation time of protons in tissue, enhancing signal to noise ratio. Contrast-enhancing agents can be classified as paramagnetic or superparamagnetic, enhancing T1 and T2 contrast, respectively. The limited sensitivity of MRI requires higher doses of contrast agents in the micro- to millimolar range as opposed to femto- and nanomolar for nuclear and optical imaging. The most commonly used contrast agents are based on the rare-earth metal gadolinium or its derivatives [186, 187]. Since free gadolinium is toxic, approved agents, such as Magnevist®, incorporate each gadolinium (Gd) atom into a chelate [188]. The most common Gd chelates are low molecular weight compounds with high T1 relaxivity, which distribute quickly into the intravascular and interstitial space, enhancing contrast according to their biodistribution. As rule of thumb, the contrast agent dose can be reduced by half when field strengths are increased from 1.5 to 3.0 T [189]. Next to the extracellular fluid agents, such as Magnevist®,

Omniscan®, and Dotarem®, Gd-based agents have been modified to preferentially improve contrast of the blood pool by binding to albumin [190, 191] or exhibit biliary excretion and uptake into hepatocytes for liver imaging [186, 192]. To achieve an increase in tumor accumulation and relaxivity as well as creating the opportunity to attach targeting molecules, macromolecular conjugates derived from conjugation of Gd-DTPA or Gd-DOTA to polymeric materials were developed [187, 193]. To decrease toxicity, linear chelators have recently been abandoned in favor of cyclic agents.

T2/T2* contrast-enhancing agents include superparamagnetic iron oxide particles (SPIO). These nano-sized iron oxide crystals, which are typically coated with polymers like dextran or carboxydextran, contain several thousand iron atoms each, causing an increase in relaxivity which can be much higher than for Gd chelates and exhibit high biocompatibility. SPIO agents accumulate in liver, spleen, bone marrow, and lymph nodes because they are subject to phagocytosis by Kupffer cells after recognition by the reticuloendothelial system. Their localization in Kupffer cells in liver parenchyma, but not in pathologic lesions, which do not contain reticuloendothelial cells, allows for imaging of benign and malignant liver lesions. A number of SPIO, e.g., Feridex® and Resovist®, received regulatory approval for liver imaging [194], but production was discontinued a few years later in the USA due to low demand. Another SPIO agent, Feraheme®, which is approved for the treatment of anemia, is being explored as imaging agent for lymph node imaging.

SPIOs are modular and allow for adjustment of the core and the coating to improve their colloidal stability, RES targeting, and relaxivity. Furthermore, in the preclinical research space, SPIO containing nanostructures are developed, which allow for modification of the hydrophilic shell, the hydrophobic core, the attachment or targeting ligands, and the loading with therapeutic drugs (see [195] for a recent overview). Diagnostic accuracy of MRI could be further improved by dual-contrast T1- and T2-weighted imaging with targeted gadolinium-labeled SPIOs [196].

Despite intense development of targeted and functionalized MRI contrast agents in the preclinical setting, clinically available contrast agents all rely on passive targeting mechanisms. The goal of imaging-specific tumor receptors with MRI in the clinic has not yet been achieved [197].

Magnetic resonance spectroscopy (MRS) is an MRI application that can detect the frequency of metabolites, especially in the brain and spine, based on chemical shift [198]; it is however limited to the same low sensitivity as MRI due to the underlying physical limitations in imaging of water protons (^{1}H). This sensitivity limit can be overcome by hyperpolarization of a material beyond thermal equilibrium conditions.

Hyperpolarization techniques allow to increase the signal of a given number of nuclear spins by more than 10^5 times, independent of the magnetic field [199]. This enables the detection of other, less abundant, nuclei beyond ^{1}H, such as ^{3}He, ^{13}C, and ^{15}N. Hyperpolarization can be achieved by artificially creating a nonequilibrium distribution of the spin states of nuclei, where the population difference between parallel and antiparallel spins is increased by several orders of magnitude. With hyperpolarized MRI visualization of transient molecular changes in metabolic processes becomes feasible, which were previously inaccessible. An important difference to conventional MRI is that the hyperpolarized agents generate the detected signal themselves, as opposed to paramagnetic agents, which shorten the relaxation time of adjacent protons. Of the different methods to create a hyperpolarized state, dynamic nuclear polarization has emerged as technique to polarize endogenous molecules (e.g., ^{13}C and ^{15}N), enabling the observation of small molecule metabolic agents and their metabolic products in action [200]. This approach allows real-time observation of fundamental metabolic processes and changes thereof, such as production of lactate and alanine from pyruvate, by injecting ^{13}C-labeled pyruvate [201]. ^{13}C-labeled pyruvate is furthermore under clinical evaluation for prostate cancer imaging, since elevated levels of lactate have been identified as tumor biomarker [202]. Preclinical investigation of the usefulness of ^{13}C-labeled molecules for tumor imaging and therapy monitoring is warranted [203–207]. Other hyperpolarization approaches, namely, the "brute force" approach and optical pumping methods, allow for hyperpolarization of noble gases (^{3}He, ^{129}Xe) [208, 209], which enabled functional MRI imaging of the lung despite its low proton density [210–212]. The lipophilic ^{129}Xe has also gained great interest for imaging of lipid-rich tissues in the body, since it readily dissolves in blood and tissue after inhalation, while ^{3}He does not [209, 213, 214].

1.2.4 Ultrasound Imaging

Ultrasound techniques hinge on the phenomenon of piezoelectric transduction to produce sound waves and subsequently detect those reflected (echoed) by physical tissue boundaries. Sound waves are generated and received by associated transducers; 2–15 MHz scanners are typical for clinical applications. The imaging technology of ultrasound has steadily improved during recent years due to the improvements in image analysis; indeed, real-time imaging with millimeter spatial resolution is now possible. For research, higher frequencies up to 100 MHz can improve resolution to less than 100 μm but at the cost of penetration depth with around 8 mm [215].

Generally, clinical ultrasound imaging is mainly used to detect and characterize lesions in the urogenital tract, liver, head and neck, and soft tissue. Though standard techniques mainly provide morphological information, assessment can be improved through application of more sophisticated elastographic or Doppler imaging techniques which inform cellularity (the higher the greater the loss in elasticity) and vascularity (by imaging the flow of blood through the Doppler Effect), respectively. 3D images can be generated by detecting ultrasound frequencies from several locations around the object [216]. As the sensitivity of the bare technology is not satisfying yet, especially for smaller vessels, those with less perfusion as well as for molecular targets, the application of contrast agents is indispensable.

Contrast agents for ultrasound imaging have historically exhibited varying degrees of sophistication, from free gas bubbles with only a short lifetime in blood first used to now state-of-the-art shelled microbubbles, of which a few, e.g., Levovist®, are clinically approved [37]. Shelled microbubbles are typically synthesized as a gas core stabilized by a lipid, protein, or polymer shell and measure only 1–4 μm in diameter, facilitating passage into even very small capillaries. After intravascular administration, vascularity of a tissue may be visualized with a very high sensitivity (picograms) and specificity. Further, microbubbles can be used as unspecific imaging agents or coupled to antibodies or peptides for more specific targeting to sites of biological relevance. In this context, microbubbles conjugated to an antibody against VEGF receptor 2 or to RGD peptide against integrins were able to accumulate in tumors in vivo [217, 218]. Recent efforts have extended the potential applications for microbubbles to initiate therapy by loading genes or drugs into the bubbles [219, 220]. Nanobubbles have been envisioned to take advantage of the enhanced permeation and retention (EPR) effect for ultrasound tumor imaging, though in practice, the decrease in size compromises the strength of the reflected ultrasound echo, limiting the usefulness of this technique presently. Therefore, ultrasound is most commonly used to image endovascular targets and to gain information on vascular structure.

A recently emerging field is optoacoustic or photoacoustic imaging. This technology is based on the emission of ultrasound after excitation with light using a nanosecond-pulsed laser and thus a transient increase in volume of the excited object [13]. This enables the localization of fluorescent probes or nanoparticles within the tissue as well as determination of the oxygenation state of hemoglobin in the blood as hemoglobin is also a strong absorber. Multispectral in vivo imaging with a resolution of approximately 100 μm and a penetration depth of several millimeters is possible through separation of different compounds using multispectral optoacoustic tomography (MSOT) [221]. Gold nanoparticles are particularly promising for optoacoustic imaging, as they offer a high absorbance and thus a relatively strong ultrasound signal [222]. Weber et al. have provided an excellent review of optoacoustic contrast agents to date [223]. By detecting the ultrasound signal from different locations around the subject simultaneously, 3D images can be generated as well.

1.2.5 Optical Imaging

Optical imaging techniques are some of the most commonly used technologies for biomedical research today; these include fluorescence- and luminescence-based approaches to visualize molecular alterations or structure. Compared to PET, SPECT or MRI, optical imaging modalities can visualize molecular alterations in a shorter time in vivo in a straightforward and cost-effective manner. Fluorescence imaging by its very nature requires excitation light which can present complications due to backscatter and autofluorescence, both of which increase signal-to-noise ratios and degrade image quality. Further, optical imaging sacrifices penetration for improved resolution and sensitivity. Because of the lower penetration depth of the light, only near-surface signals can be detected non-invasively, or minimally invasively via endoscopy. Therefore, optical imaging is currently mainly applied to detect tumors and metastases in mice, and to observe progression or regression of disease. But due to the ease of use it is also a main player in intraoperative imaging in humans.

1.2.5.1 Fluorescence Imaging: Probes and Principles

Fluorescence imaging is a rapidly growing field due to the development of techniques with higher sensitivities coupled with an increasing number of fluorescent dyes [224]. Endogenous chromophores like hemoglobin or melanin can also be detected due to their specific absorption spectra (particularly with optoacoustic imaging, see above). These endogenous and exogenous contrast molecules exhibit an absorbance maximum in the visible to near-infrared spectrum. For in vivo fluorescence imaging, the tissue is typically illuminated with a light source emitting at or near the excitation wavelength of the fluorescent agent to induce specific fluorescence. Emitted light is detected by a CCD camera enabling real-time monitoring [225, 226], which is unique to optical (and ultrasound) approaches. Depending on the camera system utilized, spatial resolution of less than 100 micrometers can be achieved in preclinical studies using near-infrared fluorescence imaging [227]. For in vivo applications, appropriate penetration depth of the light is an essential consideration when locating a structure of interest. Tissue penetration depth is a function of wavelength, scattering effects, and absorbance of endogenous components, e.g., skin or blood; scattering effects additionally alter the directionality of the emitted fluorescence photons, compromising resolution particularly at increasing depth [228, 229]. It has been shown that the near-infrared (NIR) window of light with wavelengths between 650 and 900 nm offers the highest possible penetration for optical imaging (up to 15 cm) [230]. For this reason, and unless prohibited by pharmacokinetic considerations, fluorophores are often chosen that absorb in the NIR spectrum of light. An advantage of fluorescence imaging is monitoring of different molecular targets at the same time by simultaneous application of several dyes or probes with different excitation and emission that can be deconvoluted through spectral unmixing [231]. This enables obtaining a multidimensional and more complex picture of the biology or molecular mechanisms.

The most commonly used method especially in preclinical studies is 2D-fluorescence reflectance imaging (FRI) [232]. This is a photographic technique where the emitted light is acquired from the side of the excitation illumination, making it possible to integrate camera and light source into one unit. FRI is easy to operate and can be used with high throughput, making it very popular [233]. Among others, it is used, e.g., to detect epidermal growth factor (EGF) receptor in breast cancer [234] or also protease activity in arthritis [235]. Nonetheless, FRI would benefit greatly from resolution of the drawbacks: its depth limitation, light reflection and scatter that degrades the image, the exerted effect of different tissue depths, and of the optical properties of overlying tissues onto the signal intensity and spectrum.

The molecular probes for optical imaging are generally bioconjugates consisting of a biomolecule (e.g., antibody or peptide) and fluorophore (fluorescent dye). These components facilitate specific targeting to associated overexpressed molecular receptors, and detection, respectively. To this end, small molecules for intracellular targets and specifically labeled nanoparticles are widely used as well. The advantage of antibodies is the high target affinity and specificity as well as good clinical acceptance. However, they exhibit a long blood circulation due to their large size of about 150 kDa and thus nonspecific accumulation in nontarget tissue [236]. Furthermore, they can also cause strong reactions of the immune system if the antibodies are derived from a different species (e.g., through generation of human anti-mouse antibodies if a murine antibody is used in patients) [237, 238]. On the other hand, small peptide-based optical imaging probes can offer improved pharmacokinetic properties, are less immunogenic, and show fast clearance from the blood due to their small size [239]. A specific example is the cyclic RGD peptide and its many derivatives which are routinely used in preclinical research to target $\alpha_v\beta_3$ integrins on the activated endothelium of blood vessels in tumors [224] and thus for the visualization of tumor neovasculature, one of the original hallmarks of cancer [240]. Other probes are generated to image glucose metabolism, amino acid or lipid metabolism, tumor cell proliferation, hypoxia, angiogenesis, invasiveness, apoptosis, and necrosis [224]. As an intracellular target, the DNA repair enzyme PARP1 can be visualized using the fluorescent small molecule inhibitor PARPi-FL [241, 242]. In addition, inflammation can be studied by fluorescence imaging detecting overexpressed enzyme activities in inflammatory tissue (e.g., cyclooxygenase-2 levels) or directly labeling monocytes or macrophages [243, 244].

A vast spectrum of fluorophores exists today, enabling clinicians and researchers to label targeting molecules using the optimal combination of absorption/emission properties and conjugation motif. Figure 1.4 shows chemical structures of some of the most commonly used examples; these include cyanine fluorophores Cy5.5 and Cy7, rhodamine, porphyrins, phthalocyanines, BODIPY, fluorescein isothiocyanate (FITC), and squaraines [224, 245]. The commercially available IRDye® 800CW from LI-COR® is being used in clinical trials for surgical navigation in head and neck cancer [246]. Others, like indocyanine green (ICG) are used clinically as a stand-alone contrast agent [247], predominantly for intraoperative applications, such as visualization of the ureter [248] or of sentinel lymph nodes [249, 250]. 5-aminolevulinic acid (ALA), used for delineation of glioblastoma, is an example of a widely applied non-fluorescent molecule which becomes fluorescent after it is metabolized into protoporphyrin IX [251, 252]. To obtain an optimal signal, the fluorophore should possess a high absorption coefficient at the excitation wavelength and a high fluorescence quantum yield. Within the context of specific in vivo imaging, these traits should be considered in concert with the characteristics of the targeting vector to produce a fluorescent bioconjugate with both optimal pharmacological and optical properties [253].

As mentioned previously, intraoperative fluorescence imaging is an emerging field, which moves toward molecular imaging to improve surgical success and precision [254, 255]. Until recently, mainly methodologies for preoperative planning and intraoperative delineation of important structures were used which could detect the tumor or disease but could not give a real-time guidance during the actual surgery process. Fluorescence imaging can improve the accuracy of detecting and removing tumors while simultaneously sparing healthy tissue to the largest extent possible. Compared to the human eye, intraoperative fluorescence imaging provides an ability to look under the tissue surface with high resolution and sensitivity [256]. It can further generate a high contrast between diseased and healthy surrounding tissue in real time due to the use of compact fluorescent cameras, integrating this modality into the normal workflow of the surgeon. Nonspecific fluorescent dyes like ICG

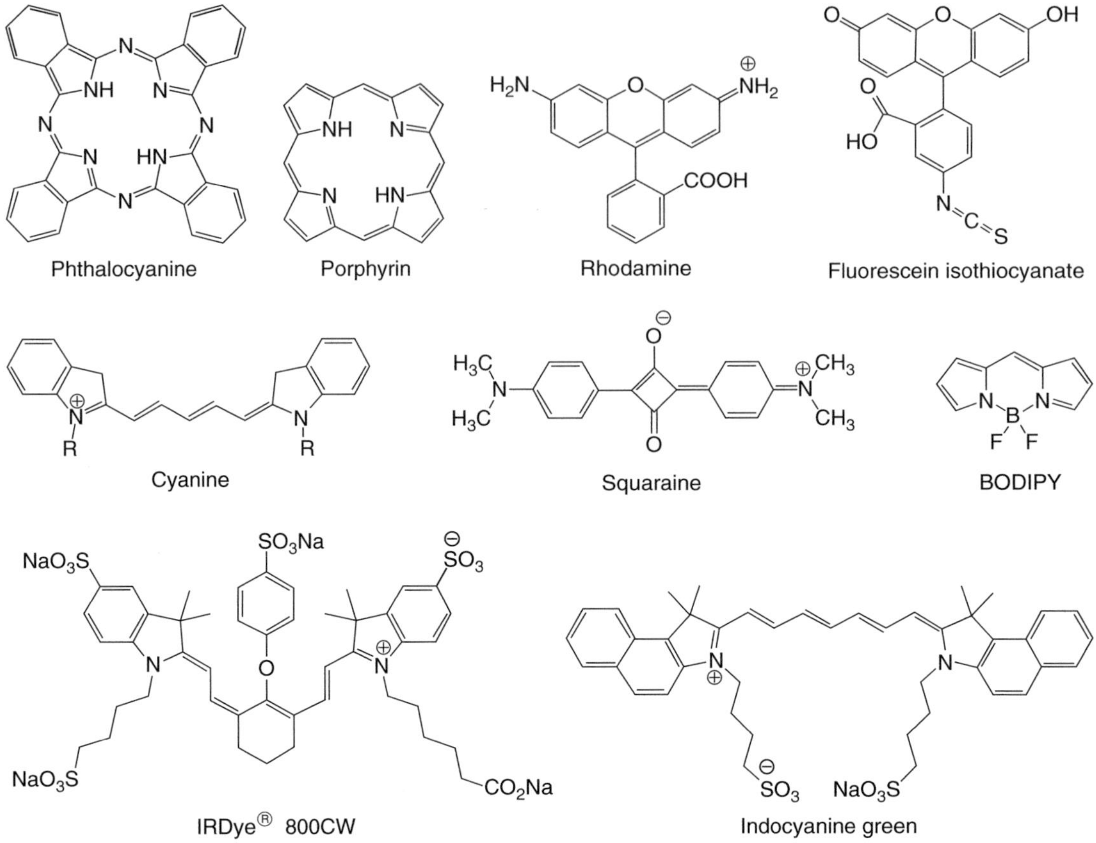

Fig. 1.4 Chemical structures of widely used fluorescent dyes

can be used to assess tissue morphology and physiology and to detect sentinel lymph nodes in real time [249, 257]. Intraoperative mapping of sentinel lymph node metastasis can be achieved using tumor-targeting inorganic ultrasmall silica nanoparticles [258]. Many additional uses of intraoperative fluorescence imaging have been reported, including targeted applications which identify molecular biomarkers upregulated in cancer, fluorescein isothiocyanate (FITC)-labeled agent targeting folate receptor-α [255], and tumor necrosis factor (TNF)-targeting antibody for visualizing TNF-positive immune cells in Crohn's disease [259]. Therapeutics including bevacizumab or cetuximab have been labeled with the NIR dye IRDye® 800CW and evaluated clinically to define tumor margins [246]. Clinical endoscopy using a fluorescently labeled peptide delineating colorectal polyps based on c-Met expression has recently been accomplished in patients as well [260].

1.2.5.2 Bioluminescence Imaging

Bioluminescence imaging is a subclass of optical imaging based on generation of light due to oxidation of a substrate by an enzyme. Hereby, the oxidation of luciferin by luciferase (from the North American firefly) is most common [46]. Within this context, the mechanism requires ATP, oxygen, and magnesium and produces light in the visible spectrum in the range of 530–640 nm. This mechanism is also used to study gene regulation by using the *luc* gene [261, 262] and specific enzymatic activities with the use of a caged, enzyme-activatable luciferin [263]. In imaging gene expression using *luc*, bioluminescence occurs when a gene of interest is switched on, while the reporter gene is under the same promoter as the gene of interest. The advantage of this methodology is that there is no background bioluminescence due to absence of internal luciferase expression in mice and humans, making it highly specific. To gain an emission with a higher wavelength and thus a better penetration depth, bioluminescence resonance energy transfer (BRET) was introduced, exciting a fluorescent molecule emitting light at up to 700 nm using the generated bioluminescence [264]. However, the required reporter gene makes this method not suitable for any clinical applications beyond benchtop assays.

1.2.5.3 Cerenkov Luminescence Imaging

Optical signals can also be generated by certain radioactive isotopes due to the generation of Cerenkov light, probably best known as the blue glow seen around the core of nuclear reactors or used fuel in cooling basins. This phenomenon occurs when charged particles (mostly electrons or positrons) travel through a dielectric medium faster than the speed of light in that medium. The emission spectrum of Cerenkov ranges from the UV to the visible and varies in intensity [14]. High-sensitivity CCD cameras for low-light conditions are generally employed for preclinical Cerenkov imaging. While Cerenkov detection has been used in applications of particle physics for many years, the first images in life science were generated in tumor-bearing mice using ^{18}F-FDG only as recently as 2009 [48]. Cerenkov from a ^{89}Zr-labeled J591 antibody was used to image prostate-specific membrane antigen (PSMA), and ^{89}Zr-labeled trastuzumab was applied in preclinical studies for intraoperative optical Cerenkov imaging during surgical resection of tumors [49, 265]. Further, the resection of sentinel lymph nodes could be performed by applying ^{18}F-FDG intradermally into mice [266]. Clinically, from patients receiving ^{18}F-FDG for routine PET/CT imaging, Cerenkov images could be acquired, enabling the detection of tumor in lymph nodes [50]; Cerenkov emission from ^{131}I in the thyroid gland of a patient was also acquired [267], both studies demonstrating the feasibility of Cerenkov luminescence imaging preclinical as well as in patients.

1.2.6 Future Perspectives

All of the mentioned modalities have benefits and limitations in their resolution, penetration depth, sensitivity, and cost-effectiveness. Significant effort has focused on combining complementary modalities to improve upon the generated images by simultaneously image structure and function [268]. For example, the combination of PET, which detects molecular processes with high sensitivity, with CT, which generates morphological images with high resolution, can afford the assessment of the presence of diseased tissue with precise anatomical localization. At the same time, CT also provides attenuation correction, required to obtain quantitative information. The same applies for the combination of PET with MR, where MR provides excellent soft tissue contrast and parametric images, while the PET provides exquisite molecular information. In this context, many multimodality imaging agents have been conceived, but translation of these agents into the clinical realm has remained slow. It remains also questionable if there is indeed more information gained from an "multimodal" agent that is capable of visualizing the same target using different modalities compared to a true multimodal agent that can indicate one molecular aspect with one modality and yet another with another modality. These will be the real agents of the future.

References

1. Mankoff DA. A definition of molecular imaging. J Nucl Med. 2007;48(6):18.
2. James ML, Gambhir SS. A molecular imaging primer: modalities, imaging agents, and applications. Physiol Rev. 2012;92(2):897–965.
3. Weissleder R, Mahmood U. Molecular imaging. Radiology. 2001;219(2):316–33.
4. Chen K, Chen X. Design and development of molecular imaging probes. Curr Top Med Chem. 2010;10(12):1227–36.
5. Weissleder R, Pittet MJ. Imaging in the era of molecular oncology. Nature. 2008;452(7187):580–9.
6. Kiessling F, et al. Targeted ultrasound imaging of cancer: an emerging technology on its way to clinics. Curr Pharm Des. 2012;18(15):2184–99.
7. Ginat DT, Gupta R. Advances in computed tomography imaging technology. Annu Rev Biomed Eng. 2014;16:431–53.
8. Bernsen MR, et al. Computed tomography and magnetic resonance imaging. Recent Results Cancer Res. 2013;187:3–63.
9. Gambhir SS. Molecular imaging of cancer with positron emission tomography. Nat Rev Cancer. 2002;2(9):683–93.
10. Rosenthal MS, et al. Quantitative SPECT imaging: a review and recommendations by the focus Committee of the Society of Nuclear Medicine

Computer and Instrumentation Council. J Nucl Med. 1995;36(8):1489–513.
11. Ntziachristos V. Fluorescence molecular imaging. Annu Rev Biomed Eng. 2006;8:1–33.
12. Paley MA, Prescher JA. Bioluminescence: a versatile technique for imaging cellular and molecular features. Medchemcomm. 2014;5(3):255–67.
13. Liu Y, Nie L, Chen X. Photoacoustic molecular imaging: from multiscale biomedical applications towards early-stage Theranostics. Trends Biotechnol. 2016;34(5):420–33.
14. Das S, Thorek DL, Grimm J. Cerenkov imaging. Adv Cancer Res. 2014;124:213–34.
15. Farwell MD, Pryma DA, Mankoff DA. PET/CT imaging in cancer: current applications and future directions. Cancer. 2014;120(22):3433–45.
16. Kim MM, et al. Non-invasive metabolic imaging of brain tumours in the era of precision medicine. Nat Rev Clin Oncol. 2016.
17. Keating J, et al. Identification of breast cancer margins using intraoperative near-infrared imaging. J Surg Oncol. 2016;113(5):508–14.
18. Bai HX, et al. Imaging genomics in cancer research: limitations and promises. Br J Radiol. 2016;89(1061):20151030.
19. Cassidy PJ, Radda GK. Molecular imaging perspectives. J R Soc Interface. 2005;2(3):133–44.
20. Patton DD. The birth of nuclear medicine instrumentation: Blumgart and Yens, 1925. J Nucl Med. 2003;44(8):1362–5.
21. Kramer-Marek G, Capala J. The role of nuclear medicine in modern therapy of cancer. Tumor Biol. 2012;33(3):629–40.
22. Verburg FA, de Keizer B, van Isselt JW. Use of radiopharmaccuticals for diagnosis, treatment, and follow-up of differentiated thyroid carcinoma. Anti Cancer Agents Med Chem. 2007;7(4):399–409.
23. Sorensen LB, Archambault M. Visualization of liver by scanning with Mo99 (Molybdate) as tracer. J Laborat Clin Med. 1963;62(2): 330.
24. Wagner HN Jr, et al. Imaging dopamine receptors in the human brain by positron tomography. Science. 1983;221(4617):1264–6.
25. Dichiro G. Positron emission tomography using [F-18] Fluorodeoxyglucose in brain-tumors - a powerful diagnostic and prognostic tool. Investig Radiol. 1987;22(5):360–71.
26. Couper GW, et al. Detection of response to chemotherapy using positron emission tomography in patients with oesophageal and gastric cancer. Br J Surg. 1998;85:31–3.
27. Andrew ER. Nuclear magnetic resonance and the brain. Brain Topogr. 1992;5(2):129–33.
28. Lauterbur PC. Image formation by induced local interactions. Examples employing nuclear magnetic resonance, 1973. Clin Orthop Relat Res. 1989;244: 3–6.
29. Damadian R, Goldsmith M, Minkoff L. NMR in cancer: XVI. FONAR image of the live human body. Physiol Chem Phys. 1977;9(1):97–100. 108
30. Laniado M, et al. First use of GdDTPA/dimeglumine in man. Physiol Chem Phys Med NMR. 1984;16(2):157–65.
31. Lohrke J, et al. 25 years of contrast-enhanced MRI: developments, current challenges and future perspectives. Adv Ther. 2016;33(1):1–28.
32. Slavkovsky P, Uhliar R. The Nobel Prize in Physiology or Medicine in 2003 To Paul C. Lauterbur, Peter Mansfield for magnetic resonance imaging. Bratisl Lek Listy. 2004; 105(7–8): 245–9.
33. Curie P, Curie J. Developpement, par pression de l'electricite polaire dans les cristaux hemiedres a faces inclinees. Comptes Rendus. 1880;91:291–5.
34. D'Amico A, Pittenger R. A brief history of active sonar. Aquat Mamm. 2009;35:426–34.
35. Dussik KT. Ultraschall-Diagnostik, insbesondere bei Gehirnerkrankungen, mittels Hyperphonographie. Phys Ther Bader Klimanheikd. 1948;1:140–5.
36. Donald I, Macvicar J, Brown TG. Investigation of abdominal masses by pulsed ultrasound. Lancet. 1958;1(7032):1188–95.
37. Paefgen V, Doleschel D, Kiessling F. Evolution of contrast agents for ultrasound imaging and ultrasound-mediated drug delivery. Front Pharmacol. 2015;6:197.
38. Renz M. Fluorescence microscopy-a historical and technical perspective. Cytometry A. 2013;83(9):767–79.
39. Zhang Y, Lovell JF. Porphyrins as theranostic agents from prehistoric to modern times. Theranostics. 2012;2(9):905–15.
40. Coons AH, Creech HJ, Jones RN. Immunological properties of an antibody containing a fluorescent group. Proc Soc Exp Biol Med. 1941;47:200–2.
41. Moore GE, et al. The clinical use of fluorescein in neurosurgery - the localization of brain tumors. J Neurosurg. 1948;5(4):392–8.
42. Shimomura O, Johnson FH, Saiga Y. Extraction, purification and properties of aequorin, a bioluminescent protein from the luminous hydromedusan. Aequorea J Cell Comp Physiol. 1962;59:223–39.
43. Harvey EN. A history of luminescence: from the earliest times until 1900. Memoirs of the American Philosophical Society 1957, Philadelphia: American Philosophical Society. xxiii, 692 p.
44. Green AA, WD ME. Biochim Biophys Acta. 1956;20:170–6.
45. Close DM, et al. In vivo bioluminescent imaging (BLI): noninvasive visualization and interrogation of biological processes in living animals. Sensors. 2011;11(1):180–206.
46. Fraga H. Firefly luminescence: a historical perspective and recent developments. Photochem Photobiol Sci. 2008;7(2):146–58.
47. L'Annunziata M. Radioactivity: introduction and history. In L'Annunziata M (ed.) Vol. 1st edn. 2007; Elsevier.
48. Robertson R, et al. Optical imaging of Cerenkov light generation from positron-emitting radiotracers. Phys Med Biol. 2009;54(16):N355–65.

49. Holland JP, et al. Intraoperative imaging of positron emission tomographic radiotracers using Cerenkov luminescence emissions. Mol Imaging. 2011;10(3):177–86. 1-3
50. Thorek DL, Riedl CC, Grimm J. Clinical Cerenkov luminescence imaging of (18)F-FDG. J Nucl Med. 2014;55(1):95–8.
51. Moses WW. Fundamental limits of spatial resolution in PET. Nucl Instrum Methods Phys Res A. 2011;648(Supplement 1):S236–40.
52. Chatziioannou AF. Molecular imaging of small animals with dedicated PET tomographs. Eur J Nucl Med Mol Imaging. 2002;29(1):98–114.
53. Myers R. The biological application of small animal PET imaging. Nucl Med Biol. 2001;28(5):585–93.
54. Meikle SR, et al. Small animal SPECT and its place in the matrix of molecular imaging technologies. Phys Med Biol. 2005;50(22):R45–61.
55. Beyer T, et al. Dual-modality PET/CT imaging: the effect of respiratory motion on combined image quality in clinical oncology. Eur J Nucl Med Mol Imaging. 2003;30(4):588–96.
56. Townsend DW, et al. PET/CT today and tomorrow. J Nucl Med. 2004;45(Suppl 1):4S–14S.
57. Judenhofer MS, et al. Simultaneous PET-MRI: a new approach for functional and morphological imaging. Nat Med. 2008;14(4):459–65.
58. Drzezga A, et al. First clinical experience with integrated whole-body PET/MR: comparison to PET/CT in patients with oncologic diagnoses. J Nucl Med. 2012;53(6):845–55.
59. Werner P, et al. Current status and future role of brain PET/MRI in clinical and research settings. Eur J Nucl Med Mol Imaging. 2015;42(3):512–26.
60. Partovi S, et al. Clinical oncologic applications of PET/MRI: a new horizon. Am J Nucl Med Mol Imaging. 2014;4(2):202–12.
61. Ter-Pogossian MM, et al. A positron-emission transaxial tomograph for nuclear imaging (PETT). Radiology. 1975;114(1):89–98.
62. Townsend DW. Physical principles and technology of clinical PET imaging. Ann Acad Med Singap. 2004;33(2):133–45.
63. Boellaard R. Standards for PET image acquisition and quantitative data analysis. J Nucl Med. 2009;50(Suppl 1):11S–20S.
64. Heiden MGV, Cantley LC, Thompson CB. Understanding the Warburg effect: the metabolic requirements of cell proliferation. Science. 2009;324(5930):1029–33.
65. Warburg O. Origin of cancer cells. Science. 1956;123(3191):309–14.
66. Warburg O, Wind F, Negelein E. The metabolism of tumors in the body. J Gen Physiol. 1927;8(6):519–30.
67. Ido T, et al. Labeled 2-Deoxy-D-glucose analogs - F-18-labeled 2-Deoxy-2-Fluoro-D-glucose, 2-Deoxy-2-Fluoro-D-mannose and C-14-2-Deoxy-2-Fluoro-D-glucose. J Label Comp Radiopharm. 1978;14(2):175–83.
68. Kuhl DE, et al. The Mark IV system for radionuclide computed tomography of the brain. Radiology. 1976;121(2):405–13.
69. Reivich M, et al. Local cerebral glucose-metabolism determination in man with 18f-2-Deoxy-2-Fluoro-D-glucose. Ann Neurol. 1977;1(5):495–6.
70. Reivich M, et al. Fluorodeoxyglucose-F-18 method for the measurement of local cerebral glucose-utilization in man. Circ Res. 1979;44(1):127–37.
71. Muehllehner G, Buchin MP, Dudek JH. Performance parameters of a positron imaging camera. IEEE Trans Nucl Sci. 1976;23(1):528–37.
72. Dichiro G, et al. F-18-2-Fluoro-2-Deoxyglucose positron emission tomography of human cerebral Gliomas. J Comput Assist Tomogr. 1981;5(6):937.
73. Patronas NJ, et al. Grading of cerebral gliomas by positron emission tomography (PET) using F-18 fluorodeoxyglucose (Fdg). J Nucl Med. 1982;23(5):P6.
74. Braun JJ, et al. 18F-FDG PET/CT in sarcoidosis management: review and report of 20 cases. Eur J Nucl Med Mol Imaging. 2008;35(8):1537–43.
75. Prager E, et al. Comparison of 18F-FDG and 67Ga-citrate in sarcoidosis imaging. Nuklearmedizin. 2008;47(1):18–23.
76. Youssef G, et al. The use of 18F FDG PET in the diagnosis of cardiac sarcoidosis: a systematic review and metaanalysis including the Ontario experience. J Nucl Med. 2012;53(2):241–8.
77. Beckers C, et al. Assessment of disease activity in rheumatoid arthritis with (18)F-FDG PET. J Nucl Med. 2004;45(6):956–64.
78. Kubota K, et al. Whole-body FDG-PET/CT on rheumatoid arthritis of large joints. Ann Nucl Med. 2009;23(9):783–91.
79. Elzinga EH, et al. 18F-FDG PET as a tool to predict the clinical outcome of infliximab treatment of rheumatoid arthritis: an explorative study. J Nucl Med. 2011;52(1):77–80.
80. Rudd JH, et al. Atherosclerosis inflammation imaging with 18F-FDG PET: carotid, iliac, and femoral uptake reproducibility, quantification methods, and recommendations. J Nucl Med. 2008;49(6):871–8.
81. Bural GG, et al. FDG-PET is an effective imaging modality to detect and quantify age-related atherosclerosis in large arteries. Eur J Nucl Med Mol Imaging. 2008;35(3):562–9.
82. Chen W, et al. Emerging role of FDG-PET/CT in assessing atherosclerosis in large arteries. Eur J Nucl Med Mol Imaging. 2009;36(1):144–51.
83. Kubota K. From tumor biology to clinical pet: a review of positron emission tomography (PET) in oncology. Ann Nucl Med. 2001;15(6):471–86.
84. Gambhir SS, et al. A tabulated summary of the FDG PET literature. J Nucl Med. 2001;42(5 Suppl):1S–93S.
85. Antoch G, et al. Accuracy of whole-body dual-modality fluorine-18-2-fluoro-2-deoxy-D-glucose positron emission tomography and computed tomography (FDG-PET/CT) for tumor staging in

solid tumors: comparison with CT and PET. J Clin Oncol. 2004;22(21):4357–68.
86. de Geus-Oei LF, et al. Monitoring and predicting response to therapy with 18F-FDG PET in colorectal cancer: a systematic review. J Nucl Med. 2009;50(Suppl 1):43S–54S.
87. Elstrom R, et al. Utility of FDG-PET scanning in lymphoma by WHO classification. Blood. 2003;101(10):3875–6.
88. Gayed I, et al. The role of 18F-FDG PET in staging and early prediction of response to therapy of recurrent gastrointestinal stromal tumors. J Nucl Med. 2004;45(1):17–21.
89. Havrilesky LJ, et al. FDG-PET for management of cervical and ovarian cancer. Gynecol Oncol. 2005;97(1):183–91.
90. Huebner RH, et al. A meta-analysis of the literature for whole-body FDG PET detection of recurrent colorectal cancer. J Nucl Med. 2000;41(7):1177–89.
91. Isasi CR, Moadel RM, Blaufox MD. A meta-analysis of FDG-PET for the evaluation of breast cancer recurrence and metastases. Breast Cancer Res Treat. 2005;90(2):105–12.
92. Keidar Z, et al. PET/CT using 18F-FDG in suspected lung cancer recurrence: diagnostic value and impact on patient management. J Nucl Med. 2004;45(10):1640–6.
93. Kelloff GJ, et al. Progress and promise of FDG-PET imaging for cancer patient management and oncologic drug development. Clin Cancer Res. 2005;11(8):2785–808.
94. Kwee TC, Kwee RM. Combined FDG-PET/CT for the detection of unknown primary tumors: systematic review and meta-analysis. Eur Radiol. 2009;19(3):731–44.
95. Shim SS, et al. Non-small cell lung cancer: prospective comparison of integrated FDG PET/CT and CT alone for preoperative staging. Radiology. 2005;236(3):1011–9.
96. Tatsumi M, et al. Initial experience with FDG-PET/CT in the evaluation of breast cancer. Eur J Nucl Med Mol Imaging. 2006;33(3):254–62.
97. van Westreenen HL, et al. Systematic review of the staging performance of 18F-fluorodeoxyglucose positron emission tomography in esophageal cancer. J Clin Oncol. 2004;22(18):3805–12.
98. Strauss LG. Fluorine-18 deoxyglucose and false-positive results: a major problem in the diagnostics of oncological patients. Eur J Nucl Med. 1996;23(10):1409–15.
99. Rosenbaum SJ, et al. False-positive FDG PET uptake-the role of PET/CT. Eur Radiol. 2006;16(5):1054–65.
100. Yu CY, et al. Comparative performance of PET tracers in biochemical recurrence of prostate cancer: a critical analysis of literature. Am J Nucl Med Mol Imaging. 2014;4(6):580–601.
101. Salminen E, et al. Investigations with FDG-PET scanning in prostate cancer show limited value for clinical practice. Acta Oncol. 2002;41(5):425–9.
102. Jadvar H, Pinski JK, Conti PS. FDG PET in suspected recurrent and metastatic prostate cancer. Oncol Rep. 2003;10(5):1485–8.
103. Shin JA, et al. Diagnostic accuracy of 18F-FDG positron emission tomography for evaluation of hepatocellular carcinoma. Korean J Hepatol. 2006;12(4):546–52.
104. Lin CY, et al. 18F-FDG PET or PET/CT for detecting extrahepatic metastases or recurrent hepatocellular carcinoma: a systematic review and meta-analysis. Eur J Radiol. 2012;81(9):2417–22.
105. Glunde K, Bhujwalla ZM, Ronen SM. Choline metabolism in malignant transformation. Nat Rev Cancer. 2011;11(12):835–48.
106. Hara T, Kosaka N, Kishi H. PET imaging of prostate cancer using carbon-11-choline. J Nucl Med. 1998;39(6):990–5.
107. Reske SN, et al. Imaging prostate cancer with 11C-choline PET/CT. J Nucl Med. 2006;47(8):1249–54.
108. Husarik DB, et al. Evaluation of [(18)F]-choline PET/CT for staging and restaging of prostate cancer. Eur J Nucl Med Mol Imaging. 2008;35(2):253–63.
109. Brogsitter C, Zophel K, Kotzerke J. F-18-choline, C-11-choline and C-11-acetate PET/CT: comparative analysis for imaging prostate cancer patients. Eur J Nucl Med Mol Imaging. 2013;40:S18–27.
110. Fanti S, et al. PET/CT with (11)C-choline for evaluation of prostate cancer patients with biochemical recurrence: meta-analysis and critical review of available data. Eur J Nucl Med Mol Imaging. 2016;43(1):55–69.
111. Umbehr MH, et al. The role of 11C-choline and 18F-fluorocholine positron emission tomography (PET) and PET/CT in prostate cancer: a systematic review and meta-analysis. Eur Urol. 2013;64(1):106–17.
112. Grassi I, et al. The clinical use of PET with 11C-acetate. Am J Nucl Med Mol Imaging. 2012;2(1):33.
113. Mohsen B, et al. Application of 11C-acetate positron-emission tomography (PET) imaging in prostate cancer: systematic review and meta-analysis of the literature. BJU Int. 2013;112(8):1062–72.
114. Oyama N, et al. 11C-acetate PET imaging of prostate cancer. J Nucl Med. 2002;43(2):181–6.
115. Mehrkens JH, et al. The positive predictive value of O-(2-[18F]fluoroethyl)-L-tyrosine (FET) PET in the diagnosis of a glioma recurrence after multimodal treatment. J Neuro-Oncol. 2008;88(1):27–35.
116. Popperl G, et al. FET PET for the evaluation of untreated gliomas: correlation of FET uptake and uptake kinetics with tumour grading. Eur J Nucl Med Mol Imaging. 2007;34(12):1933–42.
117. Floeth FW, et al. Comparison of (18)F-FET PET and 5-ALA fluorescence in cerebral gliomas. Eur J Nucl Med Mol Imaging. 2011;38(4):731–41.
118. Singhal T, et al. 11C-L-methionine positron emission tomography in the clinical management of cerebral gliomas. Mol Imaging Biol. 2008;10(1):1–18.
119. Jager PL, et al. Radiolabeled amino acids: basic aspects and clinical applications in oncology. J Nucl Med. 2001;42(3):432–45.

120. Laverman P, et al. Fluorinated amino acids for tumour imaging with positron emission tomography. Eur J Nucl Med Mol Imaging. 2002;29(5):681–90.
121. Mattoli MV, et al. Usefulness of 11C-methionine positron emission tomography in differential diagnosis between recurrent tumours and radiation necrosis in patients with glioma: an overview. Open Neurosurg J. 2012;5:8–11.
122. Weber WA, et al. O-(2-[18F]fluoroethyl)-L-tyrosine and L-[methyl-11C]methionine uptake in brain tumours: initial results of a comparative study. Eur J Nucl Med. 2000;27(5):542–9.
123. Grosu AL, et al. An interindividual comparison of O-(2-[18F]fluoroethyl)-L-tyrosine (FET)- and L-[methyl-11C]methionine (MET)-PET in patients with brain gliomas and metastases. Int J Radiat Oncol Biol Phys. 2011;81(4):1049–58.
124. Nanni C, et al. (18)F-FACBC (anti1-amino-3-(18) F-fluorocyclobutane-1-carboxylic acid) versus (11) C-choline PET/CT in prostate cancer relapse: results of a prospective trial. Eur J Nucl Med Mol Imaging. 2016;43(9):1601–10.
125. Chen W, et al. Imaging proliferation in brain tumors with 18F-FLT PET: comparison with 18F-FDG. J Nucl Med. 2005;46(6):945–52.
126. Mier W, Haberkorn U, Eisenhut M. [18F]FLT; portrait of a proliferation marker. Eur J Nucl Med Mol Imaging. 2002;29(2):165–9.
127. Wagner M, et al. 3′-[18F]fluoro-3′-deoxythymidine ([18F]-FLT) as positron emission tomography tracer for imaging proliferation in a murine B-cell lymphoma model and in the human disease. Cancer Res. 2003;63(10):2681–7.
128. Dittmann H, et al. [18F]FLT PET for diagnosis and staging of thoracic tumours. Eur J Nucl Med Mol Imaging. 2003;30(10):1407–12.
129. Smyczek-Gargya B, et al. PET with [18F]fluorothymidine for imaging of primary breast cancer: a pilot study. Eur J Nucl Med Mol Imaging. 2004;31(5):720–4.
130. Peck M, et al. Applications of PET imaging with the proliferation marker [18F]-FLT. Q J Nucl Med Mol Imaging. 2015;59(1):95–104.
131. Peeters S, et al. Hypoxia imaging with [18F]HX4 PET compared with [18F] FMISO and [18F] FAZA: from preclinical to clinical studies. Mol Cancer Therap. 2013; 12(11).
132. Servagi-Vernat S, et al. A prospective clinical study of (18) F-FAZA PET-CT hypoxia imaging in head and neck squamous cell carcinoma before and during radiation therapy. Eur J Nucl Med Mol Imaging. 2014;41(8):1544–52.
133. Bell C, et al. Hypoxia imaging in Gliomas with F-18-Fluoromisonidazole PET: toward clinical translation. Semin Nucl Med. 2015;45(2):136–50.
134. Kinoshita T, et al. Clinical impacts of tumor hypoxia imaging with FAZA and ATSM PET in NSCLC. J Thorac Oncol. 2015;10(9):S381.
135. Bollineni VR, et al. PET imaging of tumor hypoxia using F-18-Fluoroazomycin Arabinoside in stage III-IV non-small cell lung cancer patients. J Nucl Med. 2013;54(8):1175–80.
136. Holland JP, Lewis JS, Dehdashti F. Assessing tumor hypoxia by positron emission tomography with Cu-ATSM. Q J Nucl Med Mol Imag. 2009;53(2):193–200.
137. Chia K, Fleming IN, Blower PJ. Hypoxia imaging with PET: which tracers and why? Nucl Med Commun. 2012;33(3):217–22.
138. de Herder WW, et al. Somatostatin receptors in gastroentero-pancreatic neuroendocrine tumours. Endocr Relat Cancer. 2003;10(4):451–8.
139. Fischer T, et al. Reassessment of sst2 somatostatin receptor expression in human normal and neoplastic tissues using the novel rabbit monoclonal antibody UMB-1. J Clin Endocrinol Metab. 2008;93(11):4519–24.
140. Fjallskog ML, et al. Expression of somatostatin receptor subtypes 1 to 5 in tumor tissue and intratumoral vessels in malignant endocrine pancreatic tumors. Med Oncol. 2003;20(1):59–67.
141. Ginj M, et al. Radiolabeled somatostatin receptor antagonists are preferable to agonists for in vivo peptide receptor targeting of tumors. Proc Natl Acad Sci U S A. 2006;103(44):16436–41.
142. Reubi JC, Maecke HR. Peptide-based probes for cancer imaging. J Nucl Med. 2008;49(11):1735–8.
143. Breeman WA, et al. (68)Ga-labeled DOTA-peptides and (68)Ga-labeled radiopharmaceuticals for positron emission tomography: current status of research, clinical applications, and future perspectives. Semin Nucl Med. 2011;41(4):314–21.
144. Afshar-Oromieh A, et al. The diagnostic value of PET/CT imaging with the (68)Ga-labelled PSMA ligand HBED-CC in the diagnosis of recurrent prostate cancer. Eur J Nucl Med Mol Imaging. 2015;42(2):197–209.
145. Afshar-Oromieh A, et al. PET imaging with a [68Ga] gallium-labelled PSMA ligand for the diagnosis of prostate cancer: biodistribution in humans and first evaluation of tumour lesions. Eur J Nucl Med Mol Imaging. 2013;40(4):486–95.
146. Wieser G, et al. GRPR antagonist 68Ga-RM2 as PET tracer for imaging prostate cancer: initial experiences. J Nucl Med. 2014; 55.
147. Nock BA, et al. Theranostic perspectives in prostate cancer with the GRPR-antagonist NeoBOMB1—preclinical and first clinical results. J Nucl Med. 2016.
148. Zhang Y, Hong H, Cai W. PET tracers based on zirconium-89. Curr Radiopharm. 2011;4(2):131–9.
149. Wu AM. Antibodies and antimatter: the resurgence of immuno-PET. J Nucl Med. 2009;50(1):2–5.
150. van Dongen GA, et al. Immuno-PET: a navigator in monoclonal antibody development and applications. Oncologist. 2007;12(12):1379–89.
151. Verel I, Visser GW, van Dongen GA. The promise of immuno-PET in radioimmunotherapy. J Nucl Med. 2005;46(Suppl 1):164S–71S.
152. Wright BD, Lapi SE. Designing the magic bullet? The advancement of immuno-PET into clinical use. J Nucl Med. 2013;54(8):1171–4.

153. Lage E, et al. Recovery and normalization of triple coincidences in PET. Med Phys. 2015;42(3):1398–410.
154. Cal-Gonzalez J, et al. Simulation of triple coincidences in PET. Phys Med Biol. 2015;60(1):117–36.
155. Beekman FJ, et al. G -SPECT-I: a full ring high sensitivity and ultra-fast clinical molecular imaging system with < 3mm resolution. Eur J Nucl Med Mol Imaging. 2015;42:S209.
156. Hoppin JW, et al. High-resolution multi-pinhole SPECT study of arthritic hands. Eur J Nucl Med Mol Imaging. 2005;32:S259.
157. Bailey DL, Willowson KP. Quantitative SPECT/CT: SPECT joins PET as a quantitative imaging modality. Eur J Nucl Med Mol Imaging. 2014;41(Suppl 1):S17–25.
158. Nakazawa A, et al. Usefulness of dual 67Ga and 99mTc-sestamibi single-photon-emission CT scanning in the diagnosis of cardiac sarcoidosis. Chest. 2004;126(4):1372–6.
159. Weinmann P, et al. Clinical validation of simultaneous dual-isotope myocardial scintigraphy. Eur J Nucl Med Mol Imaging. 2003;30(1):25–31.
160. Richards P, Tucker WD, Srivastava SC. Technetium-99m: an historical perspective. Int J Appl Radiat Isot. 1982;33(10):793–9.
161. Khalil MM, et al. Molecular SPECT imaging: an overview. Int J Mol Imaging. 2011;2011:796025.
162. Vallabhajosula S. Molecular imaging: radiopharmaceuticals for PET and SPECT. Molecular imaging: radiopharmaceuticals for Pet and Spect. 2009; 1–371.
163. Zuckier LS, DeNardo GL. Trials and tribulations: oncological antibody imaging comes to the fore. Semin Nucl Med. 1997;27(1):10–29.
164. Laverman P, et al. Radiolabelled peptides for oncological diagnosis. Eur J Nucl Med Mol Imaging. 2012;39(Suppl 1):S78–92.
165. van der Lely AJ, et al. Octreoscan radioreceptor imaging. Endocrine. 2003;20(3):307–11.
166. de Herder WW, et al. Somatostatin receptor imaging for neuroendocrine tumors. Pituitary. 2006;9(3):243–8.
167. Kwekkeboom DJ, Krenning EP. Somatostatin receptor imaging. Semin Nucl Med. 2002;32(2):84–91.
168. Chowdhury FU, Scarsbrook AF. The role of hybrid SPECT-CT in oncology: current and emerging clinical applications. Clin Radiol. 2008;63(3):241–51.
169. Pandit-Taskar N, et al. Single photon emission computed tomography SPECT-CT improves sentinel node detection and localization in cervical and uterine malignancy. Gynecol Oncol. 2010;117(1):59–64.
170. Husarik DB, Steinert HC. Single-photon emission computed tomography/computed tomography for sentinel node mapping in breast cancer. Semin Nucl Med. 2007;37(1):29–33.
171. Uren RF, et al. SPECT/CT scans allow precise anatomical location of sentinel lymph nodes in breast cancer and redefine lymphatic drainage from the breast to the axilla. Breast. 2012;21(4):480–6.
172. Horger M, et al. Evaluation of combined transmission and emission tomography for classification of skeletal lesions. AJR Am J Roentgenol. 2004;183(3):655–61.
173. Even-Sapir E. Imaging of malignant bone involvement by morphologic, scintigraphic, and hybrid modalities. J Nucl Med. 2005;46(8):1356–67.
174. Dumas C, Schibli R, Schubiger PA. Versatile routes to C-2- and C-6-functionalized glucose derivatives of iminodiacetic acid. J Org Chem. 2003;68(2):512–8.
175. Martin WH, et al. FDG-SPECT: correlation with FDG-PET. J Nucl Med. 1995;36(6):988–95.
176. Langen KJ, et al. SPECT studies of brain tumors with L-3-[123I] iodo-alpha-methyl tyrosine: comparison with PET, 124IMT and first clinical results. J Nucl Med. 1990;31(3):281–6.
177. Weckesser M, et al. Iodine-123 alpha-methyl tyrosine single-photon emission tomography of cerebral gliomas: standardised evaluation of tumour uptake and extent. Eur J Nucl Med. 1998;25(2):150–6.
178. Kawai K, et al. A strategy for the study of cerebral amino acid transport using iodine-123-labeled amino acid radiopharmaceutical: 3-iodo-alpha-methyl-L-tyrosine. J Nucl Med. 1991;32(5):819–24.
179. Reimer P, et al. Clinical MR imaging. Springer, New York; 2010.
180. Schmidt GP, et al. High-resolution whole-body magnetic resonance image tumor staging with the use of parallel imaging versus dual-modality positron emission tomography-computed tomography - experience on a 32-channel system. Investig Radiol. 2005;40(12):743–53.
181. Lauenstein TC, et al. Whole body MR imaging for tumor staging. Radiology. 2002;225:269–70.
182. Schmidt GP, Reiser MF, Baur-Melnyk A. Whole-body MRI for the staging and follow-up of patients with metastasis. Eur J Radiol. 2009;70(3):393–400.
183. Abramson RG, et al. MR imaging biomarkers in oncology clinical trials. Magn Reson Imaging Clin N Am. 2016;24(1):11–29.
184. Golman K, et al. Silvanus Thompson Memorial lecture molecular imaging using hyperpolarized C-13. Br J Radiol. 2003;76:S118–27.
185. Edelstein WA, et al. The intrinsic signal-to-noise ratio in NMR imaging. Magn Reson Med. 1986;3(4):604–18.
186. Bellin MF, Van Der Molen AJ. Extracellular gadolinium-based contrast media: an overview. Eur J Radiol. 2008;66(2):160–7.
187. Caravan P, et al. Gadolinium(III) chelates as MRI contrast agents: structure, dynamics, and applications. Chem Rev. 1999;99(9):2293–352.
188. Kuo PH. Gadolinium-containing MRI contrast agents: important variations on a theme for NSF. J Am Coll Radiol. 2008;5(1):29–35.
189. Trattnig S, et al. The optimal use of contrast agents at high field MRI. Eur Radiol. 2006;16(6):1280–7.
190. Clarkson RB. Blood-pool MRI contrast agents: properties and characterization. Contrast Agents I. 2002;221:201–35.

191. Mohs AM, Lu ZR. Gadolinium(III)-based blood-pool contrast agents for magnetic resonance imaging: status and clinical potential. Expert Opin Drug Deliv. 2007;4(2):149–64.
192. Reimer P, Schneider G, Schima W. Hepatobiliary contrast agents for contrast-enhanced MRI of the liver: properties, clinical development and applications. Eur Radiol. 2004;14(4):559–78.
193. Cheng W, et al. Magnetic resonance imaging (MRI) contrast agents for tumor diagnosis. J Healthc Eng. 2013;4(1):23–45.
194. Wang YX. Superparamagnetic iron oxide based MRI contrast agents: current status of clinical application. Quant Imaging Med Surg. 2011;1(1):35–40.
195. Jin R, et al. Superparamagnetic iron oxide nanoparticles for MR imaging and therapy: design considerations and clinical applications. Curr Opin Pharmacol. 2014;18:18–27.
196. Yang H, et al. Targeted dual-contrast T1- and T2-weighted magnetic resonance imaging of tumors using multifunctional gadolinium-labeled superparamagnetic iron oxide nanoparticles. Biomaterials. 2011;32(20):4584–93.
197. Nunn AD, Linder KE, Tweedle MF. Can receptors be imaged with MRI agents? Q J Nucl Med. 1997;41(2):155–62.
198. Majos C, et al. Proton MR spectroscopy improves discrimination between tumor and Pseudotumoral lesion in solid brain masses. Am J Neuroradiol. 2009;30(3):544–51.
199. Coffey AM, Truong ML, Chekmenev EY. Low-field MRI can be more sensitive than high-field MRI. J Magn Reson. 2013;237:169–74.
200. Keshari KR, Wilson DM. Chemistry and biochemistry of C-13 hyperpolarized magnetic resonance using dynamic nuclear polarization. Chem Soc Rev. 2014;43(5):1627–59.
201. Golman K, In't Zandt R, Thaning M. Real-time metabolic imaging. Proc Natl Acad Sci U S A. 2006; 103(30): 11270–5.
202. Nelson SJ, et al. Metabolic imaging of patients with prostate cancer using hyperpolarized [1-(1)(3)C] pyruvate. Sci Transl Med. 2013;5(198):198ra108.
203. Keshari KR, et al. Hyperpolarized 13C-pyruvate magnetic resonance reveals rapid lactate export in metastatic renal cell carcinomas. Cancer Res. 2013;73(2):529–38.
204. Day SE, et al. Detecting tumor response to treatment using hyperpolarized 13C magnetic resonance imaging and spectroscopy. Nat Med. 2007;13(11):1382–7.
205. Gallagher FA, et al. Production of hyperpolarized [1,4-13C2]malate from [1,4-13C2]fumarate is a marker of cell necrosis and treatment response in tumors. Proc Natl Acad Sci U S A. 2009;106(47):19801–6.
206. Golman K, et al. Metabolic imaging by hyperpolarized 13C magnetic resonance imaging for in vivo tumor diagnosis. Cancer Res. 2006;66(22):10855–60.
207. Witney TH, Brindle KM. Imaging tumour cell metabolism using hyperpolarized C-13 magnetic resonance spectroscopy. Biochem Soc Trans. 2010;38:1220–4.
208. Albert MS, Balamore D. Development of hyperpolarized noble gas MRI. Nucl Instrum Methods Phys Res A. 1998;402:441–53.
209. Goodson BM. Nuclear magnetic resonance of laser-polarized noble gases in molecules, materials, and organisms. J Magn Reson. 2002;155(2):157–216.
210. Mugler JP 3rd, et al. MR imaging and spectroscopy using hyperpolarized 129Xe gas: preliminary human results. Magn Reson Med. 1997;37(6):809–15.
211. MacFall JR, et al. Human lung air spaces: potential for MR imaging with hyperpolarized He-3. Radiology. 1996;200(2):553–8.
212. Fain SB, et al. Functional lung imaging using hyperpolarized gas MRI. J Magn Reson Imaging. 2007;25(5):910–23.
213. Albert MS, et al. Hyperpolarized 129Xe MR imaging of the oral cavity. J Magn Reson B. 1996;111(2):204–7.
214. Bifone A, et al. NMR of laser-polarized xenon in human blood. Proc Natl Acad Sci U S A. 1996;93(23):12932–6.
215. Shung KK. High frequency ultrasonic imaging. J Med Ultrasound. 2009;17(1):25 30.
216. Prager RW, et al. Three-dimensional ultrasound imaging. Proc Inst Mech Eng Part H J Eng Med. 2010;224(H2):193–223.
217. Rychak JJ, et al. Microultrasound molecular imaging of vascular endothelial growth factor receptor 2 in a mouse model of tumor angiogenesis. Mol Imaging. 2007;6(5):289–96.
218. Jun HY, et al. Long residence time of ultrasound microbubbles targeted to integrin in murine tumor model. Acad Radiol. 2010;17(1):54–60.
219. Chen ZY, Liang K, Qiu RX. Targeted gene delivery in tumor xenografts by the combination of ultrasound-targeted microbubble destruction and polyethylenimine to inhibit survivin gene expression and induce apoptosis. J Exp Clin Cancer Res. 2010;29:152.
220. Li P, et al. Ultrasound triggered drug release from 10-hydroxycamptothecin-loaded phospholipid microbubbles for targeted tumor therapy in mice. J Control Release. 2012;162(2):349–54.
221. Ntziachristos V, Razansky D. Molecular imaging by means of multispectral Optoacoustic tomography (MSOT). Chem Rev. 2010;110(5):2783–94.
222. Copland JA, et al. Bioconjugated gold nanoparticles as a molecular based contrast agent: implications for imaging of deep tumors using optoacoustic tomography. Mol Imaging Biol. 2004;6(5):341–9.
223. Weber J, Beard PC, Bohndiek SE. Contrast agents for molecular photoacoustic imaging. Nat Methods. 2016;13(8):639–50.
224. Martelli C, et al. Optical imaging probes in oncology. Oncotarget. 2016;7(30):48753–87.
225. Solomon M, et al. Optical imaging in cancer research: basic principles, tumor detection, and therapeutic monitoring. Med Princ Pract. 2011;20(5):397–415.

226. Massoud TF, Gambhir SS. Molecular imaging in living subjects: seeing fundamental biological processes in a new light. Genes Dev. 2003;17(5):545–80.
227. Mahmood U, et al. Near-infrared optical imaging of protease activity for tumor detection. Radiology. 1999;213(3):866–70.
228. Arranz A, Ripoll J. Advances in optical imaging for pharmacological studies. Front Pharmacol. 2015;6:189.
229. Bradley RS, Thorniley MS. A review of attenuation correction techniques for tissue fluorescence. J R Soc Interface. 2006;3(6):1–13.
230. Mahmood U, Weissleder R. Near-infrared optical imaging of proteases in cancer. Mol Cancer Ther. 2003;2(5):489–96.
231. Mansfield JR. Distinguished photons: a review of in vivo spectral fluorescence imaging in small animals. Curr Pharm Biotechnol. 2010;11(6):628–38.
232. Etrych T, et al. Fluorescence optical imaging in anticancer drug delivery. J Control Release. 2016;226:168–81.
233. Ntziachristos V, et al. Looking and listening to light: the evolution of whole-body photonic imaging. Nat Biotechnol. 2005;23(3):313–20.
234. Ke S, et al. Near-infrared optical imaging of epidermal growth factor receptor in breast cancer xenografts. Cancer Res. 2003;63(22):7870–5.
235. Wunder A, et al. In vivo imaging of protease activity in arthritis - a novel approach for monitoring treatment response. Arthritis Rheum. 2004;50(8):2459–65.
236. Kaur S, et al. Recent trends in antibody-based oncologic imaging. Cancer Lett. 2012;315(2):97–111.
237. Hansel TT, et al. The safety and side effects of monoclonal antibodies. Nat Rev Drug Discov. 2010;9(4):325–38.
238. Nechansky A. HAHA-nothing to laugh about. Measuring the immunogenicity (human anti-human antibody response) induced by humanized monoclonal antibodies applying ELISA and SPR technology. J Pharm Biomed Anal. 2010;51(1):252–4.
239. Melendez-Alafort L, Muzzio PC, Rosato A. Optical and multimodal peptide-based probes for in vivo molecular imaging. Anti Cancer Agents Med Chem. 2012;12(5):476–99.
240. Hanahan D, Weinberg RA. Hallmarks of cancer: the next generation. Cell. 2011;144(5):646–74.
241. Reiner T, et al. Imaging therapeutic PARP inhibition in vivo through bioorthogonally developed companion imaging agents. Neoplasia. 2012;14(3):169.
242. Thurber GM, et al. Single-cell and subcellular pharmacokinetic imaging allows insight into drug action in vivo. Nat Commun. 2013;4:1504.
243. Foersch S, et al. Endomicroscopic imaging of COX-2 activity in murine sporadic and colitis-associated colorectal cancer. Diagn Ther Endosc. 2013;2013:250641.
244. Yoo JS, et al. A macrophage-specific fluorescent probe for intraoperative lymph node staging. Cancer Res. 2014;74(1):44–55.
245. Yi X, et al. Near-infrared fluorescent probes in cancer imaging and therapy: an emerging field. Int J Nanomedicine. 2014;9:1347–65.
246. Rosenthal EL, et al. Safety and tumor specificity of Cetuximab-IRDye800 for surgical navigation in head and neck cancer. Clin Cancer Res. 2015;21(16):3658–66.
247. Onda N, et al. Preferential tumor cellular uptake and retention of indocyanine green for in vivo tumor imaging. Int J Cancer. 2016;139(3):673–82.
248. Siddighi S, Yune JJ, Hardesty J. Indocyanine green for intraoperative localization of ureter. Am J Obstet Gynecol. 2014;211(4):436.
249. Toh U, et al. Navigation surgery for intraoperative sentinel lymph node detection using Indocyanine green (ICG) fluorescence real-time imaging in breast cancer. Breast Cancer Res Treat. 2015;153(2):337–44.
250. Jewell EL, et al. Detection of sentinel lymph nodes in minimally invasive surgery using indocyanine green and near-infrared fluorescence imaging for uterine and cervical malignancies. Gynecol Oncol. 2014;133(2):274–7.
251. Lau D, et al. A prospective phase II clinical trial of 5-aminolevulinic acid to assess the correlation of intraoperative fluorescence intensity and degree of histologic cellularity during resection of high-grade gliomas. J Neurosurg. 2016;124(5):1300–9.
252. Guyotat. J., et al., 5-Aminolevulinic acid-Protoporphyrin IX fluorescence-guided surgery of high-grade Gliomas: a systematic review. Adv Tech Stand Neurosurg. 2016;43(43):61–90.
253. Luo S, et al. A review of NIR dyes in cancer targeting and imaging. Biomaterials. 2011;32(29):7127–38.
254. Buchs NC, et al. Intra-operative fluorescent cholangiography using indocyanin green during robotic single site cholecystectomy. Int J Med Robot Comput Assist Surg. 2012;8(4):436–40.
255. van Dam GM, et al. Intraoperative tumor-specific fluorescence imaging in ovarian cancer by folate receptor-alpha targeting: first in-human results. Nat Med. 2011;17(10):1315–9.
256. Koch M, Ntziachristos V. Advancing surgical vision with fluorescence imaging. Annu Rev Med. 2016;67:153–64.
257. Barabino G, et al. Intraoperative near-infrared fluorescence imaging using indocyanine green in colorectal carcinomatosis surgery: proof of concept. Eur J Surg Oncol. 2016;43(1):242–3.
258. Bradbury MS, et al. Intraoperative mapping of sentinel lymph node metastases using a clinically translated ultrasmall silica nanoparticle. Wiley Interdiscip Rev Nanomed Nanobiotechnol. 2016;8(4):535–53.
259. Atreya R, et al. In vivo imaging using fluorescent antibodies to tumor necrosis factor predicts therapeutic response in Crohn's disease. Nat Med. 2014;20(3):313–8.
260. Burggraaf J, et al. Detection of colorectal polyps in humans using an intravenously administered

fluorescent peptide targeted against c-met. Nat Med. 2015;21(8):955–61.

261. Wu JC, et al. Noninvasive optical imaging of firefly luciferase reporter gene expression in skeletal muscles of living mice. Mol Ther. 2001;4(4):297–306.
262. Shah K, et al. Molecular imaging of gene therapy for cancer. Gene Ther. 2004;11(15):1175–87.
263. Li J, et al. Cage the firefly luciferin! - a strategy for developing bioluminescent probes. Chem Soc Rev. 2013;42(2):662–76.
264. Massoud TF, et al. Reporter gene imaging of protein-protein interactions in living subjects. Curr Opin Biotechnol. 2007;18(1):31–7.
265. Ruggiero A, et al. Cerenkov luminescence imaging of medical isotopes. J Nucl Med. 2010;51(7):1123–30.
266. Thorek DL, et al. Positron lymphography: multimodal, high-resolution, dynamic mapping and resection of lymph nodes after intradermal injection of 18F-FDG. J Nucl Med. 2012;53(9):1438–45.
267. Spinelli AE, et al. First human Cerenkography. J Biomed Opt. 2013;18(2):20502.
268. Singh G, et al. Nuclear and optical dual-labelled imaging agents. Design and challenges. Nuklearmedizin. 2016;55(2):41–50.

2 A Topical Report on the Design Principles of Metabolism

Christopher J. Halbrook, Ho-Joon Lee, Lewis C. Cantley, and Costas A. Lyssiotis

2.1 Metabolism: Basic Biochemical Principles and Fundamental Concepts

Physiological processes in living organisms are achieved by processing nutrients from the environment in a highly orchestrated manner. Metabolism is the collection of all the biochemical reactions and cellular processes involved in nutrient processing. Metabolic activity can be divided generally into processes that break down macromolecules to generate cellular energy (catabolism) and those that synthesize basic and complex biomolecular building blocks (anabolism) (Fig. 2.1).

The principle nutrients used in metabolism are carbohydrates, amino acids, and lipids. The central metabolic pathways within a cell that break down or synthesize these nutrients are surprisingly similar in all forms of life. They include glycolysis and gluconeogenesis, the citric acid cycle, oxidative phosphorylation, lipid biosynthesis, and nucleotide biosynthesis. They all require the transfer of energy, carbon, oxygen, nitrogen, or other chemical compounds and the maintenance of a proper chemical balance among substrates and products within all metabolic reactions for proper functioning of life. The intermediate molecules in all reaction steps are called metabolites.

The structure of metabolic pathways is diverse, varying from pathways which contain only a few reactions to complex pathways consisting of many reactions. Directionality further adds to the diversity of these pathways, as they can be linear, branched, convergent, divergent, or cyclic. Convergent or degradative pathways are called catabolic. These pathways convert large nutrient molecules into small or simple products coupled with the release of energy as heat or the storage of energy in shared chemical intermediates. Some of these important molecules include adenosine triphosphate (ATP), the reduced form of nicotinamide adenine dinucleotide (NADH), and the reduced form of nicotinamide adenine dinucleotide phosphate (NADPH) (Fig. 2.1). Divergent or biosynthetic pathways are called anabolic. These pathways function to build large and complex

Christopher J. Halbrook and Ho-Joon Lee contributed equally to this work.

C.J. Halbrook • H.-J. Lee
Department of Molecular and Integrative Physiology, University of Michigan, Ann Arbor, MI 48109, USA

L.C. Cantley
Department of Medicine, Meyer Cancer Center, Weill Cornell Medicine, New York City, NY 10065, USA

C.A. Lyssiotis (✉)
Department of Molecular and Integrative Physiology, University of Michigan, Ann Arbor, MI 48109, USA

Division of Gastroenterology, Department of Internal Medicine, University of Michigan, Ann Arbor, MI 48109, USA
e-mail: clyssiot@med.umich.edu

J.S. Lewis, K.R. Keshari (eds.), *Imaging and Metabolism*, DOI 10.1007/978-3-319-61401-4_2

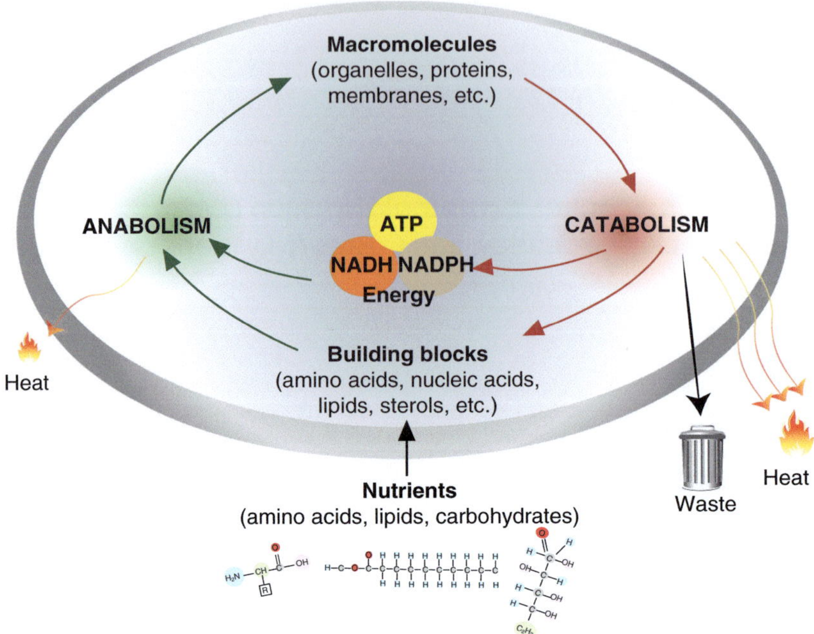

Fig. 2.1 *The basics of metabolism.* All metabolic processes can be classified as anabolic or catabolic. Anabolic metabolism uses nutrients and energy to generate basic and complex macromolecules needed to facilitate the normal functions of the cell, such as organelles, proteins, and membranes. Catabolic processes break down macromolecules and capture and store the energy from these reactions in shared chemical intermediates that can be used in anabolic reactions or to maintain the normal cellular processes. ATP, adenosine triphosphate; NADH, nicotinamide adenine dinucleotide (reduced); NADPH nicotinamide adenine dinucleotide phosphate (reduced)

molecules such as lipids, polysaccharides, proteins, and nucleic acids from small and simple precursors, utilizing energy in the process.

Biomolecules are synthesized and degraded via protein enzymes. The directionality and reversibility of these reactions are determined either through thermodynamic factors or by substrate concentration gradients. For example, anabolic and catabolic reactions that can be carried out by employing the same enzymes reversibly are typically substrate regulated. Conversely, irreversible reactions use different enzymes for anabolic and catabolic processes. These metabolic reactions tend to be thermodynamically favorable in one direction, preventing a futile cycle. Another mechanism by which cells prevent the futile use of energy is through compartmentalization of metabolic reactions. In this case, paired catabolic and anabolic reactions are localized in different cellular compartments: for example, fatty acids are synthesized in the cytosol and catabolized in the mitochondria.

The rate of metabolic regulation can be achieved instantaneously, sometimes in less than a millisecond. In such cases, intracellular messengers modify enzyme activities by various mechanisms like covalent modification (e.g., protein phosphorylation). Metabolite abundance can also regulate a metabolic pathway through substrate or product accumulation, as discussed, or by acting on a protein site that is not directly related to its enzymatic activity and thereby changing the protein activity. This is known as allosteric regulation. In contrast, when the regulatory effect is seen more slowly (in minutes or hours), cellular signaling pathways act by changing enzyme concentrations via synthesis or degradation.

In multicellular organisms, there is another important layer of metabolic regulation, where the processes summarized above can be subdivided into those that occur within a cell, the subject of the first section of this chapter, and those that occur among cells, tissues and organs, referred to as systemic metabolism, the subject of the second section of this chapter.

2.2 Cell-Autonomous Metabolism

Living organisms and cells constantly perform work for growth, movement, survival, and reproduction. These processes all require the use of energy. In order to survive, cells must maintain a pool of energy stored in chemically stable forms. This is accomplished through the uptake of nutrient fuels like carbohydrates and lipids, which are then broken down in catabolic processes to generate such energy stores. Cells can also switch from a catabolic state to an anabolic state, such as during cell division, where biomolecules must be newly synthesized to form the DNA, organelles, and cell membranes required to produce a daughter cell. There are diverse modes of molecular regulation to activate or inhibit biochemical reactions or cellular processes: allosteric regulation, posttranslational modification, and subcellular localization, among others. In the following section, we discuss anabolic and catabolic processes in several pathways from a cell-centric point of view and then discuss the mechanisms that regulate these processes.

Catabolic metabolism. Glucose is a ubiquitous fuel in biology, and its metabolism within a cell serves as an exemplary system to discuss the structure and regulation of metabolic pathways. Under normal physiological conditions in non-proliferating mammalian cells, glucose carbons are fully oxidized to carbon dioxide (CO_2). The energy generated in this process is conserved in the shared chemical intermediate adenosine triphosphate (ATP), a principle energy currency in cells. In conditions where a cell is energy replete, glucose can be stored as the glucose-polymer glycogen, to be released and metabolized when energy is required. Glucose metabolism to generate ATP is initiated in the cytosolic pathway of glycolysis, literally glucose-lysis (Fig. 2.2).

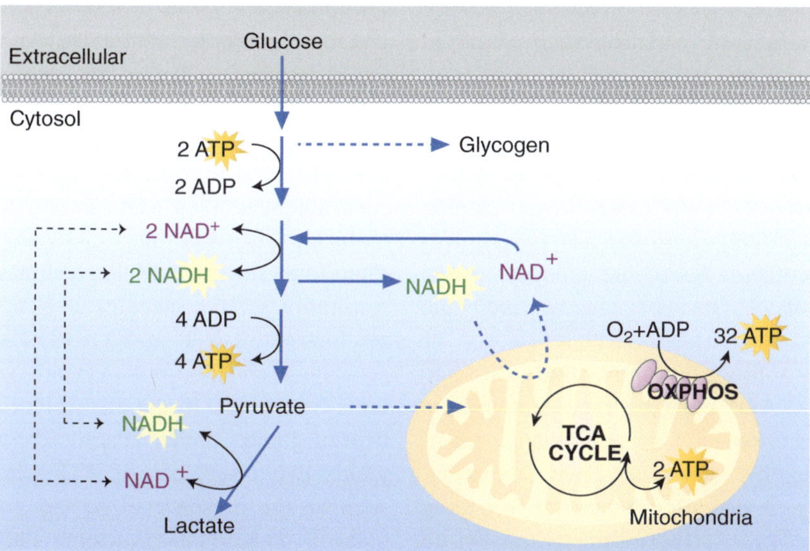

Fig. 2.2 *Glucose metabolism provides the cell with chemical energy.* Glucose is obtained from the extracellular space, where it is either catabolized to pyruvate through glycolysis or stored for later use as the glucose polymer glycogen. The initial capture of glucose in the cell costs energy in the form of ATP. Breakdown of the glucose in glycolysis returns twice the amount of energy used to capture it. Importantly, glucose metabolism into pyruvate yields reducing potential in the form of NADH. To continue glycolysis, NAD^+ must be regenerated. This can occur through pyruvate to lactate reduction or via metabolite-coupled shuttles that transfer the reducing potential stored in NADH into the mitochondria. Pyruvate transferred into the mitochondria can be used in the tricarboxylic acid (TCA) cycle, and this process together with oxidative phosphorylation (OXPHOS) can generate up to an additional 34 equivalents of ATP

Glycolysis is a universal catabolic pathway in which a series of enzyme-catalyzed reactions break down one six-carbon glucose molecule into two three-carbon molecules of pyruvate. The net energy yield of this pathway is two molecules of ATP. The direction of the penultimate step in glycolysis, pyruvate metabolism, depends on several factors; most notably is the access to molecular oxygen. In the absence of oxygen, glucose-derived carbon leaves the cell as lactate. In the presence of oxygen, glucose carbon enters the mitochondria for further metabolism. This general description of glucose metabolism is summarized in Fig. 2.2.

The process of making ATP during glycolysis requires the transfer of electrons to facilitate the enzymatic reactions. The flow of electrons is also an important form of metabolic regulation. The transfer of an electron from one molecule to another results in the oxidation of the electron-donating molecule and the reduction of the electron-accepting molecule. This form of metabolism is known as reduction-oxidation or more simply "redox" metabolism. The energy extracted from fuels by oxidation can be stored in electron carriers, which transfer electrons among metabolic intermediates in enzyme-catalyzed reactions along with the release of energy in the form of work. Examples of these molecules include NADH, NADPH, and flavin adenine dinucleotide ($FADH_2$). In glycolysis, two equivalents of the cofactor NAD^+ are reduced to two equivalents of NADH per glucose molecule (Fig. 2.2).

In order for subsequent rounds of glycolysis to proceed, the NAD^+ must be regenerated from NADH. In the absence of oxygen, this is accomplished through the reduction of pyruvate to lactate. In the presence of oxygen, the reducing potential stored in NADH is indirectly transferred to the mitochondria through small molecule-coupled shuttles for later use in ATP production. These coupled shuttles are required because the mitochondrial membrane is impervious to NAD^+ and NADH. Like pyruvate reduction to lactate, these reducing potential transfer processes stoichiometrically regenerate NAD^+ that is used to perpetuate glycolysis.

When pyruvate generated from glycolysis is transferred into the mitochondria, it is oxidized into NADH and CO_2, and the remaining carbon is ligated to coenzyme-A to make acetyl-CoA. This is used to fuel the tricarboxylic acid cycle (TCA cycle), which completely oxidizes the remaining glucose carbon into CO_2. Oxidation of carbon in the TCA cycle generates reducing potential in the form of NADH and $FADH_2$. Up to this point, the cell has now stored a large amount of electrochemical energy in NADH and $FADH_2$.

Oxidative phosphorylation (OXPHOS) is the process by which reducing potential generated in glycolysis, the TCA cycle, and fatty acid oxidation is harnessed to make ATP. This occurs through a series of five enzyme complexes located in the inner mitochondrial membrane known as the electron transport chain (ETC). The ETC makes use of the electrons stored in NADH and $FADH_2$ to pump protons out of the mitochondrial matrix into the inner membrane space of the mitochondria, forming a proton gradient (ΔpH) and an electrical gradient ($\Delta\psi_m$). The inner mitochondrial membrane is impermeable to protons, and these can only reenter the matrix by way of the last complex in the ETC, complex V (also called ATP synthase). In doing so, the energy potential is harnessed to maximize ATP production. Pumping protons across this electrochemical gradient enables ATP synthase to generate 32 molecules of ATP per molecule of glucose. Therefore, the total ATP generated by aerobic respiration is 36 molecules of ATP per molecule of glucose (32 ATP from OXPHOS, 2 ATP from glycolysis, and 2 units of ATP are recovered from the TCA cycle). In contrast, glycolytic metabolism of glucose under anaerobic conditions only yields two molecules of ATP per glucose. As such, in the presence of oxygen, mitochondrial glucose oxidation is a much more efficient way to make ATP. It is important to note that toxic reactive oxygen species (ROS) are produced in the mitochondria during this process, which are regulated by protective antioxidant enzymes, such as superoxide dismutase and glutathione peroxidase.

Anabolic metabolism. Besides its role in energy production, glucose carbon is also utilized in many anabolic reactions, such as amino acid and glycosylation precursor biosynthesis, fatty acid and sterol biosynthesis, the pentose phosphate pathway, and de novo nucleotide biosynthesis. As glucose carbon is clearly utilized for many purposes, the flux into each of these pathways needs to be tightly regulated to accommodate cellular demand.

For example, fatty acid and sterol biosynthesis both utilize glucose carbon. These two pathways share the common biosynthetic building block cytosolic acetyl-CoA. This is first generated in the mitochondria by oxidation of glucose-derived pyruvate, as described above. The mitochondrial acetyl-CoA produced in this way is then combined with oxaloacetate in the TCA cycle by citrate synthase (CS) to form citrate. When there is biosynthetic demand, the TCA cycle can act as a source of biosynthetic intermediates in a process known as anaplerosis. In this case, the citrate is anaplerotically released into the cytoplasm where it can be used in fatty acid or sterol biosynthesis. This occurs when the citrate is re-broken down into oxaloacetate and cytosolic acetyl-CoA by the enzyme ATP citrate lyase (ACL). Now in the cytosol, the acetyl-CoA can either be carboxylated into malonyl-CoA for fatty acid biosynthesis or undergo consecutive condensations into 3-hydroxy-3-methyl-glutaryl (HMG)-CoA for sterol biosynthesis. Entry of carbon into sterol biosynthesis is determined by the activity of the rate-limiting enzyme HMG-CoA reductase, which is controlled by several mechanisms including phosphorylation and a transcriptional response to low sterol levels. In a similar fashion, the levels of fatty acid biosynthesis are controlled by the rate-limiting enzyme complex acetyl-CoA carboxylase (ACC), which is subject to phosphorylation events as well as allosteric inhibition by palmitoyl-CoA, the end product of the fatty acid biosynthesis pathway. These multiple layers of regulation ensure that a cell is able to properly regulate biosynthetic activity in accordance with its needs.

Glucose carbon is also the principle source of the ribose that forms the sugar backbone of DNA and RNA. This ribose is generated in the pentose phosphate pathway following oxidation of the hexose glucose into the pentose ribose and CO_2. The energy generated from breaking a carbon-carbon bond in glucose is stored in NADPH. The regulation of glucose flux into the pentose phosphate pathway is mainly determined by the ratio of $NADP^+$ and NADPH. This is accomplished via allosteric regulation of the rate-limiting enzyme of the pentose phosphate pathway, glucose-6-phosphate dehydrogenase (G6PD), which is stimulated by $NADP^+$ and strongly inhibited by NADPH. This mechanism of pathway regulation is a classic example in which the activity of the rate-limiting enzyme is intrinsically linked to the flux through the pathway, as this changes the $NADP^+$/NADPH ratio.

Regulation of metabolic activity. As noted above, fatty acid and sterol biosynthesis and the pentose phosphate pathway are just a few of the many different processes competing for the intermediates of glucose metabolism. Indeed, at any given moment there are thousands of enzyme-catalyzed reactions occurring simultaneously in cells, many of which utilize the same substrates [1]. It is important to remember that all the metabolic reactions and pathways in a cell are inextricably interconnected. Regulation of one pathway may directly or indirectly affect other pathways, especially when sharing molecules that have many metabolic fates, such as metabolites derived from glucose carbon. The flow of metabolites must be regulated and orchestrated on multiple levels, yet be flexible enough to respond quickly to perturbations in the system. For example, yeast consumes glucose by more than tenfold in anaerobic conditions compared to aerobic conditions. However, despite this clear change in nutrient utilization, the concentrations of ATP and other metabolites derived from glucose remain similar [2]. The mechanisms by which cells are able to regulate their metabolism in response to these challenges occur on multiple levels and vary according to specific type of disturbance to the system.

To study this complexity, we simplify metabolism into pathways. To fully understand how a pathway is regulated, it is necessary to monitor all of the chemical steps involved in that pathway. However, this can be further simplified in that among multiple enzymes in a pathway, there are often a few rate-limiting enzymes that have greater control and manage metabolic flux by slow catalysis. The kinetic rates of these reactions depend on several variables beyond the catalytic efficiency of an enzyme. These include factors such as the substrate to product ratio, enzyme and cofactor concentration, the presence or absence of oxygen, and/or posttranslational regulation via cell signaling events such as insulin receptor activation. Each of these variables needs to be taken into consideration when determining the specific flux through a pathway.

Outside of the classical regulatory mechanisms listed above, another manner by which the metabolic state of a cell is controlled is through the activation or deactivation of transcription factors. The induced change in metabolic gene expression subsequently leads to changes in the proteome and ultimately the metabolome, in order for the cell to maintain or return to a steady metabolic state. As it concerns the cell's energy state, this type of regulatory mechanism often operates by controlling the levels of ATP and AMP. A prime example of this is the AMP-activated protein kinase (AMPK), which controls multiple cellular processes in response to a decrease of the [ATP]/[AMP] ratio.

An important regulatory mechanism whose importance has more recently been appreciated integrates metabolic activity and gene expression. This occurs through the regulation of the cofactors, substrates, or products of the enzymes that modify chromatin. For example, the histone proteins which pack DNA into chromatin contain numerous nutrient-sensitive modifications, including sites for acetylation, methylation, and glycosylation [3]. Given that the degree of glycosylation and acetyl-CoA biosynthesis are controlled by the rate of glucose metabolism, glucose uptake and processing can directly impact gene expression [4]. Similarly, the ratio of S-adenosylmethionine (SAM) and S-adenosylhomocysteine (SAH) is regulated by the one-carbon metabolism pathway. Recent reports have shown that enhanced SAM biosynthesis leads to gene activation and the maintenance of stem cell and cancer properties through the regulation of gene expression [5–7]. Another important metabolite pair is the TCA cycle intermediates alpha-ketoglutarate and succinate. The ratio of these molecules affects the activity of histone and DNA methyltransferases through substrate availability and product inhibition, respectively. Disruptions in this ratio have been shown to affect the stem cell state and influence cancer properties [8, 9]. This series of examples provides perspective on how metabolism, which is thought to be a consequence of gene expression, acts directly to influence and regulate gene expression.

By way of a detailed example, the type M2 isozyme of pyruvate kinase (PKM2) is a metabolic node that is regulated by several diverse mechanisms [10, 11]. PKM2 is a rate-limiting enzyme in glycolysis and acts to convert phosphoenolpyruvate (PEP) and ADP to pyruvate and ATP (Fig. 2.3). PKM2 exists largely in two homo-oligomeric states, which govern its enzymatic activity. When PKM2 is in the homo-tetrameric state, it has a high affinity for its substrate PEP and promotes pyruvate formation. In contrast, when PKM2 is in the homodimeric state, it has a very low affinity for PEP. This leads to the bottlenecking of glycolysis at PKM2 and the build-up of glycolytic metabolites upstream of PKM2. Based on the concentration gradient formed, glycolytic intermediates upstream of PKM2 can then be shunted into anabolic pathways, like the pentose phosphate pathway (to make nucleotides and NADPH) or the serine biosynthesis pathway (to make amino acids and nucleotides) (Fig. 2.3). Therefore, one can think of the tetramer to dimer ratio of PKM2 as a rheostat that toggles between a catabolic metabolic state (bioenergetics) and an anabolic state (biosynthesis).

PKM2 intrinsically prefers the homo-dimeric state and is therefore the least enzymatically active isoform among the pyruvate kinase species (i.e., PKM1 isozyme; pyruvate kinase liver, PKL; pyruvate kinase red blood cell, PKR). In proliferating cells, which includes all cancer cells, PKM2 is preferentially expressed [12]. The reasons for this have largely to do with the fact that it can be finely tuned to balance biosynthetic and energetic demands. For example, the PKM2 homo-dimer is maintained through binding to phosphorylated

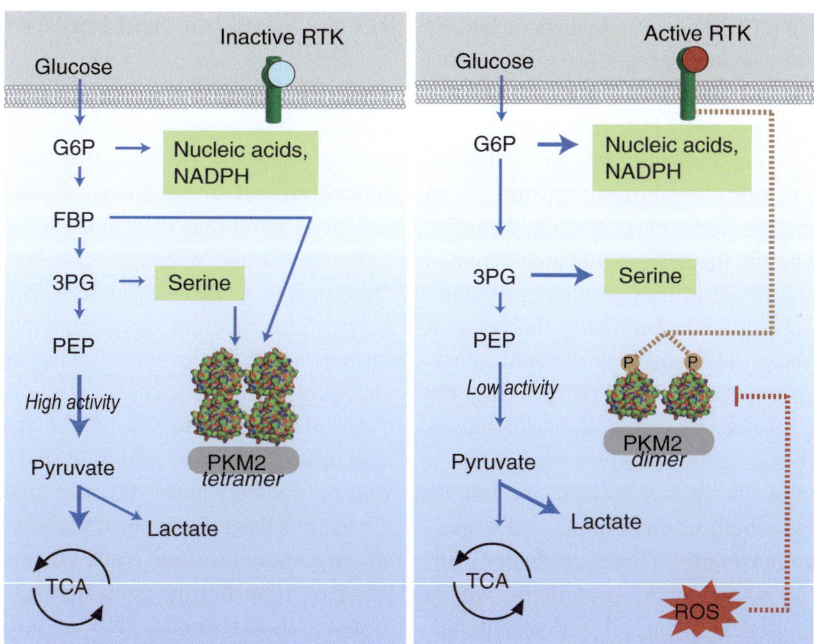

Fig. 2.3 *Mechanisms regulating the enzymatic activity of PKM2.* Pyruvate kinase isoform M2 (PKM2) is a glycolytic enzyme which catalyzes the conversion of phosphoenolpyruvate (PEP) into pyruvate. PKM2 exists in two oligomeric states, as a highly active tetramer (*left*) or a low-activity dimer (*right*). In its highly active tetrameric state, PEP is rapidly converted to pyruvate, and this is preferentially used to fuel tricarboxylic acid (TCA) cycle metabolism. In its low-activity dimeric state, the slow conversion of PEP allows for increased buildup of upstream glycolytic intermediates including 3-phosphoglycerate (3PG) and glucose 6-phosphate (G6P). In this way, the increased substrate availability promotes flux into the serine and nucleic acid biosynthetic pathways, respectively. The oligomeric state of PKM2 is influenced by several mechanisms. High concentrations of serine or the glycolytic intermediate fructose-1,6-bisphosphate (FBP) allosterically drive PKM2 tetramerization. This type of modulation is referred to as feed-forward activation. Conversely, interaction of PKM2 with phosphorylated receptor tyrosine kinases or oxidation by reactive oxygen species (ROS) inhibits tetramerization and leads to reduced activity of PKM2

growth factor receptor tyrosine kinases [13, 14]. In this way, a cell that has been instructed to grow, by growth-factor mediated receptor tyrosine kinase phosphorylation, makes use of incoming glucose carbon for biosynthetic reactions (Fig. 2.3). Similarly, reaction oxygen species (ROS) also directly inhibit PKM2 tetramerization, and thus activity, by modifying a cysteine residue that prevents homo-tetramer formation [15]. This promotes the utilization of glucose carbon in pathways that mitigate ROS, like the NADPH-generating pentose phosphate pathway and the serine biosynthesis pathway. This latter pathway makes glycine that is used in glutathione biosynthesis [16]. In fact, this important aspect of metabolic redox regulation is conserved back to yeast pyruvate kinase [17].

As the dimeric form of PKM2 allows for the preferential use of glucose carbon for biosynthetic reactions, at a given threshold, energy will be required to further facilitate biosynthesis or to prevent runaway substrate accumulation. Indeed, the buildup of upstream glycolytic intermediates and glycolysis branch pathway intermediates induces PKM2 tetramerization. This shifts the balance of glycolytic flux toward energy production, in a classic example of feed-forward pathway activation. Examples of these substrates include the glycolytic intermediate fructose-1,6-bisphosphate (FBP), serine and the purine synthesis intermediate succinyl-5-aminoimidazole-4-carboxamide-1-ribose-5′-phosphate (SAICAR) [18, 19]. In light of the complex allosteric and posttranslational regulatory mechanisms that can fine-tune glycolytic flux, it is not surprising that PKM2 is used by cancer cells as a focal point to regulate many diverse processes [20, 21] and that in certain contexts, it can endow a cell with oncogenic activity [13, 14].

Cell-autonomous metabolism, while highly conserved from early evolution onward, is an extremely complex and robust system. In order for a cell to maintain the delicate balance between anabolic and catabolic processes, there are many mechanisms of regulation built into these metabolic pathways, as the example with PKM2 illustrated. This is especially true considering the level overlap between many of these pathways which often include common substrates between competing pathways. In this section, we largely dealt with metabolism in mammalian cells operating as autonomous units. These regulatory principles hold in single-celled organisms whose nutrient availability is dictated by their extracellular environment, which is in constant flux. In the following section, we will discuss how nutrient availability is regulated and maintained in multicellular organisms by extracellular signaling, hormonal, tissue, and organ cross talk.

2.3 Systemic Metabolism

A key feature of cell-autonomous metabolism is subcellular compartmentalization. By confining a reaction spatially, the effective substrate-enzyme concentrations are greater, which increase the rate of a metabolic reaction. Furthermore, separating metabolic pathways that run in opposing directions (e.g., fatty acid biosynthesis and breakdown) into different compartments prevents the formation of futile cycles. The same concepts also apply at the level of systemic metabolism in a complex organism. Metabolic work is distributed among specialized tissues and organs to prevent redundancy and maximize efficiency.

As in cell-autonomous metabolism, glucose is an important nutrient from an organismal prospective. The tightly controlled and inter-organ systems that regulate glucose will be used as an illustrative example to describe its systemic regulation by the hormone insulin (Fig. 2.4). Glucose from the blood is the main metabolic energy source for many tissues. Organismal blood glucose homeostasis is maintained through

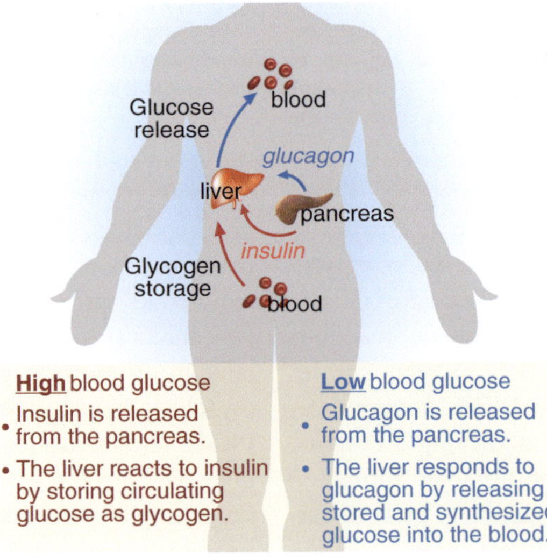

Fig. 2.4 *Regulation of systemic glucose metabolism.* The endocrine pancreas detects and responds to changes in blood glucose metabolism by secreting the hormones insulin and glucagon, which are in turn utilized by the liver to regulate the levels of blood glucose. In conditions of high blood glucose, the pancreas releases insulin into the blood. The liver responds to increases in the levels of blood insulin by storing blood glucose in the form of glycogen and increasing levels of glycolysis to utilize the high levels of glucose for energy. When blood glucose is low, the pancreas releases glucagon, which signals to the liver to switch from glycolysis to gluconeogenesis. The newly synthesized glucose, as well as glucose from stored glycogen pools, is then released into the blood

communication between the *liver*, which is the primary organ for the regulation of circulating glucose, and the *endocrine pancreas*, which secretes hormones in response to fluctuating blood glucose concentrations.

After eating a meal, glucose processed and absorbed during digestion enters portal circulation. The liver is the first stop in this process and the level of circulating glucose is determined. Based on the glucose concentration, metabolic programs in the liver are then coordinated to either synthesize or store glucose. Glucose is stored in the liver as a polymer in the form of glycogen. This process is stimulated by insulin released from the pancreas in response to high levels of circulating blood glucose. Conversely, when blood glucose levels are low, the pancreas releases glucagon, which the liver responds to by switching its metabolic processes to release glucose stored in glycogen as well as to stimulate glucose synthesis through gluconeogenesis.

In addition to the regulation of blood glucose levels by endocrine hormones (i.e., insulin and glucagon), the pancreas also plays an important role in the regulation of the exocrine digestive system by producing and releasing many catabolic enzymes into the digestive track. Pancreatic enzymes can break down proteins, amino acids, carbohydrates, and fats according to different body signals, and these aid in the digestion and absorption of nutrients.

Beyond the liver and pancreas, insulin signaling also plays important roles in adipose and muscle tissue. As insulin is released when blood sugar is high, muscle tissue responds to this signal by increasing glucose transport into the cell, as well as increasing both the rates of glycolysis and glycogen synthesis. Importantly, insulin signaling is strongly inhibitory to the activity glycogen phosphorylase in muscle cells, which prevents muscle from using glycogen stores when glucose is readily available in the bloodstream.

Insulin and glucagon are also involved in regulation of protein and lipid metabolism. For example, another important nutrient source, circulating fatty acids, is controlled by the adipose tissue in response to insulin stimulation, much in the same way insulin signaling to the liver controls levels of circulating glucose. Finally, beyond the regulation of systemic glucose and fatty acid concentrations, insulin signaling is also involved in numerous growth promoting and cellular biosynthetic processes [22–24], neuronal survival, learning, and memory [25], and disruptions of insulin signaling are at the heart of metabolic syndrome and many types of cancer [26].

2.4 How Metabolic Processes Go Wrong Leading to Disease

In the previous sections, we examined various aspects of metabolism and how these processes are regulated at a cellular and organismal level. In this section, we turn our attention to human diseases that result from dysregulation of such metabolic processes. Recent work has shown that many human diseases, like cancer and diabetes, are accompanied by metabolic defects or abnormalities that perturb normal physiology and lead to tissue dysfunction [27]. In the following section, we describe how metabolic processes can go wrong and the consequences of the deregulated metabolic state as it relates to a disease from each of three focus areas: [1] cancer as a disease of cell-autonomous metabolic dysfunction; [2] inborn errors in metabolism, which span aspects of autonomous and systemic metabolism; and [3] diabetes mellitus as a systemic disease of metabolism. While this discussion is limited to one disease per focus area, these principles are broadly applicable across many different diseases.

Cancer. Pioneering work in the past half century has illustrated clearly that cancer is a genetic disease [28]. While commonly classified as a single disease, cancer is actually many if not thousands of diseases that share a set of common features. These are referred to as the *Hallmarks of Cancer* [29, 30]. Among these ten features is the hallmark "deregulated metabolism." Despite the recognition that cancer cells have altered metabolic processes more than 100 years ago [31], only recently has it been appreciated that alterations in metabolism endow cancer cells with malignant properties, as opposed to being a consequence of the malignant phenotype. In fact, a compelling recent theory posits that the ability to capture and utilize nutrients in a cell-autonomous fashion is the most fundamental barrier limiting the transformation of a normal cell into a cancer cell [32].

In the most basic sense, metabolic processes are rewired in cancer cells to support cell growth [33]. Many of these processes are shared with normal physiological growth processes in healthy cells, like those discussed in the cell-autonomous metabolism section above. In addition, cancer cells by definition are able to persist and grow in the presence of numerous physical and oxidative stressors, nutrient and oxygen deprivation and immune cell attack. The metabolic processes reprogrammed to facilitate survival and growth under these challenging circumstances also have overlapping themes with normal metabolism. Beyond these, there are also metabolic processes that are unique to or highly overutilized in cancer cells, some of which the cancer cells become dependent upon. We have classified these as metabolic vulnerabilities [34], and much effort is now being placed on characterizing such processes to identify new cancer treatments [35].

Given the renewed interest in cancer metabolism, hallmarks of metabolic reprogramming have been recently detailed [9], and these are summarized as follows. First, cancer cells activate diverse nutrient acquisition pathways from the blood stream, extracellular space, and through communication with non-cancer cells. Second, they rewire their intracellular pathways to promote anabolic metabolism in place of catabolism. And, third, they regulate metabolic fluxes into substrates that are used by gene regulatory machinery to control gene expression, cell fate, and the tumor microenvironment.

The metabolic alterations employed by cancer cells vary widely among different types of cancer. Rather than provide a general overview, we will provide a comprehensive glimpse into the metabolic alterations that are common among pancreatic cancers. Pancreatic ductal adenocarcinoma, the most common type of pancreatic cancer, is characterized by an extremely robust fibrotic reaction where most of the epithelial tissue is replaced by a type of scar tissue composed of extracellular matrix, fibroblasts, and immune cell infiltrates. This scar tissue creates extreme pressures that collapse the vasculature and thus render these tumors nutrient and oxygen poor [36, 37]. However, in spite of the challenges imposed by this austere tumor microenvironment, pancreatic cancer remains one of the deadliest cancers [38].

To survive in this nutritionally deprived environment, pancreatic cancer cells acquire noncanonical mechanisms to scavenge nutrients (Fig. 2.5). One such mechanism is macropinocytosis, a process by which the cell nonspecifically engulfs extracellular space [39]. This is then endocytosed and fused with the lysosome to break down the contents of the fluid into basic biosynthetic building blocks. Employing this mechanism, pancreatic cancer cells have been shown to survive nutrient deprivation by breaking down proteins into constituent amino acids to fuel mitochondrial metabolism [40–42].

In addition to proteins and amino acids, pancreatic cancer cells also require a constant supply of lipids for metabolism, signaling, and proliferation. These lipids can be produced through de novo synthesis or obtained by uptake from the extracellular fluid. The majority of the fatty acids in normal cells are derived from de novo synthesis; however, oncogenic Ras signaling, observed in the vast majority of pancreatic tumors, shifts this equilibrium toward the import of fatty acids [43]. Pancreatic cancer cells have also been found to actively import cholesterol-rich low-density lipoproteins (LDL) via receptor-mediated endocytosis [44]. Inhibition of LDL import has antiproliferative effects on pancreatic cancer cells, demonstrating their reliance on such scavenging mechanisms to maintain adequate LDL pools.

Pancreatic cancer cells also make efficient use of the nutrients that are available to them through recycling processes (Fig. 2.5). Macroautophagy, usually simply referred to as autophagy, is a cellular quality control process that normal cells use to clear damaged structures and protein aggregates. As the name implies (autophagy translates to "self-eating"), in times of starvation or nutrient deprivation, cells can utilize autophagy to obtain essential nutrients from proteins and organelles to survive

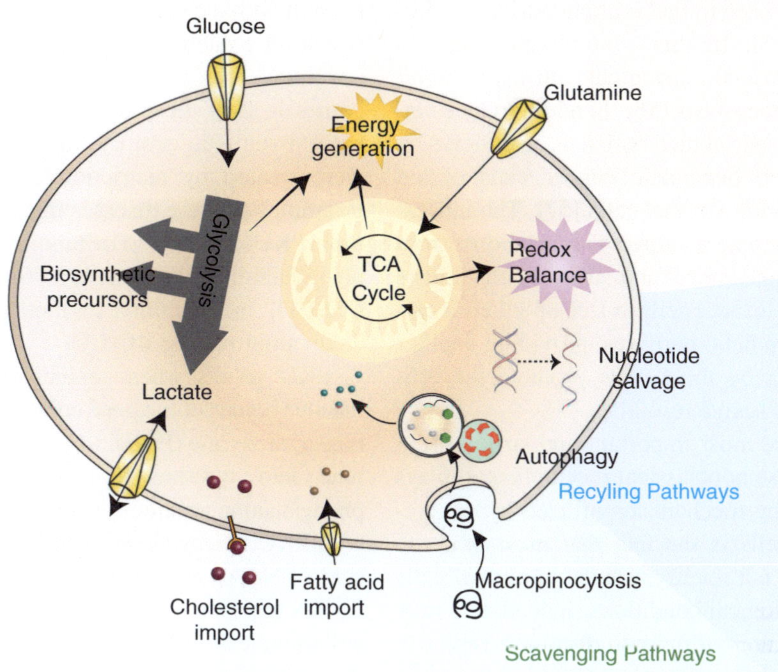

Fig. 2.5 *Nonclassical metabolic adaptations facilitate pancreatic cancer growth and survival.* Pancreatic cancer cells utilize a number of different mechanisms to survive in the nutrient-poor tumor microenvironment. These include the rewiring of intracellular metabolic pathways, the activation of recycling pathways, and the stimulation of scavenging mechanisms. First, glucose uptake is activated, which increases glycolysis and the availability of glucose carbon for biosynthetic pathways. Glutamine uptake is also activated, and this amino acid becomes an important source of carbon for the tricarboxylic acid (TCA) cycle to generate energy and biosynthetic intermediates and to maintain redox balance. Second, pancreatic cancer cells activate autophagy and nucleotide-recycling pathways. Finally, scavenging pathways are initiated to import fatty acids and cholesterol; amino acids are obtained via lysosomal breakdown of protein obtained through macropinocytosis

until resources become available. In contrast to normal cells, pancreatic cancer cells undergo elevated basal levels of autophagy, even in nutrient replete conditions. In fact, somewhat surprisingly, autophagy has been demonstrated to be required for the normal growth and proliferation of pancreatic cancer cells, providing support to both energy production and redox balance within the cell [45, 46]. Similarly, nucleotide salvage has been found to be important for the maintenance of nucleotide pools, as inhibition of nicotinamide phosphoribosyltransferase (NAMPT), a key enzyme in the NAD+ salvage pathway, leads to a drop in intracellular NAD+ pools and strongly inhibits the growth and survival of pancreatic cancer cells [47, 48].

Finally, pancreatic cancer cells also have extensively rewired metabolic pathways, as compared to normal cells, which are used to support their energetic and biosynthetic demands (Fig. 2.5). For example, pancreatic cancer cells driven by the oncogene Kras are primed for increased glucose capture and metabolism by upregulation of the glucose transporter GLUT1 and hexokinase 1/2, respectively [49]. The rate of glycolysis is also increased via the transcriptional upregulation of glycolytic gene expression by oncogenic Kras signaling, hypoxia, and a number of other mechanisms that maintain cytosolic ATP levels [50–55]. This additional flux of glucose carbon through glycolysis also provides carbon for biosynthetic needs via the pentose phosphate pathway for nucleotide biosynthesis and the hexosamine biosynthetic pathway, which produces precursor moieties for protein glycosylation.

The nonessential amino acid glutamine is another important fuel for pancreatic cancer cells, and it is used to fuel mitochondrial metabolism (Fig. 2.5). In this context, glutamine is metabolized in a non-canonical pathway to maintain redox homeostasis [56]. In addition to glutamine, mitochondrial metabolism is also fueled by alanine, which pancreatic cancer cells obtain from neighboring stromal cells [57]. The utilization of this alanine acquired via metabolic cross talk between the cancer and stromal cells allows the pancreatic cancer cells to free up glucose carbon for biosynthetic purposes, providing another example whereby these cells promote the efficient usage of scarce resources.

Perhaps the most important and striking feature of all these nonclassical metabolic pathways and scavenging mechanisms utilized by pancreatic cancer cells is the fact that most of these pathways are not readily utilized in normal cells under physiological conditions. Indeed, this may provide for an opportunity to design therapies to selectively target pancreatic cancer cells while sparing normal cells in the process. Accordingly, there are several promising strategies moving into the clinic to treat pancreatic cancer patients based on these principles, which are outlined in detail in several recent review articles [34, 35, 58, 59]. Furthermore, many of the imaging techniques currently used in the clinic are based on exploiting the differences in metabolism between normal cells and tumor cells. These techniques are currently being refined and expanded and represent one of the more promising early detection methods in the clinical pipeline.

Inborn errors of metabolism. Inborn errors of metabolism (IEM) are a large class of genetic diseases that are usually caused by defects in a single enzyme such that a vital nutrient cannot be metabolized properly [60, 61]. This can result in a nutritional deficiency or build-up of the improperly metabolized molecule in the body, which can cause a wide range of symptoms depending on the dysfunctional enzyme. These can lead to developmental delays or other serious medical problems if not properly managed.

Traditionally IEM have been classified by the nutrient class affected, for example, disorders of carbohydrate, amino acid or organic acid metabolism, or lysosomal storage. Nowadays, many more IEM have been characterized, and the classification system has been refined for greater accuracy. This is particularly relevant when it comes to how these diseases are treated. In the early twentieth century, amino acid disorders were treated by restriction of dietary protein. Examples of these diseases include phenylketonuria (PKU, inability to metabolize the amino acid phenylalanine) and maple syrup urine disease (MSUD, the inability to metabolize branched chain amino acids; BCAA).

PKU results when an individual carries two inactive copies of the gene encoding for phenylalanine hydroxylase (PAH), which converts phenylalanine into tyrosine [62]. On a normal diet, phenylalanine accumulates in the blood in patients with PKU. Phenylalanine is a large, neutral amino acid (LNAA) and enters the brain through the LNAA transporter. If phenylalanine is in excess, it will saturate the transporter and lead to a decrease in the levels of other LNAAs in the brain. These amino acids are necessary for protein and neurotransmitter synthesis, and their decreased availability is toxic to the brain. Accordingly, the primary symptoms of PKU are intellectual disability and mood disorders. In the classical treatment regime, patients on a protein-low diet become especially deficient in the amino acid tyrosine, as tyrosine is the product of the PAH-catalyzed reaction. Nowadays, PKU is considered manageable and treated entirely through dietary regulation of phenylalanine intake and tyrosine supplementation.

MSUD results when an individual carries two inactivating copies of one of the genes encoding for the mitochondrial branched-chain ketoacid dehydrogenase complex (BCKDC) [63]. This results in the inability to break down BCAAs and leucinosis. Like PKU, MSUD requires careful monitoring of the intake of dietary BCAAs. However, dietary monitoring alone is insufficient in this case, as BCAAs are released by protein breakdown in muscle, a process that is activated to meet heightened energy demands. In healthy individuals, BCAA metabolism in the mitochondria fuels the TCA cycle and leads to ATP production. This process is engaged in times of enhanced metabolic demand or during illness, for example. As such, in addition to dietary monitoring, patients with MSUD must also carefully monitor their blood chemistry during puberty and periods of rapid growth and are instructed to avoid fatigue, infections, physical stress, and exertion. Liver transplantation is another option for patients with MSUD, and this can completely reverse symptoms and the dependence on dietary and lifestyle modifications via liver-mediated regulation of BCAAs. The potential upsides of this procedure are carefully considered, as organ transplant is a nontrivial procedure that comes with many potentially life-threatening complications.

Using PKU and MSUD as case studies, these diseases provide clear examples of the well-controlled regulation of metabolic processes and how the disruption of even a single enzyme can lead to cell-autonomous and systemic metabolic catastrophe.

Diabetes mellitus. As detailed previously, the hormones secreted by the pancreas to the liver represent the primary mechanism by which blood glucose levels are regulated. Accordingly, alterations in either the ability of the pancreas to secrete insulin in response to high levels of blood glucose or an inability of the body to appropriately respond to circulating insulin levels leads to elevated circulating blood glucose levels. The resultant prolonged levels of high blood glucose carry many debilitating long-term complications due to nonspecific protein glycation, including heart disease, stroke, retinopathy, kidney failure, blindness, and amputations resulting from loss of blood flow in the limbs.

Collectively, the metabolic diseases resulting from the loss of blood glucose homeostasis are referred to as diabetes mellitus. Type 1 diabetes mellitus (T1D), occasionally referred to as juvenile diabetes, accounts for less than 10% of all cases of diabetes mellitus [64]. T1D results from the inability of the pancreas to produce sufficient insulin, usually due to the autoimmune destruction of the insulin-producing beta cells of the pancreatic islet. The exact causes driving the clinical manifestation of T1D are unknown, so no preventive treatments or cures currently exist. As a consequence, lifelong blood glucose monitoring and treatment with insulin are required.

Type 2 diabetes mellitus (T2D) represents the vast majority of the diagnosed cases of diabetes mellitus and is caused by both genetic and lifestyle factors [65]. T2D was previously referred to as adult onset diabetes; however, it is becoming increasingly common in children and young adults. Obesity, poor diet, and the lack of physical activity are among the strongest risk factors for T2D. In contrast to T1D, T2D can normally be managed with lifestyle interventions. T2D typically begins as insulin resistance, where cells lose sensitivity and fail to adequately respond to insulin stimulation. Insulin resistance of the liver has particularly important consequences, as the failure of the liver to inhibit gluconeogenesis in response to insulin leads to the continued release of glucose into the blood, even in conditions of already high blood glucose. As the severity of T2D progresses, the insulin-producing beta cells in the pancreas also lose the ability to produce sufficient insulin; therefore, insulin injections or other forms of insulin control are often required for people with severe T2D.

Understanding the mechanisms of insulin resistance requires an even broader view of systemic metabolism. While the skeletal muscles and other tissues have an important impact on insulin resistance, we will focus on the interaction between the white adipose tissue and the liver as an example. White adipose tissue stores glucose as energy in the form of triglycerides, the initiation of which is triggered by insulin signaling. Conversely, in response to low insulin levels or a lack of response to insulin signaling, white adipose tissues undergo lipolysis and release fatty acids into the blood. The increased levels of free fatty acids in the blood lead to the stimulation of gluconeogenesis in the liver [66], further potentiating the problem.

Obesity contributes to insulin resistance for several reasons. First, obese humans have a larger percentage of body mass in the form of white adipose tissue, thereby increasing the available free fatty acids pools that can be released into the blood. Secondly, obesity is correlated with increased levels of systemic inflammation [67], which has been demonstrated to increase the rate of lipolysis in the white adipose tissue [68].

Beyond these more obvious mechanisms by which obesity contributes to the development of insulin resistance, there are other interesting mechanisms linking obesity to T2D including ER stress and increased levels of circulating BCAAs [69–71].

These examples represent a simplified view of a very complex human disease to illustrate how metabolic dysregulation of one tissue type, via insulin resistance, can lead to a systemic metabolic disease. For a more detailed description of insulin resistance and diabetes, we would encourage the readers to see several excellent reviews on the topic [65, 72–75].

2.5 Concluding Remarks

Metabolism is described above in discrete pathways and processes in order to organize our understanding. It is important to remember that this is a gross oversimplification. There are thousands of metabolites and metabolic pathways in a cell concurrently communicating with each other. This complexity is even greater at the organismal level. The importance of the interconnectedness, balance, and regulation, among the pathways, is well exemplified in the disease case studies. Importantly, this fine balance and disruption by disease provide footholds to monitor metabolic homeostasis, the onset of disease, progression, and response to treatment by measuring alterations in discrete molecules related to such processes. The focus of this text book is on the field of metabolic imaging, which is devoted to monitoring alterations in metabolism. It is our hope that the principles described above provide context to understand the complexities of cellular and organismal metabolic regulation as the reader takes a deep dive into the chapters on metabolic imaging that follow.

Acknowledgments The authors would like to thank Mariana Schnell for her technical assistance preparing the figures. L.C.C. was supported by NIH Grants P01CA117969 and P01CA120964. C.A.L. is supported by grants from the American Association for Cancer Research, Pancreatic Cancer Action Network, National Pancreas Foundation, Sidney Kimmel Foundation, Damon Runyon Cancer Research Foundation, and American Gastroenterological Association.

Conflict of Interest Statement L.C.C. owns equity in, receives compensation from, and serves on the Board of Directors and Scientific Advisory Board of Agios Pharmaceuticals. Agios Pharmaceuticals is identifying metabolic pathways of cancer cells and developing drugs to inhibit such enzymes to disrupt tumor cell growth and survival.

References

1. Bennett BD, Kimball EH, Gao M, Osterhout R, Van Dien SJ, Rabinowitz JD. Absolute metabolite concentrations and implied enzyme active site occupancy in Escherichia coli. Nat Chem Biol. 2009;5(8):593–9.
2. Krebs HA. The Pasteur effect and the relations between respiration and fermentation. Essays Biochem. 1972;8:1–34.
3. Wellen KE, Thompson CB. A two-way street: reciprocal regulation of metabolism and signalling. Nat Rev Mol Cell Biol. 2012;13(4):270–6.
4. Carrer A, Wellen KE. Metabolism and epigenetics: a link cancer cells exploit. Curr Opin Biotechnol. 2015;34:23–9.
5. Shyh-Chang N, Locasale JW, Lyssiotis CA, Zheng Y, Teo RY, Ratanasirintrawoot S, et al. Influence of threonine metabolism on S-adenosylmethionine and histone methylation. Science. 2013;339(6116):222–6.
6. Yang M, Vousden KH. Serine and one-carbon metabolism in cancer. Nat Rev Cancer. 2016;16(10):650–62.
7. Zhang WC, Shyh-Chang N, Yang H, Rai A, Umashankar S, Ma S, et al. Glycine decarboxylase activity drives non-small cell lung cancer tumor-initiating cells and tumorigenesis. Cell. 2012;148(1–2):259–72.
8. Carey BW, Finley LW, Cross JR, Allis CD, Thompson CB. Intracellular alpha-ketoglutarate maintains the pluripotency of embryonic stem cells. Nature. 2015;518(7539):413–6.
9. Pavlova NN, Thompson CB. The emerging hallmarks of cancer metabolism. Cell Metab. 2016;23(1):27–47.
10. Lyssiotis CA, Anastasiou D, Locasale JW, Vander Heiden MG, Christofk HR, Cantley LC. Cellular control mechanisms that regulate pyruvate kinase M2 activity and promote cancer growth. Biomed Res-India. 2012;23:213–7.
11. Rabinowitz JD, Vastag L. Teaching the design principles of metabolism. Nat Chem Biol. 2012;8(6):497–501.
12. Israelsen WJ, Dayton TL, Davidson SM, Fiske BP, Hosios AM, Bellinger G, et al. PKM2 isoform-specific deletion reveals a differential requirement for pyruvate kinase in tumor cells. Cell. 2013;155(2):397–409.
13. Christofk HR, Vander Heiden MG, Harris MH, Ramanathan A, Gerszten RE, Wei R, et al. The M2 splice isoform of pyruvate kinase is important for cancer metabolism and tumour growth. Nature. 2008;452(7184):230–U74.

14. Christofk HR, Vander Heiden MG, Wu N, Asara JM, Cantley LC. Pyruvate kinase M2 is a phosphotyrosine-binding protein. Nature. 2008;452(7184):181–U27.
15. Anastasiou D, Poulogiannis G, Asara JM, Boxer MB, Jiang JK, Shen M, et al. Inhibition of pyruvate kinase M2 by reactive oxygen species contributes to cellular antioxidant responses. Science. 2011;334(6060):1278–83.
16. Locasale JW, Grassian AR, Melman T, Lyssiotis CA, Mattaini KR, Bass AJ, et al. Phosphoglycerate dehydrogenase diverts glycolytic flux and contributes to oncogenesis. Nat Genet. 2011;43(9):869–74.
17. Gruning NM, Rinnerthaler M, Bluemlein K, Mulleder M, Wamelink MMC, Lehrach H, et al. Pyruvate kinase triggers a metabolic feedback loop that controls redox metabolism in respiring cells. Cell Metab. 2011;14(3):415–27.
18. Chaneton B, Hillmann P, Zheng L, Martin AC, Maddocks OD, Chokkathukalam A, et al. Serine is a natural ligand and allosteric activator of pyruvate kinase M2. Nature. 2012;491(7424):458–62.
19. Keller KE, Doctor ZM, Dwyer ZW, Lee YS. SAICAR induces protein kinase activity of PKM2 that is necessary for sustained proliferative signaling of cancer cells. Mol Cell. 2014;53(5):700–9.
20. Dayton TL, Gocheva V, Miller KM, Israelsen WJ, Bhutkar A, Clish CB, et al. Germline loss of PKM2 promotes metabolic distress and hepatocellular carcinoma. Genes Dev. 2016;30(9):1020–33.
21. Luo W, Semenza GL. Emerging roles of PKM2 in cell metabolism and cancer progression. Trends Endocrinol Metab. 2012;23(11):560–6.
22. Menon S, Dibble CC, Talbott G, Hoxhaj G, Valvezan AJ, Takahashi H, et al. Spatial control of the TSC complex integrates insulin and nutrient regulation of mTORC1 at the lysosome. Cell. 2014;156(4):771–85.
23. Zhang HH, Huang JX, Duvel K, Boback B, SL W, Squillace RM, et al. Insulin stimulates adipogenesis through the Akt-TSC2-mTORC1 pathway. PLoS One. 2009;4(7)
24. Manning BD, Tee AR, Logsdon MN, Blenis J, Cantley LC. Identification of the tuberous sclerosis complex-2 tumor suppressor gene product tuberin as a target of the phosphoinositide 3-kinase/Akt pathway. Mol Cell. 2002;10(1):151–62.
25. Plum L, Belgardt BF, Bruning JC. Central insulin action in energy and glucose homeostasis. J Clin Invest. 2006;116(7):1761–6.
26. Gallagher EJ, LeRoith D. Epidemiology and molecular mechanisms tying obesity, diabetes, and the metabolic syndrome with cancer. Diabetes Care. 2013;36:S233–S9.
27. DeBerardinis RJ, Thompson CB. Cellular metabolism and disease: what do metabolic outliers teach us? Cell. 2012;148(6):1132–44.
28. Mukherjee S. The emperor of all maladies: a biography of cancer. 1st Scribner hardcover ed. New York: Scribner; 2010. xiv, 571 p., 8 p. of plates p.
29. Hanahan D, Weinberg RA. The hallmarks of cancer. Cell. 2000;100(1):57–70.
30. Hanahan D, Weinberg RA. Hallmarks of cancer: the next generation. Cell. 2011;144(5):646–74.
31. Warburg O, Posener E, Negelein E. Ueber den Stoffwechsel der Tumoren. Biochem Z. 1924;152:319–44.
32. Ward PS, Thompson CB. Metabolic reprogramming: a cancer hallmark even warburg did not anticipate. Cancer Cell. 2012;21(3):297–308.
33. Hirschey MD, DeBerardinis RJ, Diehl AM, Drew JE, Frezza C, Green MF, et al. Dysregulated metabolism contributes to oncogenesis. Semin Cancer Biol. 2015;35(Suppl):S129–50.
34. Halbrook CJ, Lyssiotis CA. Employing metabolism to improve the diagnosis and treatment of pancreatic cancer. Cancer Cell. 2017;31(1):5–19.
35. Vander Heiden MG. Targeting cancer metabolism: a therapeutic window opens. Nat Rev Drug Discov. 2011;10(9):671–84.
36. Jacobetz MA, Chan DS, Neesse A, Bapiro TE, Cook N, Frese KK, et al. Hyaluronan impairs vascular function and drug delivery in a mouse model of pancreatic cancer. Gut. 2013;62(1):112–U53.
37. Provenzano PP, Cuevas C, Chang AE, Goel VK, Von Hoff DD, Hingorani SR. Enzymatic targeting of the stroma ablates physical barriers to treatment of pancreatic ductal adenocarcinoma. Cancer Cell. 2012;21(3):418–29.
38. Siegel RL, Miller KD, Jemal A. Cancer statistics, 2016. CA Cancer J Clin. 2016;66(1):7–30.
39. Bar-Sagi D, Feramisco JR. Induction of membrane ruffling and fluid-phase pinocytosis in quiescent fibroblasts by ras proteins. Science. 1986;233(4768):1061–8.
40. Commisso C, Davidson SM, Soydaner-Azeloglu RG, Parker SJ, Kamphorst JJ, Hackett S, et al. Macropinocytosis of protein is an amino acid supply route in Ras-transformed cells. Nature. 2013;497(7451):633–7.
41. Kamphorst JJ, Nofal M, Commisso C, Hackett SR, WY L, Grabocka E, et al. Human pancreatic cancer tumors are nutrient poor and tumor cells actively scavenge extracellular protein. Cancer Res. 2015;75(3):544–53.
42. Palm W, Park Y, Wright K, Pavlova NN, Tuveson DA, Thompson CB. The utilization of extracellular proteins as nutrients is suppressed by mTORC1. Cell. 2015;162(2):259–70.
43. Kamphorst JJ, Cross JR, Fan J, de Stanchina E, Mathew R, White EP, et al. Hypoxic and Ras-transformed cells support growth by scavenging unsaturated fatty acids from lysophospholipids. Proc Natl Acad Sci U S A. 2013;110(22):8882–7.
44. Guillaumond F, Bidaut G, Ouaissi M, Servais S, Gouirand V, Olivares O, et al. Cholesterol uptake disruption, in association with chemotherapy, is a promising combined metabolic therapy for pancreatic adenocarcinoma. Proc Natl Acad Sci U S A. 2015;112(8):2473–8.
45. Yang SH, Wang XX, Contino G, Liesa M, Sahin E, Ying HQ, et al. Pancreatic cancers require autophagy for tumor growth. Genes Dev. 2011;25(7):717–29.

46. Yang A, Rajeshkumar NV, Wang X, Yabuuchi S, Alexander BM, Chu GC, et al. Autophagy is critical for pancreatic tumor growth and progression in tumors with p53 alterations. Cancer Discov. 2014;4(8):905–13.
47. Chini CC, Guerrico AM, Nin V, Camacho-Pereira J, Escande C, Barbosa MT, et al. Targeting of NAD metabolism in pancreatic cancer cells: potential novel therapy for pancreatic tumors. Clin Cancer Res. 2014;20(1):120–30.
48. Lyssiotis CA, Cantley LC. Targeting metabolic scavenging in pancreatic cancer. Clin Cancer Res. 2014;20(1):6–8.
49. Ying H, Kimmelman AC, Lyssiotis CA, Hua S, Chu GC, Fletcher-Sananikone E, et al. Oncogenic Kras maintains pancreatic tumors through regulation of anabolic glucose metabolism. Cell. 2012;149(3):656–70.
50. Gaglio D, Metallo CM, Gameiro PA, Hiller K, Danna LS, Balestrieri C, et al. Oncogenic K-Ras decouples glucose and glutamine metabolism to support cancer cell growth. Mol Syst Biol. 2011;7:523.
51. Baek G, Tse YF, ZP H, Cox D, Buboltz N, McCue P, et al. MCT4 defines a glycolytic subtype of pancreatic cancer with poor prognosis and unique metabolic dependencies. Cell Rep. 2014;9(6):2233–49.
52. Cui JJ, Shi M, Xie DC, Wei DY, Jia ZL, Zheng SJ, et al. FOXM1 promotes the warburg effect and pancreatic cancer progression via transactivation of LDHA expression. Clin Cancer Res. 2014;20(10):2595–606.
53. Shi M, Cui JJ, JW D, Wei DY, Jia ZL, Zhang J, et al. A novel KLF4/LDHA signaling pathway regulates aerobic glycolysis in and progression of pancreatic cancer. Clin Cancer Res. 2014;20(16):4370–80.
54. Chiche J, Brahimi-Horn MC, Pouyssegur J. Tumour hypoxia induces a metabolic shift causing acidosis: a common feature in cancer. J Cell Mol Med. 2010;14(4):771–94.
55. Guillaumond F, Leca J, Olivares O, Lavaut MN, Vidal N, Berthezene P, et al. Strengthened glycolysis under hypoxia supports tumor symbiosis and hexosamine biosynthesis in pancreatic adenocarcinoma. Proc Natl Acad Sci U S A. 2013;110(10):3919–24.
56. Son J, Lyssiotis CA, Ying H, Wang X, Hua S, Ligorio M, et al. Glutamine supports pancreatic cancer growth through a KRAS-regulated metabolic pathway. Nature. 2013;496(7443):101–5.
57. Sousa CM, Biancur DE, Wang X, Halbrook CJ, Sherman MH, Zhang L, et al. Pancreatic stellate cells support tumour metabolism through autophagic alanine secretion. Nature. 2016;536(7617):479–83.
58. Perera RM, Bardeesy N. Pancreatic cancer metabolism: breaking it down to build it back up. Cancer Discov. 2015;5(12):1247–61.
59. Ying HQ, Dey P, Yao WT, Kimmelman AC, Draetta GF, Maitra A, et al. Genetics and biology of pancreatic ductal adenocarcinoma. Genes Dev. 2016;30(4):355–85.
60. Erez A, DeBerardinis RJ. Metabolic dysregulation in monogenic disorders and cancer - finding method in madness. Nat Rev Cancer. 2015;15(7):440–8.
61. Sahoo S, Franzson L, Jonsson JJ, Thiele I. A compendium of inborn errors of metabolism mapped onto the human metabolic network. Mol BioSyst. 2012;8(10):2545–58.
62. NCBI. Phenylketonuria. National Center for Biotechnology Information. 1998-;Genes and Disease.
63. Strauss KA, Puffenberger EG, Morton DH. Maple syrup urine disease. In: Pagon RA, Adam MP, Ardinger HH, Wallace SE, Amemiya A, Bean LJH, et al., editors. GeneReviews(R). Seattle (WA)1993.
64. Daneman D. Type 1 diabetes. Lancet. 2006;367 (9513):847–58.
65. Polonsky KS. The past 200 years in diabetes. N Engl J Med. 2012;367(14):1332–40.
66. Perry RJ, Camporez JP, Kursawe R, Titchenell PM, Zhang D, Perry CJ, et al. Hepatic acetyl CoA links adipose tissue inflammation to hepatic insulin resistance and type 2 diabetes. Cell. 2015;160(4):745–58.
67. Weisberg SP, McCann D, Desai M, Rosenbaum M, Leibel RL, Ferrante AW, Jr. Obesity is associated with macrophage accumulation in adipose tissue. J Clin Invest 2003;112(12):1796–1808.
68. Bezaire V, Mairal A, Anesia R, Lefort C, Langin D. Chronic TNFalpha and cAMP pre-treatment of human adipocytes alter HSL, ATGL and perilipin to regulate basal and stimulated lipolysis. FEBS Lett. 2009;583(18):3045–9.
69. Newgard CB, An J, Bain JR, Muehlbauer MJ, Stevens RD, Lien LF, et al. A branched-chain amino acid-related metabolic signature that differentiates obese and lean humans and contributes to insulin resistance. Cell Metab. 2009;9(4):311–26.
70. Ozcan U, Cao Q, Yilmaz E, Lee AH, Iwakoshi NN, Ozdelen E, et al. Endoplasmic reticulum stress links obesity, insulin action, and type 2 diabetes. Science. 2004;306(5695):457–61.
71. Wang TJ, Larson MG, Vasan RS, Cheng S, Rhee EP, McCabe E, et al. Metabolite profiles and the risk of developing diabetes. Nat Med. 2011;17(4):448–U83.
72. Saini V. Molecular mechanisms of insulin resistance in type 2 diabetes mellitus. World J Diabetes. 2010;1(3):68–75.
73. Morino K, Petersen KF, Shulman GI. Molecular mechanisms of insulin resistance in humans and their potential links with mitochondrial dysfunction. Diabetes. 2006;55:S9–S15.
74. Samuel VT, Shulman GI. The pathogenesis of insulin resistance: integrating signaling pathways and substrate flux. J Clin Investig. 2016;126(1):12–22.
75. Guilherme A, Virbasius JV, Puri V, Czech MP. Adipocyte dysfunctions linking obesity to insulin resistance and type 2 diabetes. Nat Rev Mol Cell Biol. 2008;9(5):367–77.

Part II

Metabolic Imaging Approaches

3 Overview of Positron-Emission Tomography Tracers for Metabolic Imaging

Ephraim Parent and Jonathan McConathy

Abbreviations

Acetyl-CoA	Acetyl coenzyme A
ACS	Acetyl-CoA synthase
ATP	Adenosine triphosphate
BAT	Brown adipose tissue
BBB	Blood-brain barrier
BOLD	Blood-oxygen-level dependent
CDP-choline	Diphosphate-choline
ChAT	Choline acetyltransferase
CK	Choline kinase
CO_2	Carbon dioxide
CT	Computed tomography
Ctr1	Copper-transporter 1
Cu-ATSM	Copper-diacetyl-bis (*N*4-methylthiosemicarbazone)
DLBCL	Diffuse large B-cell lymphoma
DNA	Deoxyribonucleic acids
EF5	2-Nitroimidazol-[^{18}F]pentafluoropropyl acetamide
FAO	Fatty acid oxidation
FAS	Fatty acid synthesis
FASN	Fatty acid synthase
FAZA	[^{18}F]Fluoroazomycin arabinoside
FDG	2-Deoxy-2-[^{18}F]fluoro-D-glucose
FDOPA	3,4-Dihydroxy-6-[^{18}F]fluoro-L-phenylalanine
FET	*O*-(2-[^{18}F]fluoroethyl)-L-tyrosine
FGln	4-[^{18}F]-(2*S*,4*R*)-Fluoroglutamine
FHDA	16-[^{18}F]Fluorohexadecanoic acid
FLT	3′-Deoxy-3′-[^{18}F]fluorothymidine
FMISO	[^{18}F]Fluoromisonidazole
FSPG	4-(3-[^{18}F]-(2*S*,4*S*)-fluorpropyl) glutamate
GRPR	Gastrin-releasing peptide receptor
HD	Hodgkin's lymphoma
HIF-1α	Hypoxia-inducible factor-1α
LCFA	Long-chain fatty acid
MeAIB	α-[^{11}C]Methyl aminoisobutyric acid
MET	L-[^{11}C]Methionine
MIP	Maximum intensity projection
MRI	Magnetic resonance imaging
mTOR	Mammalian target of rapamycin
NADH	Nicotinamide adenine dinucleotide
NADPH	Nicotinamide adenine dinucleotide phosphate
NSCLC	Non-small cell lung cancer
PC	Phosphatidylcholine
PDC	Pyruvate dehydrogenase complex
PET	Positron-emission tomography

E. Parent
Department of Radiology, Emory University School of Medicine, Atlanta, GA 30307, USA

J. McConathy (✉)
Department of Radiology, University of Alabama at Birmingham School of Medicine, Birmingham, AL 35210, USA

Division of Molecular Imaging and Therapeutics, University of Alabama at Birmingham, 619 19th Street South, JT 773, Birmingham, AL 35249, USA
e-mail: jmcconathy@uabmc.edu

J.S. Lewis, K.R. Keshari (eds.), *Imaging and Metabolism*, DOI 10.1007/978-3-319-61401-4_3

PSA	Prostate-specific antigen
PSMA	Prostate-specific membrane antigen
RNA	Ribonucleic acid
SLC	Solute carrier
SPECT	Single photon emission computed tomography
SUV	Standardized uptake value
TCA	Tricarboxylic acid
tRNA	Transfer ribonucleic acid
UCP-1	Uncoupling protein 1

3.1 Introduction

Positron-emission tomography (PET) is a cross-sectional imaging technique that uses compounds labeled with positron-emitting radionuclides to measure the concentration and location of the radiolabeled compounds over time. PET has been used for a broad range of biomedical research and is used routinely in clinical patient care for oncologic, neurologic, and cardiac applications. PET has several properties that make this technique particularly well-suited for metabolic imaging as well as some important limitations. This chapter discusses key principles and applications of PET tracers for metabolic imaging in mammalian systems. Many of the first PET tracers developed for metabolic imaging were radiolabeled forms of naturally occurring products such as glucose and amino acids [1, 2]. Due to the wide range of metabolic PET tracers that have been developed, it is not possible to comprehensively cover this field in a single chapter. We focus primarily on small molecule PET tracers that participate in metabolic pathways and/or serve as markers for the activity of specific metabolic pathways that have been used in human imaging studies.

3.1.1 Basics of PET Imaging

A key feature of PET imaging that makes it distinct from other forms of scintigraphy is coincidence detection of annihilation photons [3]. Positron-emitting radionuclides decay through the emission of positrons which are the antiparticles to electrons. A positron travels a short distance in tissue (on the order of millimeters) determined by its kinetic energy and then interacts with an electron in the tissue to undergo an annihilation event. The distance traveled by the positron prior to annihilation differs across positron-emitting radionuclides and leads to uncertainty in localizing site of decay, reducing spatial resolution. The mass of the positron and electron are converted into energy which leads to the production of two 511 keV photons that travel at nearly 180 degrees away from each other. The paths of the annihilation photon define a line of response, and PET systems have rings of detectors that register coincidence events when two photons interact with detectors with a very short temporal window (on the order of a few nanoseconds to hundreds of picoseconds). Through coincidence detection, PET systems avoid the need for physical collimation used in planar and single photon emission computed tomography (SPECT). PET generally provides higher sensitivity as well as better temporal and spatial resolution than SPECT, although small animal SPECT systems can provide high-resolution imaging [4]. A range of PET systems are available for small animal imaging and human imaging.

An important strength of PET imaging is the quantitative nature of its measurements. The basic measurement made by PET systems is the spatial distribution and concentration of radioactivity (e.g., Bq/mL or nCi/mL) over time. Attenuation correction is performed to account for the greater probability that annihilation photons arising deep within an imaging subject will not reach the detectors than photons arising from more superficial structures. Attenuation correction can be performed using a transmission source which rotates around the imaging subject or from computed tomography (CT) or magnetic resonance imaging (MRI) data in the case of PET/CT and PET/MRI systems. For some applications, the concentration of radioactivity is converted into standardized uptake values (SUVs) which account for the amount of radioactivity administered and the mass of the subject being imaged. Expression of data as SUVs facilitates comparison across studies and across subjects where the amount of administered radioactivity and/or the mass of the subjects may vary. SUVs are calculated using the following formula:

$$\text{SUV} = \left(\frac{\text{Concentration of activity}}{\text{Injected dose}}\right) \times \left(\begin{matrix}\text{Body} \\ \text{weight}\end{matrix}\right)$$

In some cases, the lean body mass (SUV_{lean}) is used as the biodistribution of many tracers differs substantially between adipose tissue versus skeletal muscle and normal organs [5, 6]. PET quantification with SUVs is sufficient for many clinical applications, but estimation of tracer binding sites and metabolic rates often require more sophisticated methods such as kinetic modeling or graphical analysis. The exact type of analysis depends on the nature of the PET tracer, the target, and the biological parameter that is being measured [7–10].

3.1.2 Tracer Principle and Specific Activity

An important concept in nuclear medicine including PET imaging is the tracer principle. Tracers provide an adequate readout signal to provide useful information about the biological process of interest at a low enough concentration that the biological system is not perturbed by the tracer (i.e., no pharmacologic effect). The very low levels of radioactivity normally present in biological systems coupled with effective radiation detectors allow very sensitive detection of the signal arising from PET tracers at picomolar concentrations of the tracer. The term specific activity refers to the amount of radioactivity, for example, curie (Ci) or becquerel (Bq), per mass of a compound while molar activity refers to the amount of radioactivity per mole of a compound. Higher specific activity for a given compound indicates that there is more radioactivity per mass/mole. Most PET tracers can be produced in high molar activity (e.g., over 37 GBq per micromole) and act as true tracers in biological systems. For example, a 370 MBq (10 mCi) dosage of a small molecule PET tracer with a specific activity of 37 Gbq/micromole and molecular weight of 300 g/mole will have an associated administered mass of three micrograms. A typical human PET study uses on the order of 100,000- to 1,000,000-fold less mass than conventional computed tomography (CT) and magnetic resonance imaging (MRI) contrast agents.

High specific activity may be less important for certain metabolic imaging applications than for other PET studies due to the relatively high K_m of many enzymes and biological transporters (in the millimolar or micromolar range) and the presence of relatively high concentrations of competing natural substrates. An important advantage of the low mass dose associated with most PET tracers is their safety profile. Because such a small amount of material is administered in a typical PET study (on the order of micrograms or less), toxicity is rarely encountered at the mass doses required for PET studies. Thus, the vast majority of PET tracers can be translated into human use once sufficient preclinical data including dosimetry and toxicity studies have been obtained. Metabolic imaging with other modalities is possible, but the larger mass doses that must be administered may be toxic and/or cause pharmacologic effects that may interfere with data interpretation.

3.1.3 Radionuclides

The PET radionuclides carbon-11, nitrogen-13, oxygen-15, and fluorine-18 are readily accessible from medical cyclotrons. Because carbon, nitrogen, and oxygen occur in virtually all biomolecules, these radionuclides are suitable for labeling metabolic substrates for PET without changing their chemical and biological properties. However, the relatively short half-lives of C-11 (20 min), N-13 (10 min), and O-15 (2 min) impose significant limitations on the radiosynthetic methods and the maximum length of time that they can be used to produce useful data through PET imaging (typically 4–5 half-lives). The radiohalogen fluorine-18 has a longer half-life (110 min) which is advantageous for production and distribution, but fluorine is not normally present in biomolecules. Fluorine has steric requirements similar to a hydrogen atom and electronegativity similar to a hydroxyl (–OH) substituent, and fluorine-18 can often but not always be introduced into small molecules without disrupting their biological properties.

Radiometals such as Cu-64, Ga-68, and Zr-89 are well-suited to labeling larger molecules such as peptides, antibodies, and nanoparticles. Labeling with radiometals typically requires chelators that are relatively large and may carry a positive or negative charge. Incorporation of radiometal chelates in small molecules often abolishes their desired biological activities, and radiometals currently play a very limited role in most metabolic imaging with PET.

3.1.4 Limitations of PET

Although PET has many strengths, there are some important limitations that must be considered when choosing an imaging modality for metabolic imaging. PET systems detect only one signal: the annihilation photons resulting from positron-emission. Thus, it is generally not possible to image multiple probes simultaneously as can be done with some SPECT, optical, and MR spectroscopic methods. Similarly, radiolabeled metabolites cannot be distinguished from the parent PET tracer which can decrease image quality and confound quantitative analysis depending on the nature and amount of radiolabeled metabolites that are formed. In some cases, the radiolabeling position can be changed so that the radionuclide is not present in interfering metabolites. Blood sampling combined with graphical or compartmental modeling can be performed to correct for the formation of radiolabeled metabolites but adds complexity and sources of error in both preclinical and human studies. This limitation of PET is particularly relevant to metabolic imaging as it can be challenging to measure enzymatic activity with PET imaging as the substrate cannot be distinguished from the radiolabeled product of the enzymatic reaction.

Another consideration in PET studies is the use of ionizing radiation inherent to radiolabeled compounds. The radiation exposure in human studies from a typical PET study is similar to diagnostic CT studies and is generally considered safe with the major risk being a small increased risk of cancer years after the PET study [11]. The dosimetry of individual PET agents is determined primarily by their radionuclide and biodistribution over time. Longer physical and biological half-lives lead to higher radiation exposure. Also, PET tracers may concentrate in certain organs, leading to high organ radiation doses which must be taken into account for dosimetry calculations. The radiation exposure can be a significant issue for certain patient populations such as children and pregnant women, and cumulative exposures can be high if repeated imaging is required. Alternative modalities such as optical imaging and MRI do not have this limitation.

The distance traveled by the positron between emission and annihilation imposes inherent physical limitations on the spatial resolution of PET imaging systems. The spatial resolution PET is on the order of 4–6 mm for clinical human imaging systems and on the order of 1–2 mm for preclinical imaging. These resolution limits can prevent evaluation of small structures, particularly in studies using mice and other small animals.

3.2 Carbohydrates

Carbohydrates are the most abundant class of organic molecules in living systems. Carbohydrates play fundamental roles in cell biology including energy metabolism and can serve as key sources of carbon for the biosynthesis of other classes of biomolecules including nucleosides, fatty acids, amino acids, and glycoproteins. Monosaccharides have the molecular formula $(CH_2O)_n$ where $n \geq 3$, with 3–9 carbon carbohydrates being the most common in mammals. Monosaccharides are the simplest form of carbohydrates and are the building blocks of larger carbohydrates that contain two or more monosaccharides. Because carbohydrate metabolism is fundamental to so many physiologic and disease processes, carbohydrate-based PET imaging agents have been used for a wide range of research and clinical applications.

Glycolysis and the tricarboxylic acid (TCA) cycle are central pathways in the metabolism of glucose, and these pathways are critical sources of cellular energy in the form of adenosine triphosphate (ATP). The glycolytic pathway produces pyruvate under aerobic conditions which can be converted to acetyl coenzyme A (acetyl-CoA) by the pyruvate dehydrogenase complex (PDC) which enters the TCA cycle for oxidative phosphorylation to produce ATP. Under anaerobic conditions in normal tissues or aerobic glycolysis conditions in many tumors, glucose is converted to lactate through glycolysis. Metabolites derived from glucose serve as key intermediates for the synthesis of fatty acids and triglycerides, nucleosides, some amino acids, and glycoproteins. The metabolism of glucose also provides the energy to maintain the reduced form of nicotinamide adenine dinucleotide (NADH) and nicotinamide adenine dinucleotide phosphate (NADPH) [12].

3.2.1 Carbohydrate-Based PET Tracers

The most widely used PET tracer, 2-deoxy-2-[^{18}F]fluoro-D-glucose (FDG), is an analog of glucose with the 2-position hydroxyl group of D-glucose replaced with fluorine-18 as shown in Fig. 3.1. In addition to providing a positron-emitting radiolabel, this structural change limits metabolism of

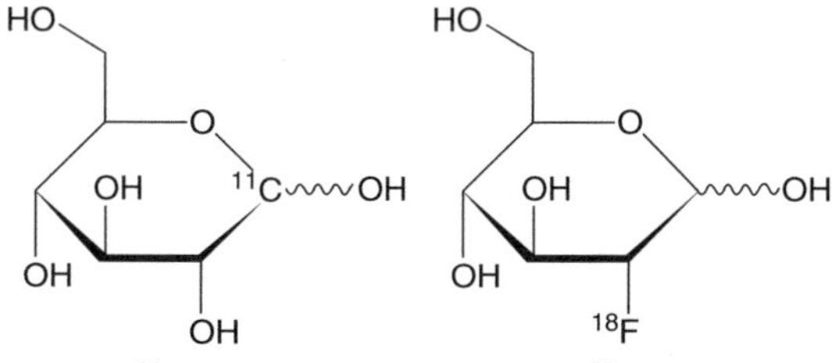

Fig. 3.1 Structures of selected carbohydrate-based PET tracers

[^{18}F]FDG to phosphorylation at the 6-position hydroxyl group. Unlike 6-phospho-D-glucose, 6-phospho-[^{18}F]FDG cannot be isomerized to proceed through the rest of the glycolytic pathway. This property leads to intracellular trapping of 6-phospho-[^{18}F]FDG in most tissues and in cancer cells, although some tissues such as the liver can enzymatically dephosphorylate 6-phospho-[^{18}F]FDG, allowing [^{18}F]FDG to be slowly released over time. The amount of uptake of [^{18}F]FDG in a tissue can serve as a measure of glycolysis and may be increased or decreased by a range of physiologic and pathophysiologic conditions.

Clinically, [^{18}F]FDG is used primarily for oncologic, neurologic, and cardiac imaging, although there is the potential for using this tracer for imaging infection and inflammation as well. The cellular uptake and retention of [^{18}F]FDG is mediated by glucose transporters and intracellular phosphorylation by hexokinase enzymes. Most studies suggest that hexokinase activity is the rate-limiting step for FDG accumulation in cancer cells [13], although the particular oncogenes and tumor suppressers active in a cancer cell may influence the balance of transport versus hexokinase activity [14–16]. The uptake of glucose and [^{18}F]FDG is tissue dependent, and in skeletal and cardiac muscle, uptake is highly regulated by insulin. PET studies performed with [^{18}F]FDG are thus typically performed under fasting conditions with low blood insulin levels to increase reproducibility and prevent high physiologic uptake of [^{18}F]FDG in skeletal muscle mediated by endogenous insulin release. Graphical analysis techniques using the Gjedde-Patlak method as well as compartment modeling methods have been developed to provide quantitative measures of [^{18}F]FDG metabolism [17].

In addition to [^{18}F]FDG, a wide range of radiolabeled carbohydrates have been developed [18, 19]. Of these, the natural form of glucose labeled with C-11 has been used most extensively, initially through photosynthetic methods and later through chemical synthesis as D-[1-^{11}C]glucose for human studies [20–22]. Advantages of [^{11}C]glucose are the chemical and biological equivalence to unlabeled glucose and the ability of this PET tracer to undergo metabolism beyond the first step of glycolysis. The term lumped constant can be used to estimate the metabolic rate of glucose using [^{18}F]FDG by correcting the fraction of [^{11}C]glucose continuing through glycolysis along with the differences in the rate constants K_m and maximum velocity V_{max} of hexokinase activity for [^{11}C]glucose and [^{18}F]FDG [23, 24]. Estimates of glycolytic rates with [^{11}C]glucose and [^{18}F]FDG using the lumped constant are generally in good agreement in the brain but can differ substantially in malignant tissues [24, 25]. These differences are attributable at least in part to differences in substrate recognition by hexokinases. Due to the intracellular trapping of the radiolabel in the case of [^{18}F]FDG but not [^{11}C]glucose, [^{18}F]FDG may provide higher tumor-to-normal tissue ratios [26].

3.2.2 Oncologic Imaging

The most widespread application of [^{18}F]FDG is for cancer imaging. Most cancer cells upregulate the glycolytic pathway with conversion of glucose to lactate even when there is adequate oxygen and mitochondrial function for oxidative phosphorylation. This phenomenon, aerobic glycolysis, is often called the Warburg effect because it was first described by Otto Warburg in the 1920s [27–29]. Regulatory pathways such as the PIK3/AKT pathway and the *Myc* oncogene drive the shift to glycolytic metabolism in many cancer cells [29]. This upregulation of glycolysis by tumor cells leads to higher uptake of [^{18}F]FDG compared to most normal tissues and is the basis of [^{18}F]FDG-PET imaging for the detection of cancer. Clinically, [^{18}F]FDG-PET is frequently used for staging a wide range of solid and hematological malignancies. [^{18}F]FDG-PET/CT can increase the detection of nodal and distant metastases compared to anatomic imaging alone with CT or MRI. Effective therapies that injure or kill tumor cells typically lead to a rapid decrease in [^{18}F]FDG uptake which can often be detected before tumor size changes as assessed with anatomic imaging modalities such as CT and MRI [30–32].

In cancer, higher [^{18}F]FDG uptake is typically associated with more aggressive malignancies and poorer prognosis [33–38]. Some cancers such as differentiated thyroid cancers, well-differentiated neuroendocrine tumors, clear cell renal cell carcinomas, prostate adenocarcinomas, and mucinous adenocarcinomas often do not have high [^{18}F]FDG uptake. Similarly, low-grade malignancies often have low [^{18}F]FDG accumulation. Because inflammatory lesions due to infection or treatment (surgery, chemotherapy and radiation) can cause increased [^{18}F]FDG uptake, these conditions can confound [^{18}F]FDG-PET studies for cancer imaging. In these settings, other metabolic or molecularly targeted PET tracers can be more effective than [^{18}F]FDG. For example, [^{11}C]choline and the amino acid [^{18}F]fluciclovine are more effective for detecting biochemically recurrent prostate cancer than [^{18}F]FDG, and these tracers are discussed later in this chapter.

A discussion of the many roles of [^{18}F]FDG-PET for research and clinical oncologic imaging is beyond the scope of this chapter, but the use of [^{18}F]FDG in the initial staging, monitoring response to therapy, and restaging after completion of therapy for lymphoma illustrates many of the useful properties of [^{18}F]FDG for oncologic imaging [39, 40]. [^{18}F]FDG has high uptake in fast-growing aggressive lymphomas such as diffuse large B-cell lymphoma (DLBCL), Hodgkin's lymphoma (HD), and Burkitt's lymphoma. [^{18}F]FDG-PET/CT can provide more accurate initial staging of aggressive lymphoma than CT alone, particularly for detection of bone marrow and organ involvement [41, 42]. Interim [^{18}F]FDG-PET imaging after two cycles of chemotherapy can provide key prognostic information in patients with HD and DLBCL; resolution of increased FDG uptake portends a good prognosis and may allow reducing the intensity of the remaining chemotherapy regimen [43]. Similarly, complete metabolic response at the end of therapy indicates a favorable prognosis, and [^{18}F]FDG-PET can be used for the detection of suspected recurrence. An example of FDG-PET/CT imaging in lymphoma before and after chemotherapy is shown in Fig. 3.2.

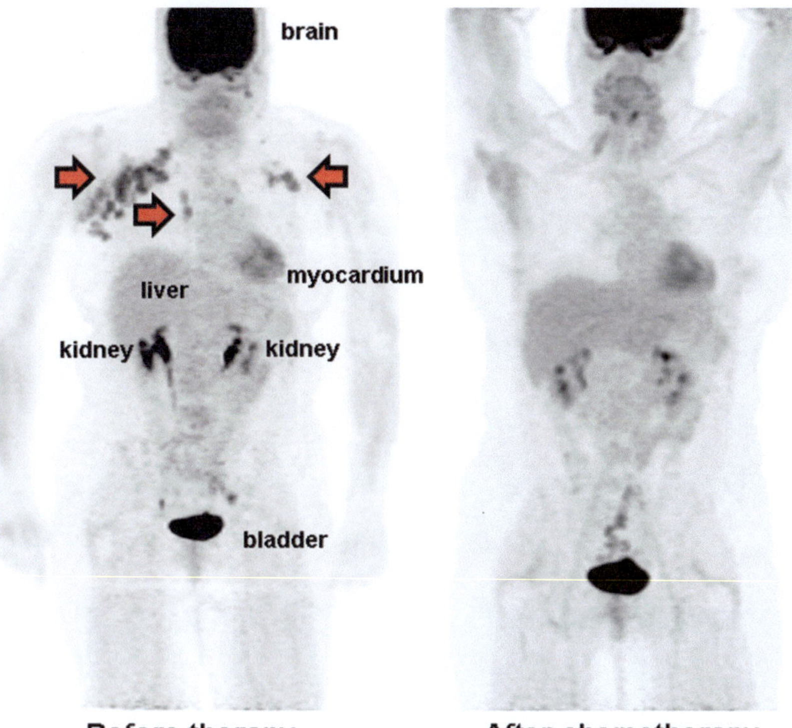

Fig. 3.2 Maximum intensity projection (MIP) images from [^{18}F] FDG-PET/CT studies before and after chemotherapy in a patient with follicular lymphoma. Metabolically active lymphoma involving lymph nodes in the axillae and the mediastinum are indicated with red arrows on the study performed before therapy. These nodes no longer have increased FDG uptake on the study performed after therapy, consistent with a complete metabolic response. Physiologic [^{18}F]FDG uptake is seen in the brain, left ventricular myocardium, liver, and urine in the kidneys and bladder

3.2.3 Neuroimaging

Glucose is the primary energy source for neurons, and [^{18}F]FDG has been used extensively as a measure of regional cerebral glucose metabolism rates. The glucose transporter 1 (GLUT1, SLC2A1) is present at the blood-brain barrier (BBB) and mediates facilitated transport of glucose and [^{18}F]FDG across the BBB [44]. Under most circumstances, glucose utilization and brain perfusion are tightly coupled and positively correlated [45]. The uptake of [^{18}F]FDG in the brain reflects both neuronal and glial cell metabolism and synaptic activity and can change rapidly with brain activity and from pathological processes such as seizures.

The most common clinical uses of [^{18}F]FDG for neuroimaging are in patients with possible dementia, epilepsy undergoing surgical evaluation or brain tumors. [^{18}F]FDG-PET has also been used in neuroimaging research of measurement of brain activation, although functional MRI using the blood-oxygen-level dependent (BOLD) method has replaced many of these PET applications [46–48]. In neurodegenerative diseases, [^{18}F]FDG uptake is decreased in characteristic brain regions due to decreased synaptic activity and neuronal loss [49, 50]. In epilepsy, [^{18}F]FDG-PET imaging is performed between seizures (interictal) and typically demonstrates decreased [^{18}F]FDG uptake in the brain region surrounding the abnormal brain tissue that is the source of seizure activity [51–53]. The use of [^{18}F]FDG-PET in neuro-oncology is limited by the high physiologic uptake of [^{18}F]FDG in gray matter which often obscures adjacent tumor tissue. [^{18}F]FDG-PET has been used for grading gliomas and for distinguishing recurrent tumor from treatment effects such as radiation necrosis as an adjunct to MRI [36, 54, 55]. Examples of [^{18}F]FDG-PET for neuroimaging in epilepsy and dementia are shown in Figs. 3.3 and 3.4, respectively.

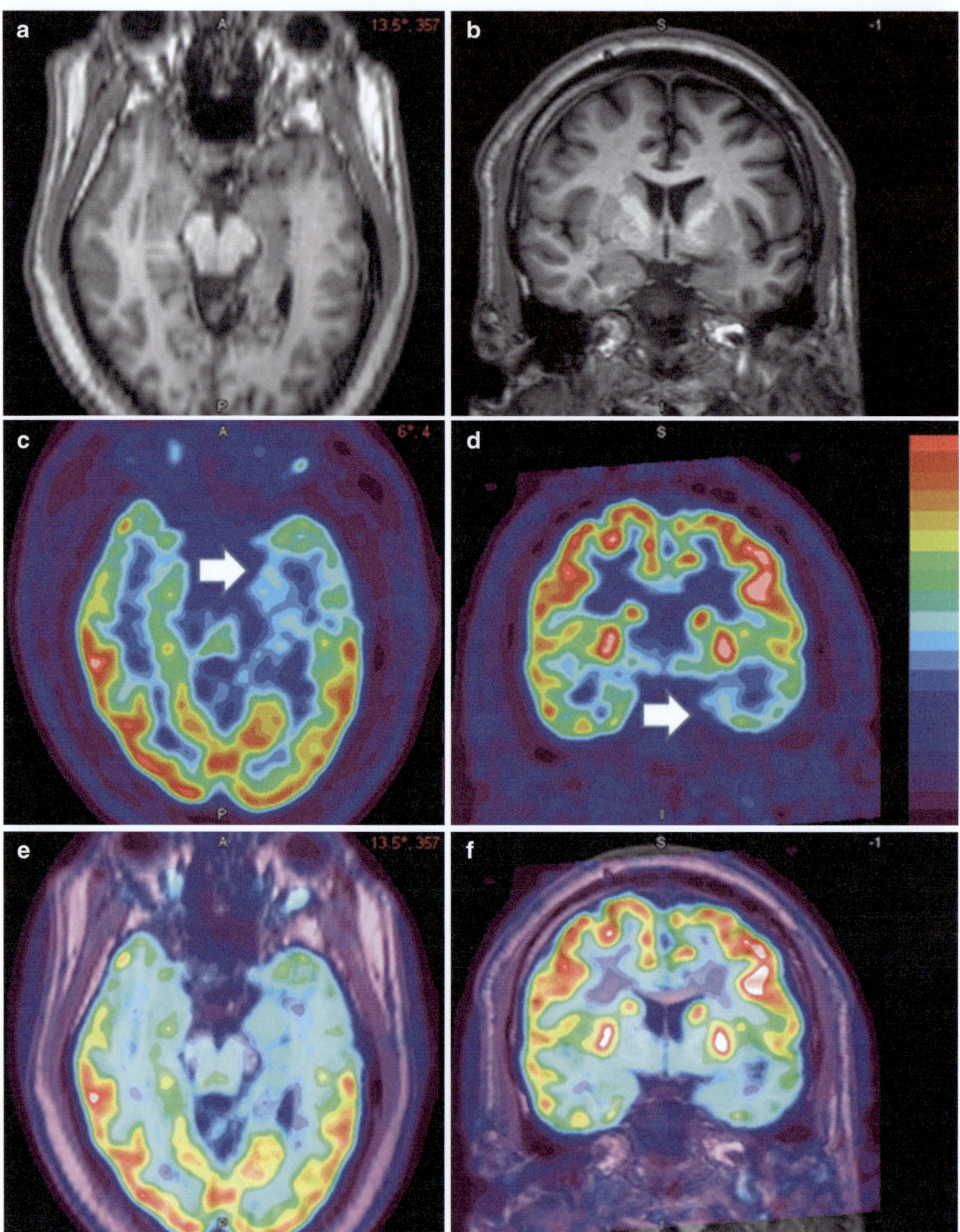

Fig. 3.3 Brain [^{18}F]FDG-PET in a patient with medically refractory epilepsy performed between seizures (interictal study). T1-weighted axial (**a**) and coronal (**b**) MR images, axial (**c**) and coronal (**d**) [^{18}F]FDG-PET, and fused PET/MR images (**e, f**) demonstrate decreased [^{18}F]FDG uptake in the left temporal lobe (*white arrows*). This regional brain hypometabolism suggests that the origin of the seizure is in the left temporal lobe which guides surgical planning

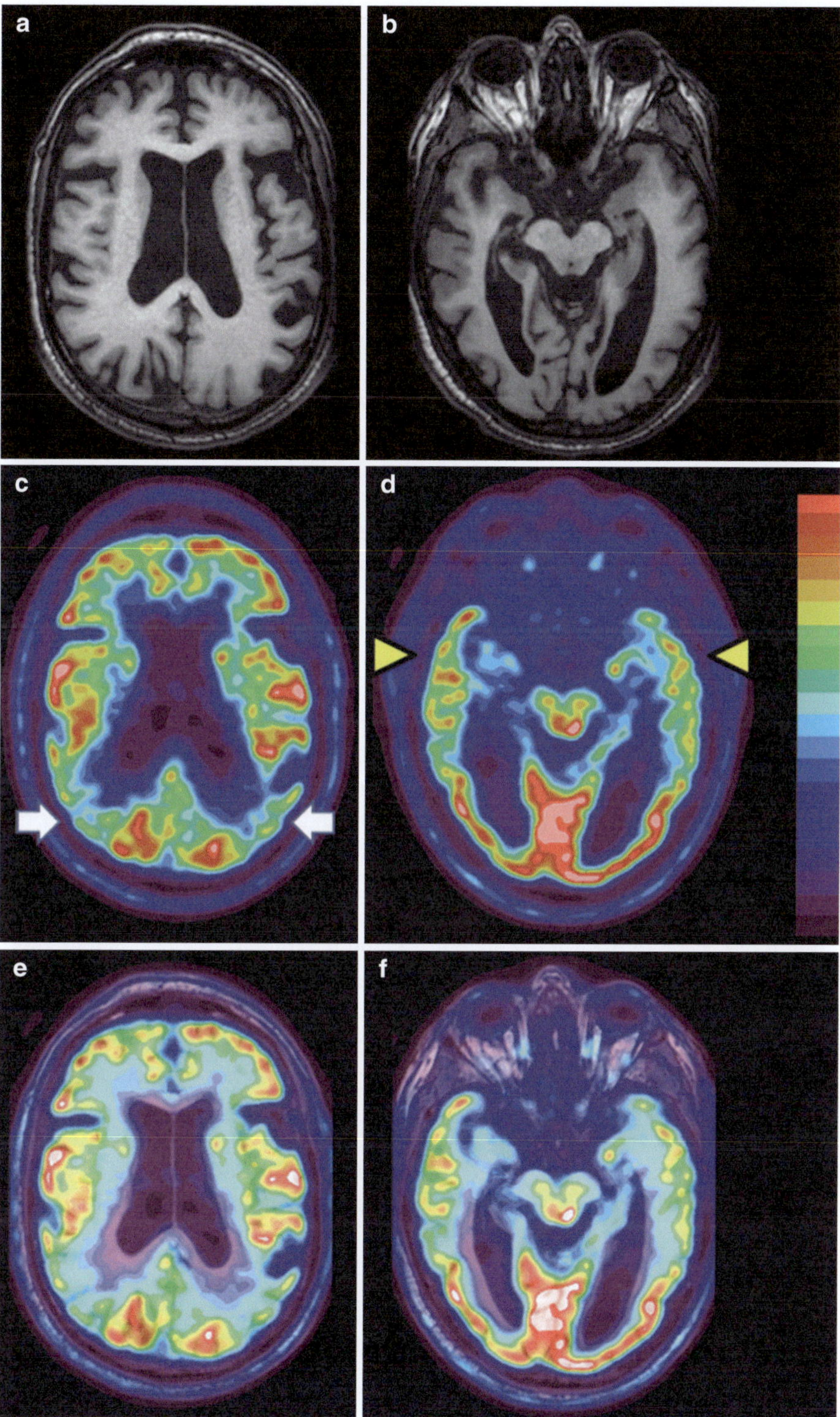

Fig. 3.4 Brain [^{18}F]FDG-PET in a patient with cognitive impairment. T1-weighted axial (**a**) and coronal (**b**) MR images, axial (**c**) and coronal (**d**) [^{18}F]FDG-PET, and fused PET/MR images (**e**, **f**) demonstrate decreased [^{18}F] FDG uptake in the parietal lobes (*white arrows*) and the temporal lobes (*yellow arrow heads*). This pattern of brain hypometabolism suggests that the patient's cognitive impairment is due to Alzheimer's dementia

3.2.4 Cardiac Imaging

Cardiac muscle (myocardium) normally utilizes glucose and fatty acids as its primary sources of energy, although myocardial cells are highly adaptable which can also use lactate, pyruvate, ketone bodies, and certain amino acids for energy metabolism. Under normal conditions, fatty acids supply most of the myocardium's energy demands. Myocardial energy metabolism is influenced by the availability of substrates. Recent ingestion of carbohydrates and higher blood insulin levels promote myocardial utilization of glucose rather than fatty acids. In contrast, prolonged fasting or consumption of a diet with high fat and very low or no carbohydrates promotes myocardial utilization of fatty acids and suppresses glucose metabolism. Myocardial ischemia (inadequate blood flow to fully meet metabolic demand) promotes glucose utilization.

Under basal conditions, glucose transport is rate limiting for glucose utilization, while ischemia and insulin stimulation lead to hexokinase phosphorylation becoming the rate-limiting step [56]. Differences in the recognition and phosphorylation of [^{18}F]FDG and [^{11}C]glucose can lead to substantial differences in estimates of myocardial glucose metabolism with [^{11}C]glucose providing more accurate measurements but requiring more complicated modeling and sampling techniques [57, 58]. Patient preparation is critical for performing myocardial imaging with [^{18}F]FDG or [^{11}C]glucose imaging, and depending on the application, either glucose or fatty acid metabolism may be desired.

The heart does not maintain a significant depot of stored fuel substrates, and without a continual supply of fuel and oxygen, myocardial cells are able to sustain metabolism for only a few minutes. During ischemia, myocardial fatty acid catabolism is affected in a matter of seconds with reciprocal utilization of glucose and fatty acids. The studies that have used fatty acid tracers to evaluate the ischemic heart have provided complementary findings when compared to those measuring glucose, with ischemic myocardium preferentially metabolizing glucose [59, 60]. Under ischemic conditions, cardiac myocyte glucose utilization is quickly upregulated, which allows sufficient ATP for maintenance of ionic gradients through anaerobic glycolysis but does not supply sufficient ATP for full contractile function. This pattern of decreased fatty acid use and enhanced glucose use is characteristic of ischemic myocardium.

Clinically, [^{18}F]FDG-PET has two major uses: (1) to assess for myocardial viability when chronic resting ischemia is suspected and (2) to assess for active inflammation due to sarcoidosis. Chronic resting ischemia leads to decreased myocardial contractility and is not readily distinguished from infarction through myocardial perfusion imaging. This condition is referred to as hibernating myocardium, and the presence of maintained [^{18}F]FDG uptake indicated viable myocardium that may benefit from revascularization [61–63]. For viability studies, patient preparation that promotes myocardial glucose metabolism is necessary. In contrast, assessment for inflammation due to myocardial involvement by sarcoidosis, an idiopathic systemic inflammatory condition that can cause life-threatening arrhythmias through myocardial involvement, requires suppression of normal myocardial uptake of [^{18}F]FDG. An example of myocardial imaging with [^{18}F]FDG-PET is shown in Fig. 3.5.

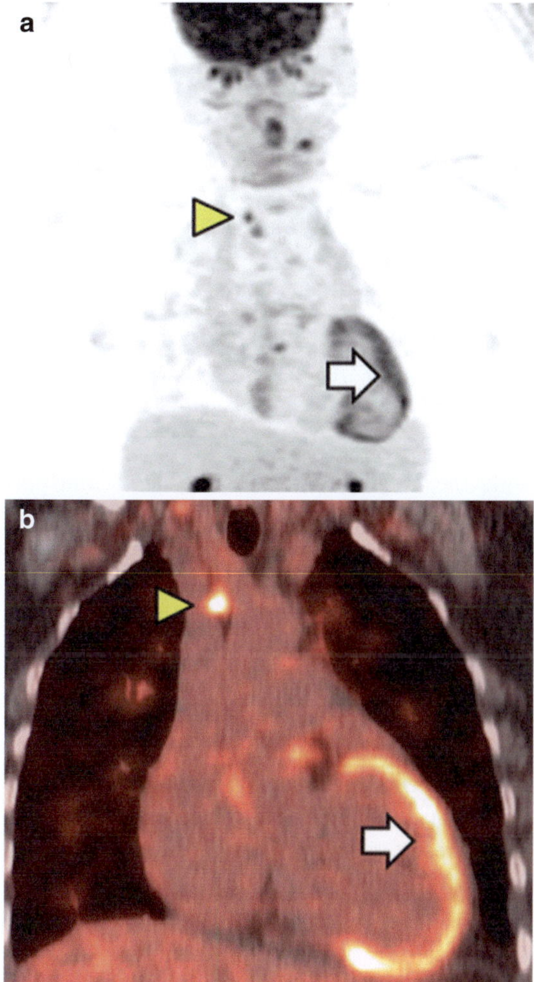

Fig. 3.5 Maximum intensity projection (MIP) image (**a**) and coronal PET/CT (**b**) images from a myocardial [^{18}F]FDG-PET/CT study performed in a patient with suspected sarcoidosis. Increased activity is seen in the left ventricular myocardium (*white arrow*) despite suppression of glucose metabolism, indicating active inflammation due to sarcoidosis. Additionally, mediastinal lymph nodes with increased [^{18}F]FDG uptake are present, and one of these nodes involved by sarcoidosis is indicated by a *yellow arrow head*

3.2.5 Brown Adipose Tissue

Brown adipose tissue (BAT) is a metabolically active form of fat with adipocytes that contain the uncoupling protein 1 (UCP-1) which can uncouple electron transport in the mitochondria leading to the generation of heat rather than ATP production. BAT can be activated through sympathetic innervation and is a source of thermogenesis during cold exposure. In humans, BAT is typically located in the neck, the supraclavicular region, and the intrathoracic fat of the posterior intercostal spaces and mediastinum. In oncologic [^{18}F]FDG-PET studies, BAT can interfere with detection of malignant tissue. There is growing evidence that higher amounts of BAT are associated with better glucose homeostasis, better blood lipid profiles, and decreased vascular inflammation [64, 65]. Increased [^{18}F]FDG uptake can be used to estimate BAT metabolic activity, and recently standardized patient preparation, PET acquisition parameters, and quantitative measures for human studies have been proposed [66].

3.3 Amino Acids

α-Amino acids are small polar molecules with amino and carboxylic acid groups attached to the same carbon (the α-carbon). Amino acid side chains arising from the α-carbon determine the physiochemical and biological properties of an individual amino acid. Amino acids are the building blocks of proteins, and there are 21 standard amino acids in humans which are incorporated into proteins via transfer ribonucleic acids (tRNAs). Many other amino acids are formed through biosynthetic pathways, metabolic intermediates, and posttranslational modification of

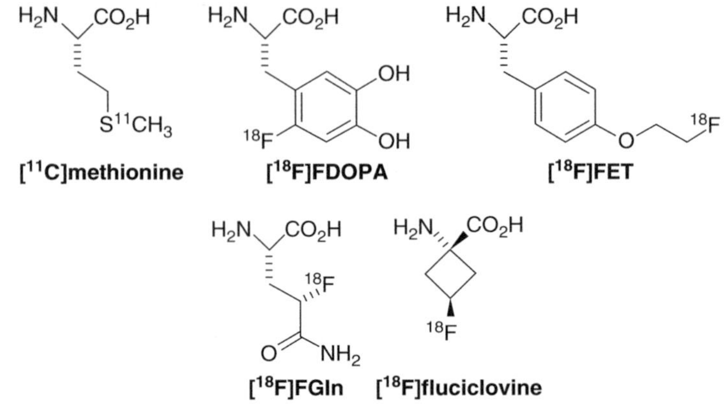

Fig. 3.6 Structures of selected radiolabel amino acids for PET imaging

[^{11}C]methionine [^{18}F]FDOPA [^{18}F]FET [^{18}F]FGln [^{18}F]fluciclovine

proteins. In addition to their role in protein synthesis, amino acids play a wide range of key roles in cellular metabolism including sources of energy (particularly glutamine), carbon sources for anabolic pathways, and neurotransmission (e.g., glycine, glutamate, and precursors to the monoamines dopamine, norepinephrine, and serotonin) [12].

Amino acids cross cell membranes through carrier proteins called amino acid transporters that are members of a family of biological transporters called solute carrier (SLC) proteins [67, 68]. Over 20 amino acid transporter families have been identified in mammalian cells that differ in terms of their mechanisms of transport, tissue distributions, substrate specificity, and regulation. Most PET imaging performed with radiolabeled amino acids primarily measures amino acid transporter rather than intracellular metabolism with some important exceptions. Amino acid transport and metabolism is altered in many cancer cells, and the major application of radiolabeled amino acids in humans has been for oncologic imaging. An important unanswered question is whether amino acid transport can be used as a reliable surrogate for intracellular metabolism/utilization of specific amino acids. Several amino acid transporters including LAT1 and ASCT2 play important roles in cellular signaling through the mammalian target of rapamycin (mTOR) pathway [69–71]. Amino acid-based PET tracers are currently not as widely applicable as [^{18}F]FDG but play key roles for certain types of tumors.

Naturally occurring amino acids can be labeled with N-13 and C-11 and are compatible with the relatively fast amino acid transport kinetics that typically lead to peak uptake within 10–20 min after intravenous administration. The rapid metabolism of most naturally occurring amino acids coupled with the desirability of longer physical half-lives for batch production and remote distribution has motivated the development of nonnatural amino acids labeled with fluorine-18. In some cases, nonnatural amino acids are metabolically stable and may be more selective for specific amino acid transporters [72, 73]. Structures of some radiolabeled amino acids used for PET imaging are shown in Fig. 3.6.

3.3.1 Neuro-Oncology

One of the best established uses of radiolabeled amino acids is for neuro-oncology. Although [^{18}F]FDG is effective for imaging most malignancies, the high physiological glucose metabolic rate leads to high uptake of [^{18}F]FDG which can obscure lesions in the brain. Amino acids with large neutral side chains such as L-[^{11}C]methionine (MET), *O*-(2-[^{18}F]fluoroethyl)-L-tyrosine (FET), and 3,4-dihydroxy-6-[^{18}F]fluoro-L-phenylalanine (FDOPA) are system L substrates that have been used extensively for imaging brain tumors. System L is composed of four family members: LAT1 (SLC7A5), LAT2 (SLC7A8), LAT3 (SLC43A1), and LAT4 (SLC43A2). Because LAT1 is active at the blood-brain barrier (BBB), substrates for system L transport can cross the intact BBB and reach the entire tumor volume. Unlike [^{18}F]FDG, system L amino acids have relatively low uptake in normal brain tissue. These property allows tracers like [^{11}C]MET, [^{18}F]FET, and [^{18}F]FDOPA to reach the entire brain tumor volume unlike CT and MRI contrast agents and many PET tracers that do not cross the BBB. An example of brain tumor imaging with a radiolabeled amino acid is shown in Fig. 3.7. Additionally, higher levels of LAT1 are associated with worse prognosis in gliomas and many other human cancers [71, 74–76]. This class of amino acids has proven utility for diagnosis, surgical and biopsy planning, monitoring response to chemotherapy, and detecting recurrent disease [77–79]. There is recent data suggesting that faster washout of [^{18}F]FET is associated with high tumor grade and may predict more aggressive behavior in lower-grade gliomas [80, 81].

One of the limitations of system L transport is the reversible mechanism of transport (exchange for LAT1 and LAT2; facilitated diffusion for LAT3 and LAT4). This limits to the tumor-to-brain ratios that can be achieved with pure system L substrates. Other radiolabeled amino acids that are not primarily substrates for system L including 4-[^{18}F]-(2*S*,4*R*)-fluoroglutamine (FGln), 4-(3-[^{18}F]-(2*S*,4*S*)-fluorpropyl)glutamate (FSPG), and *anti*-3-[^{18}F]FACBC have demonstrated high uptake in the enhancing regions of brain tumors, but their ability to visualize the entire tumor volume as has been demonstrated with system L substrates has not been fully evaluated [82–84].

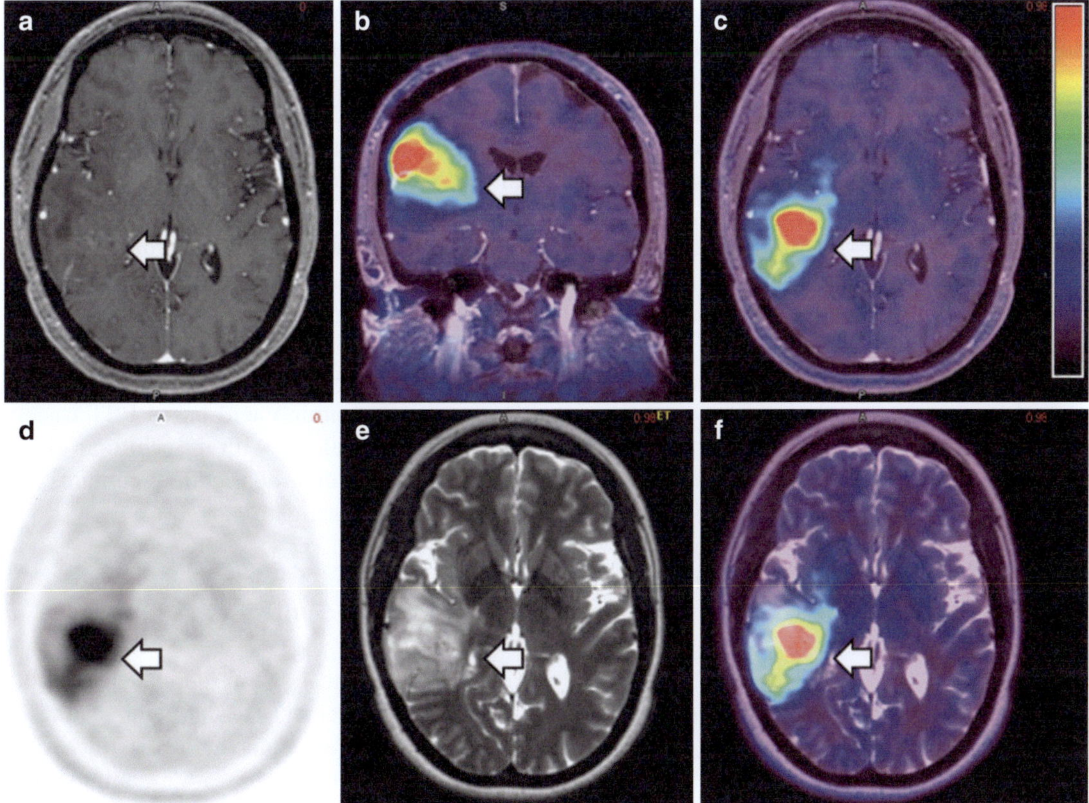

Fig. 3.7 Selected images from an [^{18}F]FDOPA-PET/MRI study performed in a patient with a high-grade glioma. The tumor is indicated with *white arrows*. The axial T1-weighted post-contrast MR image (**a**) shows minimal contrast enhancement in this region of the tumor, while the [^{18}F]FDOPA-PET image (**d**) shows increased activity relative to normal brain. Fused coronal (**b**) and axial (**c**) T1-weighted post-contrast images also demonstrate increased [^{18}F]FDOPA uptake in the tumor. The axial T2-weighted MR image (**e**) shows both tumor and edema, most of which overlaps with but is not identical to the [^{18}F]FDOPA uptake seen on the PET/MR fusion image (**f**)

3.3.2 Prostate Cancer

A variety of PET tracers have been developed and applied to prostate cancer imaging including metabolic tracers such as [^{11}C]choline and [^{11}C]acetate that are discussed in other sections of this chapter. Other PET tracers targeting cell surface proteins including prostate-specific membrane antigen (PSMA) and the gastrin-releasing peptide receptor (GRPR) are promising agents for prostate cancer imaging but are beyond the scope of this discussion [85–87]. The detection and localization of recurrent prostate cancer is a common clinical scenario, and [^{18}F]FDG and anatomic imaging with CT and MRI have limited sensitivity. The expression of several amino acid transporters is upregulated in human prostate cancer cells and can be targeted with radiolabeled amino acids [88, 89]. In May 2016, the nonnatural amino acid *anti*-3-[^{18}F]FACBC (fluciclovine) received FDA approval for clinical use for the detection of biochemically recurrent prostate cancer. The cellular uptake of [^{18}F]fluciclovine is mediated by several amino acid transporters with ASCT2 (SLC1A5) as the major transporter in prostate cancer cells with minor contributions by LAT1 and by SNAT2 (SLC38A2). ASCT2 is a neutral amino acid transporter which is a key transporter of glutamine in cancer, and SNAT2 is a transporter for small neutral amino acids. These amino acid transporters have high expression in human prostate cancer although they are not specific to prostate cancer. Limited human data suggest that [^{11}C]methionine and the selective system A substrate, α-[^{11}C]methyl aminoisobutyric acid (MeAIB), may also have applications for imaging prostate cancer [90, 91].

3.3.3 Neuroendocrine Tumors

Certain amino acids, particularly [^{18}F]FDOPA and ^{11}C- and ^{18}F-labeled analogs of tryptophan, have shown useful imaging properties for neuroendocrine tumors. These amino acids enter cells through system L transport but appear to have better imaging properties than other system L substrates, presumably due to intracellular metabolism of [^{18}F]FDOPA and tryptophan analogs. PET tracers that target somatostatin receptors such as ^{68}Ga-labeled DOTATATE, DOTATOC, and DOTANOC generally have superior diagnostic accuracy for well-differentiated neuroendocrine tumors, although there is data suggesting that [^{18}F]FDOPA may be more effective for carcinoid tumors that are hormonally active [92–94].

3.3.4 Glutaminolysis

Like glucose metabolism, many human cancers upregulate the utilization of the amino acid glutamine [95–97]. Therapeutics that interfere with glutamine metabolism represent a promising approach to cancer treatment, and there is great interest in developing imaging agents to measure glutamine metabolism. A major focus has been glutaminolysis which is the intracellular conversion of glutamine to glutamate with subsequent metabolism to other compounds including pyruvate, citrate, and alanine which can be used for energy or carbon sources for anabolism. A number of PET tracers have been developed that are substrates for glutamine transport including [^{11}C]glutamine, ^{18}F-labeled analogs of glutamine (e.g., [^{18}F]FGln), and the alicyclic amino acid [^{18}F]fluciclovine [88, 98–102]. Currently, it is not clear that the uptake and retention of amino acid-based PET tracers is positively correlated with intracellular glutaminolysis, and this application remains an active area of investigation.

3.3.5 Protein Synthesis

An obvious application of radiolabeled amino acids is measurement of protein synthesis. However, only a few amino acid PET tracers are well-suited for this purpose. Many amino acids have multiple potential metabolic fates other than incorporation into proteins which confounds PET image analysis, and many nonnatural amino acids do not participate in protein synthesis. The best established PET tracer for protein synthesis is L-[^{11}C]leucine labeled at the carboxylic acid position [103–105]. When L-[^{11}C]leucine is incorporated into proteins through amide bond formation, the C-11 label is retained. The other primary metabolic fate of leucine is conversion into α-ketoisocaproic acid which leads to decarboxylation and loss of the C-11 label as [^{11}C]carbon dioxide (CO_2). Other amino acids that have been used to estimate protein synthesis include [1-^{11}C]-L-tyrosine and 2-[^{18}F]fluoro-L-tyrosine [106, 107]. Measurement of protein synthesis with L-[^{11}C]leucine requires kinetic modeling and cannot be done through simple SUV measurements alone.

3.4 Nucleoside Analogs

Cellular proliferation is a fundamental process in cell biology and is dysregulated in neoplastic cells. Cell division requires the synthesis of deoxyribonucleic acids (DNA), and thus nucleosides and nucleoside analogs have been developed as PET tracers for measuring proliferation rates. This class of tracers have increased uptake in cells during the S-phase of the cell cycle when DNA synthesis is occurring but not during other cell cycle phases (G_1, M, and G_2 phases). Because thymidine is present in DNA but not in ribonucleic acid (RNA), tracer development for proliferation imaging with nucleosides has focused on thymidine analogs. Other strategies, notable sigma-2 receptor ligands, have been developed for imaging cellular proliferation but are not discussed in this chapter [108–110].

Initial proliferation imaging with nucleoside analogs was performed with [^{11}C]thymidine [111–113], but the rapid metabolism of this tracer made estimation of proliferation rates challenging. Currently, the most well-established PET tracer in this class is 3′-deoxy-3′-[^{18}F]fluorothymidine (FLT). In a fashion analogous to [^{18}F]FDG, the 3′-hydroxyl group on the deoxyribose portion of thymidine is replaced with F-18 in [^{18}F]FLT. This substitution provides a PET radionuclide for imaging and also prevents incorporation of [^{18}F]FLT into DNA. Other ^{18}F-labeled analogs of thymidine have been developed including [^{18}F]FMAU that are substituted with F-18 at the 2′-position and can be incorporated into DNA. However, it is not clear that radiolabeled nucleosides that are incorporated into DNA provide more accurate assessment of proliferation or superior image quality than non-incorporated nucleosides. Examples of radiolabeled nucleosides and nucleoside ana logs are shown in Fig. 3.8.

Thymidine and its analogs are transported across cell membranes by facilitated transport by the type 1 equilibrative nucleoside transporters (ENT1) followed by phosphorylated by thymidine kinases [114, 115]. Both thymidine and [^{18}F]FLT are substrates for phosphorylation by cytosolic thymidine kinase 1. In the case of [^{18}F]FLT, phosphorylation is the rate-limiting step determining cellular retention under most circumstances [116]. In contrast, incorporation of [^{11}C]thymidine triphosphate into DNA is the rate-limiting step for retention [117]. In some tissues, dephosphorylation of [^{18}F]FLT occurs which can lead to [^{18}F]FLT leaving the cell over time [118, 119].

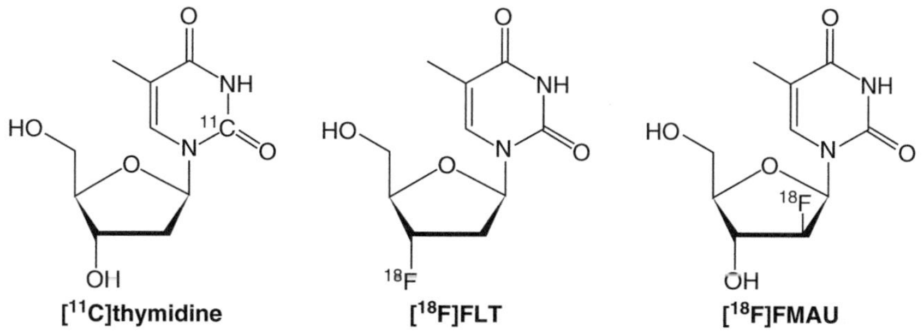

[^{11}C]thymidine [^{18}F]FLT [^{18}F]FMAU

Fig. 3.8 Structures of selected nucleoside-based PET tracers for proliferation imaging

3.4.1 Oncologic Imaging

The primary use of [^{18}F]FLT-PET has been for cancer imaging, particularly for assessing response to therapy [120–123]. Because effective anticancer therapies stop or slow cancer cell proliferation, PET tracers that accurately measure cellular proliferation in vivo are expected to be effective for a wide range of cancers and therapeutics. The use of nucleoside analogs such as [^{18}F]FLT may be particularly valuable early in the course of therapy and may be useful as a surrogate endpoint in early-phase clinical trials of experimental therapeutics. Although [^{18}F]FLT is not currently used for routine clinical imaging, there is the potential to use [^{18}F]FLT-PET to stop futile treatment regimens and switch to alternative therapies earlier than is possible with [^{18}F]FDG-PET and/or anatomic imaging alone. Studies indicate that [^{18}F]FLT has lower uptake in the setting of inflammation than [^{18}F]FDG which is an advantage when treatments such as chemotherapy, radiation, and immunotherapies often induce inflammatory responses in tumors [124–126]. An important limitation that has been observed with [^{18}F]FLT and other nucleoside-based agents is relatively low sensitivity for detecting metastases [127–129], suggesting that [^{18}F]FLT-PET cannot replace staging using [^{18}F]FDG-PET, CT, and/or MRI.

A number of relatively small imaging trials have been performed using [^{18}F]FLT-PET in a range of cancer types including lymphoma, non-small cell lung cancer (NSCLC), squamous cell head and neck cancer, breast cancer, acute myelogenous leukemia, gastrointestinal malignancies, and glioblastoma [123]. The majority of these studies demonstrate that [^{18}F]FLT-PET can serve as an early predictor of response to therapy, and decreases in [^{18}F]FLT uptake in tumors are correlated with progression-free and disease-free survival. Larger prospective trials demonstrating that [^{18}F]FLT-PET can provide earlier and/or more accurate assessment of response to therapy than other imaging techniques that improves patient management are needed.

An important consideration when using [^{18}F]FLT-PET to monitor response to therapy is the potential for alterations in [^{18}F]FLT metabolism in the liver due to chemotherapeutic agents, and some investigators have advocated blood sampling to avoid incorrectly interpreting [^{18}F]FLT-PET studies due to metabolic changes rather than changes in tumor proliferation [122]. Additionally, simple SUV measurements may not be optimal for assessing response using [^{18}F]FLT [119, 122]. Although [^{18}F]FLT-PET has shown promising results for measuring proliferation and evaluating response to therapy in glioma [130–134], the poor brain availability of [^{18}F]FLT prevents assessment of non-enhancing tumor regions [135, 136] . These added elements of complexity make the use and standardization of this tracer in the routine clinical setting more challenging.

3.5 Fatty Acids

Fatty acids are utilized in many cellular processes for energy and production of ATP. When compared to carbohydrates and proteins, fatty acids yield the most ATP on an energy per gram basis and are completely oxidized to CO_2 and water by β-oxidation and the TCA cycle. Additionally, fatty acids are essential components of phospholipids that form the phospholipid bilayers of all cell membranes. Some lipids such as arachidonic acid are involved in signaling pathways. Molecular imaging using fatty acids has taken advantage of both lipogenesis and oxidation to evaluate tumor growth and cellular metabolism, respectively.

Fatty acids can either be incorporated from the extracellular media or obtained from hydrolyzed triglycerides by neutral hydrolases in the cytoplasm or acid hydrolases in an autophagic pathway [137]. Fatty acid synthesis (FAS) is an anabolic process that converts acetyl-CoA to malonyl-CoA via acetyl-CoA carboxylase. Malonyl-CoA is in turn committed to FAS and is involved in the elongation of fatty acids through fatty acid synthase (FASN). Additional modifications of fatty acids are subsequently performed by elongases and desaturases.

Fatty acids are also catabolized by the fatty acid oxidation (FAO; β-oxidation) pathway. Fatty acids provide twice as much ATP as carbohydrates and are the preferred form of storage (e.g., triglycerides in adipose tissue) under conditions of nutrient abundance. Fatty acids are abundant in blood under fasting conditions and under aerobic conditions; the heart primarily utilizes β-oxidation of fatty acids for fuel. The uptake of fatty acids by the heart is dependent on many factors including the concentration of fatty acids in blood, the albumin-to-fatty acid ratio, the fatty acid chain length, and the availability of oxygen, which is required for β-oxidation to proceed [138]. After a carbohydrate load and insulin release, the metabolism of the heart shifts remarkably. Insulin decreases lipolysis from adipocytes, lowering blood fatty acid concentration, and induces translocation of glucose transporters from the cardiac sarcolemma. A decline in fatty acid concentration results in a shift of myocardial metabolism from fatty acids to glucose. Lactate and ketones can also be alternatively used by the heart when they are abundant in blood.

All fatty acids that normally exist in humans are even-chain fatty acids which break down to CO_2. Straight chain FAs labeled at the C-1 position (e.g., [^{11}C]acetate, [1-^{11}C]palmitate) most accurately reflect physiologic oxidation because all of the other carbons in the chain can undergo other metabolic fates [139]. Fatty acids labeled at the omega end of the chain (opposite the carboxylic acid moiety) have a longer residence half-life in the myocardium because β-oxidation proceeds from the carboxylic acid (C-1) end. Ketone body synthesis is another metabolic pathway that uses acetyl-CoA. This involves the formation of acetoacetate mediated by the cooperative action of acetyl-CoA transferase and acetoacetyl-CoA thiolase followed by succinyl coenzyme A/acetoacetate coenzyme transferase, an initiator of ketone body utilization in tumor cells [140].

Acetate is catabolized via the TCA cycle to produce CO_2 and water. [^{11}C]Acetate, a 2-carbon fatty acid labeled in the C-1 position, is esterified and enters the TCA cycle where the C-1 (labeled) carbon leaves as $^{11}CO_2$. Acetate does not easily cross the blood-brain barrier and is not extracted from the blood stream as a substrate for neuronal energy metabolism. [^{11}C]Acetate is rapidly cleared from circulation resulting in high initial retention in organs with high basal metabolism, as expected in the brain. [^{18}F]Fluoroacetate demonstrated a much longer half-life in blood and no evidence of specific retention [141]. The structures of [^{11}C]acetate and [^{18}F]fluoroacetate are shown in Fig. 3.9.

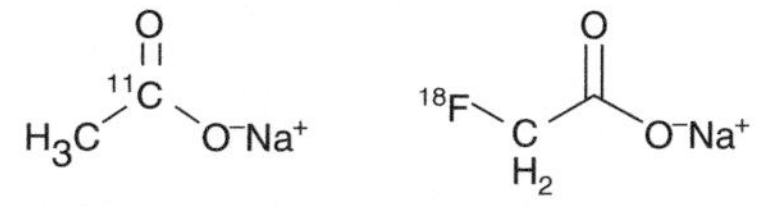

[^{11}C]acetate **[^{18}F]fluoroacetate**

Fig. 3.9 Structures of [^{11}C]acetate and [^{18}F]fluoroacetate

3.5.1 Oncologic Imaging

Fatty acids are major substrates for catabolic and anabolic processes with cancer cells often demonstrating high levels of lipid accumulation [142], fatty acid oxidation [143], and de novo fatty acid synthesis [144] and have been identified as a potential therapeutic target in multiple cancers [145, 146]. Fatty acids labeled with both C-11 and F-18 have been developed as PET traces for studying fatty acid synthesis and β-oxidation [147]. Cancer cells often demonstrate a lipogenic phenotype requiring that fatty acids be synthesized de novo to maintain cell proliferation and viability [148] and survival [149].

[^{11}C]Acetate has been shown to act as a marker of fatty acid synthesis [150–152]. The majority of studies analyzing the efficacy of [^{11}C]acetate in oncologic imaging have focused on the detection of prostate cancer [153], with several additional cancers demonstrating high tumor-to-background uptake including hepatocellular carcinoma, thymomas, renal cancers, brain tumors, and lung malignancies [154, 155]. FASN enzymes are upregulated in virtually all prostate cancers [156], and several studies have confirmed that accumulation of [^{11}C]acetate in prostate cancer cells is associated with upregulation of enzymes involved in lipogenesis [151,

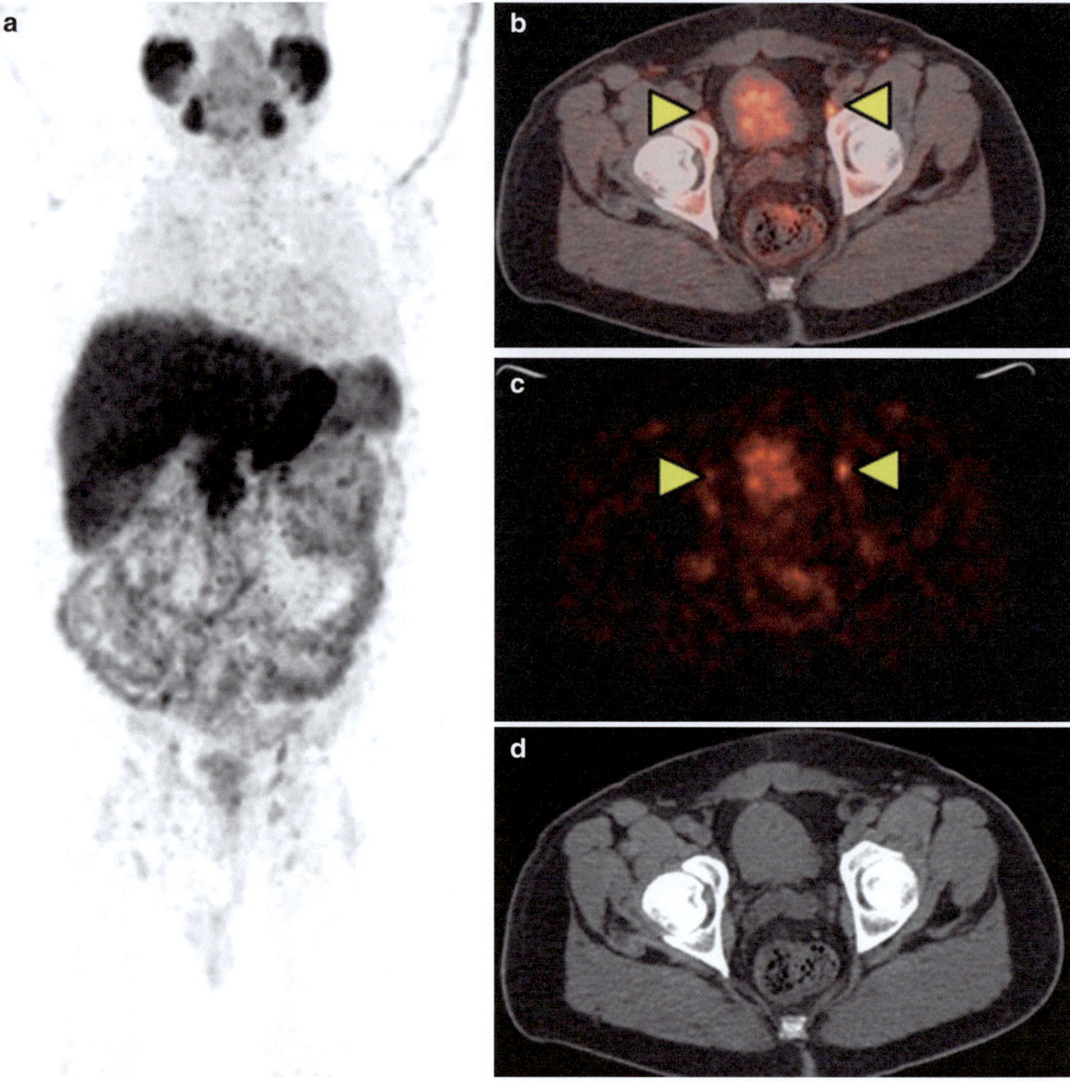

Fig. 3.10 [11C]Acetate-PET/CT in a man with recently diagnosed prostate cancer involving the left lobe of the prostate. A whole-body maximum intensity projection (MIP) image (**a**) and fused PET/CT (**b**) and PET (**c**) images demonstrate increased activity in bilateral external iliac lymph nodes, consistent with nodal metastases. The corresponding non-contrast CT image (**d**) shows that the lymph nodes are not pathologically enlarged and thus would not be identified as metastases by CT alone

157]. Accumulation of [11C]acetate is highly correlated with FASN expression, and the FASN inhibitor orlistat, an antiobesity drug, is shown to have anticancer activity in relation to [11C] acetate uptake [158]. Recently, [11C]acetate SUV_{max} accurately identified patients at increased risk and was directly and linearly correlated with survival time [159]. [11C]Acetate-PET imaging has also been shown to be effective in determining response to therapy in men with bone metastatic prostate cancer before and after androgen deprivation therapy, or after first-line chemotherapy [160]. An example of a [11C]acetate-PET/CT study in prostate cancer is shown in Fig. 3.10.

A major problem with using [11C]acetate as a marker of FASN activity (tumorigenesis) is that both oxidative and fatty acid synthesis pathways compete for [^{11}C]acetate, and the short half-life of carbon-11 may possibly be too short to actually detect the synthetic component. Several fluorinated acetate analogs have been synthesized to take advantage of the longer half-life of fluorine-18 to attempt to produce PET tracers capable of measuring FASN activity. [^{18}F]Fluoroacetate has been synthesized and evaluated as a tracer for fatty acid synthesis, but in vivo studies have demonstrated that it is not a substrate for the fatty acid synthesis pathway. [^{18}F]Fluoroacetate is transported through cell membranes by either monocarboxylate transporters and/or by diffusion and is subsequently converted to fluoroacetyl-CoA by the enzyme acetyl-CoA synthases 1 (ACS1; cytoplasmic) and 2 (ACS2; mitochondrial) [161, 162]. Unlike acetate, fluoroacetyl-CoA is not an efficient substrate for FASN, and therefore the fluoroacetyl moiety is not incorporated into de novo synthesized fatty acids. Additionally, while citrate can be utilized by the ATP citrate lyase, which is one of the key lipogenic enzymes that is overexpress in many cancer cells for fatty acid synthesis, fluorocitrate cannot be utilized by ATP citrate lyase because it is irreversibly bound to aconitase. Therefore, [^{18}F]fluorocitrate is accumulated in cells until it degrades radiochemically. However, it is conceivable that fluoroacetate in tracer dosages may be converted in part to fluoroacetoacetate, which would reflect de novo ketone synthetic activity in cancer cells which utilize ketone bodies for energy production [163], and may explain the increased uptake and accumulation of [^{18}F]fluoroacetate in prostate cancer [164].

3.5.2 Cardiac Imaging

As discussed in the carbohydrate section of this chapter, the heart does not maintain a substantial energy reserve and thus requires nutrients from the blood for function and survival. Under ischemic conditions, anaerobic glycolysis is the primary energy source for myocytes. The response of the heart to reperfusion is complex, likely reflecting the duration and severity of ischemia and the timing and adequacy of reperfusion, as well as the amount of collateral blood flow. Postischemic studies have shown recovery of fatty acid metabolism directly associated with recovery of perfusion [165]. Some studies have used fatty acid imaging to evaluate reperfusion and the benefit of novel anti-ischemic treatment approaches [166]. Conversely, in both nonischemic and ischemic heart failure, there are variable changes in myocardial fatty acid uptake. The majority of studies demonstrate increased fatty acid uptake, whether the underlying problem is ischemia [167], nonischemic cardiomyopathy [168], or diabetic cardiomyopathy. It is not known whether these various causes of heart failure produce altered fatty acid utilization via the same mechanism and whether increased fatty acid transport relates to the impairment of function [169].

In the heart, the TCA acid cycle is closely coupled to oxidative phosphorylation, and several studies have demonstrated that the efflux of labeled CO_2 after the administration of [^{11}C]acetate reflects myocardial oxygen consumption [170, 171]. Conversely, myocardial [^{18}F]fluoroacetate retention does not relate to blood flow or oxidative metabolism. These findings are consistent with the finding that [^{18}F]fluoroacetate is not a preferred substrate for monocarboxylate transporters and that minimal conversion of [^{18}F]fluoroacetate to [^{18}F]acetyl-CoA occurs. Thus, [^{18}F]fluoroacetate is not useful as a tracer of mitochondrial ACS2 activity. Additionally, unlike acetate, fluoroacetate stops the TCA cycle from completion after the formation of fluorocitrate [172, 173]. Fluorocitrate acts as an irreversible inhibitor of aconitase [174], which is the catalytic enzyme for the conversion of citrate to *cis*-cistrate, a necessary intermediate for the successful completion of the TCA cycle. Comparison of [^{11}C]acetate to [^{18}F]fluoroacetate found little similarity in the distribution and retention of the two radiotracers in clinical trials.

3.5.3 Long-Chain Fatty Acid Cardiac Imaging

The 16-carbon chain fatty acid [1-^{11}C]palmitate has been studied extensively in cardiovascular PET research studies to monitor changes in metabolism in response to physiologic and pathologic conditions [175, 176]. Long-chain fatty acids are rapidly and avidly extracted by the heart, but uptake and subsequent metabolism are complex. Compartmental modeling of myocardial time-activity curves allows for estimation of [^{11}C]palmitate uptake, esterification, and oxidation [177]. Studies have shown that under certain circumstances, washout of [^{11}C]palmitate from the myocardium correlated with myocardial oxygen consumption [178], allowed delineation of zones of myocardial infarction [179], and was able to characterize the efficacy of reperfusion strategies [180]. However, under myocardial ischemia conditions, back-diffusion of unoxidized [^{11}C]palmitate is confounded with metabolic clearance of β-oxidized [^{11}C]palmitate. For quantitative imaging of fatty acid metabolism, most studies are done in the fasting state to optimize tracer uptake, because plasma fatty acid levels are high. Glucose loading markedly affects the residence time of palmitate in the heart (prolonging it) because long-chain fatty acids are shunted into triglycerides and phospholipids with glucose loading.

^{18}F-labeled long-chain fatty acid (LCFA) analogs were developed to take advantage of the longer half-life of F-18. The odd-chain length LCFA analog, 17-[^{18}F]fluoroheptadecanoic acid, was found to have a rapid uptake in the heart similar to [^{11}C]palmitate with biphasic clearance from the myocardium. The even-chain LCFA analog, 16-[^{18}F]fluorohexadecanoic acid (FHDA), also showed similar biphasic clearance from the heart, but with different clearance rates and different labeled metabolites in the heart. For FHDA, the primary putative metabolite is 2-[^{18}F]fluoroacetyl-CoA, which undergoes a variety of metabolic transformations, including defluorination. The complex metabolic handling of the ^{18}F-labeled LCFA analogs, in addition to their in vivo defluorination, complicates the development of quantitative modeling strategies.

To simplify the myocardial kinetics of radiolabel LCFAs, structural modifications have been investigated to impede oxidation or esterification. These structural modifications include branched chain analogs [181–183], heteroatom substitution [184–186], and cyclopropyl group incorporation [187]. While a few of these compounds have been evaluated in small clinical studies [169], none are currently in routine clinical use. Structures of representative LCFA PET tracers are show in Fig. 3.11.

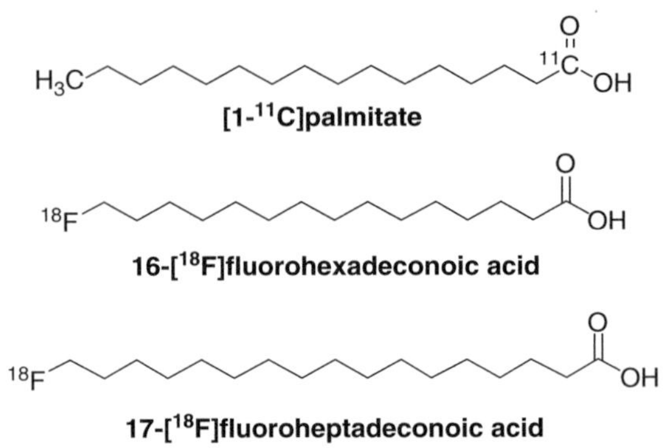

Fig. 3.11 Structures of selected long-chain fatty acids (LCFAs) used for PET imaging

3.6 Membrane Synthesis

Choline is a quaternary ammonium organic base that is an essential component of phospholipids and cell membranes and is involved in three major metabolic pathways: (A) phosphorylation, (B) oxidation, and (C) acetylation [188]. The phosphorylation pathway in mammalian cells starts with choline and results in the synthesis and incorporation of phosphatidylcholine (PC) into cell membranes via the Kennedy pathway. Choline kinase (CK) catalyzes choline phosphorylation to produce phosphocholine, which acts as an intracellular storage pool of choline and is the rate-limiting step in the Kennedy pathway. Phosphocholine is modified to diphosphate-choline (CDP-choline) by the enzyme cytidylyltransferase and then to other intermediates before being incorporated into cell membrane phospholipids as phosphatidylcholine [189]. Malignant transformation is associated with enhanced choline transport and utilization, characterized by increased choline kinase α (CHKα) expression, which leads to a phenotype characterized by increased radiolabeled choline uptake [190, 191].

Fig. 3.12 Structure of [^{11}C]choline and selected fluorinated analogs

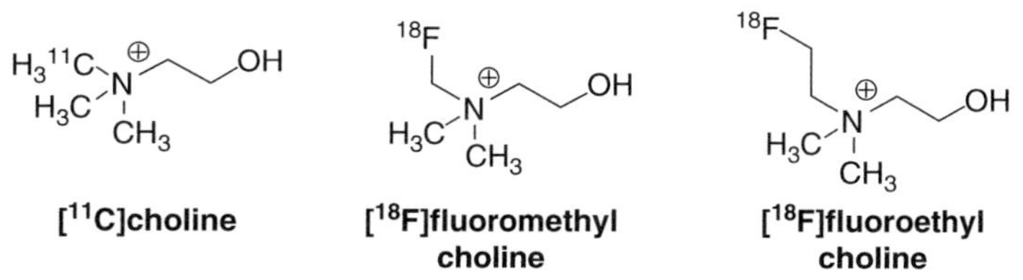

The choline oxidation pathway mainly occurs in the liver and kidneys where the choline oxidase system (choline dehydrogenase and betaine aldehyde dehydrogenase) catalyzes the formation of betaine. Betaine can act either as an organic intracellular osmolyte regulator or can be used as a methyl group donor to produce methionine from homocysteine [192]. [^{11}C]Choline and the fluoro-analogs are readily oxidized to betaines by choline oxidase, mainly in the kidney and liver, with metabolites detectable in plasma soon after injection of the radiotracer [193, 194]. The acetylation pathway involves choline acetyltransferase (ChAT) catalyzing the reaction of acetyl coenzyme A with choline to produce acetylcholine which acts as a neurotransmitter. The structure of choline and selected ^{18}F-labeled analogs are shown in Fig. 3.12.

3.6.1 Oncologic Imaging

Choline metabolism has been shown to be directly related to proliferation and oncogenic signaling [195]. Choline is taken up into cells via specific choline-transporting transmembrane systems, and total choline-containing phospholipid metabolite levels have been shown to increase as cells progress from normal to immortalized tumor cells [196]. Several studies have shown that alteration of lipid metabolism occurs in breast [196], colon [197], ovarian [198], and prostate cancers [199]. An altered lipogenic phenotype allows cancer cells to synthesize new membranes [200], store energy, and generate modules involved in cell signaling regulation and invasion [201]. Additionally, upregulation and increased activity of lipogenic enzymes (including fatty acid synthase and choline kinase) have specifically been shown to occur throughout the various stages of prostate cancer and correlate with poor prognosis and survival [199].

Cell membrane fatty acid composition differs between normal and malignant cells [202]. The relative amount of choline phospholipids, which are predominately distributed in the membrane outer leaflets, is reduced in all malignant tumor membranes [191, 203]. Malignant cells are found to have an upregulation of choline kinase, which leads to an upregulation of phosphatidylcholine that is then incorporated into and trapped in tumor cell membranes [204]. However, several studies have also demonstrated that hypoxia alters the choline uptake profile in malignancies with reduced choline phosphorylation observed in hypoxic cancer cells [205, 206]. Hypoxia-inducible factor (HIF)-1α regulates the glycolytic activity by promoting the expression of both glucose transporters and glycolytic enzymes, leading to decreased oxidative phosphorylation and increased lactate production via lactate dehydrogenase. This effect leads to an overall increase in FDG uptake and decreased [^{11}C]choline uptake in hypoxic prostate cancer cells.

PET radiopharmaceuticals targeting choline metabolism and uptake have utilized [^{11}C]choline or ^{18}F-labeled choline analogs. The choline analogs, [^{18}F]fluoromethylcholine and [^{18}F]fluoroethylcholine, have been used extensively for imaging several malignancies but primarily for detection of prostate cancer [207, 208]. The mechanism of choline accumulation in tumors is not completely understood and may reflect either the activity of the de novo phosphatidylcholine synthesis pathway or oxidative metabolism via the betaine-sarcosine-glycine pathway which was recently demonstrated to be highly active in prostate cancer [189, 209]. In 2012, the US Food and Drug Administration announced approval of [^{11}C]choline for clinical PET imaging in recurrent prostate cancer (Fig. 3.13).

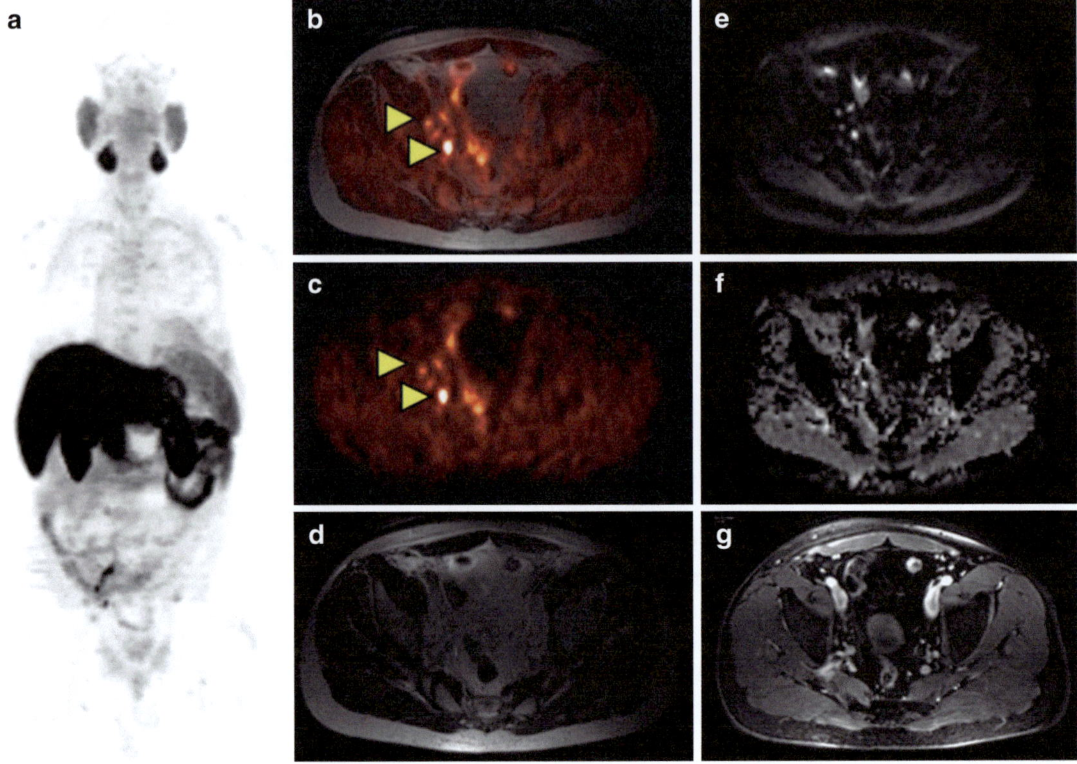

Fig. 3.13 [11C]choline-PET/MR in a man with recurrent prostate cancer based on rising serum prostate-specific antigen (PSA) after prostatectomy. Right iliac chain lymph nodes with increased activity are seen on the maximum intensity projection (MIP) image (**a**) and on the axial fused PET/MRI (**b**) and PET only (**c**) images as indicated with *yellow arrow heads*. The nodes are also seen on the axial T2-weighted (**d**), diffusion-weighted (**e**), apparent diffusion coefficient, (**f**) and post-contrast fat saturation T1-weighted images (**g**)

While [11C]choline requires an on-site cyclotron due to the short half-life of carbon-11, this PET tracer has benefits such as rapid blood clearance (<5 min), rapid uptake within prostate tissue (3–5 min), and substantially less urinary elimination when compared to both [18F]FDG and fluorinated choline analogs [205]. [11C]Choline demonstrates the highest physiological tissue uptake in the renal cortex, followed by the liver and pancreas, with variable intestinal uptake. While there is early vascular uptake, there is low-to-absent physiological uptake in the cerebral cortex. Fluorinated choline analogs are excreted via the urinary system with a high accumulation in the urinary bladder, which is not ideal for assessment of the pelvic region for prostate nodal metastases. However, the longer half-life of fluorinated choline analogs allows for delayed acquisition which may provide a high tumor-to-background ratio.

The differentiation between benign prostatic hyperplasia (BPH), prostatitis, and high-grade intraepithelial neoplasia is not always possible in primary staging of prostate cancer using choline-PET/CT as these conditions also demonstrate high choline uptake [210–212]. Additionally, there is decreased choline uptake in patients in response to androgen deprivation therapy [213, 214] with reported significant differences between [11C]choline and [18F]fluorocholine imaging in patients undergoing androgen deprivation therapy [215]. Choline uptake in prostate nodal metastases has been shown to decrease in response to chemotherapy and radiotherapy [216]. In addition to prostate cancer, radiolabeled choline has been utilized in other tumor models including head and neck

[217, 218] and breast cancers [219] which have also shown decreased choline uptake in response to chemotherapy and radiotherapy.

3.7 Hypoxia

Hypoxia is a common feature of malignant tumors resulting from a functional disturbance in microcirculation and increased oxygen consumption. Tumor hypoxia is heterogeneous in time and space and not only accounts for tissue necrosis, but it also has a strong impact on tumor biology with negative prognostic outcomes. Hypoxia causes resistance to chemotherapy [220] (i.e., decreased tumor concentration of the chemotherapeutic agent, loss of sensitivity to p53-mediated apoptosis, and loss of decreased cell proliferation by metabolic stress) and radiotherapy (i.e., reducing free radical damage by intracellular reactive oxygen species when hypoxic). Beyond its role in neovascularization as a mechanism for tumor adaptation to nutrient and oxygen deprivation, hypoxia has also been shown to lead to an elongated cellular life span and immortality, metabolism changes, and stem cell proliferative deregulation and inflammation [221]. Below a certain critical oxygen concentration threshold, hypoxia-inducible factor 1 (HIF-1) is activated which upregulates a variety of genes controlling metabolic pathways, pH regulation, angiogenesis, metastatic potential, DNA replication, protein synthesis, and treatment resistance [222, 223].

Hypoxia also regulates the proliferation and differentiation of different types of stem-like cancer cells [224]. Tumors have been shown to have subpopulations of cells with characteristics similar to nonmalignant stem cells called "cancer stem cells" [225, 226]. The cancer stem cell model proposes that this cancer cell population is ultimately responsible for tumor initiation, progression, and recurrence. To evaluate for a hypoxic microenvironment, a commercially available oxygen electrode permits oxygen partial pressure levels (pO2) in human tumors. This method is inherently limited due to its invasive nature and is only pertinent for easily accessible tumors of sufficient size. An additional invasive method is histologic cytological coloration of the excised tumor with nitroimidazole compounds (i.e., pimonidazole or EF5) or immunohistochemical analysis of hypoxia marker proteins (i.e., HIF-1α or carbonic anhydrase IV).

Several molecular imaging agents have been evaluated as a means to noninvasively assess for hypoxia in the tumor microenvironment, and the structures of several of these tracers are shown in Fig. 3.14. An ideal hypoxia imaging agent should have high membrane permeability for easy access to intracellular mitochondria and a low redox potential to allow stability in

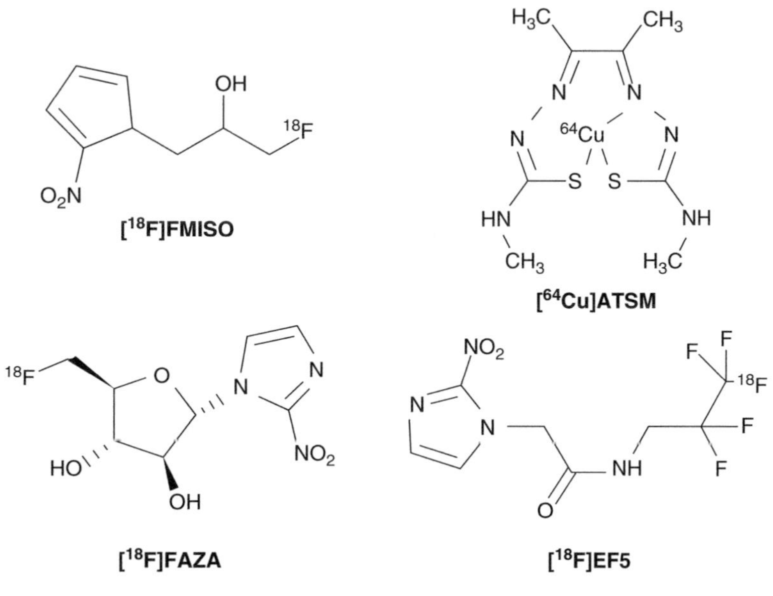

Fig. 3.14 Structure of selected PET tracers for hypoxia imaging

normoxic conditions. Copper (Cu)-diacetyl-bis(*N*4-methylthiosemicarbazone) (Cu-ATSM) is a hypoxic marker that is selectively retained in hypoxic tissues [227–229]. It is believed that Cu-ATSM undergoes bioreductive trapping under hypoxic conditions. After cellular entry, Cu(II)-ATSM in reduced to an unstable Cu(I)-ATSM species, which when protonated at the *N*3 and *N*6 positions, will lead to the complex dissociating and subsequent irreversible trapping of Cu(I) within the cellular copper metabolic processes [230]. Cellular trapping of the copper is nondependent on oxygen, pH, and NADH which is an essential cofactor [231]. In vitro studies found that the Cu-ATSM lipophilic molecule may diffuse into cells by combined passive and facilitated (protein-carrier-mediated) mechanisms with no evidence to support a role for copper-transporter 1 (Ctr1) facilitated uptake [232]. The reduced Cu(I)-ATSM is charged and less lipophilic and is therefore retained in the cell. In a normoxic cell, Cu(I)-ATSM can be reoxidized and diffuse out of the cell [233]. There is controversy in the field regarding the nature of Cu-ATSM retention and how well it correlates with tissue hypoxia versus accumulation due to blood flow and copper transport [234].

^{64}Cu-ATSM hypoxia imaging has been explored in various in vitro and in vivo preclinical models, with variable in vivo hypoxia mapping (likely related to cell lineage and acquisition time after injection). This heterogeneity of ^{64}Cu-ATSM uptake has led to a complicated interpretation of tumor hypoxia mapping with a need to further clarify whether radiotracer distribution is more defined by perfusion (early time) or $_{p}O_2$ levels (late time). Only a few clinical studies have been performed with Cu-ATSM; however, they have shown a predictive response to traditional cancer therapies in patients with rectal [235], lung [236], and uterine cervical cancer [237, 238] where higher Cu-ATSM uptake portended a worse prognosis.

Nitroimidazole compounds are used for imaging oxygen-deprived hypoxic cells, based on the intracellular accumulation of radicals formed after the reductive reaction by nitroreductases. Under hypoxic conditions, nitroimidazole compounds are reduced by intracellular nitroreductases at low oxygen levels, < 10 mmHg, with the metabolites subsequently serving as electron acceptors. The reduced metabolites form covalent bonds with macromolecules and become biochemically trapped in the hypoxic cells [239]. The metabolism of nitroimidazoles relies on active electron transport enzymes and functional nitroreductase enzymes; thus, trapping does not occur in necrotic tissues. In normoxic tissues, the metabolites are reoxidized and cleared from cells by back-diffusion. Hypoxic tissues can thus be delineated as an area of high tracer uptake after allowing a sufficient period of time for the non-trapped parent radiotracer to be excreted from the cells [240].

[^{18}F]Fluoromisonidazole (FMISO) is a derivative of nitroimidazole and is the most studied nitroimidazole for hypoxia imaging [241]. [^{18}F]FMISO enters cells by passive diffusion where it is metabolized and trapped in hypoxic cells. Time activity curves show that [^{18}F]FMISO achieves equilibrium within plasma within 30 min, with selective retention of [^{18}F]FMISO observed in hypoxic tissue by 1 h after injection and retention observed starting around 2.5 h [239]. The long uptake time and low tumor-to-background ratios are the main drawbacks of [^{18}F]FMISO imaging which may limit the applicability of the tracer in clinical practice. Several studies correlating direct oxygen measurements with [^{18}F]FMISO have been performed, demonstrating that [^{18}F]FMISO retention requires a hypoxic level of <10 mm Hg [242]. The need for severe hypoxia for [^{18}F]FMISO retention will likely limit the use of this tracer for evaluating nonneoplastic hypoxic conditions where milder hypoxia is typically present. Hypoxic imaging with [^{18}F]FMISO has been evaluated in many solid tumors including glioma [243], head and neck cancer [244], lung cancer [245], breast cancer [246], colorectal cancer [247], and renal cell carcinoma [248] with the majority confirming [^{18}F]FMISO demonstrates selective uptake in hypoxic tumors. Studies comparing [^{18}F]FMISO with [^{18}F]FDG in head and neck cancers found good correlation between [^{18}F]FMISO and pO_2, but no correlation between pO_2 measurements and FDG uptake [249]. Conversely however, in a study of sarcomas, no correlation was found between [^{18}F]FMISO and pO_2 [250].

The slow uptake of [^{18}F]FMISO in target tissue and slow clearance of unbound [^{18}F]FMISO from non-hypoxic areas stimulated the development of other tracers with improved pharmacokinetics, such as [^{18}F]fluoroazomycin arabinoside ([^{18}F]FAZA). Compared to [^{18}F]FMISO, the biodistribution of [^{18}F]FAZA is improved through the addition of a sugar moiety, making it less lipophilic [251]. Several clinical and preclinical studies have demonstrated overall superior pharmacokinetics and higher contrast with nontarget tissues when compared to [^{18}F]FMISO [252, 253]. 2-Nitroimidazol-[^{18}F]pentafluoropropyl acetamide ([^{18}F]EF5) and 2-nitroimidazol-[^{18}F]trifluoropropyl acetamide ([^{18}F]EF3) are examples of another class of hypoxia-sensitive radiopharmaceuticals which are more lipophilic than [^{18}F]FMISO and have possible advantages over [^{18}F]FMISO in clinical trials [254, 255].

3.8 Summary

A broad range of small molecule PET tracers have been developed and applied to the metabolic imaging of physiologic and disease processes. PET-based approaches take advantage of the tracer principle and the diversity of radiosynthetic methods for incorporating carbon-11 and fluorine-18 into small molecules. The well-established preclinical, translational, and clinical applications of PET imaging will continue to play key roles in metabolic imaging. Important limitations of PET include the potential formation of radiolabeled metabolites, exposure to ionizing radiation, and the need for blood sampling and modeling for certain applications. Other imaging modalities including MRI and optical techniques can complement PET for metabolic imaging and are discussed in other chapters.

References

1. Ter-Pogossian MM. The origins of positron emission tomography. Semin Nucl Med. 1992;22(3):140–9.
2. Welch MJ, Redvanly CS. Handbook of radiopharmaceuticals: radiochemistry and applications, vol. xiv. Chichester, England: Wiley; 2003. p. 848.
3. Vaquero JJ, Kinahan P. Positron emission tomography: current challenges and opportunities for technological advances in clinical and preclinical imaging systems. Annu Rev Biomed Eng. 2015;17:385–414.
4. Cherry SR, Sorenson JA, Phelps ME. Physics in nuclear medicine. 4th ed. Philadelphia: Elsevier/Saunders; 2012. p. 523.
5. Nakamoto Y, Zasadny KR, Minn H, Wahl RL. Reproducibility of common semi-quantitative parameters for evaluating lung cancer glucose metabolism with positron emission tomography using 2-deoxy-2-[^{18}F]fluoro-D-glucose. Mol Imaging Biol. 2002;4(2):171–8.
6. Devriese J, Beels L, Maes A, Van De Wiele C, Gheysens O, Pottel H. Review of clinically accessible methods to determine lean body mass for normalization of standardized uptake values. Q J Nucl Med Mol Imaging. 2016;60(1):1–11.
7. Watabe H, Ikoma Y, Kimura Y, Naganawa M, Shidahara M. PET kinetic analysis—compartmental model. Ann Nucl Med. 2006;20(9):583–8.
8. Schmidt KC, Turkheimer FE. Kinetic modeling in positron emission tomography. Q J Nucl Med. 2002;46(1):70–85.
9. Price JC. Principles of tracer kinetic analysis. Neuroimaging Clin N Am. 2003;13(4):689–704.
10. Tonietto M, Rizzo G, Veronese M, Fujita M, Zoghbi SS, Zanotti-Fregonara P, et al. Plasma radiometabolite correction in dynamic PET studies: insights on the available modeling approaches. J Cereb Blood Flow Metab. 2016;36(2):326–39.
11. Hricak H, Brenner DJ, Adelstein SJ, Frush DP, Hall EJ, Howell RW, et al. Managing radiation use in medical imaging: a multifaceted challenge. Radiology. 2011;258(3):889–905.
12. Devlin TM. Textbook of biochemistry: with clinical correlations. 7th ed. Hoboken, NJ: Wiley; 2011. p. 1204.
13. Smith TA. The rate-limiting step for tumor [^{18}F]fluoro-2-deoxy-D-glucose (FDG) incorporation. Nucl Med Biol. 2001;28(1):1–4.
14. Morani F, Phadngam S, Follo C, Titone R, Aimaretti G, Galetto A, et al. PTEN regulates plasma membrane expression of glucose transporter 1 and glucose uptake in thyroid cancer cells. J Mol Endocrinol. 2014;53(2):247–58.
15. Gwak H, Haegeman G, Tsang BK, Song YS. Cancer-specific interruption of glucose metabolism by resveratrol is mediated through inhibition of Akt/GLUT1 axis in ovarian cancer cells. Mol Carcinog. 2015;54(12):1529–40.
16. Alvarez JV, Belka GK, Pan TC, Chen CC, Blankemeyer E, Alavi A, et al. Oncogene pathway activation in mammary tumors dictates FDG-PET uptake. Cancer Res. 2014;74(24):7583–98.
17. Patlak CS, Blasberg RG, Fenstermacher JD. Graphical evaluation of blood-to-brain transfer constants from multiple-time uptake data. J Cereb Blood Flow Metab. 1983;3(1):1–7.
18. Barrios-Lopez B, Bergstrom K. Radiolabeled sugars used for PET and SPECT imaging: mini-review. Curr Radiopharm. 2015.

19. Mun J. Radiofluorinated carbohydrates for positron emission tomography. Curr Top Med Chem. 2013;13(8):944–50.
20. Ehrin E, Stone-Elander S, Nilsson JL, Bergstrom M, Blomqvist G, Brismar T, et al. C-11-labeled glucose and its utilization in positron-emission tomography. J Nucl Med. 1983;24(4):326–31.
21. Lifton JF, Welch MJ. Preparation of glucose labeled with 20-minute half-lived carbon-11. Radiat Res. 1971;45(1):35–40.
22. Shiue C-Y, Wolf AP. The syntheses of 1-[^{11}C]-D-glucose and related compounds for the measurement of brain glucose metabolism. J Label Compd Radiopharm. 1985;22(2):171–82.
23. Sokoloff L, Reivich M, Kennedy C, Des Rosiers MH, Patlak CS, Pettigrew KD, et al. The [^{14}C] deoxyglucose method for the measurement of local cerebral glucose utilization: theory, procedure, and normal values in the conscious and anesthetized albino rat. J Neurochem. 1977;28(5):897–916.
24. Krohn KA, Mankoff DA, Muzi M, Link JM, Spence AM. True tracers: comparing FDG with glucose and FLT with thymidine. Nucl Med Biol. 2005;32(7):663–71.
25. Graham MM, Muzi M, Spence AM, O'Sullivan F, Lewellen TK, Link JM, et al. The FDG lumped constant in normal human brain. J Nucl Med. 2002;43(9):1157–66.
26. Spence AM, Muzi M, Graham MM, O'Sullivan F, Krohn KA, Link JM, et al. Glucose metabolism in human malignant gliomas measured quantitatively with PET, 1-[C-11]glucose and FDG: analysis of the FDG lumped constant. J Nucl Med. 1998;39(3):440–8.
27. Liberti MV, Locasale JW. The Warburg effect: how does it benefit cancer cells? Trends Biochem Sci. 2016;41(3):211–8.
28. Potter M, Newport E, Morten KJ. The Warburg effect: 80 years on. Biochem Soc Trans. 2016;44(5):1499–505.
29. Vander Heiden MG, Cantley LC, Thompson CB. Understanding the Warburg effect: the metabolic requirements of cell proliferation. Science. 2009;324(5930):1029–33.
30. Grigsby PW, Siegel BA, Dehdashti F, Rader J, Zoberi I. Posttherapy [^{18}F] fluorodeoxyglucose positron emission tomography in carcinoma of the cervix: response and outcome. J Clin Oncol. 2004;22(11):2167–71.
31. Wahl RL, Jacene H, Kasamon Y, Lodge MA. From RECIST to PERCIST: evolving considerations for PET response criteria in solid tumors. J Nucl Med. 2009;50(Suppl 1):122S–50S.
32. Goudarzi B, Jacene HA, Wahl RL. Measuring the "unmeasurable": assessment of bone marrow response to therapy using FDG-PET in patients with lymphoma. Acad Radiol. 2010;17(9):1175–85.
33. Liu J, Dong M, Sun X, Li W, Xing L, Yu J. Prognostic value of ^{18}F-FDG PET/CT in surgical non-small cell lung cancer: a meta-analysis. PLoS One. 2016;11(1):e0146195.
34. Kubo T, Furuta T, Johan MP, Ochi M. Prognostic significance of ^{18}F-FDG PET at diagnosis in patients with soft tissue sarcoma and bone sarcoma; systematic review and meta-analysis. Eur J Cancer. 2016;58:104–11.
35. Padma MV, Said S, Jacobs M, Hwang DR, Dunigan K, Satter M, et al. Prediction of pathology and survival by FDG PET in gliomas. J Neuro-Oncol. 2003;64(3):227–37.
36. Yoon JH, Kim JH, Kang WJ, Sohn CH, Choi SH, Yun TJ, et al. Grading of cerebral glioma with multiparametric MR imaging and ^{18}F-FDG-PET: concordance and accuracy. Eur Radiol. 2014;24(2):380–9.
37. Ulaner GA, Eaton A, Morris PG, Lilienstein J, Jhaveri K, Patil S, et al. Prognostic value of quantitative fluorodeoxyglucose measurements in newly diagnosed metastatic breast cancer. Cancer Med. 2013;2(5):725–33.
38. Park SY, Cho A, WS Y, Lee CY, Lee JG, Kim DJ, et al. Prognostic value of total lesion glycolysis by ^{18}F-FDG PET/CT in surgically resected stage IA non-small cell lung cancer. J Nucl Med. 2015;56(1):45–9.
39. Cheson BD, Fisher RI, Barrington SF, Cavalli F, Schwartz LH, Zucca E, et al. Recommendations for initial evaluation, staging, and response assessment of Hodgkin and non-Hodgkin lymphoma: the Lugano classification. J Clin Oncol. 2014;32(27):3059–68.
40. Fallanca F, Alongi P, Incerti E, Gianolli L, Picchio M, Kayani I, et al. Diagnostic accuracy of FDG PET/CT for clinical evaluation at the end of treatment of HL and NHL: a comparison of the Deauville criteria (DC) and the international harmonization project criteria (IHPC). Eur J Nucl Med Mol Imaging. 2016;
41. Valls L, Badve C, Avril S, Herrmann K, Faulhaber P, O'Donnell J, et al. FDG-PET imaging in hematological malignancies. Blood Rev. 2016;30(4):317–31.
42. Gallamini A, Hutchings M, Ramadan S. Clinical presentation and staging of Hodgkin lymphoma. Semin Hematol. 2016;53(3):148–54.
43. Press OW, Li H, Schoder H, Straus DJ, Moskowitz CH, LeBlanc M, et al. US intergroup trial of response-adapted therapy for stage III to IV Hodgkin lymphoma using early interim fluorodeoxyglucose-positron emission tomography imaging: Southwest Oncology Group S0816. J Clin Oncol. 2016;34(17):2020–7.
44. Nalecz KA. Solute carriers in the blood-brain Barrier: safety in abundance. Neurochem Res. 2016;
45. Paulson OB, Hasselbalch SG, Rostrup E, Knudsen GM, Pelligrino D. Cerebral blood flow response to functional activation. J Cereb Blood Flow Metab. 2010;30(1):2–14.
46. Nenov VI, Halgren E, Smith ME, Badier JM, Ropchan J, Blahd WH, et al. Localized brain metabolic response correlated with potentials evoked by words. Behav Brain Res. 1991;44(1):101–4.

47. Kushner MJ, Rosenquist A, Alavi A, Rosen M, Dann R, Fazekas F, et al. Cerebral metabolism and patterned visual stimulation: a positron emission tomographic study of the human visual cortex. Neurology. 1988;38(1):89–95.
48. Krings T, Schreckenberger M, Rohde V, Spetzger U, Sabri O, Reinges MH, et al. Functional MRI and ^{18}F FDG-positron emission tomography for presurgical planning: comparison with electrical cortical stimulation. Acta Neurochir. 2002;144(9):889–99; discussion 99
49. Foster NL, Heidebrink JL, Clark CM, Jagust WJ, Arnold SE, Barbas NR, et al. FDG-PET improves accuracy in distinguishing frontotemporal dementia and Alzheimer's disease. Brain. 2007;130(Pt 10):2616–35.
50. Panegyres PK, Rogers JM, McCarthy M, Campbell A, Wu JS. Fluorodeoxyglucose-positron emission tomography in the differential diagnosis of early-onset dementia: a prospective, community-based study. BMC Neurol. 2009;9:41.
51. Goffin K, Dedeurwaerdere S, Van Laere K, Van Paesschen W. Neuronuclear assessment of patients with epilepsy. Semin Nucl Med. 2008;38(4):227–39.
52. Gok B, Jallo G, Hayeri R, Wahl R, Aygun N. The evaluation of FDG-PET imaging for epileptogenic focus localization in patients with MRI positive and MRI negative temporal lobe epilepsy. Neuroradiology. 2013;55(5):541–50.
53. Kumar A, Juhasz C, Asano E, Sood S, Muzik O, Chugani HT. Objective detection of epileptic foci by ^{18}F-FDG PET in children undergoing epilepsy surgery. J Nucl Med. 2010;51(12):1901–7.
54. Dankbaar JW, Snijders TJ, Robe PA, Seute T, Eppinga W, Hendrikse J, et al. The use of ^{18}F-FDG PET to differentiate progressive disease from treatment induced necrosis in high grade glioma. J Neuro-Oncol. 2015;125(1):167–75.
55. Nihashi T, Dahabreh IJ, Terasawa T. Diagnostic accuracy of PET for recurrent glioma diagnosis: a meta-analysis. AJNR Am J Neuroradiol. 2013;34(5):944–50. s1-11
56. Southworth R. Hexokinase-mitochondrial interaction in cardiac tissue: implications for cardiac glucose uptake, the ^{18}FDG lumped constant and cardiac protection. J Bioenerg Biomembr. 2009;41(2):187–93.
57. Herrero P, Sharp TL, Dence C, Haraden BM, Gropler RJ. Comparison of 1-^{11}C-glucose and ^{18}F-FDG for quantifying myocardial glucose use with PET. J Nucl Med. 2002;43(11):1530–41.
58. Herrero P, Kisrieva-Ware Z, Dence CS, Patterson B, Coggan AR, Han DH, et al. PET measurements of myocardial glucose metabolism with 1-^{11}C-glucose and kinetic modeling. J Nucl Med. 2007;48(6):955–64.
59. Renstrom B, Rommelfanger S, Stone CK, DeGrado TR, Carlson KJ, Scarbrough E, et al. Comparison of fatty acid tracers FTHA and BMIPP during myocardial ischemia and hypoxia. J Nucl Med. 1998;39(10):1684–9.
60. Schelbert HR. Evaluation of "metabolic fingerprints" of myocardial ischemia. Can J Cardiol. 1986;Suppl A:121A–30A.
61. Uebleis C, Hellweger S, Laubender RP, Becker A, Sohn HY, Lehner S, et al. The amount of dysfunctional but viable myocardium predicts long-term survival in patients with ischemic cardiomyopathy and left ventricular dysfunction. Int J Cardiovasc Imaging. 2013;29(7):1645–53.
62. Wiggers H, Nielsen SS, Holdgaard P, Flo C, Norrelund H, Halbirk M, et al. Adaptation of nonrevascularized human hibernating and chronically stunned myocardium to long-term chronic myocardial ischemia. Am J Cardiol. 2006;98(12):1574–80.
63. Abraham A, Nichol G, Williams KA, Guo A, deKemp RA, Garrard L, et al. ^{18}F-FDG PET imaging of myocardial viability in an experienced center with access to ^{18}F-FDG and integration with clinical management teams: the Ottawa-FIVE substudy of the PARR 2 trial. J Nucl Med. 2010;51(4):567–74.
64. Takx RA, Ishai A, Truong QA, MacNabb MH, Scherrer-Crosbie M, Tawakol A. Supraclavicular Brown adipose tissue ^{18}F-FDG uptake and cardiovascular disease. J Nucl Med. 2016;57(8):1221–5.
65. Ozguven S, Ones T, Yilmaz Y, Turoglu HT, Imeryuz N. The role of active brown adipose tissue in human metabolism. Eur J Nucl Med Mol Imaging. 2016;43(2):355–61.
66. Chen KY, Cypess AM, Laughlin MR, Haft CR, HH H, Bredella MA, et al. Brown adipose reporting criteria in imaging studies (BARCIST 1.0): recommendations for standardized FDG-PET/CT experiments in humans. Cell Metab. 2016;24(2):210–22.
67. Hediger MA, Clemencon B, Burrier RE, Bruford EA. The ABCs of membrane transporters in health and disease (SLC series): introduction. Mol Asp Med. 2013;34(2-3):95–107.
68. Cesar-Razquin A, Snijder B, Frappier-Brinton T, Isserlin R, Gyimesi G, Bai X, et al. A call for systematic research on solute carriers. Cell. 2015;162(3):478–87.
69. Rosario FJ, Kanai Y, Powell TL, Jansson T. Mammalian target of rapamycin signalling modulates amino acid uptake by regulating transporter cell surface abundance in primary human trophoblast cells. J Physiol. 2013;591(Pt 3):609–25.
70. Dodd KM, Tee AR. Leucine and mTORC1: a complex relationship. Am J Physiol Endocrinol Metab. 2012;302(11):E1329–42.
71. Fuchs BC, Bode BP. Amino acid transporters ASCT2 and LAT1 in cancer: partners in crime? Semin Cancer Biol. 2005;15(4):254–66.
72. Huang C, McConathy J. Radiolabeled amino acids for oncologic imaging. J Nucl Med. 2013;54(7):1007–10.
73. McConathy J, Yu W, Jarkas N, Seo W, Schuster DM, Goodman MM. Radiohalogenated nonnatural amino acids as PET and SPECT tumor imaging agents. Med Res Rev. 2012;32(4):868–905.

74. Haining Z, Kawai N, Miyake K, .Okada M, Okubo S, Zhang X, et al. Relation of LAT1/4F2hc expression with pathological grade, proliferation and angiogenesis in human gliomas. BMC Clin Pathol 2012;12:4.
75. Kobayashi K, Ohnishi A, Promsuk J, Shimizu S, Kanai Y, Shiokawa Y, et al. Enhanced tumor growth elicited by L-type amino acid transporter 1 in human malignant glioma cells. Neurosurgery. 2008;62(2):493-503; discussion –4.
76. Nawashiro H, Otani N, Shinomiya N, Fukui S, Ooigawa H, Shima K, et al. L-type amino acid transporter 1 as a potential molecular target in human astrocytic tumors. Int J Cancer. 2006;119(3):484–92.
77. Rapp M, Floeth FW, Felsberg J, Steiger HJ, Sabel M, Langen KJ, et al. Clinical value of *O*-(2-[^{18}F]-fluoroethyl)-L-tyrosine positron emission tomography in patients with low-grade glioma. Neurosurg Focus. 2013;34(2):E3.
78. Galldiks N, Langen KJ, Pope WB. From the clinician's point of view - what is the status quo of positron emission tomography in patients with brain tumors? Neuro-Oncology. 2015;17(11):1434–44.
79. Glaudemans AW, Enting RH, Heesters MA, Dierckx RA, van Rheenen RW, Walenkamp AM, et al. Value of ^{11}C-methionine PET in imaging brain tumours and metastases. Eur J Nucl Med Mol Imaging. 2013;40(4):615–35.
80. Thon N, Kunz M, Lemke L, Jansen NL, Eigenbrod S, Kreth S, et al. Dynamic ^{18}F-FET PET in suspected WHO grade II gliomas defines distinct biological subgroups with different clinical courses. Int J Cancer. 2015;136(9):2132–45.
81. Lohmann P, Herzog H, Rota Kops E, Stoffels G, Judov N, Filss C, et al. Dual-time-point *O*-(2-[^{18}F] fluoroethyl)-L-tyrosine PET for grading of cerebral gliomas. Eur Radiol. 2015;25(10):3017–24.
82. Venneti S, Dunphy MP, Zhang H, Pitter KL, Zanzonico P, Campos C, et al. Glutamine-based PET imaging facilitates enhanced metabolic evaluation of gliomas in vivo. Sci Transl Med. 2015;7(274):274ra17.
83. Mittra ES, Koglin N, Mosci C, Kumar M, Hoehne A, Keu KV, et al. Pilot preclinical and clinical evaluation of (4*S*)-4-(3-[^{18}F]Fluoropropyl)-L-glutamate (^{18}F-FSPG) for PET/CT imaging of intracranial malignancies. PLoS One. 2016;11(2):e0148628.
84. Kondo A, Ishii H, Aoki S, Suzuki M, Nagasawa H, Kubota K, et al. Phase IIa clinical study of [^{18}F]fluciclovine: efficacy and safety of a new PET tracer for brain tumors. Ann Nucl Med. 2016;30(9):608–18.
85. Rowe SP, Gorin MA, Allaf ME, Pienta KJ, Tran PT, Pomper MG, et al. PET imaging of prostate-specific membrane antigen in prostate cancer: current state of the art and future challenges. Prostate Cancer Prostatic Dis. 2016;19(3):223–30.
86. Wibmer AG, Burger IA, Sala E, Hricak H, Weber WA, Vargas HA. Molecular imaging of prostate cancer. Radiographics. 2016;36(1):142–59.
87. Minamimoto R, Hancock S, Schneider B, Chin FT, Jamali M, Loening A, et al. Pilot comparison of ^{68}Ga-RM2 PET and ^{68}Ga-PSMA-11 PET in patients with biochemically recurrent prostate cancer. J Nucl Med. 2016;57(4):557–62.
88. Oka S, Okudaira H, Yoshida Y, Schuster DM, Goodman MM, Shirakami Y. Transport mechanisms of *trans*-1-amino-3-fluoro[1-^{14}C]cyclobutanecarboxylic acid in prostate cancer cells. Nucl Med Biol. 2012;39(1):109–19.
89. Schuster DM, Nanni C, Fanti S. Evaluation of prostate cancer with radiolabeled amino acid analogs. J Nucl Med. 2016;57(Suppl 3):61S–6S.
90. Shiiba M, Ishihara K, Kimura G, Kuwako T, Yoshihara H, Sato H, et al. Evaluation of primary prostate cancer using ^{11}C-methionine-PET/CT and ^{18}F-FDG-PET/CT. Ann Nucl Med. 2012;26(2):138–45.
91. Arimoto MK, Higashi T, Nishii R, Kagawa S, Takahashi M, Kishibe Y, et al. ^{11}C-methylaminoisobutyric acid (MeAIB) PET for evaluation of prostate cancer: compared with ^{18}F-fluorodeoxyglucose PET. Ann Nucl Med. 2016;30(8):553–62.
92. Ambrosini V, Morigi JJ, Nanni C, Castellucci P, Fanti S. Current status of PET imaging of neuroendocrine tumours ([^{18}F]FDOPA, [^{68}Ga]tracers, [^{11}C]/[^{18}F]-HTP). Q J Nucl Med Mol Imaging. 2015;59(1):58–69.
93. Imperiale A, Rust E, Gabriel S, Detour J, Goichot B, Duclos B, et al. ^{18}F-fluorodihydroxyphenylalanine PET/CT in patients with neuroendocrine tumors of unknown origin: relation to tumor origin and differentiation. J Nucl Med. 2014;55(3):367–72.
94. Janssen I, Chen CC, Taieb D, Patronas NJ, Millo CM, Adams KT, et al. ^{68}Ga-DOTATATE PET/CT in the localization of head and neck paragangliomas compared with other functional imaging modalities and CT/MRI. J Nucl Med. 2016;57(2):186–91.
95. Wise DR, Thompson CB. Glutamine addiction: a new therapeutic target in cancer. Trends Biochem Sci. 2010;35(8):427–33.
96. Villar VH, Merhi F, Djavaheri-Mergny M, Duran RV. Glutaminolysis and autophagy in cancer. Autophagy. 2015;11(8):1198–208.
97. Jin L, Alesi GN, Kang S. Glutaminolysis as a target for cancer therapy. Oncogene. 2016;35(28):3619–25.
98. Wu Z, Zha Z, Li G, Lieberman BP, Choi SR, Ploessl K, et al. [^{18}F](2*S*,4*S*)-4-(3-Fluoropropyl) glutamine as a tumor imaging agent. Mol Pharm. 2014;11(11):3852–66.
99. Qu W, Oya S, Lieberman BP, Ploessl K, Wang L, Wise DR, et al. Preparation and characterization of L-[5-^{11}C]-glutamine for metabolic imaging of tumors. J Nucl Med. 2012;53(1):98–105.
100. Ploessl K, Wang L, Lieberman BP, Qu W, Kung HF. Comparative evaluation of ^{18}F-labeled glutamic acid and glutamine as tumor metabolic imaging agents. J Nucl Med. 2012;53(10):1616–24.
101. Qu W, Zha Z, Ploessl K, Lieberman BP, Zhu L, Wise DR, et al. Synthesis of optically pure 4-fluoro-glutamines as potential metabolic imaging agents for tumors. J Am Chem Soc. 2011;133(4):1122–33.

102. Okudaira H, Nakanishi T, Oka S, Kobayashi M, Tamagami H, Schuster DM, et al. Kinetic analyses of *trans*-1-amino-3-[^{18}F]fluorocyclobutanecarboxylic acid transport in Xenopus laevis oocytes expressing human ASCT2 and SNAT2. Nucl Med Biol. 2013;
103. Sundaram SK, Muzik O, Chugani DC, Mu F, Mangner TJ, Chugani HT. Quantification of protein synthesis in the human brain using L-[1-^{11}C]-leucine PET: incorporation of factors for large neutral amino acids in plasma and for amino acids recycled from tissue. J Nucl Med. 2006;47(11):1787–95.
104. Smith CB, Schmidt KC, Qin M, Burlin TV, Cook MP, Kang J, et al. Measurement of regional rates of cerebral protein synthesis with L-[1-^{11}C]leucine and PET with correction for recycling of tissue amino acids: II. Validation in rhesus monkeys. J Cereb Blood Flow Metab. 2005;25(5):629–40.
105. Schmidt KC, Cook MP, Qin M, Kang J, Burlin TV, Smith CB. Measurement of regional rates of cerebral protein synthesis with L-[1-^{11}C]leucine and PET with correction for recycling of tissue amino acids: I. Kinetic modeling approach. J Cereb Blood Flow Metab. 2005;25(5):617–28.
106. Pruim J, Willemsen AT, Molenaar WM, van Waarde A, Paans AM, Heesters MA, et al. Brain tumors: L-[1-C-11] tyrosine PET for visualization and quantification of protein synthesis rate. Radiology. 1995;197(1):221–6.
107. Coenen HH, Kling P, Stocklin G. Cerebral metabolism of L-[2-^{18}F]fluorotyrosine, a new PET tracer of protein synthesis. J Nucl Med. 1989;30(8):1367–72.
108. Xu J, Zeng C, Chu W, Pan F, Rothfuss JM, Zhang F, et al. Identification of the PGRMC1 protein complex as the putative sigma-2 receptor binding site. Nat Commun. 2011;2:380.
109. Shoghi KI, Xu J, Su Y, He J, Rowland D, Yan Y, et al. Quantitative receptor-based imaging of tumor proliferation with the sigma-2 ligand [^{18}F]ISO-1. PLoS One. 2013;8(9):e74188.
110. Mach RH, Dehdashti F, Wheeler KT. PET radiotracers for imaging the proliferative status of solid tumors. PET Clin. 2009;4(1):1–15.
111. Christman D, Crawford EJ, Friedkin M, Wolf AP. Detection of DNA synthesis in intact organisms with positron-emitting (methyl-^{11}C)thymidine. Proc Natl Acad Sci U S A. 1972;69(4):988–92.
112. Poupeye EM, Goethals PP, Dams RF, De Leenheer AP, van Eijkeren ME. Evaluation of [^{11}C]thymidine for measurement of cell proliferation in fast dividing tissues. Nucl Med Biol. 1993;20(3):359–62.
113. Shields AF, Larson SM, Grunbaum Z, Graham MM. Short-term thymidine uptake in normal and neoplastic tissues: studies for PET. J Nucl Med. 1984;25(7):759–64.
114. Kostakoglu L. Novel PET radiotracers for potential use in management of lymphoma. PET Clin. 2012;7:83–117.
115. Plotnik DA, Emerick LE, Krohn KA, Unadkat JD, Schwartz JL. Different modes of transport for ^{3}H-thymidine, ^{3}H-FLT, and ^{3}H-FMAU in proliferating and nonproliferating human tumor cells. J Nucl Med. 2010;51(9):1464–71.
116. Grierson JR, Schwartz JL, Muzi M, Jordan R, Krohn KA. Metabolism of 3′-deoxy-3′-[F-18]fluorothymidine in proliferating A549 cells: validations for positron emission tomography. Nucl Med Biol. 2004;31(7):829–37.
117. Mankoff DA, Muzi M, Krohn KA. Quantitative positron emission tomography imaging to measure tumor response to therapy: what is the best method? Mol Imaging Biol. 2003;5(5):281–5.
118. Muzi M, Vesselle H, Grierson JR, Mankoff DA, Schmidt RA, Peterson L, et al. Kinetic analysis of 3′-deoxy-3′-fluorothymidine PET studies: validation studies in patients with lung cancer. J Nucl Med. 2005;46(2):274–82.
119. Muzi M, Mankoff DA, Grierson JR, Wells JM, Vesselle H, Krohn KA. Kinetic modeling of 3′-deoxy-3′-fluorothymidine in somatic tumors: mathematical studies. J Nucl Med. 2005;46(2):371–80.
120. Tehrani OS, Shields AF. PET imaging of proliferation with pyrimidines. J Nucl Med. 2013;54(6):903–12.
121. Herrmann K, Buck AK. Proliferation imaging with ^{18}F fluorothymidine PET/computed tomography: physiologic uptake, variants, and pitfalls. PET Clin. 2014;9(3):331–8.
122. Peck M, Pollack HA, Friesen A, Muzi M, Shoner SC, Shankland EG, et al. Applications of PET imaging with the proliferation marker [^{18}F]-FLT. Q J Nucl Med Mol Imaging. 2015;59(1):95–104.
123. Bollineni VR, Kramer GM, Jansma EP, Liu Y, Oyen WJ. A systematic review on [^{18}F]FLT-PET uptake as a measure of treatment response in cancer patients. Eur J Cancer. 2016;55:81–97.
124. van Waarde A, Jager PL, Ishiwata K, Dierckx RA, Elsinga PH. Comparison of sigma-ligands and metabolic PET tracers for differentiating tumor from inflammation. J Nucl Med. 2006;47(1):150–4.
125. Lee TS, Ahn SH, Moon BS, Chun KS, Kang JH, Cheon GJ, et al. Comparison of ^{18}F-FDG, ^{18}F-FET and ^{18}F-FLT for differentiation between tumor and inflammation in rats. Nucl Med Biol. 2009;36(6):681–6.
126. Tan Y, Liang J, Liu D, Zhu F, Wang G, Ding X, et al. ^{18}F-FLT PET/CT imaging in a Wister rabbit inflammation model. Exp Ther Med. 2014;8(1):69–72.
127. Dittmann H, Dohmen BM, Paulsen F, Eichhorn K, Eschmann SM, Horger M, et al. [^{18}F]FLT PET for diagnosis and staging of thoracic tumours. Eur J Nucl Med Mol Imaging. 2003;30(10):1407–12.
128. Cobben DC, Elsinga PH, Hoekstra HJ, Suurmeijer AJ, Vaalburg W, Maas B, et al. Is ^{18}F-3′-fluoro-3′-deoxy-L-thymidine useful for the staging and restaging of non-small cell lung cancer? J Nucl Med. 2004;45(10):1677–82.
129. van Westreenen HL, Cobben DC, Jager PL, van Dullemen HM, Wesseling J, Elsinga PH, et al. Comparison of ^{18}F-FLT PET and ^{18}F-FDG PET in esophageal cancer. J Nucl Med. 2005;46(3):400–4.

130. Zhao F, Cui Y, Li M, Fu Z, Chen Z, Kong L, et al. Prognostic value of 3′-deoxy-3′-^{18}F-fluorothymidine ([^{18}F] FLT PET) in patients with recurrent malignant gliomas. Nucl Med Biol. 2014;41(8):710–5.
131. Mitamura K, Yamamoto Y, Kudomi N, Maeda Y, Norikane T, Miyake K, et al. Intratumoral heterogeneity of ^{18}F-FLT uptake predicts proliferation and survival in patients with newly diagnosed gliomas. Ann Nucl Med. 2016;
132. Ma DJ, Galanis E, Anderson SK, Schiff D, Kaufmann TJ, Peller PJ, et al. A phase II trial of everolimus, temozolomide, and radiotherapy in patients with newly diagnosed glioblastoma: NCCTG N057K. Neuro-Oncology. 2015;17(9):1261–9.
133. Lodge MA, Holdhoff M, Leal JP, Bag AK, Nabors LB, Mintz A, et al. Repeatability of ^{18}F-FLT PET in a multi-center study of patients with high grade glioma. In: J Nucl Med; 2016.
134. Chen W, Cloughesy T, Kamdar N, Satyamurthy N, Bergsneider M, Liau L, et al. Imaging proliferation in brain tumors with ^{18}F-FLT PET: comparison with ^{18}F-FDG. J Nucl Med. 2005;46(6):945–52.
135. Nowosielski M, DiFranco MD, Putzer D, Seiz M, Recheis W, Jacobs AH, et al. An intra-individual comparison of MRI, [^{18}F]-FET and [^{18}F]-FLT PET in patients with high-grade gliomas. PLoS One. 2014;9(4):e95830.
136. Tripathi M, Sharma R, D'Souza M, Jaimini A, Panwar P, Varshney R, et al. Comparative evaluation of F-18 FDOPA, F-18 FDG, and F-18 FLT-PET/CT for metabolic imaging of low grade gliomas. Clin Nucl Med. 2009;34(12):878–83.
137. Singh R, Cuervo AM. Lipophagy: connecting autophagy and lipid metabolism. Int J Cell Biol 2012;2012:282041.
138. Camici P, Ferrannini E, Opie LH. Myocardial metabolism in ischemic heart disease: basic principles and application to imaging by positron emission tomography. Prog Cardiovasc Dis. 1989;32(3):217–38.
139. Bergmann SR. Imaging of myocardial fatty acid metabolism with PET. J Nucl Cardiol. 2007;14(3 Suppl):S118–24.
140. Lopes-Cardozo M, Mulder I, van Vugt F, Hermans PG, van den Bergh SG, Klazinga W, et al. Aspects of ketogenesis: control and mechanism of ketone-body formation in isolated rat-liver mitochondria. Mol Cell Biochem. 1975;9(3):155–73.
141. Lindhe O, Sun A, Ulin J, Rahman O, Langstrom B, Sorensen J. [^{18}F]Fluoroacetate is not a functional analogue of [^{11}C]acetate in normal physiology. Eur J Nucl Med Mol Imaging. 2009;36(9):1453–9.
142. Bozza PT, Viola JP. Lipid droplets in inflammation and cancer. Prostaglandins Leukot Essent Fatty Acids. 2010;82(4-6):243–50.
143. Carracedo A, Cantley LC, Pandolfi PP. Cancer metabolism: fatty acid oxidation in the limelight. Nat Rev Cancer. 2013;13(4):227–32.
144. Deberardinis RJ, Sayed N, Ditsworth D, Thompson CB. Brick by brick: metabolism and tumor cell growth. Curr Opin Genet Dev. 2008;18(1):54–61.
145. Mashimo T, Pichumani K, Vemireddy V, Hatanpaa KJ, Singh DK, Sirasanagandla S, et al. Acetate is a bioenergetic substrate for human glioblastoma and brain metastases. Cell. 2014;159(7):1603–14.
146. Lyssiotis CA, Cantley LC. Acetate fuels the cancer engine. Cell. 2014;159(7):1492–4.
147. Iozzo P, Bucci M, Roivainen A, Nagren K, Jarvisalo MJ, Kiss J, et al. Fatty acid metabolism in the liver, measured by positron emission tomography, is increased in obese individuals. Gastroenterology. 2010;139(3):846-56, 56 e1-6.
148. Swinnen JV, Brusselmans K, Verhoeven G. Increased lipogenesis in cancer cells: new players, novel targets. Curr Opin Clin Nutr Metab Care. 2006;9(4):358–65.
149. Daniels VW, Smans K, Royaux I, Chypre M, Swinnen JV, Zaidi N. Cancer cells differentially activate and thrive on de novo lipid synthesis pathways in a low-lipid environment. PLoS One. 2014;9(9):e106913.
150. Lewis DY, Boren J, Shaw GL, Bielik R, Ramos-Montoya A, Larkin TJ, et al. Late imaging with [1-^{11}C]acetate improves detection of tumor fatty acid synthesis with PET. J Nucl Med. 2014;55(7):1144–9.
151. Vavere AL, Kridel SJ, Wheeler FB, Lewis JS. 1-^{11}C-acetate as a PET radiopharmaceutical for imaging fatty acid synthase expression in prostate cancer. J Nucl Med. 2008;49(2):327–34.
152. Yoshii Y, Waki A, Furukawa T, Kiyono Y, Mori T, Yoshii H, et al. Tumor uptake of radiolabeled acetate reflects the expression of cytosolic acetyl-CoA synthetase: implications for the mechanism of acetate PET. Nucl Med Biol 2009;36(7):771-7.
153. Mohsen B, Giorgio T, Rasoul ZS, Werner L, Ali GR, Reza DK, et al. Application of C-11-acetate positron-emission tomography (PET) imaging in prostate cancer: systematic review and meta-analysis of the literature. BJU Int. 2013;112(8):1062–72.
154. Grassi I, Nanni C, Allegri V, Morigi JJ, Montini GC, Castellucci P, et al. The clinical use of PET with ^{11}C-acetate. Am J Nucl Med Mol Imaging. 2012;2(1):33–47.
155. Menendez JA, Lupu R. Fatty acid synthase and the lipogenic phenotype in cancer pathogenesis. Nat Rev Cancer. 2007;7(10):763–77.
156. Rossi S, Graner E, Febbo P, Weinstein L, Bhattacharya N, Onody T, et al. Fatty acid synthase expression defines distinct molecular signatures in prostate cancer. Mol Cancer Res. 2003;1(10):707–15.
157. Dimitrakopoulou-Strauss A, Strauss LG. PET imaging of prostate cancer with ^{11}C-acetate. J Nucl Med. 2003;44(4):556–8.
158. Yoshii Y, Furukawa T, Oyama N, Hasegawa Y, Kiyono Y, Nishii R, et al. Fatty acid synthase is a key target in multiple essential tumor functions of prostate cancer: uptake of radiolabeled acetate as a predictor of the targeted therapy outcome. PLoS One. 2013;8(5):e64570.
159. Regula N, Haggman M, Johansson S, Sorensen J. Malignant lipogenesis defined by ^{11}C-acetate PET/CT predicts prostate cancer-specific survival

in patients with biochemical relapse after prostatectomy. Eur J Nucl Med Mol Imaging. 2016;

160. EY Y, Muzi M, Hackenbracht JA, Rezvani BB, Link JM, Montgomery RB, et al. C11-acetate and F-18 FDG PET for men with prostate cancer bone metastases: relative findings and response to therapy. Clin Nucl Med. 2011;36(3):192–8.
161. Muir D, Berl S, Clarke DD. Acetate and fluoroacetate as possible markers for glial metabolism in vivo. Brain Res. 1986;380(2):336–40.
162. Clarke DD. Fluoroacetate and fluorocitrate: mechanism of action. Neurochem Res. 1991;16(9):1055–8.
163. Nishii R, Tong W, Wendt R, 3rd, Soghomonyan S, Mukhopadhyay U, Balatoni J, et al. Pharmacokinetics, metabolism, biodistribution, radiation dosimetry, and toxicology of ^{18}F-fluoroacetate (^{18}F-FACE) in non-human primates. Mol Imaging Biol 2012;14(2):213-224.
164. Ponde DE, Dence CS, Oyama N, Kim J, Tai YC, Laforest R, et al. ^{18}F-fluoroacetate: a potential acetate analog for prostate tumor imaging—in vivo evaluation of ^{18}F-fluoroacetate versus ^{11}C-acetate. J Nucl Med. 2007;48(3):420–8.
165. Miyabe H, Ohte N, Iida A, Narita H, Yoshida T, Kimura G. Evaluation of fatty acid beta-oxidation in patients with prior myocardial infarction in relation to myocardial blood flow, total oxidative metabolism, and left ventricular wall motion. Circ J. 2005;69(12):1459–65.
166. Bessi VL, Labbe SM, Huynh DN, Menard L, Jossart C, Febbraio M, et al. EP 80317, a selective CD36 ligand, shows cardioprotective effects against post-ischaemic myocardial damage in mice. Cardiovasc Res. 2012;96(1):99–108.
167. Ishida Y, Nagata S, Uehara T, Yasumura Y, Fukuchi K, Miyatake K. Clinical analysis of myocardial perfusion and metabolism in patients with hypertrophic cardiomyopathy by single photon emission tomography and positron emission tomography. J Cardiol. 2001;37(Suppl 1):121–8.
168. Taylor M, Wallhaus TR, Degrado TR, Russell DC, Stanko P, Nickles RJ, et al. An evaluation of myocardial fatty acid and glucose uptake using PET with [^{18}F]fluoro-6-thia-heptadecanoic acid and [^{18}F]FDG in patients with congestive heart failure. J Nucl Med. 2001;42(1):55–62.
169. Mather KJ, DeGrado TR. Imaging of myocardial fatty acid oxidation. Biochim Biophys Acta. 2016;
170. Brown MA, Myears DW, Bergmann SR. Noninvasive assessment of canine myocardial oxidative metabolism with carbon-11 acetate and positron emission tomography. J Am Coll Cardiol. 1988;12(4):1054–63.
171. Brown MA, Myears DW, Bergmann SR. Validity of estimates of myocardial oxidative metabolism with carbon-11 acetate and positron emission tomography despite altered patterns of substrate utilization. J Nucl Med. 1989;30(2):187–93.
172. Peters R, Wakelin RW. Biochemistry of fluoroacetate poisoning; the isolation and some properties of the fluorotricarboxylic acid inhibitor of citrate metabolism. Proceedings of the Royal Society of London Series B, Biological sciences. 1953;140(901):497–507.
173. Proudfoot AT, Bradberry SM, Vale JA. Sodium fluoroacetate poisoning. Toxicol Rev. 2006;25(4):213–9.
174. Lauble H, Kennedy MC, Emptage MH, Beinert H, Stout CD. The reaction of fluorocitrate with aconitase and the crystal structure of the enzyme-inhibitor complex. Proc Natl Acad Sci U S A. 1996;93(24):13699–703.
175. Lerch RA, Ambos HD, Bergmann SR, Welch MJ, Ter-Pogossian MM, Sobel BE. Localization of viable, ischemic myocardium by positron-emission tomography with ^{11}C-palmitate. Circulation. 1981;64(4):689–99.
176. Bergmann SR. Use and limitations of metabolic tracers labeled with positron-emitting radionuclides in the identification of viable myocardium. J Nucl Med. 1994;35(4 Suppl):15S–22S.
177. Bergmann SR, Weinheimer CJ, Markham J, Herrero P. Quantitation of myocardial fatty acid metabolism using PET. J Nucl Med. 1996;37(10):1723–30.
178. Schon HR, Schelbert HR, Robinson G, Najafi A, Huang SC, Hansen H, et al. C- 11 labeled palmitic acid for the noninvasive evaluation of regional myocardial fatty acid metabolism with positron-computed tomography. I. Kinetics of C- 11 palmitic acid in normal myocardium. Am Heart J. 1982;103(4 Pt 1):532–47.
179. Lerch R, Tamm C, Papageorgiou I, Benzi RH. Myocardial fatty acid oxidation during ischemia and reperfusion. Mol Cell Biochem. 1992;116(1-2):103–9.
180. Knabb RM, Rosamond TL, Fox KA, Sobel BE, Bergmann SR. Enhancement of salvage of reperfused ischemic myocardium by diltiazem. J Am Coll Cardiol. 1986;8(4):861–71.
181. Livni E, Elmaleh DR, Levy S, Brownell GL, Strauss WH. Beta-methyl[1-^{11}C]heptadecanoic acid: a new myocardial metabolic tracer for positron emission tomography. J Nucl Med. 1982;23(2):169–75.
182. Takahashi T, Nishimura S, Ido T, Ishiwata K, Iwata R. Biological evaluation of 5-methyl-branched-chain omega-[^{18}F]fluorofatty acid: a potential myocardial imaging tracer for positron emission tomography. Nucl Med Biol. 1996;23(3):303–8.
183. Goodman MM, Kirsch G, Knapp FF, Jr. Synthesis and evaluation of radioiodinated terminal p-iodophenyl-substituted alpha- and beta-methyl-branched fatty acids. J Med Chem 1984;27(3):390-397.
184. Knapp FF, Jr., Ambrose KR, Callahan AP, Ferren LA, Grigsby RA, Irgolic KJ. Effects of chain length and tellurium position on the myocardial uptake of Te-123*m* fatty acids. J Nucl Med 1981;22(11):988-993.
185. DeGrado TR, Coenen HH, Stocklin G. 14(*R*,*S*)-[^{18}F]fluoro-6-thia-heptadecanoic acid (FTHA): evaluation in mouse of a new probe of myocardial utilization of long chain fatty acids. J Nucl Med. 1991;32(10):1888–96.

186. DeGrado TR, Wang S, Holden JE, Nickles RJ, Taylor M, Stone CK. Synthesis and preliminary evaluation of ^{18}F-labeled 4-thia palmitate as a PET tracer of myocardial fatty acid oxidation. Nucl Med Biol. 2000;27(3):221–31.
187. Shoup TM, Elmaleh DR, Bonab AA, Fischman AJ. Evaluation of trans-9-^{18}F-fluoro-3,4-Methyleneheptadecanoic acid as a PET tracer for myocardial fatty acid imaging. J Nucl Med. 2005;46(2):297–304.
188. Roivainen A, Forsback S, Gronroos T, Lehikoinen P, Kahkonen M, Sutinen E, et al. Blood metabolism of [methyl-^{11}C]choline; implications for in vivo imaging with positron emission tomography. Eur J Nucl Med. 2000;27(1):25–32.
189. Gibellini F, Smith TK. The Kennedy pathway—de novo synthesis of phosphatidylethanolamine and phosphatidylcholine. IUBMB Life. 2010;62(6):414–28.
190. Ackerstaff E, Pflug BR, Nelson JB, Bhujwalla ZM. Detection of increased choline compounds with proton nuclear magnetic resonance spectroscopy subsequent to malignant transformation of human prostatic epithelial cells. Cancer Res. 2001;61(9):3599–603.
191. Glunde K, Bhujwalla ZM, Ronen SM. Choline metabolism in malignant transformation. Nat Rev Cancer. 2011;11(12):835–48.
192. Lever M, Slow S. The clinical significance of betaine, an osmolyte with a key role in methyl group metabolism. Clin Biochem. 2010;43(9):732–44.
193. Bansal A, Shuyan W, Hara T, Harris RA, Degrado TR. Biodisposition and metabolism of [^{18}F]fluorocholine in 9L glioma cells and 9L glioma-bearing fisher rats. Eur J Nucl Med Mol Imaging. 2008;35(6):1192–203.
194. Smith G, Zhao Y, Leyton J, Shan B, Nguyen QD, Perumal M, et al. Radiosynthesis and pre-clinical evaluation of [^{18}F]fluoro-[1,2-$^{2}H_{4}$]choline. Nucl Med Biol. 2011;38(1):39–51.
195. Cantor JR, Sabatini DM. Cancer cell metabolism: one hallmark, many faces. Cancer Discov. 2012;2(10):881–98.
196. Aboagye EO, Bhujwalla ZM. Malignant transformation alters membrane choline phospholipid metabolism of human mammary epithelial cells. Cancer Res. 1999;59(1):80–4.
197. Accioly MT, Pacheco P, Maya-Monteiro CM, Carrossini N, Robbs BK, Oliveira SS, et al. Lipid bodies are reservoirs of cyclooxygenase-2 and sites of prostaglandin-E2 synthesis in colon cancer cells. Cancer Res. 2008;68(6):1732–40.
198. Nomura DK, Long JZ, Niessen S, Hoover HS, Ng SW, Cravatt BF. Monoacylglycerol lipase regulates a fatty acid network that promotes cancer pathogenesis. Cell. 2010;140(1):49–61.
199. Zadra G, Photopoulos C, Loda M. The fat side of prostate cancer. Biochim Biophys Acta. 2013;1831(10):1518–32.
200. DeBerardinis RJ, Lum JJ, Hatzivassiliou G, Thompson CB. The biology of cancer: metabolic reprogramming fuels cell growth and proliferation. Cell Metab. 2008;7(1):11–20.
201. Fackler OT, Grosse R. Cell motility through plasma membrane blebbing. J Cell Biol. 2008;181(6):879–84.
202. de Castro LF, Maycas M, Bravo B, Esbrit P, Gortazar A. VEGF receptor 2 (VEGFR2) activation is essential for osteocyte survival induced by mechanotransduction. J Cell Physiol. 2015;230(2):278–85.
203. Meng X, Riordan NH, Riordan HD, Mikirova N, Jackson J, Gonzalez MJ, et al. Cell membrane fatty acid composition differs between normal and malignant cell lines. P R Health Sci J. 2004;23(2):103–6.
204. Yoshimoto M, Waki A, Obata A, Furukawa T, Yonekura Y, Fujibayashi Y. Radiolabeled choline as a proliferation marker: comparison with radiolabeled acetate. Nucl Med Biol. 2004;31(7):859–65.
205. Hara T, Kosaka N, Kishi H. PET imaging of prostate cancer using carbon-11-choline. J Nucl Med. 1998;39(6):990–5.
206. Bansal A, Harris RA, DeGrado TR. Choline phosphorylation and regulation of transcription of choline kinase alpha in hypoxia. J Lipid Res. 2012;53(1):149–57.
207. DeGrado TR, Coleman RE, Wang S, Baldwin SW, Orr MD, Robertson CN, et al. Synthesis and evaluation of ^{18}F-labeled choline as an oncologic tracer for positron emission tomography: initial findings in prostate cancer. Cancer Res. 2001;61(1):110–7.
208. Umbehr MH, Muntener M, Hany T, Sulser T, Bachmann LM. The role of ^{11}C-choline and ^{18}F-fluorocholine positron emission tomography (PET) and PET/CT in prostate cancer: a systematic review and meta-analysis. Eur Urol. 2013;64(1):106–17.
209. de Vogel S, Ulvik A, Meyer K, Ueland PM, Nygard O, Vollset SE, et al. Sarcosine and other metabolites along the choline oxidation pathway in relation to prostate cancer—a large nested case-control study within the JANUS cohort in Norway. Int J Cancer. 2014;134(1):197–206.
210. Schmid DT, John H, Zweifel R, Cservenyak T, Westera G, Goerres GW, et al. Fluorocholine PET/CT in patients with prostate cancer: initial experience. Radiology. 2005;235(2):623–8.
211. Sutinen E, Nurmi M, Roivainen A, Varpula M, Tolvanen T, Lehikoinen P, et al. Kinetics of [^{11}C]choline uptake in prostate cancer: a PET study. Eur J Nucl Med Mol Imaging. 2004;31(3):317–24.
212. Yoshida S, Nakagomi K, Goto S, Futatsubashi M, Torizuka T. ^{11}C-choline positron emission tomography in prostate cancer: primary staging and recurrent site staging. Urol Int. 2005;74(3):214–20.
213. Fuccio C, Schiavina R, Castellucci P, Rubello D, Martorana G, Celli M, et al. Androgen deprivation therapy influences the uptake of ^{11}C-choline in patients with recurrent prostate cancer: the preliminary results of a sequential

PET/CT study. Eur J Nucl Med Mol Imaging. 2011;38(11):1985–9.

214. Giovacchini G, Picchio M, Coradeschi E, Scattoni V, Bettinardi V, Cozzarini C, et al. [^{11}C]choline uptake with PET/CT for the initial diagnosis of prostate cancer: relation to PSA levels, tumour stage and anti-androgenic therapy. Eur J Nucl Med Mol Imaging. 2008;35(6):1065–73.
215. Buchegger F, Garibotto V, Zilli T, Allainmat L, Jorcano S, Vees H, et al. First imaging results of an intraindividual comparison of ^{11}C-acetate and ^{18}F-fluorocholine PET/CT in patients with prostate cancer at early biochemical first or second relapse after prostatectomy or radiotherapy. Eur J Nucl Med Mol Imaging. 2014;41(1):68–78.
216. Casamassima F, Masi L, Menichelli C, Bonucci I, Casamassima E, Lazzeri M, et al. Efficacy of eradicative radiotherapy for limited nodal metastases detected with choline PET scan in prostate cancer patients. Tumori. 2011;97(1):49–55.
217. Parashar B, Wernicke AG, Rice S, Osborne J, Singh P, Nori D, et al. Early assessment of radiation response using a novel functional imaging modality—[^{18}F]fluorocholine PET (FCH-PET): a pilot study. Discov Med. 2012;14(74):13–20.
218. Panagiotidis E, Shankar A, Afaq A, Bomanji J. Assessing therapy response of secreting pineal germ cell tumor on simultaneous ^{18}F-choline PET/MRI. Clin Nucl Med. 2014;39(9):e387–8.
219. Al-Saeedi F, Welch AE, Smith TA. [methyl-^{3}H] choline incorporation into MCF7 tumour cells: correlation with proliferation. Eur J Nucl Med Mol Imaging. 2005;32(6):660–7.
220. Harrison L, Blackwell K. Hypoxia and anemia: factors in decreased sensitivity to radiation therapy and chemotherapy? Oncologist. 2004;9(Suppl 5):31–40.
221. Carnero A, Lleonart M. The hypoxic microenvironment: a determinant of cancer stem cell evolution. BioEssays. 2016;38(Suppl 1):S65–74.
222. Fleming IN, Manavaki R, Blower PJ, West C, Williams KJ, Harris AL, et al. Imaging tumour hypoxia with positron emission tomography. Br J Cancer. 2015;112(2):238–50.
223. Semenza GL. Hydroxylation of HIF-1: oxygen sensing at the molecular level. Physiology (Bethesda). 2004;19:176–82.
224. Keith B, Simon MC. Hypoxia-inducible factors, stem cells, and cancer. Cell. 2007;129(3):465–72.
225. Huntly BJ, Gilliland DG. Leukaemia stem cells and the evolution of cancer-stem-cell research. Nat Rev Cancer. 2005;5(4):311–21.
226. Reya T, Morrison SJ, Clarke MF, Weissman IL. Stem cells, cancer, and cancer stem cells. Nature. 2001;414(6859):105–11.
227. Lewis JS, Herrero P, Sharp TL, Engelbach JA, Fujibayashi Y, Laforest R, et al. Delineation of hypoxia in canine myocardium using PET and copper(II)-diacetyl-*bis*(*N*(4)-methylthiosemicarbazone). J Nucl Med. 2002;43(11):1557–69.
228. Lewis JS, Sharp TL, Laforest R, Fujibayashi Y, Welch MJ. Tumor uptake of copper-diacetyl-*bis*(*N*(4)-methylthiosemicarbazone): effect of changes in tissue oxygenation. J Nucl Med. 2001;42(4):655–61.
229. Lapi SE, Voller TF, Welch MJ. Positron emission tomography imaging of hypoxia. PET Clin. 2009;4(1):39–47.
230. Obata A, Yoshimi E, Waki A, Lewis JS, Oyama N, Welch MJ, et al. Retention mechanism of hypoxia selective nuclear imaging/radiotherapeutic agent cu-diacetyl-*bis*(*N*4-methylthiosemicarbazone) (cu-ATSM) in tumor cells. Ann Nucl Med. 2001;15(6):499–504.
231. Dearling JL, Packard AB. Some thoughts on the mechanism of cellular trapping of cu(II)-ATSM. Nucl Med Biol. 2010;37(3):237–43.
232. Price KA, Crouch PJ, Volitakis I, Paterson BM, Lim S, Donnelly PS, et al. Mechanisms controlling the cellular accumulation of copper *bis*(thiosemicarbazonato) complexes. Inorg Chem. 2011;50(19):9594–605.
233. Lewis JS, McCarthy DW, McCarthy TJ, Fujibayashi Y, Welch MJ. Evaluation of ^{64}Cu-ATSM in vitro and in vivo in a hypoxic tumor model. J Nucl Med. 1999;40(1):177–83.
234. Colombie M, Gouard S, Frindel M, Vidal A, Cherel M, Kraeber-Bodere F, et al. Focus on the controversial aspects of ^{64}Cu-ATSM in tumoral hypoxia mapping by PET imaging. Front Med (Lausanne). 2015;2:58.
235. Dietz DW, Dehdashti F, Grigsby PW, Malyapa RS, Myerson RJ, Picus J, et al. Tumor hypoxia detected by positron emission tomography with ^{60}Cu-ATSM as a predictor of response and survival in patients undergoing Neoadjuvant chemoradiotherapy for rectal carcinoma: a pilot study. Dis Colon Rectum. 2008;51(11):1641–8.
236. Dehdashti F, Mintun MA, Lewis JS, Bradley J, Govindan R, Laforest R, et al. In vivo assessment of tumor hypoxia in lung cancer with ^{60}Cu-ATSM. Eur J Nucl Med Mol Imaging. 2003;30(6):844–50.
237. Lewis JS, Laforest R, Dehdashti F, Grigsby PW, Welch MJ, Siegel BA. An imaging comparison of ^{64}Cu-ATSM and ^{60}Cu-ATSM in cancer of the uterine cervix. J Nucl Med. 2008;49(7):1177–82.
238. Dehdashti F, Grigsby PW, Lewis JS, Laforest R, Siegel BA, Welch MJ. Assessing tumor hypoxia in cervical cancer by PET with ^{60}Cu-labeled diacetyl-*bis*(*N*4-methylthiosemicarbazone). J Nucl Med. 2008;49(2):201–5.
239. Koh WJ, Rasey JS, Evans ML, Grierson JR, Lewellen TK, Graham MM, et al. Imaging of hypoxia in human tumors with [F-18]fluoromisonidazole. Int J Radiat Oncol Biol Phys. 1992;22(1):199–212.
240. Jerabek PA, Patrick TB, Kilbourn MR, Dischino DD, Welch MJ. Synthesis and biodistribution of ^{18}F-labeled fluoronitroimidazoles: potential in vivo markers of hypoxic tissue. Int J Rad Appl Instrum A. 1986;37(7):599–605.
241. Rasey JS, Koh WJ, Evans ML, Peterson LM, Lewellen TK, Graham MM, et al. Quantifying

regional hypoxia in human tumors with positron emission tomography of [18F]fluoromisonidazole: a pretherapy study of 37 patients. Int J Radiat Oncol Biol Phys. 1996;36(2):417–28.
242. Lawrentschuk N, Poon AM, Foo SS, Putra LG, Murone C, Davis ID, et al. Assessing regional hypoxia in human renal tumours using 18F-fluoromisonidazole positron emission tomography. BJU Int. 2005;96(4):540–6.
243. Hatano T, Zhao S, Zhao Y, Nishijima K, Kuno N, Hanzawa H, et al. Biological characteristics of intratumoral [F-18]fluoromisonidazole distribution in a rodent model of glioma. Int J Oncol. 2013;42(3):823–30.
244. Troost EG, Laverman P, Philippens ME, Lok J, van der Kogel AJ, Oyen WJ, et al. Correlation of [18F] FMISO autoradiography and pimonidazole [corrected] immunohistochemistry in human head and neck carcinoma xenografts. Eur J Nucl Med Mol Imaging. 2008;35(10):1803–11.
245. Lee ST, Scott AM. Hypoxia positron emission tomography imaging with 18F-fluoromisonidazole. Semin Nucl Med. 2007;37(6):451–61.
246. Cheng J, Lei L, Xu J, Sun Y, Zhang Y, Wang X, et al. 18F-fluoromisonidazole PET/CT: a potential tool for predicting primary endocrine therapy resistance in breast cancer. J Nucl Med. 2013;54(3):333–40.
247. Cheng X, Bayer C, Maftei CA, Astner ST, Vaupel P, Ziegler SI, et al. Preclinical evaluation of parametric image reconstruction of [18F]FMISO PET: correlation with ex vivo immunohistochemistry. Phys Med Biol. 2014;59(2):347–62.
248. Murakami M, Zhao S, Zhao Y, Chowdhury NF, Yu W, Nishijima K, et al. Evaluation of changes in the tumor microenvironment after sorafenib therapy by sequential histology and 18F-fluoromisonidazole hypoxia imaging in renal cell carcinoma. Int J Oncol. 2012;41(5):1593–600.
249. Zimny M, Gagel B, DiMartino E, Hamacher K, Coenen HH, Westhofen M, et al. FDG—a marker of tumour hypoxia? A comparison with [18F]fluoromisonidazole and pO_2-polarography in metastatic head and neck cancer. Eur J Nucl Med Mol Imaging. 2006;33(12):1426–31.
250. Bentzen L, Keiding S, Nordsmark M, Falborg L, Hansen SB, Keller J, et al. Tumour oxygenation assessed by 18F-fluoromisonidazole PET and polarographic needle electrodes in human soft tissue tumours. Radiother Oncol. 2003;67(3):339–44.
251. Busk M, Horsman MR, Jakobsen S, Bussink J, van der Kogel A, Overgaard J. Cellular uptake of PET tracers of glucose metabolism and hypoxia and their linkage. Eur J Nucl Med Mol Imaging. 2008;35(12):2294–303.
252. Halmos GB, Bruine de Bruin L, Langendijk JA, van der Laan BF, Pruim J, Steenbakkers RJ. Head and neck tumor hypoxia imaging by 18F-fluoroazomycin-arabinoside (18F-FAZA)-PET: a review. Clin Nucl Med. 2014;39(1):44–8.
253. Sorger D, Patt M, Kumar P, Wiebe LI, Barthel H, Seese A, et al. [18F]Fluoroazomycinarabinofuranoside (18FAZA) and [18F]fluoromisonidazole (18FMISO): a comparative study of their selective uptake in hypoxic cells and PET imaging in experimental rat tumors. Nucl Med Biol. 2003;30(3):317–26.
254. Evans SM, Judy KD, Dunphy I, Jenkins WT, Nelson PT, Collins R, et al. Comparative measurements of hypoxia in human brain tumors using needle electrodes and EF5 binding. Cancer Res. 2004;64(5):1886–92.
255. Evans SM, Fraker D, Hahn SM, Gleason K, Jenkins WT, Jenkins K, et al. EF5 binding and clinical outcome in human soft tissue sarcomas. Int J Radiat Oncol Biol Phys. 2006;64(3):922–7.

Introduction: MRI/MRS as Metabolic Imaging Tools

4

David Wilson and Michael Ohliger

Metabolic imaging using magnetic resonance has its roots in a relatively obscure technology, used by physicists in the late 1940s to study the nuclear magnetic moments of nuclei. This technique was nuclear magnetic resonance (NMR), based on the original observations of Bloch and Purcell in 1946 that nuclei with a given spin could be studied by applying an oscillating radiofrequency field, at a frequency corresponding to energy difference between nuclear orientations. When this so-called "resonance" frequency is applied to matter, the resulting emitted signal is the basis for NMR and magnetic resonance imaging (MRI). The discovery most relevant to metabolic imaging was that of chemical shift, described in several publications in 1949–1950, and the consequence of the subtle changes in local magnetic field, resulting from electric shell interactions. This remarkable finding is the fundamental principle of magnetic resonance spectroscopy (MRS), whereby nuclei can be identified reliably depending on their chemical structure, independent of magnetic field strength. Today in the clinic, several key metabolites present in the brain are easily identified using MRS techniques. Changes in the frequency-specific metabolic map or "spectrum" are used to diagnose disease and monitor the effects of medical treatments, in cancer and other illnesses.

In this chapter, we will describe the theoretical basis and physics behind MRI/MRS and their application to clinical imaging. MRS especially using ^{1}H nuclei will garner the bulk of our attention, a metabolic technique studied in a large number of diseases and organs, including the brain and prostate. Metabolic study using MRS has progressed beyond the study of nuclei in situ (^{1}H, ^{23}Na, and ^{31}P) and may be applied to introduced MR-active nuclei containing a net one-half spin, for example, via infusion of an enriched ^{13}C or ^{15}N drug or metabolic substrate. Site-specific enrichment is one strategy used to track the metabolism of these so-called "insensitive" nuclei, hindered by their low natural abundance and gyromagnetic ratio (γ). Recently, a revolutionary technology has been used to markedly increase the SNR of introduced, low γ nuclei, namely, hyperpolarized (HP) MRS. The physical basis of this technique as well as its application to metabolism will be described. Finally, we will address other exciting new MR techniques applied to metabolism including chemical exchange saturation transfer (CEST) imaging and relaxivity-based strategies.

D. Wilson • M. Ohliger
Department of Radiology, University of California
San Francisco, San Francisco, CA 94143, USA
e-mail: David.M.Wilson@ucsf.edu

J.S. Lewis, K.R. Keshari (eds.), *Imaging and Metabolism*, DOI 10.1007/978-3-319-61401-4_4

4.1 Basics of MRI/MRS Techniques

Magnetic resonance imaging (MRI) techniques exploit the magnetic properties of materials to form detailed images of biological tissues and to extract molecular information. Unlike computed tomography (CT), MRI does not rely on ionizing radiation to form an image. In addition, MRI is very flexible, permitting pulse sequences to be designed to yield images with different types of soft tissue contrast. The majority of magnetic resonance techniques that are used clinically are sensitive to the spatial distribution of water molecules (the most ubiquitous NMR-visible molecules) and the chemical environment of those molecules. Using MR spectroscopy (MRS), numerous other biological compounds can be detected in situ. These compounds often give important metabolic information about the tissue being imaged. In addition, there is growing interest in imaging the metabolism of exogenously administered compounds in order to probe different biological processes. The first part of this chapter describes the physical principles of MRI and MRS, focusing on the different ways the magnetic properties of tissues can be exploited to obtain diverse types of image contrast. The second part of this chapter describes specific examples of how MRI/MRS are used to assess metabolism in basic science and in the clinic.

4.1.1 Magnetic Resonance

All particles have intrinsic angular momentum, or "spin." Because of quantum mechanics, the spin of a particle is constrained to discrete integer or half-integer values. The most common particle used in magnetic resonance imaging is the hydrogen nucleus, which consists of a single proton that can take on spin values of either +1/2 or −1/2. The angular momentum of the proton in conjunction with its positive charge causes it also to behave like a small magnetic dipole, producing a small magnetic field similar to a bar magnet with the north and south poles aligned according to the direction of the spin. At room temperature and without any external magnetic field, all of the proton spins within a sample will point in random directions, and therefore the total magnetic field emanating from the sample is zero. However, when the sample is placed in a strong magnetic field, the protons will align with their spins preferentially parallel or antiparallel to the applied field (Fig. 4.1). Because the protons have lower energy when their spins are parallel to the magnetic field, at room temperature there is a small excess of proton spins aligned parallel to the applied magnetic field. Although this population difference is quite small (approximately three per million at 3 T), when summed over the large number of protons in any biological sample, a macroscopic net magnetization is created that can be detected through the phenomenon of magnetic resonance described below. An expanded review of magnetic resonance can be found in several references [1–3].

In most descriptions of NMR and MRI, the word "spin" is used in two ways. First, it refers to the angular momentum quantum number described in the paragraph above. Second, the word spin is used generically to refer to whichever nuclear particle (^{1}H, ^{23}Na, ^{31}P) that is being investigated using NMR. We follow the same practice here.

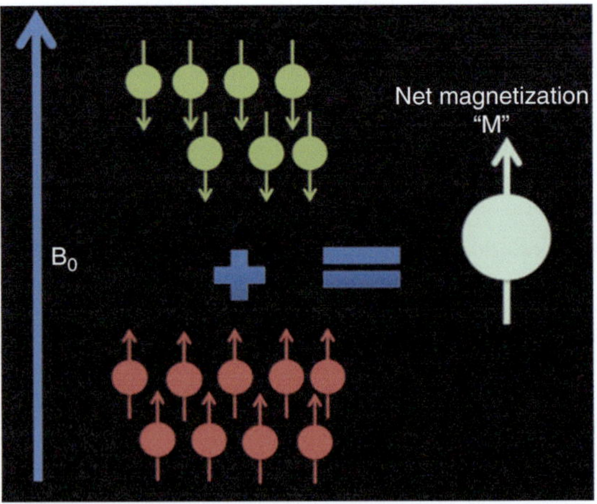

Fig. 4.1 Spins placed within a large magnetic field (B0) align themselves parallel or antiparallel with respect to that field. Because the parallel alignment has lower energy, slightly more spins will be in that state. This yields a small net macroscopic magnetization

MRI scanners that are used for clinical and preclinical imaging consist of four main components: (1) a strong main magnetic field, B_0, that is typically generated by a superconducting magnet and never changes; (2) a radiofrequency transmitter coil that is responsible for NMR excitation; (3) gradient coils that create small linearly varying fields and allow for spatial localization; and (4) radiofrequency receiver coils that detect the MRI signal arising from the sample. Sometimes, the same radiofrequency coil is used for excitation as well as signal reception.

When a sample such as a human patient or animal is placed in an MRI scanner, the spins within that sample become preferentially aligned with the strong main magnetic field, creating a small macroscopic magnetization. At equilibrium, this magnetization is static and therefore not detectable. When the proton spins are excited using the radiofrequency transmitter coil, they are rotated into a plane transverse to the main magnetic field. While they are in this transverse plane, the spins begin to precess around the axis of the main magnetic field (Fig. 4.2). The precession of these charged particles in turn creates a time-varying radiofrequency field that is detected outside of the sample. The frequency of precession, known as the *Larmor frequency*, is determined by the equation:

$$\omega = B\gamma,$$

where B is the strength of the main magnetic field and γ is the gyromagnetic ratio, which is a constant that is different for every type of nucleus. The simplicity of this formula underlies many of the principal strengths of magnetic resonance imaging. The local magnetic field experienced by the proton is often slightly different from the main magnetic field because of electromagnetic screening and other effects that occur in the proton's local environment. Therefore, the detected resonance frequency is a sensitive measure of the local chemical environment of the protons within a sample. Different molecules will have different characteristic "chemical shifts."

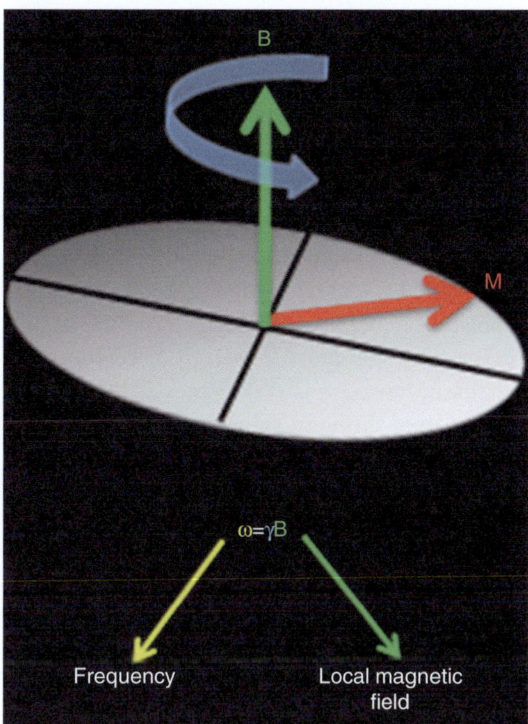

Fig. 4.2 Spins in the plane transverse to the main magnetic field process with the Larmor frequency, which is proportional to the gyromagnetic ratio, g, and the local magnetic field sensed by the spin. This frequency is therefore sensitive to the local chemical environment

4.1.2 Relaxation and Tissue Contrast

In magnetic resonance imaging, information is derived about the composition of tissues (e.g., tissue contrast) by three main mechanisms. First the MR signal is in general proportional to the number of precessing protons, and therefore tissue with more protons will give higher signal. In practice, this "spin density" contrast is of limited utility because the water density of most tissues is uniform. The second method of deriving chemical information about tissues is using the frequency of precession described above, where protons in different chemical environments (i.e., belonging to different molecules) have slightly different resonance frequencies. The shifts in frequencies between different molecules are typically well known and can be used to determine which molecules are present. This "chemical shift" contrast underlies many specialized MR spectroscopy techniques described below. One common application of chemical shift contrast is the separation of fat and water, which have a resonance frequency difference of approximately 220 Hz at 1.5 T (440 Hz at 3.0 T). This chemical separation underlies many "fat saturation" techniques that allow imaging without contamination of fat and also techniques that are sensitive to fat deposition in organs such as the liver [4].

The third and most frequently used source of soft tissue contrast is differences in the rate of relaxation of different spins toward equilibrium. As discussed above, spins that are aligned with the large external magnetic field tend to stay in the same orientations, with a small excess of spins aligned with the field rather than against it. When protons are excited into the transverse plane, the equilibrium is altered and fewer protons are left aligned with the external field. As the protons precess in the transverse plane, they give off energy and eventually relax toward equilibrium. This relaxation occurs with two different time constants (Fig. 4.3). The time constant with which the transverse magnetization decays is known as T_2, and the time constant with which the longitudinal magnetization (i.e., spins aligned with the field) reappears is known as T_1. The rate at which magnetization within tissue returns to equilibrium is very sensitive to the local chemical and physical interactions and therefore gives information about the local chemical environment. MRI techniques can be designed to emphasize either the T_1 or T_2 of a tissue.

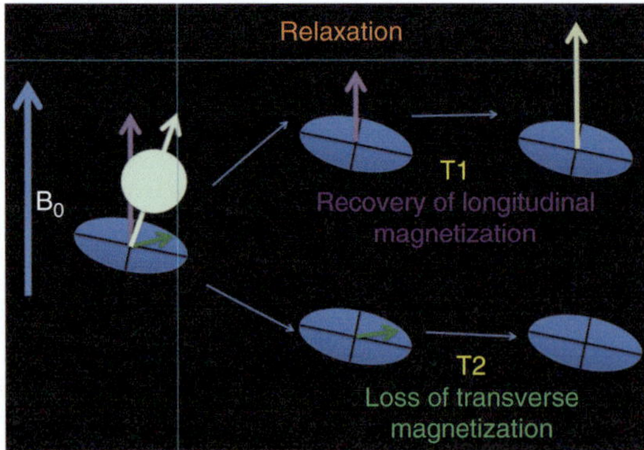

Fig. 4.3 Two relaxation time constants in NMR. T1 is the time constant for recovery of longitudinal magnetization. T2 is the time constant for decay of transverse magnetization

This relaxation-based contrast underlies the majority of routine clinical imaging. As a general rule, molecules that are in isotropic environments such as fluid collections have very long relaxation times (long T_1 and T_2), while semisolid tissues such as tendons that exist in anisotropic environments have very short relaxation times. Areas of iron deposition or blood products tend to create local magnetic field inhomogeneities that shorten T_2 [5].

In addition to being the dominant source of intrinsic tissue contrast, relaxation rates are the principal mechanism for exogenously administered contrast. Gadolinium-based (Gd^{3+}) contrast agents have an outer shell that rapidly exchanges with protons from surrounding water molecules, dramatically shortening the T_1 of surrounding water. Iron-based nanoparticles (e.g., SPIOs), which are accumulated in macrophages and can also be designed to target certain tissues, also lead to a shortening of T_1 but predominantly cause a shortening of T_2.

4.1.3 Spatial Encoding and MRI

The focus of this chapter is on the chemical and molecular sensitivity of MRI and MR spectroscopy. We will briefly discuss the ways in which MRI is able to extract information about the spatial distribution of protons and other spins within tissues, although a detailed discussion of this complex topic is beyond the scope of the chapter. Excellent review articles [2, 6] are available for further information on this subject. Spatial information is obtained in MRI through the application of magnetic field "gradients," which are specialized magnetic fields that point in the same direction as the main magnetic field but vary linearly in magnitude along either the x-, y-, or z-axis (off-axis gradients can be created by combining one or more of these basic gradients). When a gradient is applied, each part of the sample "sees" a different magnetic field, with the resonance frequency then mapped to spatial position. This is known as "frequency encoding." This basic technique only works along a single axis. In order to obtain information perpendicular to the axis used for frequency-encode gradient, an alternative encoding scheme called "phase encoding" must be used in which successively larger gradients are applied in a step-by-step fashion so that the relative phases of protons in adjacent voxels change at each step. Because phase encoding requires multiple repetitions for each phase-encoding step, imaging time is chiefly determined by the number of phase-encoding steps that are necessary to acquire an image.

The MR signal that is obtained in both the frequency-encode and phase-encode directions is not a direct image of the sample. Rather, it is a representation of the relative amplitude of various spatial frequencies that occur within the image. This spatial frequency-based representation of an image, or "k-space," is similar to the way sound can be decomposed into various auditory frequencies or light can be decomposed into different colors [7]. The properties of k-space are such that data that occur at the center of k-space are slowly varying and contribute most to the overall SNR of the image and the overall image contrast. Data that occur at the periphery of k-space contain information about the rapidly varying edges within an image and contribute most to spatial resolution.

4.1.4 Combining Spatial Encoding and Chemical Information: MR Spectroscopic Imaging

Magnetic resonance spectroscopic imaging is a method of combining the chemical shift molecular information of different molecules resonating at different frequencies with the spatial information obtained using magnetic field gradients described above. There are two main strategies of spectroscopic imaging. "Single-voxel techniques" are those in which only a single voxel is excited and an NMR spectrum is obtained from that voxel. These techniques have the advantage that they are relatively fast. However, they tend to be limited in signal to noise because only a small sample is being excited. Chemical shift imaging techniques integrate the spectroscopic step into the phase-encoding methodology described above. Instead of frequency encoding using spatially varying magnetic field gradients, NMR spectra are acquired during each phase-encoding step where the resonance frequency is determined not by spatial position but by chemical composition [8]. The penalty for using this approach is that there is no longer a spatial frequency-encode direction. All spatial dimensions must be acquired using phase encoding. The time required to obtain extra phase encoding greatly slows down acquisition. Numerous strategies have been developed to try to avoid some of this penalty in acquisition time, and this is an active field of research.

Practical methods for spatial localization in clinical MR spectroscopy fall into two main categories [9, 10]. In point-resolved spectroscopy (PRESS), a single volume is excited by using three frequency-selective RF pulses in three planes that intersect within the volume of interest. An alternative scheme is known as the stimulated echo acquisition mode (STEAM), which is based on the acquisition of stimulated echoes. Broadly speaking, STEAM allows for shorter echo times and acquisition of spectral metabolites with short-T_2 relaxation times but suffers from lower baseline signal to noise than PRESS [11].

Regardless of the acquisition method for spectroscopic imaging, there are several important technical considerations. First, when acquiring proton spectroscopic imaging, the signals from molecules present in small concentration can be obscured by the predominant signal that comes from water or even lipid. Therefore, specialized water saturation or lipid saturation schemes are needed. Second, in order to acquire high-quality spectroscopic images, it is important that the magnetic field in the sample be as uniform as possible. This uniformity is typically obtained by applying small additional "shim" magnetic fields to compensate for nonuniformity of the main magnetic field. Undesired variations in the main magnetic field will cause protons to precess at slightly different frequencies, eventually becoming out of phase and suppressing the observable peaks.

4.1.5 Magnetic Resonance Spectroscopy Beyond Protons

MRI can be used to image many nuclei other than protons. Several other nuclei of biological interest that have half-integer spin necessary to be visible by MRI include ^{13}C, ^{13}P, and ^{23}Na as summarized in Table 4.1 [12]. These atoms are of interest because they are often contained in molecules that are important in metabolism or cellular energetics. Although the basic physical principles of magnetic resonance using these nuclei are the same as for protons, there are several important practical challenges. First, because these nuclei resonate at different frequencies from protons, specialized hardware is required to image these nuclei, including RF coils and amplifiers. Second, these atoms tend to be present at relatively low levels. For example, natural abundance ^{13}C is only 1% of the total carbon in the body, the majority of which is ^{12}C that is not visible by MRI. Third, the gyromagnetic ratio of these compounds is lower than ^{1}H, which leads to decreased overall signal received from a single nucleus. Finally, several of these nuclei have long-T_1 relaxation times compared to protons. T_1 relaxation is necessary to recover the longitudinal magnetization before the next data point is acquired. Waiting for this additional T_1 recovery greatly lengthens scan time.

Because of these limitations, non-proton MRI is not typically performed on a routine basis clinically, but there are numerous research applications. These applications can use introduced half-integer spin nuclei. While ^{1}H, ^{23}Na, and ^{31}P MRS studies have focused on nuclei in situ, several other nuclei have been investigated following long infusions of small molecules containing MR-active nuclei, for example, ^{2}H and ^{19}F. For example, the metabolism of the chemotherapeutic agent 5-fluorouracil has been studied using ^{19}F MRI.

4.2 Magnetic Resonance Spectroscopy: Clinical Application and Innovation

Over the last several decades, MRS has evolved to become a robust technique, frequently used in clinical studies and in most cases available to MR technologists at the push of a button. Although MRS was first applied to endogenous ^{31}P nuclei, the vast majority of patient studies use the ^{1}H nuclei of abundant biomolecules—most notably choline (Ch), creatine (Cr), and N-acetylaspartate (NAA) in the normal brain and citrate (Cit) in the normal prostate. To reliably detect and quantify these and other metabolites, MRS exploits their different ^{1}H chemical shifts. Several technical advances have allowed the proliferation of ^{1}H

Table 4.1 NMR-active nuclei typically used for biomedical applications

Nuclei	m (spin)	Natural abundance (%)	γ (rel to ^{1}H)	$\Delta\delta$ (ppm)	T_1 range	Example biomedical application
$_{1}H$	1/2	99.98	1	13	0.1–2 s	Total body MRI and MRSI
$_{2}H$	1	0.02	0.1535	13	<1 s	Metabolic tracer injection using MRSI
$_{13}C$	1/2	1.11	0.2515	200	0.1–100 s	Metabolic tracer injection using MRSI
$_{15}N$	1/2	0.37	0.1013	900	0.1–400s	Metabolic tracer injection using MRSI
$_{17}O$	5/2	0.04	0.1355	1160	5–50 ms	Oxidative metabolism using MRSI
$_{19}F$	1/2	100.00	0.9409	700	0.1–1 s	Tracer injection of therapies using MRSI
$_{23}Na$	3/2	100.00	0.2645	72	10–50 ms	Neurodegeneration and cardiac using MRI
$_{31}P$	1/2	100.00	0.4048	430	0.05–2 s	Bioenergetics and pH using MRSI

MRI magnetic resonance imaging, *MRSI* magnetic resonance spectroscopic imaging, *m* quantum spin number, γ gyromagnetic ratio, $\Delta\delta$ chemical shift

MRS as a metabolic imaging tool, most notably the introduction of superconducting magnets, the use of the Fourier transform (FT) for signal processing, the introduction of high-sensitivity surface RF coils, and the ever-increasing field strength of modern clinical MRI systems. MRS is now widely available, used to study both common diseases (cancer, neurodegenerative disease) and rare metabolic disorders. Most properties of ^{1}H make it the ideal nucleus for MRS study, especially its high natural abundance (99%), large gyromagnetic ratio (γ), and inherent compatibility with routine clinical MRI exams. In most cases, the same hardware can be used for study of anatomy (^{1}H MRI) and metabolism (^{1}H MRS). We will begin by discussing ^{1}H MRS and then discuss the motivations for pursuing other spin-1/2 nuclei.

4.2.1 First Application: Nuclei In Situ

Studies of biological tissues using NMR spectroscopy culminated in the first use of MRS in patients, used to study ^{31}P in situ. The major advantages of ^{1}H were soon recognized, and in 1983 Behar et al. reported *in vivo* ^{1}H MRS of the human brain. Several advances were required for robust ^{1}H MRS including improvements in magnetic field homogeneity and water suppression techniques. The latter methods were needed to overcome the water signal that would otherwise dominate the ^{1}H spectrum and prohibit the study of low-concentration metabolites. Currently, spatially localized ^{1}H spectroscopy can be performed for a variety of tissues, including the brain, prostate, muscle, and liver. In the brain, ^{1}H MRS is often performed with anatomic imaging to allow co-localization of structural and metabolic abnormalities. Using 3D magnetic resonance shift imaging (MRSI), the brain can be parcelated into individual volume elements (voxels), which may be evaluated independently for relative metabolite concentrations. ^{1}H MRS can be performed on voxel volumes as low as 1 cm^3, a relatively high spatial resolution for a metabolic technique.

What metabolites can be studied using ^{1}H MRS? In general, to be visible by ^{1}H MRS, metabolites need to [1] have a high steady-state concentration, [2] exhibit a large fraction that is not membrane or protein bound, [3] have a long spin-spin relaxation constant (T_2), and [4] have distinct upfield resonances in the 1–4 ppm range. The resonances observed also depend on the part of the brain studied and the imaging parameters applied in particular the echo time (TE). Spectra may be acquired using a short or long echo time depending on the clinical question. Examples of short-TE (in this case 6 ms) and long-TE (288 ms) ^{1}H spectra acquired in the normal brain are shown in Fig. 4.4, showing the simplification of the spectrum seen at the longer echo time [13]. At longer echo times, short-T_2 nuclei are not seen—in the normal brain, only choline (Ch), creatine (Cr), and N-acetylaspartate (NAA) are visualized. This simplification is useful for derangements such as cancer, for which these (and lactate) are the most relevant resonances. However, some applications

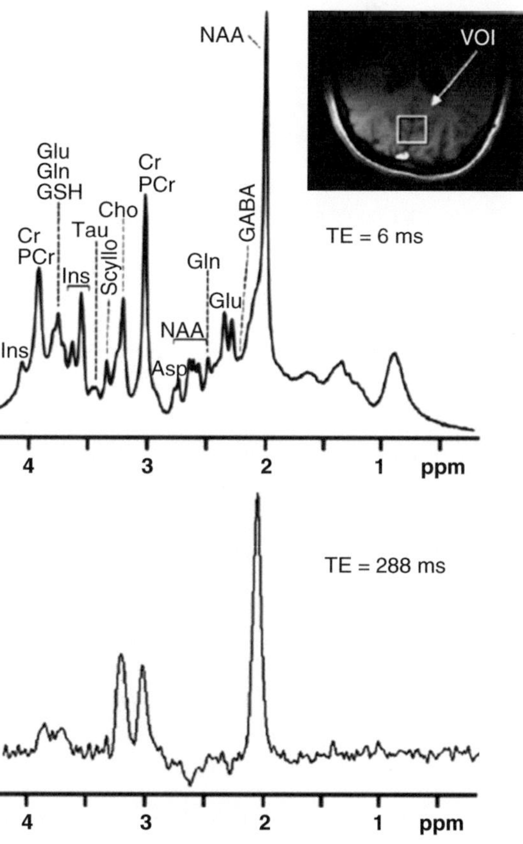

Fig. 4.4 ^{1}H NMR spectrum from a gray matter-rich 8 cm^3 voxel in the occipital lobe of a volunteer acquired with an optimized SE-based acquisition scheme at 3 T (TE = 6 ms), compared with a spectrum obtained at TE = 288 ms. Inset: transverse T1-weighted GRE image showing voxel location

require a more granular analysis of additional metabolites, for example, the search for inborn errors of metabolism in pediatric neuroimaging. When certain resonances are present in ^{1}H MRS, these are highly specific for metabolic disorders. For example, the diagnosis of maple syrup urine disease, also called branched-chain ketoaciduria, is clinched by ^{1}H MRS as shown in Fig. 4.5. This disease of newborns is caused by genetic defects of the branched-chain alpha-keto acid dehydrogenase complex, preventing the breakdown of the amino acids leucine, isoleucine, and valine. As a result, these amino acids accumulate at high concentrations in the brain, and their hydrophobic (water-repelling) side chains result in unique upfield resonances, easily identified by their chemical shifts.

In the simplified, long-TE spectrum, the major metabolites identified in the adult brain are, in order of decreasing ppm, Ch, Cr, NAA, and sometimes Lac. Choline has been extensively studied as a tumor-specific metabolite, and both brain and prostate tumors have a larger than expected Ch resonance. The Ch peak is assigned at 3.22 ppm and represents the sum of choline and other choline-containing compounds (e.g., phosphocholine) with near-identical chemical shift. Ch is a marker of phospholipid synthesis and degradation, reflecting cellular proliferation. Figure 4.6 shows the 3D MRSI of a patient with brain cancer (glioblastoma multiforme)

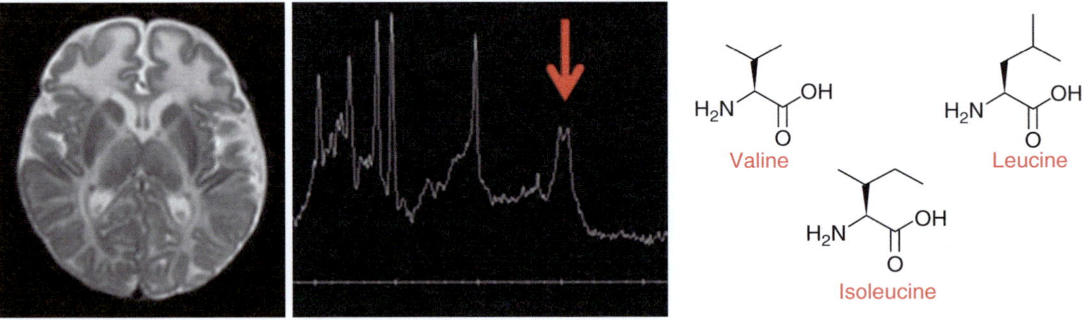

Fig. 4.5 On the left, T_2-weighted MRI of a neonatal brain showing increased fluid signal in the frontal white matter. Short-TE ^{1}H MRS was performed, demonstrating resonances around 1 ppm corresponding to the side chains of the branched-chain amino acids valine, leucine, and isoleucine. In this case the abnormal ^{1}H MRS is highly specific for maple syrup urine disease

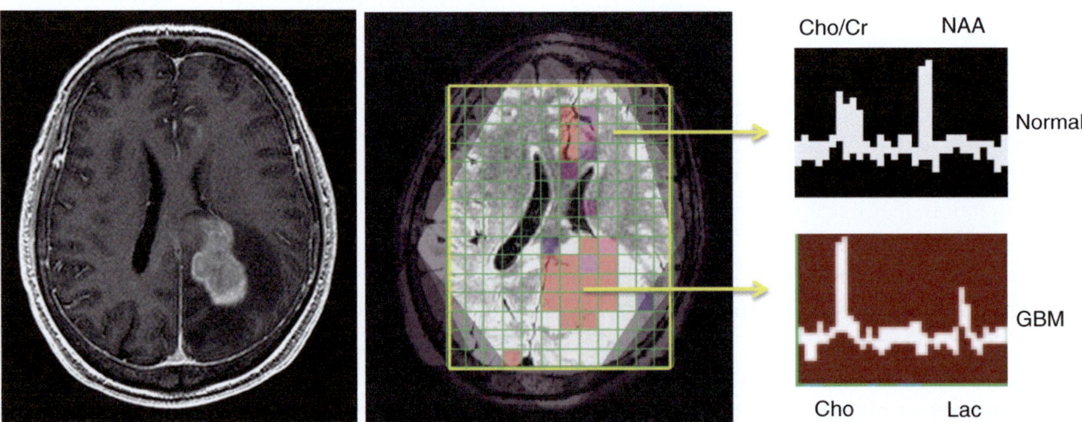

Fig. 4.6 3D ^{1}H MRSI performed on a patient with glioblastoma multiforme, the most common malignant primary brain tumor. On the left, postgadolinium T_1-weighted imaging reveals a large enhancing tumor. Spectroscopic imaging revealed significant metabolic derangement in voxels corresponding to tumor, with marked elevation of Ch, loss of NAA, and visualization of Lac, all features of a high-grade lesion. Sample voxels for normal and tumor regions are shown on the right

showing increased choline in voxels corresponding to tumor. The MRS observable protons in Cr resonate at 3.02 ppm, representing a combination of creatine and phosphocreatine. Cr is a phosphate source and marker of energy metabolism. The concentration of Cr is relatively constant, and thus it is often used as an internal reference for calculating metabolite ratios. In brain tumors, Cr signal may be reduced. The largest peak observed in the water-suppressed ^{1}H MRS spectrum is NAA, seen at 2.02 ppm. NAA is a nervous system-specific metabolite and is detected in both gray and white matter. The exact physiologic role of NAA is controversial, but it has been postulated to be an important acetate source and may play a role as a cerebral osmolyte. It is a marker of neuronal and axonal viability/density, and reduced magnitude of this peak in ^{1}H MRS is seen in numerous intracranial diseases, from cancer to multiple sclerosis. Finally, the Lac peak is not usually seen in the normal brain, occurring at 1.33 ppm. The concentration of Lac increases under anaerobic metabolism as seen in hypoxic-ischemic injury, metabolic disorders, and seizures. It is also seen in several tumors, an important product of the metabolic programming seen in cancer. According to the Warburg hypothesis, tumors use accelerated glycolysis as a primitive energy mechanism, in the process making significant quantities of lactate. This derangement is summarized in Fig. 4.7a [14].

Importantly, the lactate resonance observed by ^{1}H MRS reflects the steady-state, in situ concentration of this metabolite. This is in contrast to the metabolic information gleaned from hyperpolarized ^{13}C MRS, whereby the conversion of introduced ^{13}C pyruvate to ^{13}C lactate is observed in real time.

The discussion in this chapter largely focuses on brain ^{1}H MRS, but prostate spectroscopy has also evolved into a highly informative technique, commonly performed in conjunction with anatomic imaging during a prostate MR exams. This technique allows visualization of the metabolic reprogramming seen in malignant prostate cancer cells. Three-dimensional MR spectroscopic imaging (MRSI) allows metabolic evaluation of the entire prostate gland, with resonances corresponding to citrate, creatine, choline, and polyamines readily visualized. As shown in Fig. 4.7b, the spectra taken from regions of prostate cancer show significantly reduced or absent citrate (Cit) and polyamines (PA) relative to those seen in the normal surrounding gland. These changes in citrate are attributed to a shift from citrate-producing to citrate-oxidizing metabolism. Because choline is elevated in prostate cancer, the choline-to-citrate ratio ([choline + creatine]/citrate) is commonly used for spectral analysis since the choline and creatine peaks are poorly resolved.

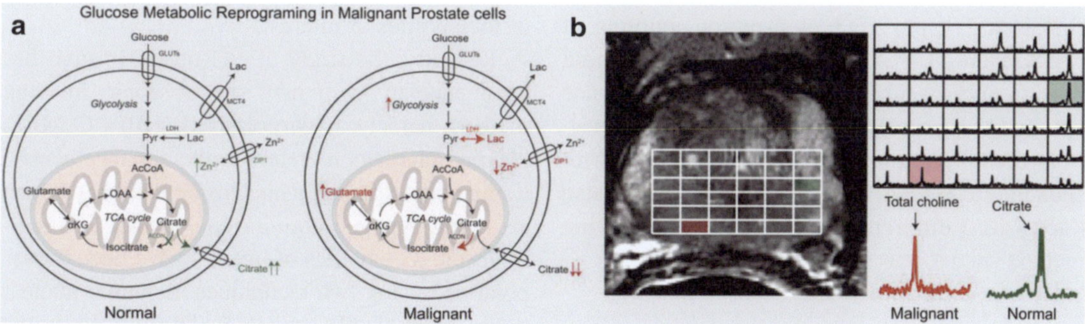

Fig. 4.7 Metabolic reprogramming in prostate cancer, observed by ^{1}H MRS. (**a**) Change in glucose metabolism when comparing normal prostate glandular epithelial cells and malignant cells. (**b**) Representative T_2-weighted imaging and corresponding three-dimensional MRSI array in patient with Gleason 3 + 4 cancer in the right base of the prostate gland. Inlaid spectra corresponding to normal and malignant voxel demonstrate differences in metabolism for these regions, with large citrate resonance observed in normal prostate tissue and abnormal choline peak in cancer. *GLUTs* glucose transporters, *ZIP1* zinc transporter, *AcCoA* acetyl-CoA, *ACCH* acetylcholine, *αKG* α-ketoglutarate, *Lac* lactate, *LDH* lactate dehydrogenase, *MCT4* monocarboxylate transporter 4, *OAA* oxaloacetate, *Pyr* pyruvate, *TCA* tricarboxylic acid

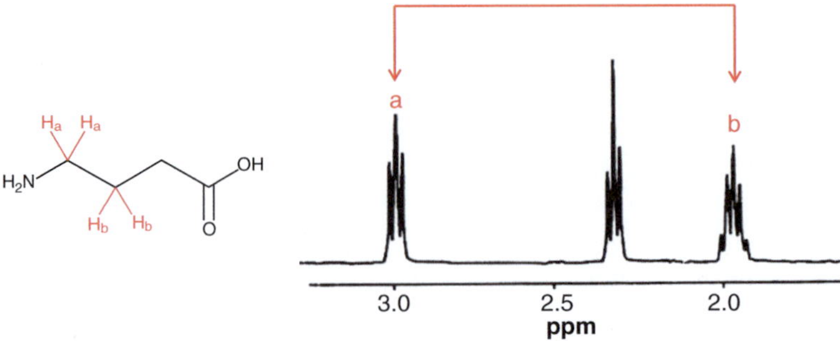

Fig. 4.8 The chemical structure of gamma-aminobutyric acid (GABA) is displayed with its corresponding ^{1}H NMR in solution, showing the coupled ^{1}H resonances at 3.0 and 1.9 ppm that are used for identifying this metabolite in an "edited" ^{1}H MRS in vivo spectrum

Finally, spectral editing and 2D techniques can allow identification of numerous metabolites, not identified on simple ^{1}H MRS spectra. For example, analyses of vitamin C, glutathione (GSH/GSSG), and gamma-aminobutyric acid (GABA) are possible, even though these small molecules are not visible using routine clinical acquisitions. GABA is the main inhibitory neurotransmitter in the human central nervous system, reducing neuronal excitability. Using spectral editing, the frequency-specific coupling of GABA can be used to detect it. The GABA signal at 3.0 ppm is coupled to the signal at 1.9 ppm, whereas the signals of other metabolites at 3.0 ppm (e.g., Cr) are not coupled to signals at 1.9 ppm. The structure of GABA and the coupled spins used are shown in Fig. 4.8. If a frequency-selective pulse is applied at 1.9 ppm, this will have an indirect effect on the signals at 3.0 ppm, via proton-proton coupling. If two sequences are performed, with and without this frequency-selective pulse, the difference between these spectra will yield an "edited" spectrum containing only the coupled signals corresponding to GABA. This editing approach is also known as J-difference editing and was the first method used to specifically detect GABA.

4.2.2 Ramping Up the Signal: Hyperpolarized MRS

Despite the success of ^{1}H MRS in studying basic metabolism and its perturbations, there are some limitations of this technique. As one can see looking at the *in vivo* brain ^{1}H spectrum in Fig. 4.4a, one concern is that it's a bit crowded, with most metabolites of interest falling into a narrow range (approximately 3 ppm). This overlap of key resonances has been addressed by spectral editing as previously discussed, as well as by 2D MRS studies, analogous to those used in solution NMR to study proteins and other biomolecules. One approach is to consider other half-spin nuclei, whose sensitivity can be enhanced by enrichment and hyperpolarized techniques. In particular, ^{13}C is of special relevance in studying the flux through glycolysis and other basic metabolic pathways. However, study of ^{13}C nuclei in situ is not possible at clinically relevant imaging times, due to low natural abundance (1.1% of C is the NMR-detectable ^{13}C nucleus), gyromagnetic ratio, and concentrations of metabolites of interest.

Recently, the study of ^{13}C nuclei in vivo has been enabled by a new spectroscopic imaging method, namely, hyperpolarized (HP) ^{13}C MRS. "Hyperpolarization" refers to the enhancement of a spin polarization of a nucleus beyond that is seen at thermodynamic equilibrium. Nuclei in small-molecule metabolites of interest have been hyperpolarized using two techniques, dynamic nuclear polarization (DNP) and PASADENA. While the PASADENA method has the benefit of rapid polarization times, the DNP technique has the advantage of being applicable to a broad range of chemistries and metabolites.

The physics of DNP are beyond the scope of this chapter and are discussed elsewhere [15].

As early as 1953, Overhauser described the key finding of DNP, namely, that the heating of one spin system could lead to cooling of another. In the solid state at low temperatures, high electron polarizations could be transferred to nuclei via microwave irradiation, at frequencies close to the resonance frequency of the electron spin. Subsequently, de Boer demonstrated that through thermal contact between nuclear and electronic spins, dynamic nuclear polarization is produced. The mechanism requires an unpaired electron source or electron paramagnetic agent (EPA), often an organic free radical. In comparison to thermal equilibrium polarization, approximately 2.47 ppm (0.000247%) for a ^{13}C sample in a 3 T clinical magnet, very high polarizations can be obtained in the solid state using this method, up to 50%. The hyperpolarization field was revolutionized by technology allowing fast heating/melting of the frozen sample (dissolution), with retention of spin polarization in solution. This was accomplished only recently by Ardenkjaer-Larsen et al. [16]. Following this development, the hyperpolarized ^{13}C MRS field has progressed rapidly, used to explore transient chemical phenomena in solution and complex biologic systems.

In the DNP polarizer, at moderate magnetic field strength (up to 5 T) and liquid helium temperatures (1 K), electron spin polarization is at unity. Using microwave irradiation, transfer of electron spin polarization is accomplished by microwave irradiation, with the solid-state polarization reaching a maximum in 1–2 h for most samples. Following dissolution, *in vitro* and *in vivo* applications must be performed rapidly to minimize T_1-dependent loss of signal. At a time corresponding to the T_1 of the polarized nucleus, only 37% of the original hyperpolarized signal is present. For example, the T_1 of the C_1 carbon of pyruvate is approximately 60 s; thus, there is 37% of the original signal present at 60 s and 14% at 120 s. Therefore, the kinetics of the interrogated system must be extremely rapid, and most solution and *in vivo* HP ^{13}C MR studies are performed the first 1–2 min following dissolution. For *in vivo* MR studies, special hardware is required to transmit and receive radiofrequency signals at the ^{13}C frequency. These exams are often performed using a dual-tuned coil used to acquire ^{1}H anatomical imaging, for correlation of ^{13}C spectra to organs/tissues of interest.

There are many unique features of HP ^{13}C studies, which are inaccessible using routine spectroscopic imaging. First, due to the extremely low signal of thermally polarized ^{13}C in situ, there is essentially no background. Second, this technology allows visualization of metabolism in real time, with introduced hyperpolarized substrate A being converted to its metabolic product B, detected by chemical shift. As stated previously, differences in chemical shift are highly specific and reproducible. Both dynamic and single-time-point studies are typically performed, as shown in Fig. 4.9 [17]. In this example, hyperpolarized [1-^{13}C] pyruvate was hyperpolarized and injected into a rat with a brain tumor orthotopic xenograft. First, a dynamic experiment was conducted where a 15 cm axial slab was excited with a low-flip-angle (5°) pulse and a 3 s repetition time. HP pyruvate then underwent enzymatic conversion and its metabolic products (lactate 183 ppm, and alanine 176.5 ppm) observed as they formed in real time. This type of experiment is used to determine the timing of single-time-point studies. Here the researchers chose to initiate the 2D MRSI sequence at 20 s after the start of the pyruvate injection. Analysis of the 2D data shows differential metabolism to HP lactate corresponding to the site of tumor implantation. This abnormal flux of HP pyruvate to HP lactate is consistent with the Warburg mechanism and correlates with the higher concentrations of steady-state lactate often seen in tumor, observed in situ using ^{1}H MRS.

A decade after the first demonstration of dissolution-DNP by Ardenkjaer-Larsen et al. [16], metabolic imaging using hyperpolarized ^{13}C pyruvate was accomplished in prostate cancer patients [18]. Importantly, this study showed that injection of hyperpolarized ^{13}C pyruvate was safe in 31 patients with biopsy-proven localized prostate cancer with a median age of 63 y. Safety was important to establish, given the difference in pharmacologic dose between ^{13}C hyperpolarized MR and other metabolic imaging technologies such as PET (the difference between

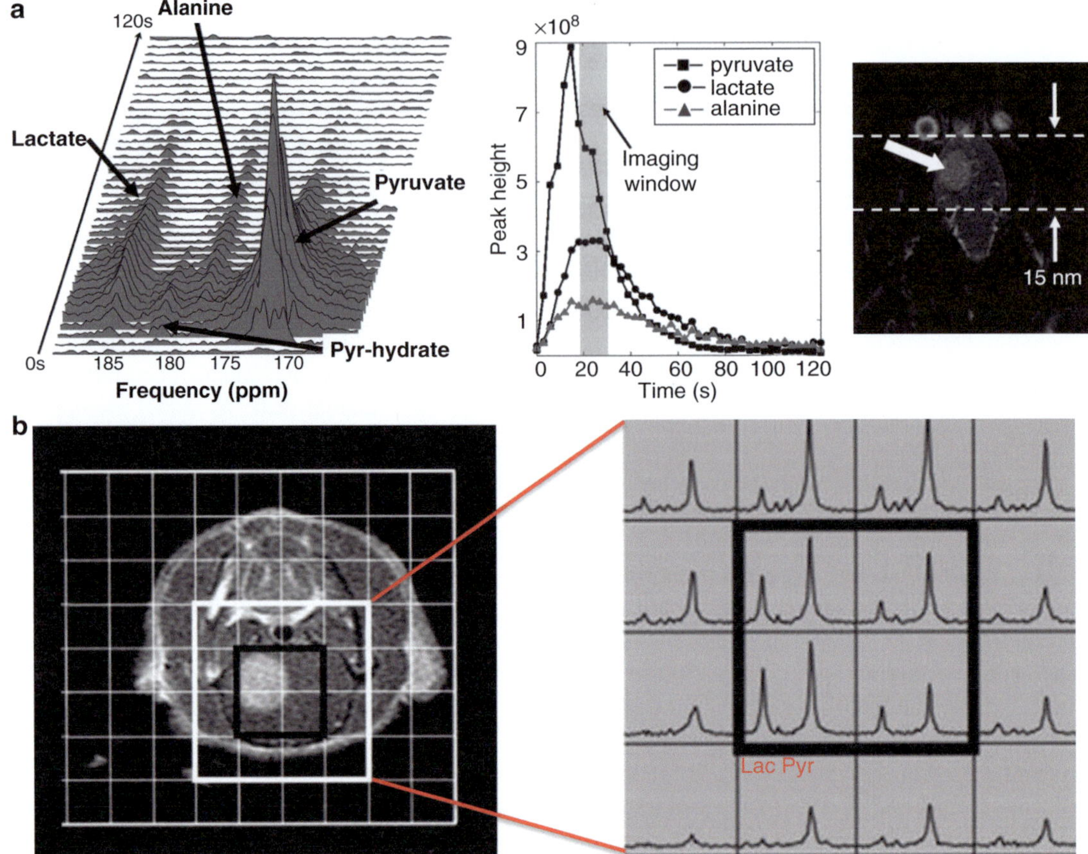

Fig. 4.9 Metabolic imaging of a brain tumor in a rat using hyperpolarized ^{13}C spectroscopy. In all cases HP ^{13}C pyruvate was injected intravenously and its metabolic products ^{13}C lactate and ^{13}C alanine observed. (**a**) Dynamic ^{13}C spectra (obtained every 3 s) obtained through a 15 mM slab of a tumor-bearing rat brain. These data showed the ^{13}C Lac signal reaching a maximum around 20–30; thus, this time window was chosen for spatially resolved studies. (**b**) The anatomic location of the ^{13}C pyruvate to ^{13}C lactate conversion was investigated using 2D CSI. In this case increased ^{13}C lactate was seen in voxels corresponding to tumor

hyperpolarized ^{13}C pyruvate and ^{18}F-FDG doses is on the order of 10^7). Both two-dimensional dynamic MRSI and single-time-point MRSI were demonstrated, showing that in many cases the observed hyperpolarized ^{13}C lactate metabolite accurately reflected the presence, location, and size of cancer relative to surrounding benign tissues. A study performed using the highest hyperpolarized ^{13}C pyruvate dose is depicted in Fig. 4.10. Significantly, in several cases hyperpolarized ^{13}C MRS revealed regions of the prostate that were previously missed by state-of-the-art ^{1}H multiparametric imaging that was performed as part of the clinical trial. This study was highly promising and demonstrated the potential to use hyperpolarized MR in a variety of clinical contexts with altered glycolysis.

4.3 Chemical Exchange Saturation Transfer (CEST)

One of the main limitations of MR at thermal equilibrium is its low sensitivity compared to nuclear techniques such as PET. Until recently, MR agents used in vivo have been largely limited to limiting to relaxation agents (discussed later in this chapter). A new approach was reported by Ward et al. in 2000, describing the use of exchangeable protons to image diamagnetic species [19]. In this

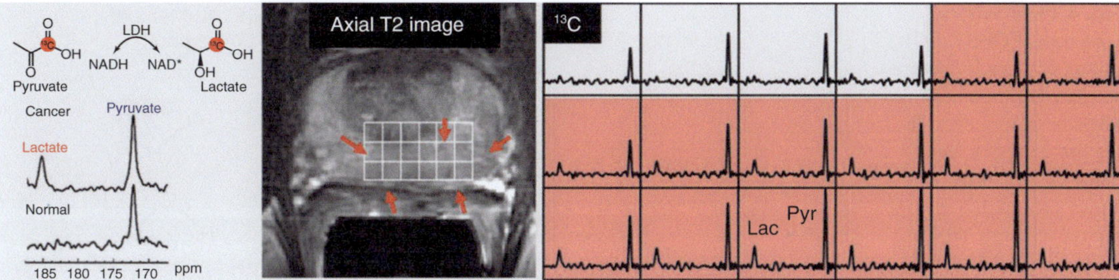

Fig. 4.10 Hyperpolarized 13C MRS study in human patient with biopsy-proven Gleason grade 3 + 3 prostate cancer using three-dimensional MRSI at a single time point. This patient received highest dose of hyperpolarized ^{13}C pyruvate (0.43 mL/kg). Axial T2-weighted image through malignant region is juxtaposed with corresponding ^{13}C spectral array, with area of putative tumor highlighted by pink shading. Increased conversion to hyperpolarized ^{13}C lactate was seen in this region, consistent with abnormalities found on multiparametric ^{1}H staging examination. *Lac* lactate, *Pyr* pyruvate, *LDH* lactate dehydrogenase, *NAD* nicotinamide adenine dinucleotide, *NADH* reduced nicotinamide adenine dinucleotide

approach, selective radiofrequency (RF) saturation of the protons of interest is used to generate contrast, detected changes in the water signal. This approach was called "chemical exchange saturation transfer" or "CEST." CEST imaging has a simple premise, as shown in Fig. 4.11 [20]. Exchangeable protons of small-molecule metabolites are selectively saturated using RF irradiation. When this saturation is subsequently transferred to bulk water via exchange, the water signal becomes slightly attenuated. Due to the low concentration of metabolite protons (at most in the mM range), a single saturation transfer event would not show any discernable effect on the bulk water (110 M) resonance. However, if a sufficiently fast metabolite exchange rate and long saturation time allow for numerous saturation events to occur, the resulting enhancement produces a discernible effect on the water signal, allowing low-concentration metabolites to be detected indirectly.

The reported applications of CEST imaging are numerous and include pH imaging and the detection of metals, enzymes, nucleic acids, and molecular recognition events. An example of an exciting recent CEST approach is glucoCEST, reported recently as an MR-based technology to rival other methods used to image glycolytic tissues, namely, ^{18}F-FDG-PET. Analogous to other CEST methods, glucose and water with thermal equilibrium magnetization are irradiated with a narrow-bandwidth radiofrequency pulse corresponding to the –OH resonant frequency, saturating their magnetization. The basic method is described in Fig. 4.12a [21]. Following rapid exchange with water protons, the transferred magnetization can be measured as a decreased water signal. This difference is amplified by continuous saturation. The resulting "glucoCEST enhancement" or GCE could be mapped as shown in Fig. 4.12b, showing GCE maps from a cross section through two mouse xenografts (SW1222), with arrows pointing to the tumor (T) and paraspinal muscle (M) regions. These studies showed significantly increased glucose uptake in the tumor relative to muscle, a finding that recapitulated the accumulation of ^{18}F-FDG.

For clinical translation of CEST, several obstacles need to be overcome in particular toxicity of exogenously administered agents and potentially high RF power deposition in magnetization transfer experiments. Clinical application requires the investigators to address the danger of too much RF power deposition when performing magnetization transfer experiments. To protect patients, the FDA has established recommended specific absorption rate (SAR) requirements, which limit the application of certain MR sequences with high power deposition. To address the toxicity problem, several endogenous molecules may be used to generate CEST contrast. Use of these endogenous compounds is a major advantage of CEST imaging. For example, the waste product urea has been imaged *in vivo*, as have exchangeable amide protons seen in mobile proteins and peptides.

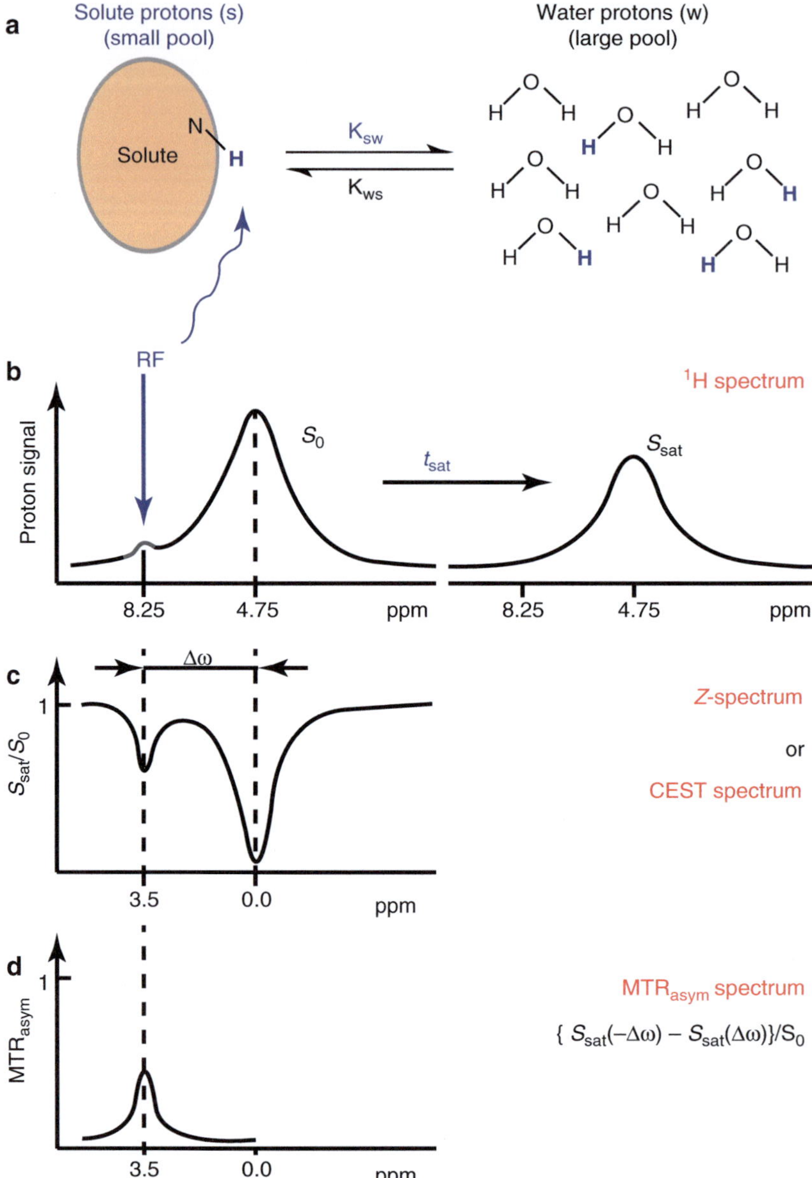

Fig. 4.11 Basic principle of CEST. (**a**, **b**) Solute protons (*blue*) are saturated at their specific resonance frequency in the proton spectrum (here 8.25 ppm for amide protons). Via rapid exchange, this saturation is transferred to water (4.75 ppm) with corresponding effect on the water signal (**b**, *right*). (**c**) Measurement of normalized water saturation (*S*sat/*S*0) as a function of irradiation frequency, generating a so-called Z-spectrum (or CEST spectrum or MT spectrum). (**d**) Result of magnetization transfer ratio (MTR = 1 – *S*sat/*S*0) asymmetry analysis of the Z-spectrum with respect to the water frequency

4.4 Metabolic Imaging: Other MR Techniques

In general, other MR-based molecular imaging methods are not targeted at metabolism per se. Other than the spectroscopic technologies previously described, clinical molecular imaging techniques are largely relaxivity-based, using perturbations of T_1 relaxation or T_2/T_2^* relaxation. There are two main types of MR contrast agents available. The first are Gd(III)-chelates and other paramagnetic compounds, used to generate positive contrast in T_1-weighted imaging. Currently, gadolinium chelates such as gadopentetate dimeglumine (Gd-DTPA, Magnevist) are widely used in MR imaging particularly in oncologic applications. These chelates have low molecular weight (<1000 Da) allowing their extravasation into tumor across leaky capillaries, producing the imaging finding of "enhancement." Since Gd-DTPA cannot traverse the blood-brain

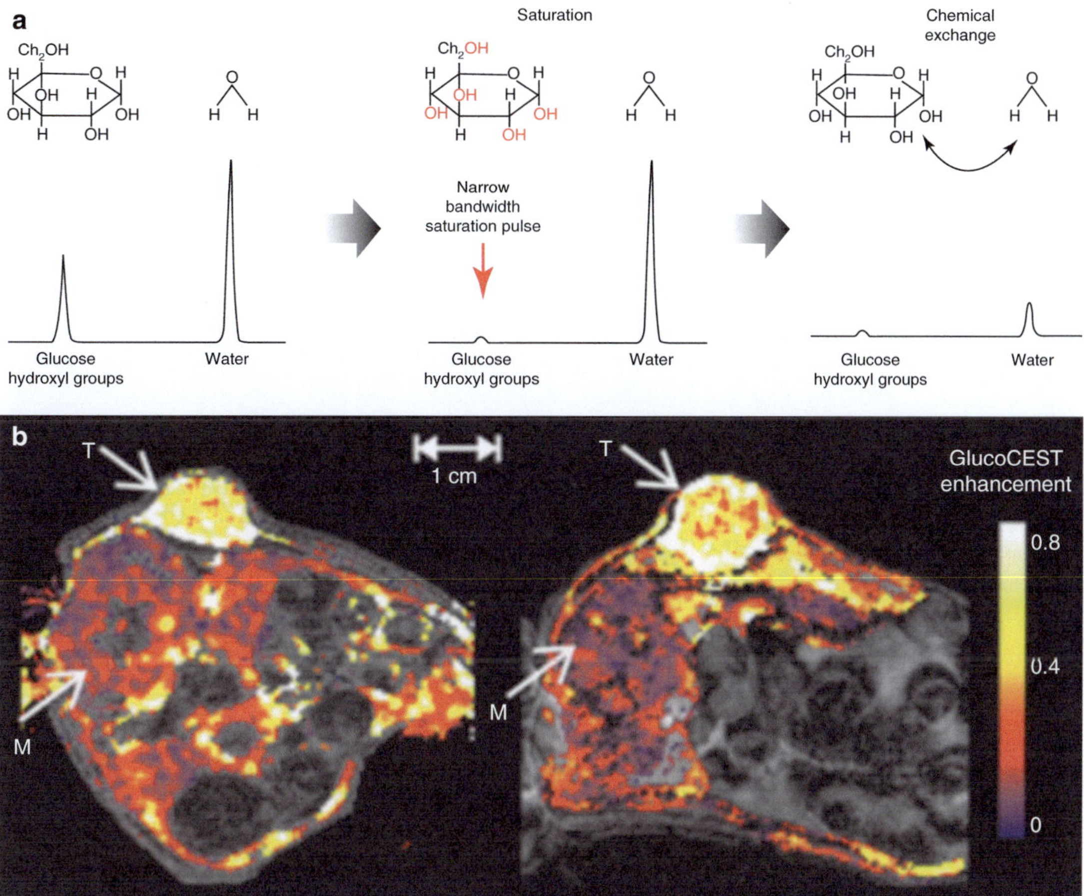

Fig. 4.12 (**a**) Simulated magnetic resonance frequency spectra with peaks corresponding to glucose (hydroxyl groups) and water. Glucose pools are irradiated with a narrow-bandwidth radiofrequency pulse centered at the hydroxyl group resonant frequency, which saturates their magnetization. These protons then exchange with water protons, transferring their magnetization and reducing the corresponding water signal. By continuously saturating the water signal, glucoCEST provides an amplification process for the glucose signal. (**b**) GCE maps from a cross section through two mouse xenografts (SW1222), with arrows pointing to the tumor (T) and paraspinal muscles (M). The color scale represents the amount of GCE, with glucose uptake higher in the tissues compared to the surrounding muscles

barrier (BBB) in the normal brain, lesion areas are easily visible in many diseases. These include areas of tumor, active demyelination, and infection (Fig. 4.13). Another type of contrast agent employs Fe_2O_3- and Fe_3O_4-derived superparamagnetic iron oxide (SPIO) nanoparticles, mainly producing *T*2-weighted imaging (*T*2WI) with negative contrast. An example is ferumoxytol, an intravenous iron preparation for treatment of the anemia of chronic kidney disease (CKD). SPIO particles potentially address some of the toxicity concerns arising from the toxicity of free Gd (III), believed to cause nephrogenic systemic fibrosis (NSF), a rare systemic disorder. In contrast to Gd-derived chelates, SPIO nanoparticles can be degraded in the normal iron recycling pathways. In addition, SPIO structures may allow for better targeting, via packaging with receptor-specific ligands.

Numerous recently developed MR approaches may allow better elucidation of metabolic pathways. These include sensors for analytes and metabolism-relevant small molecules and enzyme-sensitive MR probes. The concentrations of several analytes are tightly regulated and critical in both normal physiology and metabolic disease.

These include metals, reactive oxygen species, H^+ (protons), and others. One approach to MR-based pH sensing involves incorporation of a moiety that undergoes pH-dependent protonation and deprotonation, altering the interaction between this group and other contrast agent components. Figure 4.14 shows a reported relaxivity-based approach for pH sensing [22]. The pH-sensing MRI contrast agent NP-DO3A has a phenol group attached that when protonated results in dissociation from gadolinium. The pH- dependent relaxivity profile for NP-DO3A is shown in Fig. 4.14b, showing increasing relaxivity with decreasing pH (filled diamonds). Sensors of pH are of high interest in

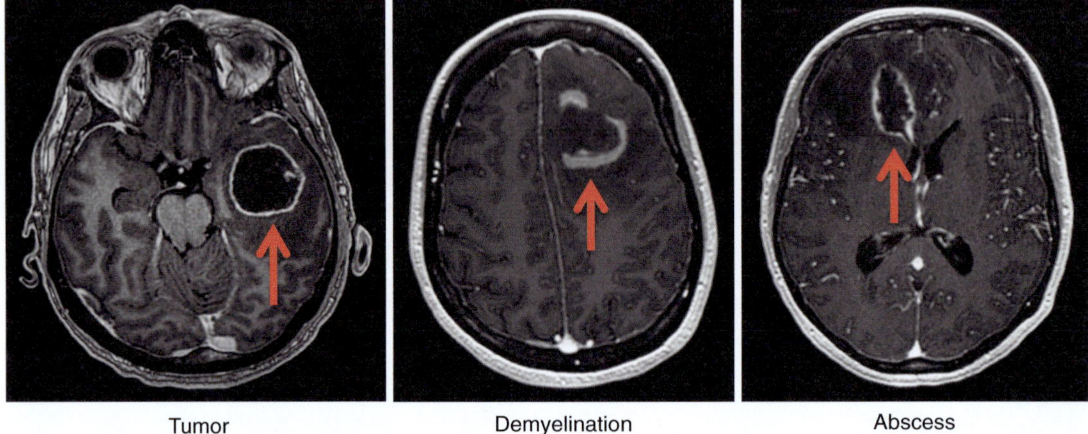

Fig. 4.13 Imaging the brain using Gd-chelates. All MR sequences are T_1-weighted, performed after administration of Gd contrast. For many processes in the brain, the blood-brain barrier is disrupted resulting in significant Gd accumulation, causing focal T_1 shortening and the imaging finding of "enhancement." These exams show three different pathologies, namely, high-grade tumor (glioblastoma multiforme), acute demyelinating disease, and bacterial abscess. These processes can sometimes be difficult to distinguish using routine ^1H methods, motivating the development of targeted approaches

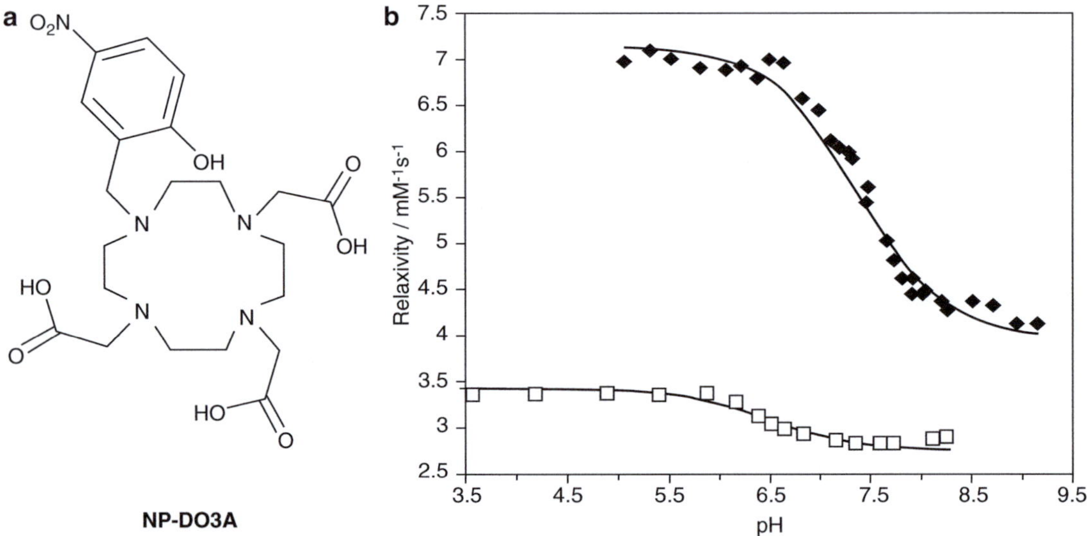

Fig. 4.14 (**a**) Structure of pH-sensing MRI contrast agent NP-DO3A. The phenol –OH dissociates from Gd when protonated (lower pH), markedly increasing relaxivity. (**b**) Relaxivity pH profile for NP-DO3A. Filled diamonds show increasing relaxivity at more acidic pH

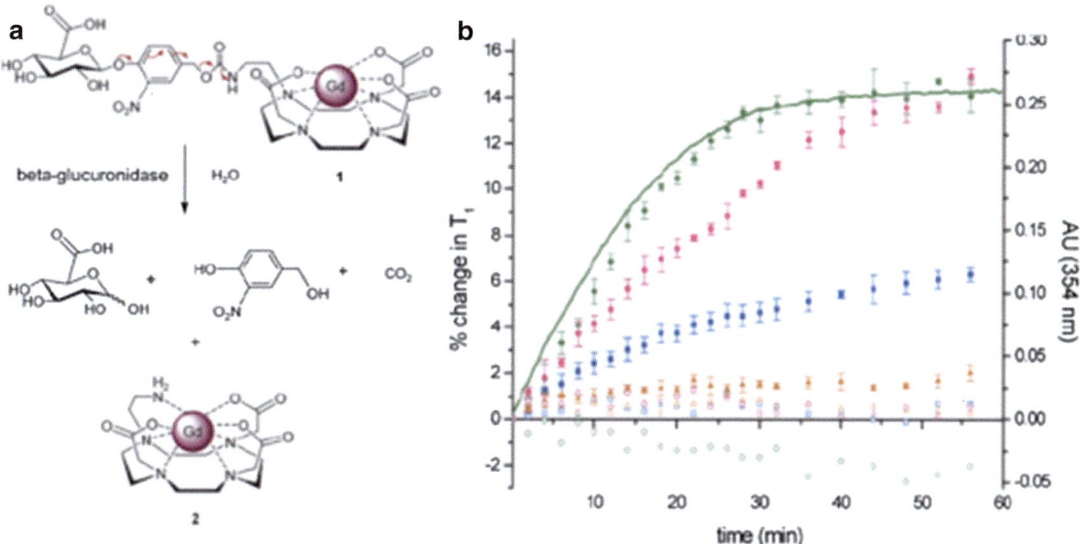

Fig. 4.15 (**a**) Strategy for sensing beta-glucuronidase activity using a gadolinium-based probe. (**b**) Hydrolysis of the agent in different buffers. No enzyme was present for all unfilled symbols. *Green* = acetate buffer, pH 5.0; *pink* = male human blood serum; *blue* = phosphate buffer with 0.01% (w/v) bovine serum albumin (BSA), pH 7.4; *orange* = phosphate buffer with 0.01% (w/v) bovine serum albumin (BSA) and 24 mM NaHCO3, pH 7.4. The effect on T1 was largest for human blood serum (*pink*)

several diseases especially cancer, for which local invasion and metastases are highly correlated with acidification of the extracellular matrix (ECM). There are several pathways for H^+ export from the cytosol into the extracellular space, which serve to maintain a stable intracellular pH, or pH_i, in cancer cells despite a greater pH gradient across the cell membrane. Important proteins involved in H^+ export and pH_i maintenance include monocarboxylate transporters (MCTs), particularly MCT4, which co-export lactate and H^+; Na^+/H^+ exchanger 1 (NHE1); vacuolar H^+-ATPases (V-ATPases); and outward-facing carbonic anhydrase (CA) isoforms, particularly CAIX and CAXII. Thus, imaging extracellular pH may provide a readout of these mechanisms, highly relevant in the metabolic reprogramming seen in cancer and other diseases.

Several of the first activatable MRI probes reported were enzyme-activated. The basic concept is relatively simple—a portion of the probe mimics an endogenous substrate, and cleavage results in a change in properties of the probe. One strategy is to develop an MR-based sensor whose degree of hydration is modulated in an enzyme-dependent way, thus affecting hydration. For example, a beta-glucuronidase sensor was reported by Duimstra et al., depicted in Fig. 4.15 [23]. This sensor consists of GdDOTA coupled to a β-glucuronic acid moiety. The enzyme-catalyzed hydrolysis of the agent is shown in different buffers, with and without the presence of enzyme. Again, the resulting change in Gd (III) chelating affects relaxivity. The β-glucuronic acid moiety is released in the presence of the β-glucuronidase, providing additional binding sites for water to the probe.

Conclusions

Magnetic resonance is a powerful molecular imaging tool and will be increasingly applied to *in vivo* biochemistry. The current interest in limiting ionizing radiation, the proliferation of high-field clinical MR magnets, and the recent development of highly innovative MR techniques will all enforce this trend. Importantly, both clinicians and researchers are realizing the synergy between MR and other imaging modalities, resulting in the development of dual imaging technologies such as PET-MR. Advanced MR methods will be developed in concert with discoveries from other fields and benefit patients suffering from a variety of disorders.

References

1. Gibby WA. Basic principles of magnetic resonance imaging. Neurosurg Clin N Am. 2005;16:1–64. doi:10.1016/j.nec.2004.08.017.
2. Plewes DB, Kucharczyk W. Physics of MRI: a primer. J Magn Reson Imaging. 2012;35:1038–54. doi:10.1002/jmri.23642.
3. Pooley RA. AAPM/RSNA physics tutorial for residents: fundamental physics of MR imaging. Radiographics. 2005;25:1087–99. doi:10.1148/rg.254055027.
4. Perman WH, Balci NC, Akduman I. Review of magnetic resonance spectroscopy in the liver and the pancreas. Top Magn Reson Imaging. 2009;20:89–97. doi:10.1097/RMR.0b013e3181c422f1.
5. Bottomley PA, Foster TH, Argersinger RE, Pfeifer LM. A review of normal tissue hydrogen NMR relaxation times and relaxation mechanisms from 1-100 MHz: dependence on tissue type, NMR frequency, temperature, species, excision, and age. Med Phys. 1984;11:425–48. doi:10.1118/1.595535.
6. Bitar R, et al. MR pulse sequences: what every radiologist wants to know but is afraid to ask. Radiographics. 2006;26:513–37. doi:10.1148/rg.262055063.
7. Gallagher TA, Nemeth AJ, Hacein-Bey L. An introduction to the Fourier transform: relationship to MRI. AJR Am J Roentgenol. 2008;190:1396–405. doi:10.2214/AJR.07.2874.
8. Skoch A, Jiru F, Bunke J. Spectroscopic imaging: basic principles. Eur J Radiol. 2008;67:230–9. doi:10.1016/j.ejrad.2008.03.003.
9. van der Graaf M. In vivo magnetic resonance spectroscopy: basic methodology and clinical applications. Eur Biophys J. 2010;39:527–40. doi:10.1007/s00249-009-0517-y.
10. Haase A, et al. MR imaging using stimulated echoes (STEAM). Radiology. 1986;160:787–90. doi:10.1148/radiology.160.3.3737918.
11. Moonen CT, et al. Comparison of single-shot localization methods (STEAM and PRESS) for in vivo proton NMR spectroscopy. NMR Biomed. 1989;2:201–8.
12. Keshari KR, Wilson DM. Chemistry and biochemistry of C-13 hyperpolarized magnetic resonance using dynamic nuclear polarization. Chem Soc Rev. 2014;43:1627–59.
13. Mekle R, et al. MR spectroscopy of the human brain with enhanced signal intensity at ultrashort echo times on a clinical platform at 3T and 7T. Magn Reson Med. 2009;61:1279–85. doi:10.1002/mrm.21961.
14. Wilson DM, Kurhanewicz J. Hyperpolarized 13C MR for molecular imaging of prostate cancer. J Nucl Med. 2014;55:1567–72. doi:10.2967/jnumed.114.141705.
15. Abragam A, Goldman M. Principles of dynamic nuclear-polarization. Rep Prog Phys. 1978;41:395–467.
16. Ardenkjaer-Larsen JH, et al. Increase in signal-to-noise ratio of > 10,000 times in liquid-state NMR. Proc Natl Acad Sci U S A. 2003;100:10158–63. doi:10.1073/pnas.1733835100.
17. Park I, et al. Hyperpolarized 13C magnetic resonance metabolic imaging: application to brain tumors. Neuro-Oncology. 2010;12:133–44. doi:10.1093/neuonc/nop043.
18. Nelson SJ, et al. Metabolic imaging of patients with prostate cancer using hyperpolarized [1-(1)(3)C]pyruvate. Sci Transl Med. 2013; 5:198ra108, doi:10.1126/scitranslmed.3006070
19. Ward KM, Aletras AH, Balaban RS. A new class of contrast agents for MRI based on proton chemical exchange dependent saturation transfer (CEST). J Magn Reson. 2000;143:79–87. doi:10.1006/jmre.1999.1956.
20. van Zijl PC, Yadav NN. Chemical exchange saturation transfer (CEST): what is in a name and what isn't? Magn Reson Med. 2011;65:927–48. doi:10.1002/mrm.22761.
21. Walker-Samuel S, et al. In vivo imaging of glucose uptake and metabolism in tumors. Nat Med. 2013;19:1067–72. doi:10.1038/nm.3252.
22. Woods M, et al. Synthesis, relaxometric and photophysical properties of a new pH-responsive MRI contrast agent: the effect of other ligating groups on dissociation of a p-nitrophenolic pendant arm. J Am Chem Soc. 2004;126:9248–56. doi:10.1021/ja048299z.
23. Duimstra JA, Femia FJ, Meade TJ. A gadolinium chelate for detection of beta-glucuronidase: a self-immolative approach. J Am Chem Soc. 2005;127:12847–55. doi:10.1021/ja042162r.

5 Metabolic Imaging Approaches: Optical Imaging

Matthew A. Wall, Tiffany M. Heaster, Karissa Tilbury, Woo June Choi, Darren Roblyer, Ruikang Wang, Melissa Skala, and Jonathan T.C. Liu

Throughout history, humans have been observing biomedical processes through optical imaging with their eyes and, more recently, through various optical imaging devices and recording media. Optical imaging is fast, relying upon the interaction of photons with tissues and chemicals, and can be sensitive to a wide range of contrast mechanisms. However, one of the shortcomings of optical imaging is the limited penetration depth of optical photons in most tissues. Nevertheless, a wide range of optical techniques have been developed to observe biological processes and structures at various depths and spatial scales, in which these two parameters typically must trade off with each other [1]. While optical imaging is most often utilized for visualizing morphological structures and their changes over time, techniques have recently been developed for the direct optical imaging of metabolic processes.

In this chapter, we review three major classes of optical imaging of metabolism: (1) the imaging of oxygenation (Sect. 5.1), which correlates with metabolic activity (here, we will separately consider methods for wide-field imaging of tissue oxygenation (Sect. 5.1.1) and high-resolution imaging of vascular oxygenation (Sect. 5.1.2)); (2) the autofluorescence imaging of redox ratios that are a direct readout of cellular respiration (Sect. 5.2); and (3) the imaging of exogenous contrast agents that report on various

M.A. Wall
Institute for Systems Biology, Seattle, WA, USA

T.M. Heaster
Department of Biomedical Engineering, University of Wisconsin-Madison, Madison, WI, USA

K. Tilbury
Department of Chemical and Biological Engineering, University of Maine, Orono, ME, USA

W.J. Choi
Department of Bioengineering, University of Washington, Seattle, WA, USA

D. Roblyer
Department of Biomedical Engineering, Boston University, Boston, MA, USA
e-mail: roblyer@bu.edu

R. Wang
Department of Bioengineering, University of Washington, Seattle, WA, USA
e-mail: wangrk@uw.edu

M. Skala
Department of Biomedical Engineering, University of Wisconsin-Madison, Madison, WI, USA

Morgridge Institute for Research, Madison, WI, USA
e-mail: m.skala@vanderbilt.edu

J.T.C. Liu (✉)
Department of Mechanical Engineering, University of Washington, Seattle, WA, USA
e-mail: jonliu@uw.edu

J.S. Lewis, K.R. Keshari (eds.), *Imaging and Metabolism*, DOI 10.1007/978-3-319-61401-4_5

metabolic parameters such as nutrient uptake, enzyme activity, local chemical environment, and cell signaling (Sect. 5.3).

5.1 Imaging Oxygenation

5.1.1 Deep-Tissue Optical Imaging of Oxygenation

5.1.1.1 Introduction

While the ability of optical microscopy to image with subcellular resolution at relatively superficial tissue depths (typically <1 mm) is well documented, optical methods are also capable of imaging deep tissue (several centimeters) under certain conditions. Practically, imaging more than several hundred microns in tissue depth requires dealing with photons that have scattered tens, hundreds, or thousands of times during their traverse through a dense matrix of cellular and extracellular materials including cellular organelles, matrix structures, and many other components, each with different optical indices of refraction (IOR). Each transition from a material of one IOR to a different IOR alters the direction of photon travel, and the aggregate outcome of these multiple scattering events is a generalized blurring effect and degradation of the ability to resolve tissue structures. In fact, optical scattering plays such a dominant role in tissue that after a short photon travel distance (called the transport mean free path (MFP), typically ~1–2 mm in human tissues), photons *diffuse* nearly isotropically, losing the memory of their initial trajectory into the tissue [2]. Because of this, the study of multiply scattered photons in biological tissue is called *diffuse optics*, and although there is a continuing challenge to extract higher-resolution spatial information with diffuse optical techniques (see section 5.1.2.1 on photoacoustic microscopy), there are also enormous benefits to utilizing these deep traveling photons to probe and monitor human tissue. Some of these benefits include the ability to interrogate tissue up to several centimeters below the skin and the ability to extract key metabolic and molecular information from tissue without the use of exogenous probes. Additionally, light-tissue interactions are generally safe as visible and near-infrared photons are nonionizing and light levels are typically well below thermal damage thresholds. Finally, instrumentation is generally cost-effective and portable, and sometimes even wearable. A brief overview of the key aspects of diffuse optical spectroscopy, imaging, and tomography (DOS, DOI, and DOT) is covered here as well as an overview of two emerging application areas: chemotherapy monitoring in breast cancer patients and functional activation mapping in the brain.

5.1.1.2 Diffuse Optical Imaging and Spectroscopy

As photons travel through biological tissue, they encounter two fundamental physical processes, optical absorption and optical scattering. Optical absorption converts photon energy to other forms of energy (e.g., thermal/vibrational). Optical scattering alters the directional vector of photon paths. In the visible and near-infrared (NIR), together spanning a wavelength range of approximately ~400–1300 nm, scattering effects dominate over absorption effects by a factor of 10 or more in human tissue [2]. Due to the highly scattering nature of biological tissue at these wavelengths, photon propagation can be modeled as a diffusive process, where the diffusion coefficient is a property of both optical absorption (specified by the coefficient μ_a (mm^{-1})) and optical reduced scattering (specified by the coefficient μ_s' (mm^{-1})). The NIR region is particularly useful for in vivo measurements as the relatively low absorption by important tissue chromophores (e.g., hemoglobin and water) allows for deep photon penetration. In breast tissue, for example, research groups have been able to use diffuse optical techniques to measure transmission through 10 cm or more of tissue [3, 4].

One of the key features of diffuse optical technologies is the ability to separate or otherwise account for the differential effects of absorption and scattering on overall optical attenuation. For some versions of diffuse optical techniques, this allows for the extraction of μ_a values from tissue in vivo. If μ_a is extracted at multiple wavelengths spanning the visible and NIR, then it is possible to extract tissue molar concentrations of key metabolic parameters, specifically oxyhemoglobin (ctO_2Hb), deoxyhemoglobin (ctHHb), water (ctH_2O), and bulk lipid. ctO_2Hb and ctHHb can be used to extract total blood volume (i.e., ctO_2Hb + ctHHb) and tissue oxygen saturation (i.e., $ctO_2Hb/(ctO_2Hb + ctHHb)$). These parameters can be determined without the use of exogenous contrast agents, and because they are quantitative, these tissue chromophore concentrations can be tracked over time and compared between patients for diagnostic and prognostic applications.

Diffuse optical technologies may be referred to by the terms diffuse optical imaging (DOI), diffuse optical tomography (DOT), or diffuse optical spectroscopy (DOS) depending on specific measurement configuration (i.e., the number of sources and detectors and their placement on the subject and the number of wavelengths utilized) and the analysis techniques used to process raw data. Instruments vary greatly in footprint size and measurement geometry, ranging from small and flexible wearable probes to much larger setups that require an immobilized human subject during measurements. Optical light sources and detectors may be placed directly on the skin or may be directed to and from the patient using optical fibers. Diffuse optical technologies are broadly classified into three variants: continuous wave (CW), frequency domain (FD), and time domain (TD). CW techniques utilize light sources that provide a constant output intensity during measurements, while FD and TD utilize light sources that are modulated in time or space. CW techniques are generally the simplest to implement as they do not require modulated laser sources, and the requirements for optical detector sensitivity are relaxed compared to other techniques. A major limitation of CW techniques is the inability to directly separate absorption and scattering, although relative changes in ctO_2Hb and ctHHb can be determined if assumptions or prior knowledge of the wavelength dependence of scattering are available. Figure 5.1a shows an example of a wearable CW probe that's being developed for monitoring tumor hemodynamics during chemotherapy in breast cancer patients with locally advanced disease [5]. The device was designed to be placed above a known tumor location and provide continuous measurements of ctO_2Hb and ctHHb changes over several hours over a fairly large area (approximately 6 cm × 6 cm). Surface-mount packaging of LEDs and photodiodes helps to reduce device footprint and facilitates the design of flexible optical probes that can be used in direct contact with the skin. Several previous wearable CW devices have been developed and applied for studies related to cardiology, blood oxygen saturation, and cerebral activities in human body [7, 8].

FD and TD diffuse optical techniques provide improved separation of absorption and scattering, and more direct extractions of tissue chromophore concentrations, but typically require modulated or pulsed laser sources and more sensitive detectors. TD methods require time-gated detectors and ultrafast pulsed sources. FD methods utilize laser sources intensity-modulated at single frequencies or swept through a range of RF frequencies (generally 50 MHz–1 GHz). By measuring the amplitude decay and phase shift induced by tissue at each

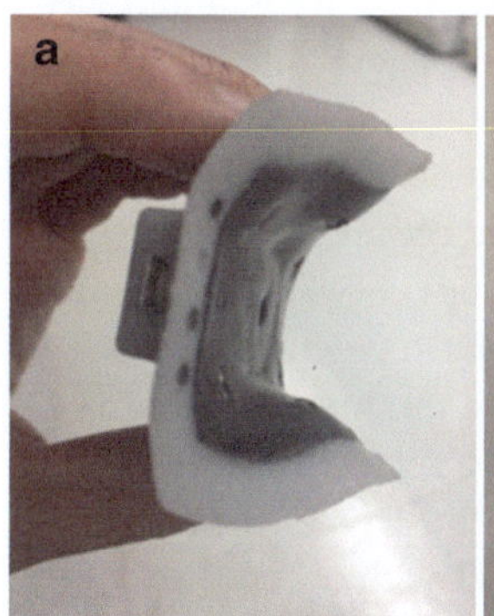

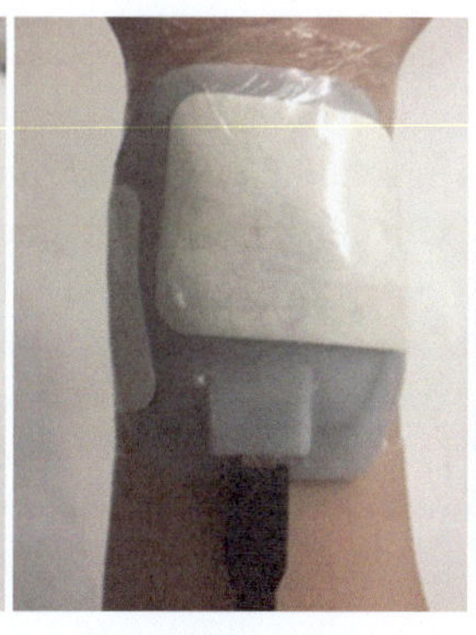

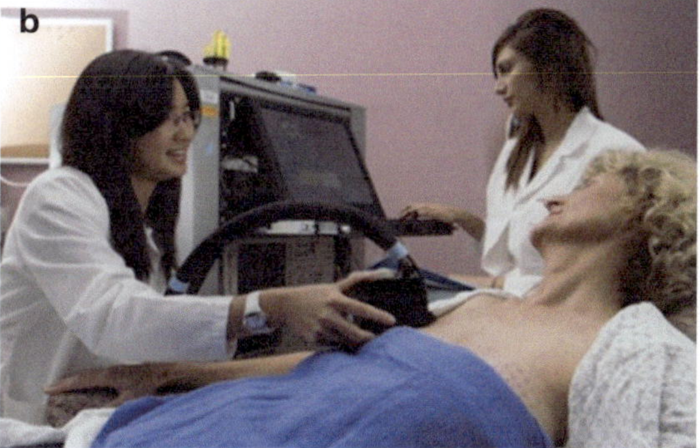

Fig. 5.1 Diffuse optical technologies have been developed for a wide range of applications. Instrument footprint varies depending on the requirements of each application. (**a**) A CW wearable probe developed for in vivo monitoring of chemotherapy response in the infusion suite for patients with breast cancer. The probe is thin and flexible to conform to the patient's anatomy. The probe is secured to the subject's skin using IV tape, demonstrated here on the wrist of a normal volunteer. Adapted from Teng et al. [5]. (**b**) A handheld CW + FD DOS probe used for monitoring breast cancer patients over weeks and months of chemotherapy. Adapted from Tromberg et al. [6]

laser wavelength and modulation frequency, μ_a and μ_s' at each of these wavelengths can be extracted. Figure 5.1b shows an example of a combined FD + CW instrument that utilizes a handheld probe that's placed on the skin of subject [6]. Point measurements take several seconds and the probe can be scanned over a known tumor location or region of interest. Topographic images of extracted chromophore concentrations can be made by interpolation between discrete measurement points. Other groups have utilized parallel-plate measurement geometries or circumferential source and detector fiber geometries for breast measurements using CW, TD, and FD modalities, often allowing for tomographic reconstructions of spatially varying chromophore concentrations throughout the breast [3, 9–12]. Diffuse optical technologies have also been combined with anatomic imaging modalities including MRI, US, and mammography to better combine spatial and functional information [11, 13, 14]. Recently there has been a growing interest in utilizing digital micromirror devices (DMDs) to spatially modulate light projected onto tissue. This mode of light modulation can be used for tomographic reconstructions in thick tissue or for mapping spatially varying optical properties over a wide-field area using a technique called spatial frequency-domain imaging (SFDI) [15, 16]. For an excellent in-depth discussion of diffuse optical instrumentation and techniques, we refer the reader to the recent review by Durduran et al. [17].

5.1.1.3 Diffuse Optics for Monitoring Metabolic Tumor Response to Chemotherapy in Breast Cancer

There is significant interest in applying diffuse optical technologies to tracking the metabolic response of breast tumors during chemotherapy. The optical absorption of breast tissue in the NIR is sufficiently low to allow for tracking of tumors embedded deep (several centimeters) within the breast. Diffuse optical measurements reveal metabolic information relating to tissue vascularity, oxygen utilization, tissue density, and biochemical composition, and in contrast to other medical imaging technologies, such as computed tomography (CT) and positron emission tomography (PET), diffuse optical spectroscopic imaging (DOSI) uses nonionizing radiation, has fast acquisition times, requires no external contrast agents, and is relatively inexpensive. These advantages allow for longitudinal studies in which subjects can be imaged weekly or even daily, suggesting diffuse optical technologies may be beneficial in the clinical care and management of these patients, especially at the bedside.

There are a growing number of studies showing that diffuse optical techniques are capable of tracking and predicting outcomes based on oxygenation and other metabolic changes in breast cancer patients receiving neoadjuvant (presurgical) chemotherapy (NAC). Patients treated with NAC are typically diagnosed with locally advanced tumors approximately 2 cm in diameter or larger. Treatment regimens vary in length and in the specific drug cocktails utilized, but most patients are treated for several months with a combination of cytotoxic drugs as well as targeted agents dependent on molecular biomarker status (e.g., Herceptin is given to HER2/neu-positive patients). A variety of diffuse optical instruments have been employed to track tumor hemoglobin, water, and lipid changes during treatment, including FD techniques [18–21], TD techniques [22], and CW techniques [23]. Most studies have found that drops in ctO_2Hb, ctHHb, and total hemoglobin are predictive of a pathologic complete response (pCR) [22, 24, 25]. pCR is an important study endpoint as it has been shown to correlate with longer-term survival [26]. Figure 5.2 shows a single patient tracked over 8 weeks of NAC with a TD DOT system. A substantial decrease in ctO_2Hb is visually apparent by week 4 and week 8, a trend that was consistent among patients achieving pCR in the study [22]. Several studies have indicated that decreases in tumor water content and increases in lipid content are predictive of pCR [27]. A recent study of 41 subjects also found that baseline tumor oxygenation was substantially different in the tumors of patients who went on to achieve pCR versus those that had a partial or no response [28]. Higher tissue oxygen saturation was correlated with a better response, and when tumor oxygen saturation was combined with estrogen receptor status in a statistical model, a high classification accuracy was achieved for discriminating pCR versus non-pCR (sensitivity 100%, specificity 85.7%). Similar results by other groups have also been reported [20, 23].

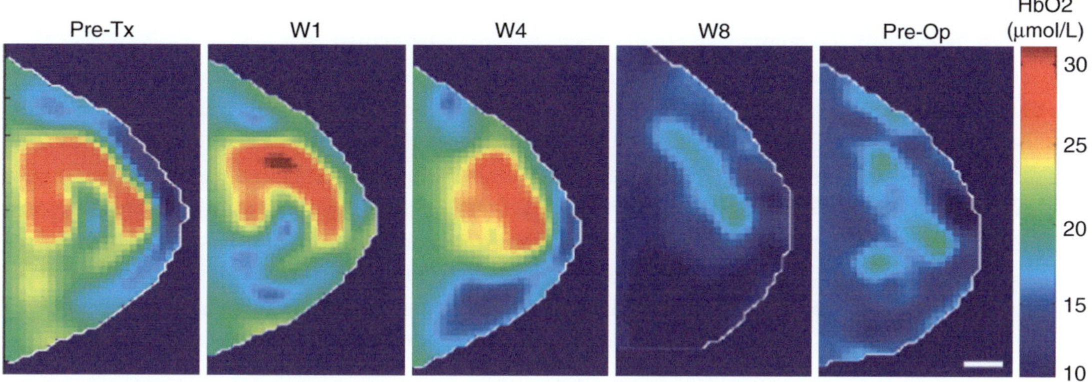

Fig. 5.2 Tomographic reconstructions of a breast cancer patient undergoing neoadjuvant chemotherapy. TD DOT measurements were taken prior to the start of treatment and then at weeks 1, 4, and 8 and prior to surgery. Tumor oxyhemoglobin levels drop substantially by weeks 4 and 8 and prior to surgery. This is a common observation in patients who respond favorably to treatment. Adapted from Falou et al. [22]

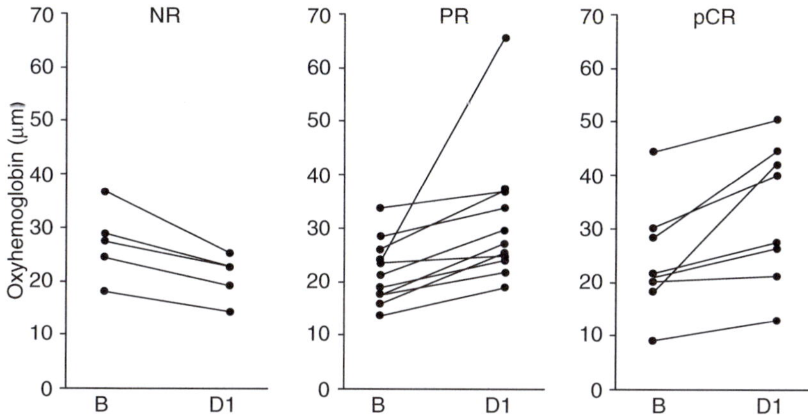

Fig. 5.3 Changes in oxyhemoglobin levels from baseline to 24 h after a first chemotherapy infusion in 24 tumors from 23 breast cancer patients receiving neoadjuvant chemotherapy. Patients who did not respond (NR) to treatment (i.e., less than 50% reduction in tumor size over the entire course of chemotherapy) had a drop in oxyhemoglobin on Day 1. Patients with a more favorable response (i.e., either a partial response (PR) or pathologic complete response (pCR)) had an increase, or flare, in oxyhemoglobin levels on Day 1. Adapted from Roblyer et al. [29]

While most prior studies have been focused on changes in tissue chromophore concentrations occurring after several weeks of treatment, newer studies have reported that changes in oxygenation and hemoglobin concentration earlier during treatment may correlate with response [18, 29]. A recent study reported that ctO_2Hb changes on the first day after an initial chemotherapy infusion could statistically differentiate responders from nonresponders (see Fig. 5.3) [29]. Patients that went on to achieve a favorable response (partial or pCR) had an increase, or flare, in tumor oxygenation 24 h after infusion. This highlights the potential importance of tracking tumor oxygenation during treatment.

5.1.1.4 Diffuse Optics for Tracking Oxygenation Levels in the Brain

DOI and DOT have been used extensively in the brain. It should be noted that NIR diffuse optical technologies are often referred to by the term near-infrared spectroscopy, or NIRS, for applications in the brain. NIR light can penetrate the skull and into the cortex and has been used for a substantial number of functional studies of the human visual cortex, auditory cortex, sensorimotor regions, and others [30–33]. Diffuse optical technologies provide oxygenation information that expands upon the information content available with the blood oxygen-level dependent (BOLD) signal achieved with fMRI. The BOLD signal is primarily dependent on ctHHb levels, while diffuse optical measurements provide ctO_2Hb, ctHHb, total blood volume, and tissue oxygen saturation levels. Figure 5.4 shows an instrumentation setup for a CW DOT system with 24 sources (LED pairs) and 28 detectors designed to measure fast functional activation in the human visual cortex with high spatial resolution [34]. The system provides 13.2 × 6.6 cm functional maps of visual cortex activation at a 12-Hz frame rate and provided data in good agreement with fMRI and PET retinotopic maps.

5.1.1.5 Diffuse Optics for Small Animal Imaging

There is an effort to reproduce the clinical observations described in the prior sections in small animal models to better control experimental setups and to help determine the molecular and cellular correlates of these observations. Both probe- and imaging-based diffuse optical systems have been used to track oxygenation and metabolism in small animal tumor models during chemotherapy [35]. Figure 5.5 shows an

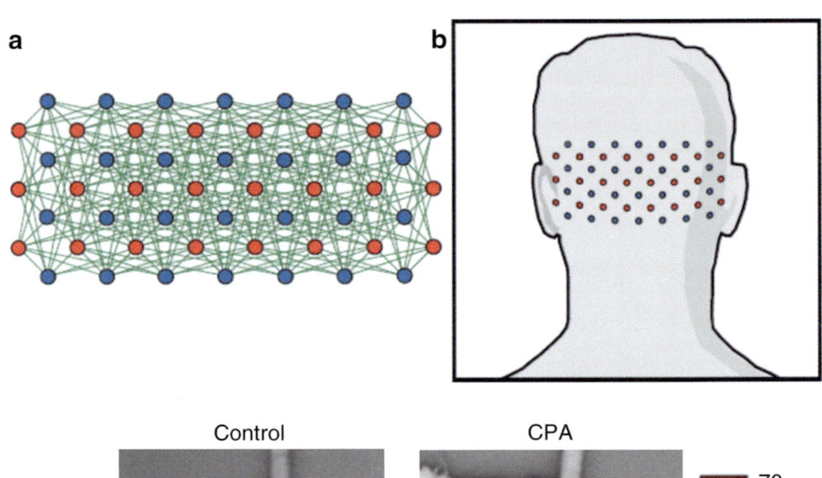

Fig. 5.4 A CW DOT measurement configuration for retinotopic mapping of the visual cortex. This system has 24 sources (LED pairs) and 28 detectors and collects data at a 12-Hz frame rate. Adapted from Zeff et al. [34]

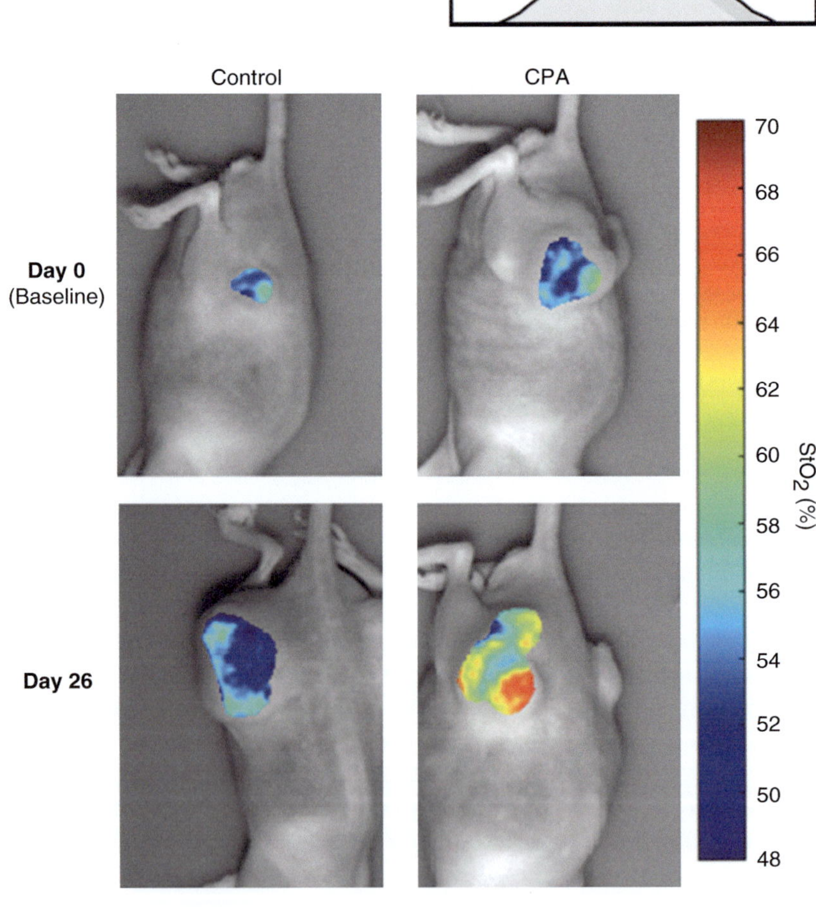

Fig. 5.5 Prostate xenograft tumor models longitudinally tracked during chemotherapy using spatial frequency-domain imaging (SFDI). Hemodynamic information is only shown on the tumor region. In untreated mice, tumor oxygen saturation (StO_2) decreased as tumors grew larger. Treated mice were given three cycles of cyclophosphamide over a period of 18 days. Day 26 is shown in the figure, which corresponds to treatment rebound. Compared to controls, treated mice had a substantial increase in tumor oxygen saturation (StO_2) in this time period

example of a small animal prostate tumor xenograft model before and after treatment with the cytotoxic/antiangiogenic cyclophosphamide/DC101. Spatial frequency-domain imaging (SFDI) was used to collect wide-field maps of tumor oxygenation. Significant changes in oxygenation are apparent after multiple cycles of treatment. SFDI has also been used for tracking drug delivery in the brain and for oxygenation monitoring in mouse models of Alzheimer's disease [36, 37].

5.1.2 High-Resolution Imaging of Blood Oxygenation *In Vivo*

Functional blood carries oxygen to cells and tissues to maintain their metabolic activities. Blood oxygen levels are an important indicator of how effectively oxygen is carried by hemoglobin and consumed due to tissue metabolic demands. Hemoglobin oxygen saturation (sO_2) is one of the key parameters to describe the amount of oxygen in the blood. More specifically, it is defined as the percentage of oxygenated hemoglobin (HbO_2) compared to the total amount of hemoglobin (HbT) in the blood (oxygenated hemoglobin (HbO_2) + deoxygenated hemoglobin (HbR)). Imaging sO_2 is important for understanding tissue metabolism and hemodynamics. It is also invaluable for many applications such as evaluating brain activities, the healing process of wounds, and the effects of chemotherapy on tumors. In this chapter, we provide an overview of three types of high-resolution optical imaging modalities to image blood oxygenation in functional vessels. The abilities of noninvasive optical imaging techniques to visualize and quantify the chromophore concentration in single blood vessels are described and demonstrated through *ex vivo* and *in vivo* experimental findings.

5.1.2.1 Photoacoustic Microscopy

Photoacoustic microscopy (PAM) is a label-free functional imaging technique that utilizes optical absorption contrast along with ultrasonic detection through the photoacoustic (PA) effect that was first discovered by Alexander G. Bell in 1880 [38]. PAM imaging detects wideband (50 MHz) acoustic waves emitted as a result of transient thermoelastic expansion due to short pulses (pulse duration of 6 ~ 7 ns) of optical energy (~100 nJ) that is absorbed by certain molecules (hemoglobin or melanin) in biological tissues [39]. The acoustic waves are then detected with a focused ultrasonic transducer. As the magnitude of the photoacoustic wave is proportional to the local optical energy deposition (optical absorption), the detected PA signals provide image contrast based on the distribution of optical absorbers. Typically, the axial resolution and lateral resolution of PAM are determined by the central frequency and bandwidth, as well as the NA (focal diameter) of the ultrasonic transducer [39]. Using a high central frequency, wideband ultrasonic focused transducer, PAM has achieved spatial resolution in the range of tens of micrometers with an imaging depth of ~3 mm in live animals [38, 39].

Based on endogenous optical absorption contrast, PAM is well suited for blood vessel imaging because HbO_2 and HbR in the blood are two major absorbers in mammalian tissues, where their optical absorption in the visible spectrum is typically orders of magnitude higher than the absorption from surrounding tissue (http://omlc./ogi.edu/spectra/hemoglobin/index.html). Moreover, recent studies have shown that photoacoustic imaging can be used for sO_2 imaging *in vivo* [40]. Measurement of sO_2 using PAM is similar to near-infrared spectroscopy (NIRS) [41], where the blood absorption coefficient $\mu_a(\lambda_i)(cm^{-1})$ usually can be expressed as:

$$\mu_a(\lambda_i) = \varepsilon_{HbR}(\lambda_i)[HbR] + \varepsilon_{HbO_2}(\lambda_i)[HbO_2]. \tag{5.1}$$

Here, $\varepsilon_{HbR}(\lambda_i)$ and $\varepsilon_{HbO_2}(\lambda_i)$ are the known molar extinction coefficients ($cm^{-1}mM^{-1}$) of HbR and HbO_2 at a given wavelength λ_i. $[HbR]$ and $[HbO_2]$ are the concentrations (mM^{-1}) of the two forms of hemoglobin, respectively. Since the PA signal amplitude $\Phi(\lambda_i)$ is proportional to the optical energy deposition (optical absorption), it can be expressed with a blood absorption coefficient $\mu_a(\lambda_i)$ as:

$$\Phi(\lambda_i) \propto \mu_a(\lambda_i)F(\lambda_i) = \begin{Bmatrix} \varepsilon_{HbR}(\lambda_i)[HbR] \\ +\varepsilon_{HbO_2}(\lambda_i)[HbO_2] \end{Bmatrix} F(\lambda_i). \tag{5.2}$$

Here, $F(\lambda_i)$ is the optical fluence at wavelength λ_i. In Eq. (5.2), the PA signal is related to the unknown concentrations of HbR and HbO_2 at a specific wavelength. As blood oxygen saturation (sO_2) is the fraction of HbO_2 relative to total hemoglobin (HbO_2 + HbR), the PA measurements need to be performed at two wavelengths (at least) to differentiate [*HbR*] and [HbO_2]. Assuming that the optical fluence *F* is wavelength independent, we can calculate [*HbR*] and [HbO_2] using two independent PA signal amplitudes acquired at two wavelengths (λ_1 and λ_2):

$$[HbO_2] = K \cdot \frac{\Phi(\lambda_1)\varepsilon_{HbR}(\lambda_2) - \Phi(\lambda_2)\varepsilon_{HbR}(\lambda_1)}{\varepsilon_{HbO_2}(\lambda_1)\varepsilon_{HbR}(\lambda_2) - \varepsilon_{HbO_2}(\lambda_2)\varepsilon_{HbR}(\lambda_1)}, \quad (5.3)$$

and

$$[HbR] = K \cdot \frac{\Phi(\lambda_1)\varepsilon_{HbO_2}(\lambda_2) - \Phi(\lambda_2)\varepsilon_{HbO_2}(\lambda_1)}{\varepsilon_{HbO_2}(\lambda_2)\varepsilon_{HbR}(\lambda_1) - \varepsilon_{HbO_2}(\lambda_1)\varepsilon_{HbR}(\lambda_2)}, \quad (5.4)$$

where *K* is a predetermined constant. Finally, sO_2 can be calculated as

$$sO_2 = \frac{[HbO_2]}{[HbO_2]+[HbR]} = \frac{\Phi(\lambda_1)\varepsilon_{HbR}(\lambda_2) - \Phi(\lambda_2)\varepsilon_{HbR}(\lambda_1)}{\Phi(\lambda_1)\left[\varepsilon_{HbR}(\lambda_2) - \varepsilon_{HbO_2}(\lambda_2)\right] - \Phi(\lambda_2)\left[\varepsilon_{HbR}(\lambda_1) - \varepsilon_{HbO_2}(\lambda_1)\right]}. \quad (5.5)$$

The optical wavelengths are often chosen within the visible spectral region between 570 nm and 600 nm where the published molar extinction coefficients of HbR and HbO_2 at the selected wavelengths are known [40]. At the conclusion of a dual-wavelength measurement, the relative concentration of HbR and HbO_2, as well as the sO_2 value, can be calculated. Although two wavelengths are enough to determine sO_2 in principle, the use of multiwavelengths can be beneficial for reducing measurement error [40].

In 2006, sO_2 imaging with PAM was first performed on subcutaneous vessels of adult Sprague-Dawley rats using four wavelengths (578, 584, 590, and 596 nm) as shown in Fig. 5.6 [39]. In Fig. 5.6a, the static sO_2 levels were mapped for each vessel with pseudo-coloring ranging from blue to red. The blood vessels with high (0.97 ± 0.02) and low (0.77 ± 0.04) sO_2 levels in Fig. 5.6a were confirmed to be arterioles (red) and venules (blue) in a red fluorescent microsphere-perfusion image (Fig. 5.6b). This indicates that PAM is able to discern between arterial and venous blood based upon the measured sO_2 values and that PAM can quantify variations in sO_2 in different physiological states

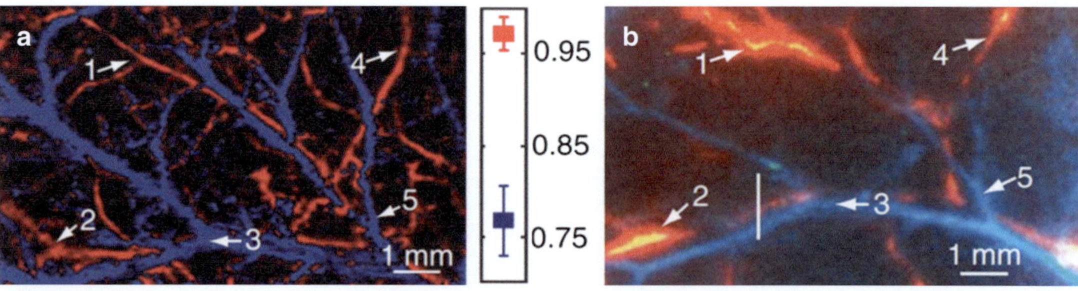

Fig. 5.6 *In vivo* functional imaging of sO_2 by PAM in a Sprague-Dawley rat [39]. (**a**) sO_2 image of subcutaneous vessels. Calculated sO_2 for each vessel is pseudo-colored to indicate high sO_2 (*red*) and low sO_2 (*blue*) values. (**b**) Microsphere-perfusion image showing arterioles (*red*) and venules (*blue*). Vessels numbered 1–5 are correctly matched with those in (**a**)

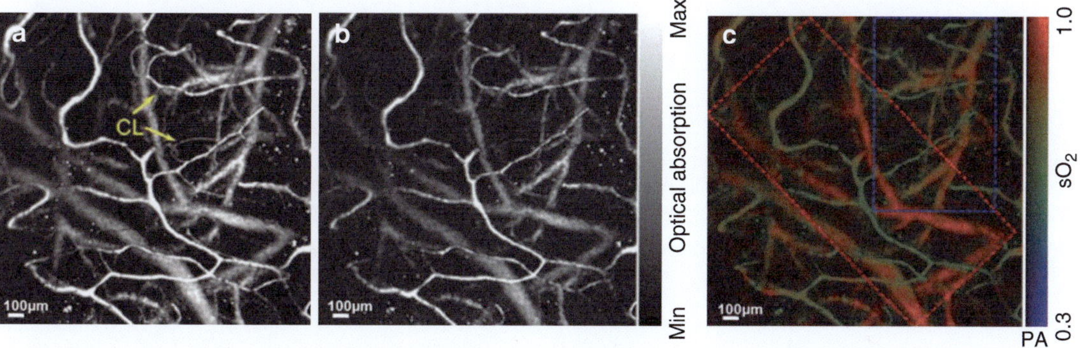

Fig. 5.7 *In vivo* transcranial OR-PAM imaging of mouse brain microvasculature under normoxia condition [43]. (**a**) and (**b**) Maximum amplitude projection (MAP) images of mouse brain acquired at 570 nm and 578 nm, respectively. (**c**) Corresponding sO_2 image. The *red* and *green* vessels are believed to be arterioles and venules, respectively. *PA*: photoacoustic signal amplitude, *CL*: single capillaries

(e.g., hyperoxia, normoxia, and hypoxia) in single blood vessels [39].

The advent of optical-resolution PAM (OR-PAM), utilizing diffraction-limited optical focusing, has enabled the imaging of hemoglobin absorption contrast at the capillary level [42]. In 2009, for the first time, OR-PAM was shown to achieve *in vivo* imaging of microvascular morphology and blood oxygenation in single microvessels of the mouse brain within an intact skull using dual-wavelength imaging (570 nm and 578 nm) (Fig. 5.7) [43].

Most recently, fast OR-PAM has been developed for volumetric, high-resolution, high-speed imaging [44]. This new embodiment of PAM, which incorporates a customized MEMS scanner and a single-wavelength pulse-width-based method, has allowed blood oxygenation imaging with capillary-level resolution at a 2-D frame rate of 400 Hz over a 3-mm scanning range and a volumetric rate of 1 Hz over a 3 × 2 mm^2 field of view [44]. Figure 5.8 shows an example of fast OR-PAM imaging of a living mouse brain through an intact skull with the scalp removed. Brain vasculature in a 5 × 10 mm^2 region of the brain was visualized at an optical focal plane located 250 μm below the skull surface. Dynamic focusing in the brain tissue, with a 100-μm z-step increment, enabled a volumetric imaging depth of 0.8 mm (Fig. 5.8b). A sO_2 image of the same mouse brain was achieved using the pulse-width-based method mentioned previously (Fig. 5.8c). Furthermore, functional OR-PAM was used to image variations in sO_2 levels in a mouse brain evoked by external stimuli as shown in Fig. 5.8d. For a 20-s long electrical stimulation of the left hind limb of the mouse, sO_2 levels in the hemisphere contralateral to the left hind limb substantially increased in the deep capillary beds (see subregions (i, ii) in (**d**)). The sO_2 increase was less pronounced in the veins and insignificant in the arteries [44]. Further estimation of the oxygen metabolism was possible with supplementary metabolic parameters derived from the PAM measurements such as the fractional change of cerebral blood flow (CBF), oxygen extraction fraction (OEF), and cerebral metabolic rate of oxygen ($CMRO_2$) as shown in Fig. 5.8e.

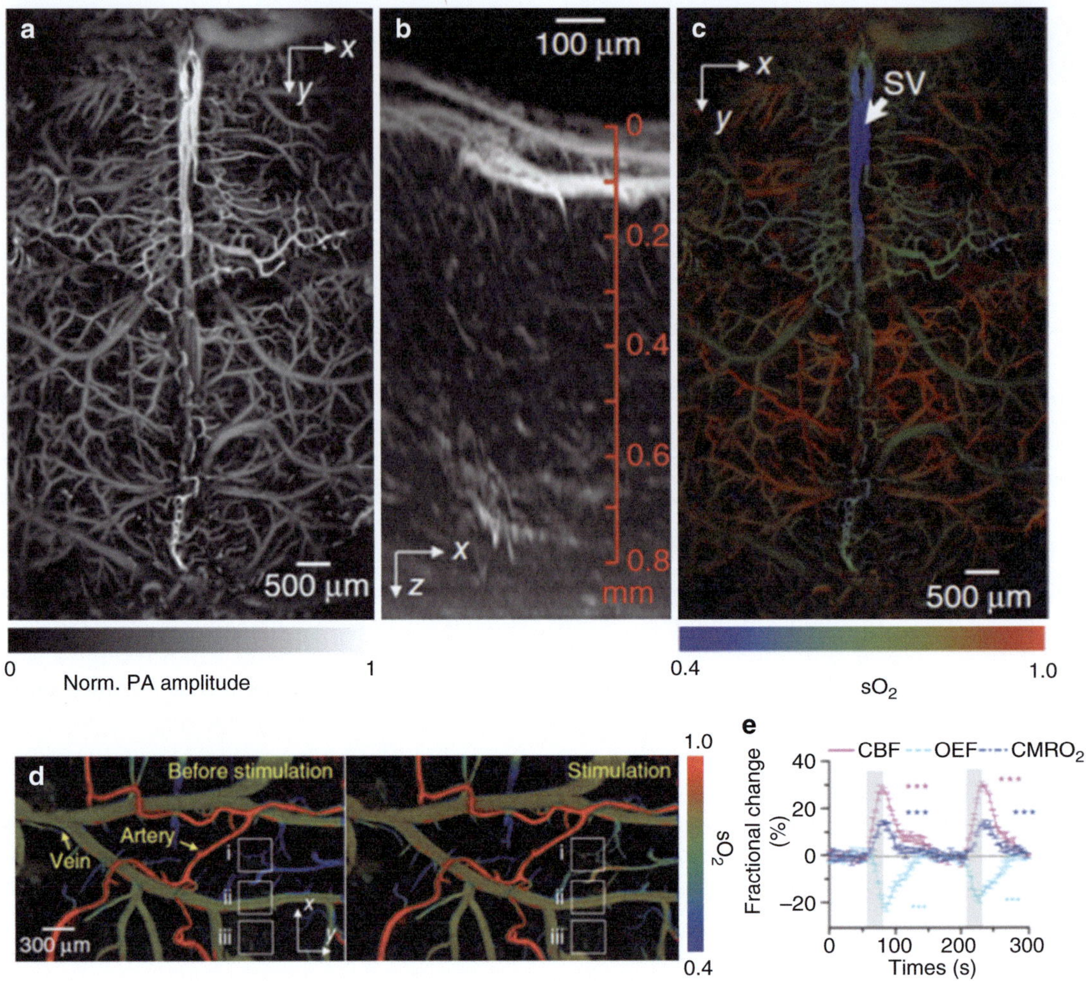

Fig. 5.8 Fast OR-PAM imaging of a mouse brain *in vivo* [44]. (**a**) XY image projection (5 × 10 mm^2) of brain vasculature through the intact skull (acquisition time: 15 s). (**b**) XZ image projection (0.6 × 0.6 mm^2) of brain vasculature. (**c**) Representation of blood oxygen saturation (sO_2) in the same mouse brain, mapped using a single-wavelength pulse-width-based method (acquisition time: 40 s). (**d**) Fast sO_2 imaging before (*left*) and during (*right*) stimulations of the left hind limb of a mouse. (**e**) Time course of the fractional changes in the cerebral blood flow (CBF), oxygen extraction fraction (OEF), and cerebral metabolic rate of oxygen ($CMRO_2$) in the core responding region that was located 100 µm below the cortical surface. The *gray* bars outline the stimulation periods (20 s)

5.1.2.2 Two-Photon and Confocal Microscopy

Fluorescence microscopic imaging techniques have also been exploited for high-resolution measurements of partial oxygen pressure (pO_2) in the cerebral microvessels of living rodents. pO_2 is another key component of the physiological state of an organ, resulting from the balance between oxygen delivery and its consumption. Disturbances in the oxygenation of tissues and organs are associated with several pathological conditions such as cancer, diabetes, stroke, etc. For pO_2 measurements, phosphorescence quenching technique has often been used in time- or frequency-domain modes [45]. This technique relies on the changes in the phosphorescence lifetime of O_2-sensitive phosphorescent probes as they are quenched by oxygen. The exogenous O_2-sensitive probes are intravenously administered as a bolus injection and confined to the vessel. Phosphorescence lifetimes typically range from 20 to 620 µs depending on the pO_2 levels (159-0 mmHg) in blood [46].

The detected phosphorescence decay signal can be expressed with a simple exponential function as [46]

$$I(t) = I_0 \exp\left(-\frac{t}{\tau}\right) + c. \tag{5.6}$$

Here, the first term represents the phosphorescence decay of oxygen dyes, containing the amplitude of the phosphorescence signal I_0 and decay time τ. The second term is a background signal that may be due to residual excitation light but is typically negligible compared to the first term [46]. Consequently, the phosphorescence decay can be calculated by applying a nonlinear least squares fitting to Eq. (5.6).

Recently, it has been suggested that combining two-photon (2P) excitation with pO_2 quantification via phosphorescence quenching could lead to a new method well suited for high-resolution pO_2 measurements [47]. *In vivo* pO_2 measurements using two-photon microscopy (TPM) were first demonstrated in the brain of small animals in 2008 [47]. Multiple points within individual vessels were selected for pO_2 measurements with two-photon microscopy, and phosphorescence decay curves were recorded at each location. As a phosphorescent probe, a commercially available porphyrin-based oxygen probe (Oxyphor R2) was excited by a 13-ns Ti-sapphire pulsed laser at a wavelength of 780 nm.

TPM has enabled depth-resolved microvascular pO_2 measurements of rat cortical vessels down to a depth of 120 μm below the cortical surface as shown in Fig. 5.9a, b [47]. The figures depict an arteriole with measured intravascular pO_2 values indicated for normoxic vessels (normal level of O_2) and hyperoxic vessels (excess supply of O_2), respectively. The pO_2 values agreed well with previously published values [48] (~40 mmHg in the normoxia case and ~60 mmHg in the hyperoxia case). Figure 5.9c is a curve fitting of the phosphorescence signals detected from the pO_2 measurement points (solid boxes) in the arterioles in Fig. 5.9a, b. The results show a quicker phosphorescence decay for the hyperoxia case relative to the normoxia case, which is due to more significant phosphorescence quenching at higher pO_2 levels (66.7 mmHg).

Confocal microscopy also has been utilized for pO_2 measurements with similar methodology as TPM [46]. Although both two-photon and confocal microscopy have offered high spatial resolution in probing pO_2 in single microvessels, the latter method was particularly effective for fast data acquisition because the single-photon excitation efficiency of phosphorescence is higher than the two-photon efficiency. In 2009, the first pO_2 measurements were reported using confocal laser scanning microscopy (CLSM) of Oxyphor R2 [46]. Figure 5.10a shows a color-coded CLSM angiogram (400 × 400 μm²) of pial vessels in the rat brain *in vivo*, obtained by integrating Oxyphor R2 phosphorescence signals. pO_2 measurements were conducted at selected

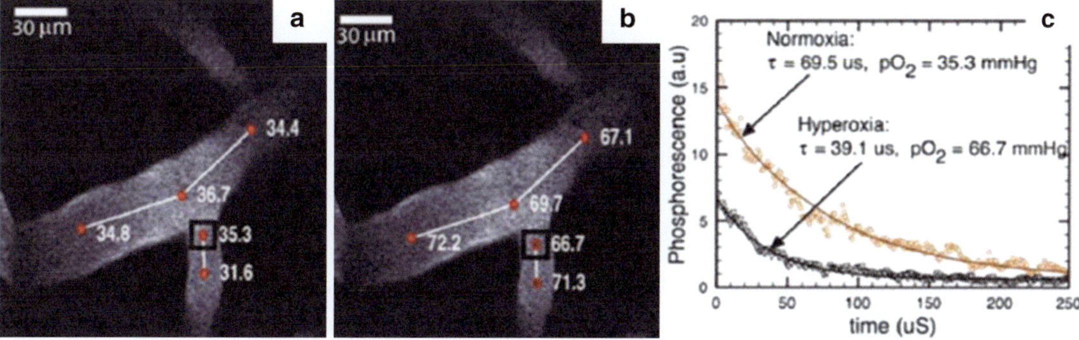

Fig. 5.9 *In vivo* pO_2 measurement of rat cortical vessels using two-photon microscopy (TPM) [47]. (**a**) and (**b**) Images of an arteriole network 120 μm below the cortical surface with intravascular pO_2 values corresponding to normoxia and hyperoxia conditions, respectively. (**c**) The phosphorescence decay profiles with best-fit curves for the highlighted points (*solid boxes*) in (**a**) and (**b**)

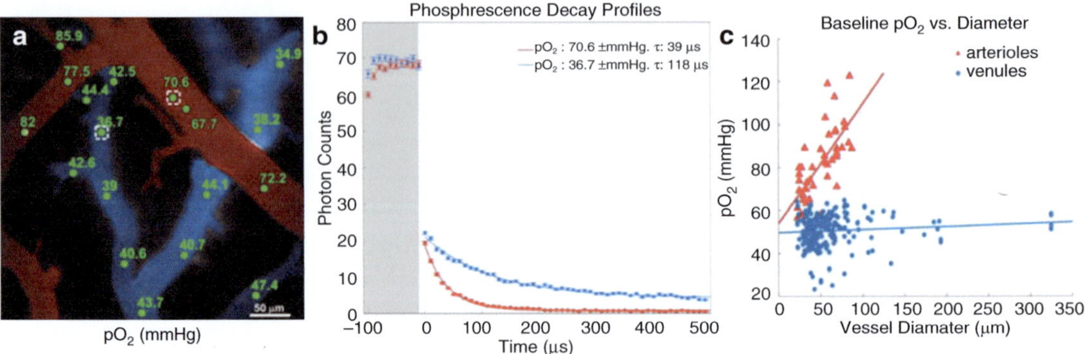

Fig. 5.10 *In vivo* pO_2 measurement of rat cortical vessels under normoxia condition using confocal laser scanning microscopy (CLSM) [46, 49]. (**a**) Color-coded CLSM angiogram (400 × 400 μm^2) of pial vessels through an open-skull cranial window. Arterioles are indicated in *red*, and venules are *blue*. (**b**) Phosphorescence decay profiles measured at the points indicated by the *dashed boxes* in (**a**). Higher O_2 concentrations in the arterioles induce more quenching of phosphorescence signal, leading to faster decay times (*red* profile). (**c**) Distribution of pO_2 values in arterioles and venules as a function of vessel diameters, measured in ten animals, showing that pO_2 varies with vessel diameter for pial arterioles but is relative constant for venules

points in the pial vessel locations (green dots), and the corresponding pO_2 levels (green values) are displayed in Fig. 5.10a. The pO_2 values could be calculated from the measured phosphorescence decay profiles shown in Fig. 5.10b. The shaded region in Fig. 5.10b represents the time frame (100 μs) during which the excitation light (at 532 nm) was transmitted to the rat brain. The graph shows that the phosphorescence decay in arterioles (red profile) has a shorter lifetime (39 μs) than the lifetime in the venules (118 μs, blue profile), corresponding to pO_2 values of 70.6 and 36.7 mmHg for the arterioles and venules, respectively [50]. The difference in the pO_2 values between the arterioles and venules is apparent in Fig. 5.10c [49]. Interestingly, arteriolar pO_2 values dramatically decreased with vessel diameter as opposed to the venules, for which pO_2 were insensitive to diameter.

For both TPM and CLSM measurements, the phosphorescence quenching techniques that are utilized can induce reactive single oxygen molecules as a reaction by-product. Care must be taken to avoid photo-oxidative damage to the vasculature and tissue from excessive single oxygen. Exposure to ambient light should be minimized by enclosing the whole system to rule out background noise from external environment.

5.1.2.3 Optical Coherence Tomography

Optical coherence tomography (OCT) is a noninvasive optical imaging technique that can measure backscattered light signals from internal tissue layers of living samples [51]. With the advantages of being able to achieve label-free, high-speed, high-resolution imaging, OCT has provided microstructural information of organs and tissues as well as functional or physiological information [52]. In 2003, OCT imaging of blood oxygenation was pioneered through the use of time-domain (TD) spectroscopic OCT (SOCT). In the SOCT measurement, a single A-scan (depth scan) was performed on whole blood solutions saturated at 0% and 100% using an oxygenator, and the absorption coefficients of HbO_2 and HbR were calculated using Beer's law [53]. Then, the same research group proposed a SOCT method to assess sO_2 by measuring the saturation-dependent differential attenuation coefficient $\Delta\mu_t$ at a pair of wavelengths (780 nm and 820 nm) within the source bandwidth [54]. They experimentally showed a negative linear correlation between $\Delta\mu_t$ of whole blood sample and sO_2.

Since the advent of Fourier domain OCT (FD-OCT), there have been several attempts to measure sO_2 that have benefited from the improved signal sensitivity and data acquisition speed of FD-OCT over TD-OCT [55–57]. Kagemann *et al.* proposed a SOCT method to assess sO_2 of human retinal blood *in vivo* with optical density ratios (ODRs) that was calculated at oxygen-sensitive (855 nm) and oxygen-insensitive (805 nm, isosbestic point) wavelengths, respectively. The optical density was defined as a measure of light absorbance from a vessel relative to the absorbance from tissue surrounding the blood vessel [55]. Unlike previous studies that utilized the crossover feature of the optical absorption spectra of oxy- and deoxy-Hb at around 800-nm wavelengths, Yi *et al.* demonstrated the feasibility of estimating sO_2 from single red blood cells (RBCs) *in vitro* in the visible wavelength band using SOCT [56]. sO_2 measurements with SOCT in the visible range are desirable because the absorption of hemoglobin is much stronger [56], but comes at the expense of limited penetration depth (a few hundred microns in tissue). Recently, this group has reported the first application of visible SOCT for the *in vivo* mapping of sO_2 in rodent retinal blood vessels [57].

While most SOCT methods are quite effective in dealing with specular reflections from surface vessels, such methods are challenging to apply to biological tissues because of wavelength-dependent speckle patterns resulting from multiple scattering events within a single resolution element, which eventually prevent reliable estimations of blood oxygenation. In spite of this, Chong *et al.* have developed a SOCT analysis method for quantitative mapping of blood oxygenation in the brain and retina of rodents using OCT angiography (OCTA) [58]. Figure 5.11 shows images of oxygen saturation, cumulative deoxyhemoglobin (LC_{Hb}), cumulative oxyhemoglobin (LC_{HbO2}), and cumulative total hemoglobin concentration (LC_{HbT}), for brain vasculature both before (a–d) and after (e–h) cardiac arrest.

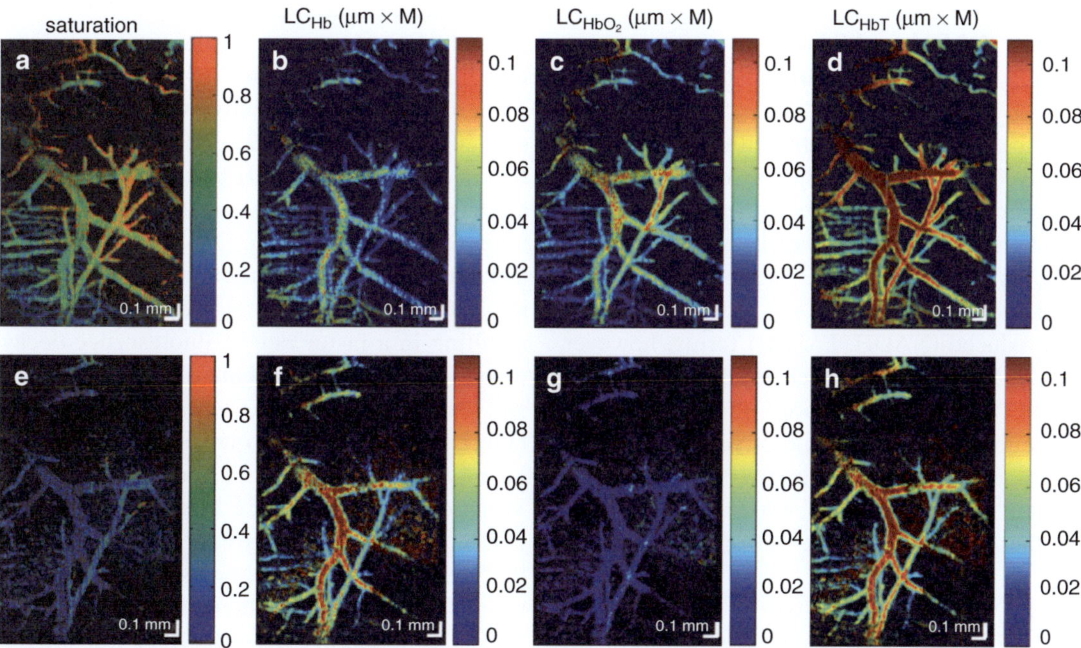

Fig. 5.11 Mapping of blood oxygenation in the mouse brain *in vivo* [58]. (**a**, **e**) Oxygen saturation. (**b**, **f**) Cumulative deoxyhemoglobin map (LC_{Hb}). (**c**, **g**) Cumulative oxyhemoglobin map (LC_{HbO_2}). (**d**, **h**) Cumulative total hemoglobin map (LC_{HbT}). Panels (**a–d**) are images obtained at baseline conditions and panels (**e–h**) are images obtained after cardiac arrest

5.2 Autofluorescence Microscopy of Metabolism

5.2.1 Introduction

Coupling microscopy with autofluorescence is appealing for studying metabolism in living tissues. This approach is advantageous because it is nondestructive and provides high-resolution structural and functional information without the need for exogenous labels that interfere with the biochemical and physiological state of the sample. Chance and colleagues completed seminal studies to characterize the autofluorescence of nicotinamide adenine dinucleotide (NADH) and flavin adenine dinucleotide (FAD) in isolated cells, and later in brain, liver, and bladder tissues [59–64]. More recently, the fluorescence lifetimes of the metabolic coenzymes NADH and FAD have been investigated in human tissues to image the heterogeneity of cellular metabolism in normal and diseased states [65–71].

5.2.2 NADH and FAD Autofluorescence Properties

NADH and FAD are intracellular coenzymes involved in adenosine triphosphate (ATP) production through oxidative phosphorylation and reactions that feed oxidative phosphorylation (e.g., glycolysis, Krebs cycle). In the cell, NADH and FAD exist in oxidized (FAD, NAD+) and reduced (NADH, $FADH_2$) forms; however, only NADH and FAD yield significant fluorescence [62, 72–74]. Notably, the efficiency of autofluorescence from both NADH and FAD is dependent on the surrounding microenvironment of the molecule (i.e., bound vs. unbound to another molecule). These molecules are generally measured in concert, due to their complementary roles in metabolism and their spectral separation. Specifically, NADH is optimally excited at 350 nm and has an emission maximum at 460 nm, whereas FAD is optimally excited at 435 nm and has an emission maximum at 535 nm. NADH has a greater quantum yield in comparison to FAD; therefore, it is associated with a greater overall fluorescence intensity. The molecules NADH and NADPH are both autofluorescent, with overlapping excitation/emission spectra and fluorescence lifetimes [65]. Previous studies have established that the autofluorescence is dominated by NADH (due to its greater quantum yield) and that metabolic perturbations due to cancer progression and drug treatment are mostly attributed to NADH [6, 8–13]. However, for accuracy, this autofluorescence is usually denoted as NAD(P)H.

Since both NAD(P)H and FAD have different fluorescent properties and vital roles in metabolism, researchers have measured these fluorophores to characterize the "optical redox ratio" (ratio of fluorescence intensities of NAD(P)H and FAD). These techniques have been used as indicators of physiological change within a cell, tissue, or organism [61, 65–71, 73, 75–77]. Recently, studies have also incorporated the NAD(P)H and FAD fluorescence lifetimes, or the time that the molecule remains in the excited state before decaying back to the ground state, to extract additional biological information. The lifetime of the fluorophore is more sensitive to the microenvironment and is able to differentiate between free and protein-bound states of NAD(P)H and FAD. Primarily, conformational changes in these molecules upon enzymatic binding result in modified decay rates. NADH in an unbound state exhibits partial quenching of its adenine side chain, resulting in a faster rate of fluorescence decay than in the unquenched, bound form. The opposite trend is observable with FAD, with its bound form undergoing quenching and, subsequently, exhibiting a faster fluorescence decay. Variations in fluorescence lifetime can also be correlated to microenvironmental changes in the presence of oxygen, tyrosine, and tryptophan or, alternatively, fluctuation in the local temperature and pH [78–80]. To appreciate the metabolic information provided by imaging NAD(P)H and FAD autofluorescence, the roles of NADH and FAD in cellular metabolism must be understood [81].

5.2.3 Role of NADH and FAD in Cellular Respiration

Cells break down glucose and other substrates in the cell to produce energy in the form of ATP through glycolysis, Krebs cycle (also known as the citric acid cycle or the tricarboxylic acid cycle), and oxidative phosphorylation [82]. Glycolytic reactions in the cell produce two molecules of NADH to serve as electron donors for the mitochondrial respiratory chain. These reactions break the initial glucose molecule into two pyruvate molecules. Pyruvate is then further converted into acetyl-CoA to enter the Krebs cycle, and FAD is reduced to $FADH_2$ during pyruvate decarboxylation. The breakdown of a single glucose molecule in glycolysis and the Krebs cycle can result in ten NADH molecules, which then donate their electrons in the electron transport chain. Maintaining an appropriate pool of NADH is critical for maintaining the required proton gradient across the inner and outer membranes of the mitochondria for ATP synthesis. Cells with elevated NAD(P)H levels have a greater potential to produce ATP through oxidative phosphorylation due to the prevalence of electron donors. Conversely, cells with high FAD and low NAD(P)H fluorescence signals have an increased demand for ATP generation and require increased oxidative phosphorylation to meet these energy demands (Fig. 5.12).

Due to the autofluorescent properties of both NAD(P)H and FAD and their role in metabolism, the ratio of NAD(P)H/FAD, known as the optical redox ratio, can be used to monitor cellular metabolism. The optical redox ratio was first demonstrated by Chance and colleagues in the 1950s and 1960s [62, 64, 72, 83–85]. This metric examines the relative abundance of NAD(P)H and FAD per cell by calculating the ratio of the NAD(P)H intensity to FAD intensity given by Eq. (5.7).

$$Redox\ Ratio = \frac{\mathrm{NAD(P)H}}{\mathrm{FAD}} \quad (5.7)$$

The redox ratio provides a global assessment of intracellular metabolic activity and can be indicative of generalized variations in metabolism across cell types and in response to perturbations [86]. For example, increased redox ratio values correlate with increased glycolytic metabolism [66, 87]. Increases in oxidative metabolism cause simultaneous consumption of NAD(P)H and production of FAD, thus resulting in a decreased redox ratio [66, 87].

In addition to the redox ratio, the fluorescence lifetimes of NAD(P)H and FAD provide a more detailed perspective of the binding state of NAD(P)H and FAD. NAD(P)H disassociation from protein provokes partial quenching of nicotinamide by the adenine moiety of the

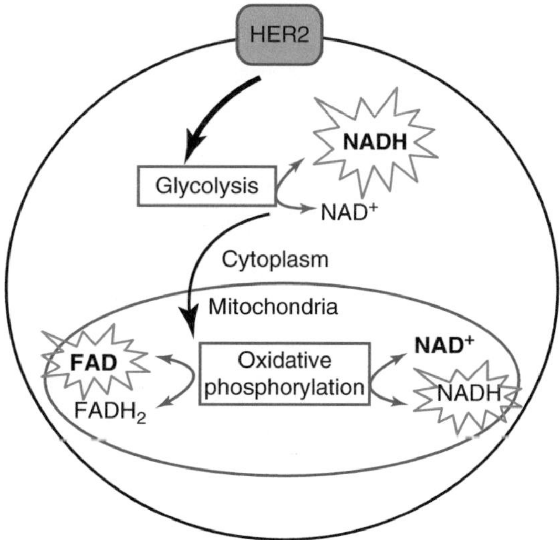

Fig. 5.12 Simplified diagram of cellular respiration to visualize the roles of the coenzymes NAD(P)H and FAD in glycolysis and oxidative phosphorylation. Specifically, this diagram shows the effect of a HER2 receptor mutation, which will drive an increase in glycolysis resulting in increased NADH. Net direction of reactions is represented here in *bold*. Figure adapted from [67]

molecule, resulting in a shorter fluorescence lifetime. When NAD(P)H is bound to a protein, the distance between the adenine and nicotinamide moieties increases, resulting in less fluorescence quenching and a longer fluorescence lifetime. The converse is true for FAD (short lifetime in the protein-bound state, long lifetime in the free state). Thus, the fluorescence lifetimes of NAD(P)H and FAD are distinct for the free and protein-bound forms of the molecule. FAD and NADH bind to several enzymes in metabolic reactions (i.e., lactate dehydrogenase, malate dehydrogenase, succinate dehydrogenase, etc.), suggesting the application of these biomarkers to identify active enzymes via lifetime signatures. However, the enzyme-specific effects on fluorescence lifetime are currently under investigation. A two-component fluorescence decay model given by Eq. (5.8) provides optimal fitting of the fluorescence decays of NAD(P)H and FAD in cells:

$$I(t) = \alpha_1 e^{-t/\tau_1} + \alpha_2 e^{-t/\tau_2} + C \tag{5.8}$$

Here, α_1 and α_2 are the fractional components of the short and long lifetimes, respectively. The long lifetime, τ_2, is the protein-bound component for NAD(P)H and the free component for FAD. The short lifetime, τ_1, is the free component for NAD(P)H and the protein-bound component for FAD. The bound component of FAD decreases in the presence of NAD+ due to increased intramolecular dynamic quenching; therefore, the FAD lifetime is sensitive to the level of NAD+ in a cell [33]. Furthermore, the mean lifetime, τ_{m}, functions as a representative metric of protein binding on fluorescence decay kinetics. This can be calculated as a weighted average of the short and long lifetime components, given in Eq. (5.9).

$$\tau_m = \alpha_1 \tau_1 + \alpha_2 \tau_2 \tag{5.9}$$

Altogether, the redox ratio and the fluorescence lifetimes provide a method to quantify dynamic changes in cellular metabolism that are useful for disease diagnosis, monitoring response to therapy, and monitoring cell function.

5.2.4 Physiological Origins of Variations in NADH and FAD

In contrast to current biochemical assays (e.g., mass spectrometry and flow cytometry), autofluorescence imaging of NAD(P)H and FAD can resolve single-cell behavior within live, intact samples without any preparation (e.g., fixing, dying). This allows for observation and quantification of metabolic changes in response to environmental stimuli. A well-defined example of this can be observed from increased redox ratios during hypoxia due to the production of NAD(P)H during anaerobic glycolysis [65, 88, 89]. NAD(P)H and FAD fluorescence are also dependent on the functional state of the cells. The fluorescence of NAD(P)H and FAD are different in proliferative and quiescent cells, terminally differentiated cells, as well as diseased cells [34, 35]. Warburg and colleagues described a preference on glycolysis in cancer cells with adequate oxygen in the 1920s, and this effect has also been noted in differentiating stem cells [65, 76, 77, 88, 90–92]. This reliance on glycolysis is also exhibited by healthy, proliferating cells, in contrast to quiescent cells. Ultimately, large changes in baseline redox ratios and lifetime components are likely more related to the ratio of catabolic to anabolic metabolism rather than simply the rate of ATP production in cells.

Cancerous cells can be characterized by distinct metabolism and response to metabolic perturbations, including anticancer drugs. Recently, consideration has been given to the effects of metabolic dysfunction and cancer onset. Inhibition of respiration pathways along with increased glycolysis correlates with cancer cell growth [92]. Past studies have examined levels of NAD(P)H autofluorescence between various cancer cell lines to determine that NAD(P)H concentration could function as a biomarker for all cancer types [65–71, 76, 77, 81]. Characteristic of tumor metabolism, decreases in protein-bound NAD(P)H were observed in the presence of dysplasia, attributed to a transition of active metabolic pathways from oxidative phosphorylation to glycolysis. These fluctuations in protein-bound

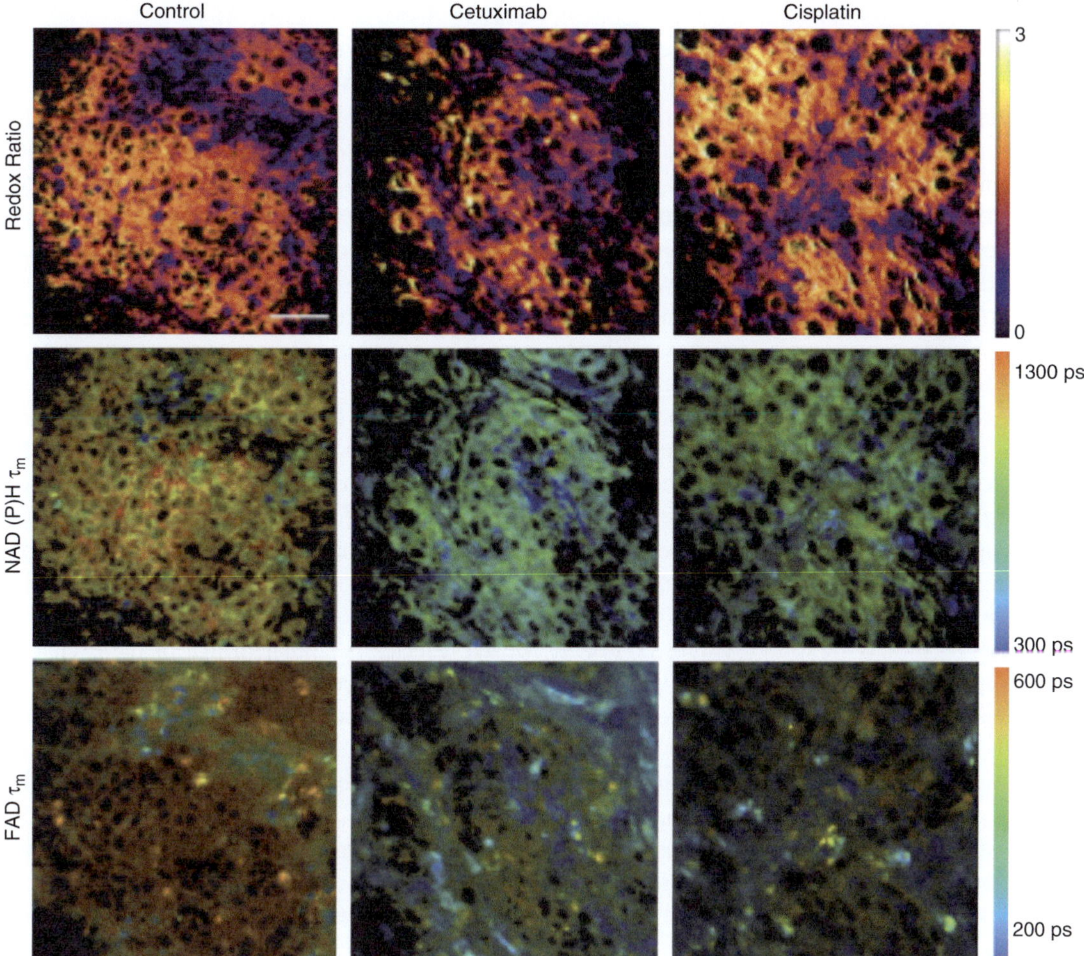

Fig. 5.13 Representative in vivo images of the optical redox ratio, NAD(P)H τ_m and FAD τ_m, of a FaDu xenograft model for head and neck cancer. The xenografts were untreated or underwent cetuximab or cisplatin treatment. The autofluorescence of NAD(P)H and FAD at this 48-h time point indicate a differential response to anticancer drugs within a treatment group, as well as a heterogeneous cellular response to treatment. Scale bar = 50 μm. Figure adapted from [71]

NAD(P)H also correlate with the severity of precancerous tissue, allowing differentiation between normal, low-grade, and high-grade dysplasia [65, 76, 92, 93]. Notably, early stage cancer growth has been identified with autofluorescence imaging of NAD(P)H and FAD [65–71, 76]. Additionally, changes in NAD(P)H and FAD fluorescence intensities and lifetimes have been quantified in response to drug treatment in cancer [67–71]. As seen in Fig. 5.13, in vivo autofluorescence imaging of NAD(P)H and FAD (or "optical metabolic imaging") in head and neck cancer demonstrates the capability of this technique to monitor heterogeneous cellular responses to anticancer therapies. These studies have identified optical metabolic imaging as a promising tool to monitor cancer progression and to assess anticancer drug efficacy.

5.2.5 Instrument Requirements for Redox Ratio Imaging

Confocal microscopy has been a widely accepted approach in the field of autofluorescence imaging of NAD(P)H and FAD, due to its enhanced resolution and capacity for optical sectioning. This technique uses a laser excitation source, typically an argon/krypton laser, with an initial pinhole aperture in the light path, to ensure a high-quality intensity profile for the excitation light. The excitation beam can then be directed via dichroic mirrors and subsequent optical components through the objective to illuminate a single point (typically) within the sample (this point is scanned to construct an image). Fluorescence emission passes back through the objective for transmission through the dichroic mirror and collection optics. A second pinhole positioned in front of the detector (e.g., photomultiplier tube) blocks the out-of-focus light from reaching the detector. This setup promotes the isolation of fluorescence signal from individual fluorophores, which is beneficial for quantifying relative concentrations of fluorophore within a sample. Overall, confocal microscopy is optimized for thin samples with high fluorophore concentrations (e.g., cell monolayers).

Multiphoton microscopy is attractive for imaging thick samples (e.g., in vivo, 3D cultures) and uses near- infrared excitation, thereby avoiding the damaging ultraviolet light that is often used for autofluorescence confocal microscopy [65]. Multiphoton microscopy uses focused infrared laser pulses to promote nonlinear excitation of photons at a localized point (voxel) within a sample, typically using a femtosecond pulsed laser (e.g., titanium-sapphire laser). As with conventional point-scanned confocal microscopy, two-dimensional images of the sample are generated by raster scanning the excitation beam and subsequently collecting fluorescence emission point-by-point via a photomultiplier tube. Due to the use of nonlinear excitation, in which fluorescence excitation is limited to a small focal volume, multiphoton microscopy achieves reduced photodamage and photobleaching compared to confocal microscopy [94, 95]. Additionally, the use of infrared laser pulses, with localized signal generation, results in deeper image penetration, an important improvement for in vivo imaging [78].

5.2.6 Instrumentation Requirements for FLIM Imaging

Recently, fluorescence lifetime imaging has gained popularity due to its sensitivity to the fluorophore conformational state and environment [65–71, 76, 77, 93]. Fluorescence lifetime measurements require (1) an excitation source that is intensity-modulated or pulsed and (2) time-resolved fluorescence detection. Fluorescence lifetime measurements can be recorded in either the Fourier (frequency) domain or the time domain, each with their respective advantages. Fourier domain fluorescence allows for shorter acquisition times and thus enhanced data collection rates [96]. Fourier domain measurements require a frequency-modulated beam for sample excitation and a frequency-modulated photomultiplier tube for detection. If the modulation frequency of the detector is similar to that of the excitation beam, the amplitude and phase shift of the fluorescence signal can be measured, which allows for calculation of fluorescence lifetimes. Time-domain fluorescence measurements typically exhibit increased sensitivity to low signal intensity and are therefore well suited for weak autofluorescence from NAD(P)H and FAD [65, 69, 86]. In time-domain fluorescence microscopy, the time difference between the excitation pulse and the emitted photons is resolved. Practically, this is done using time-correlated single-photon counting (TCSPC) [97]. Here, the arrival time of the first photon after the pulse is monitored with high resolution. However, it is assumed that no more than one photon is emitted per laser pulse (80-MHz repetition rate), which is true in almost all cases when performing autofluorescence microscopy and imaging samples with fluorescent labels [78]. A decay curve is built up after detection of a large number of photons. The decay curve is deconvolved with the instrument response to provide a direct measurement of the fluorescence decay of the fluorophore.

5.2.7 Summary

Autofluorescence imaging of metabolism is attractive because it provides nondestructive measures of single-cell metabolism. This approach is particularly useful for the study of dynamic changes within intact samples and for studies of spatial relationships between cells within a relevant physiological context. This approach is also accessible because it does not require transfections or the use of exogenous contrast agents. Limitations include imaging depth, which can be overcome with window chamber models for in vivo imaging [6, 8, 13]. Overall, as new microscopy technologies are developed, added functional measures of NAD(P)H and FAD can be incorporated into commercial microscopes for improved functionality (e.g., anisotropy, combined spectral and lifetime imaging, etc.) [36, 37].

5.3 Optical Metabolic Contrast Agents

5.3.1 Introduction

Optical metabolic imaging with exogenous contrast agents has advanced our understanding of processes that make life possible and continues to illuminate phenomena that are difficult or impossible to study with alternative technologies. A fundamental advantage of optical metabolic imaging with exogenous contrast agents is the combination of high spatial and temporal resolution with molecular-scale information. Unlike alternative contrast-enhanced modalities like positron emission tomography (PET) or magnetic resonance imaging (MRI), optical imaging is capable of high-resolution imaging in real time (even subcellular resolution, if needed), such that metabolic processes can be tracked inter- and intracellularly.

An exhaustive survey of optical metabolic contrast agents (OMCA) cannot be achieved in a single book, let alone a chapter. Instead, we provide in the following subsections a brief overview of four major branches of OMCA and refer the interested reader to recent literature reviews for more comprehensive detail [32, 98, 99]. The four branches presented herein—imaging of nutrient uptake, enzyme activity, local chemical environment, and cell signaling—highlight the breadth of basic scientific phenomena that can be studied and clinically translatable discoveries that are possible with OMCA (Fig. 5.14). Myriad contrast agents exist for metabolic imaging but typically fall into one of five classes (Fig. 5.15).

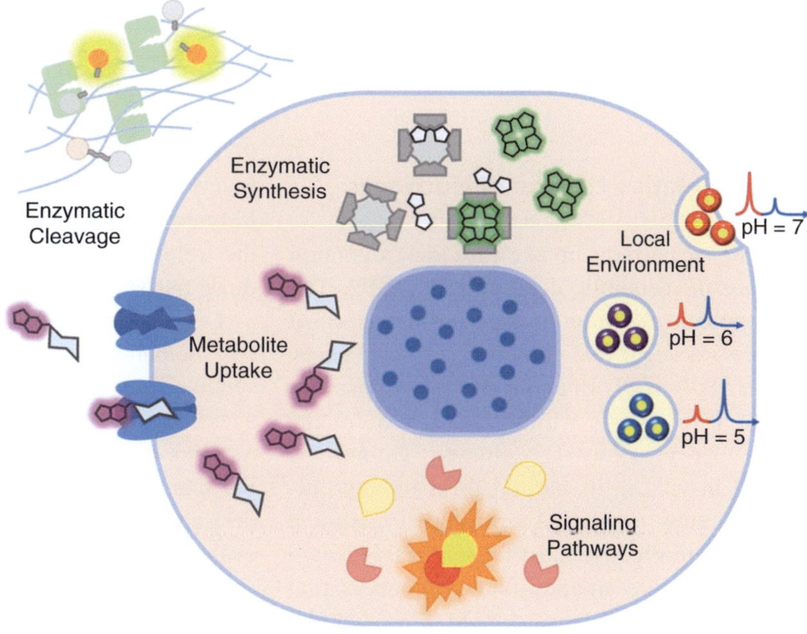

Fig. 5.14 Metabolic processes imaged with exogenous contrast agents. The five classes of optical metabolic contrast agents excel in imaging four fundamental aspects of metabolism: metabolite uptake, enzyme activity, local chemical environment, and cell signaling

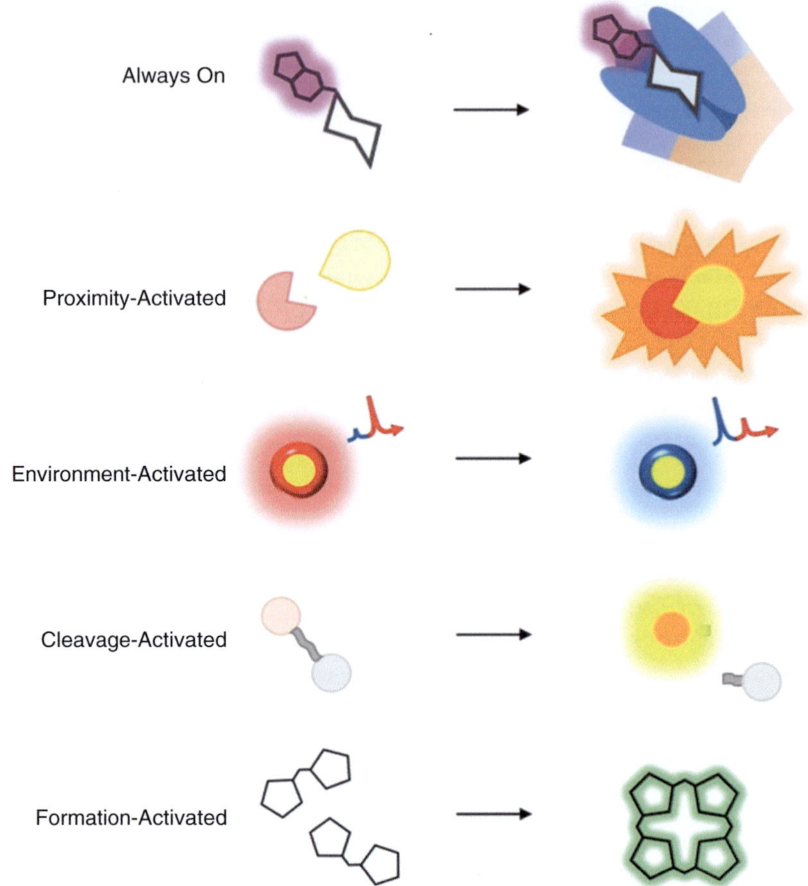

Fig. 5.15 Classes of optical metabolic contrast agents. Exogenous contrast agents employed in metabolic imaging can be broadly categorized by their mechanism of signal production. The simplest examples are non-activatable reporter molecules that are always "on," such as fluorescent metabolite analogues. The remaining four classes have signals which are activated or deactivated by specific events, such as the co-localization of two species (proximity-activated), changes in chemical environment (environment-activated), cleavage of peptide sequences (cleavage-activated), or intracellular synthesis of a detectable species (formation-activated)

Representative examples are provided throughout; however, they only constitute a fraction of the library currently available.

5.3.2 Relative Uptake of Nutrients

The rate of nutrient uptake provides a general measure of metabolic demand [100, 101]. The prototypical example is the consumption of glucose—a sugar and common cellular energy source [102–104]. Imaging glucose consumption in vivo reveals which tissues require the most energy. However, glucose cannot be tracked in vivo in its natural form by any current imaging device. Accordingly, chemical analogues to glucose must be synthesized such that they possess an additional component that can be traced by some instrument. For example, substituting an ^{18}F radionuclide for the 2′-hydroxyl group yields the ubiquitous glucose analogue fluorodeoxyglucose ([18]FDG) that is used as an exogenous contrast agent for PET imaging [104, 105]. Cancer imaging and functional studies of the brain are two particularly common applications of [18]FDG, due to the relatively high glucose consumption in those tissues [104–108].

Despite the success of PET for assessing glucose demand in vivo, the burden and expense of synthesizing and handling radioactive contrast agents makes them non-ideal for high-throughput research applications like drug discovery [109]. For this reason, optical analogues of glucose are desirable. Fluorescent glucose analogues, for example, enable cancer imaging as well as screening of glucose consumption rates in the presence of various therapeutics in order to assess their therapeutic efficacy [109–111]. The drawback to fluorescent glucose analogues, however, is that the fluorescent moiety alters the chemical properties of the analogue relative to natural glucose because it is large and typically hydrophobic [112]. Therefore, the consumption of the analogue may not reflect the true consumption of glucose.

A Raman-active chemical substitution is an example of an alternative optical labeling technique that has been pioneered to minimize the alterations that are often induced in the process of making metabolites traceable. Stimulated Raman scattering (SRS) requires only that an alkyne group (i.e., carbon-carbon triple bond) be attached to a metabolite in order for in vivo tracking to be performed [112–115]. The vibrational motion of the alkyne bond imparts an optical "barcode" in the light scattered from the analogue, such that it can be unambiguously detected [115]. Although SRS requires two lasers and generates a weaker signal than fluorescence, some modern devices can perform in vivo SRS imaging in real time [116]. Heterogeneous uptake patterns in cancer and brain tissue were demonstrated by SRS imaging of glucose analogues [112].

5.3.3 Enzyme Activity

The extraordinarily complex balance of chemical reactions involved in metabolism is maintained by the relative activity of enzymes. The concentration and state (i.e., active or inactive for catalyzing reactions) of enzymes determine the metabolism of a cell or tissue [117]. The importance of a precise balance of enzymes for healthy metabolism is reflected in the multitude of diseases associated with changes in the degree of enzyme expression. Sensitive imaging of enzymatic activity is therefore essential for the detection and diagnosis of disease [99]. This is particularly true for cancer, where changes in the expression of certain enzymes, such as proteases, can provide opportunities for early detection and offer a measure of the cancer's aggressiveness [118–120].

The most successful approach to imaging the activity of proteases has been the implementation of cleavage-activated fluorescent probes [119, 121, 122]. These exogenous contrast agents comprise one or more fluorophores in a quenched state tethered to a peptide sequence that is uniquely cleaved by the protease to be imaged. As soon as the protease cleaves the peptide, the fluorescence can be detected. Activatable fluorescent probes have demonstrated great success for optical imaging of specific proteases such as matrix metalloproteinases and cathepsin [123, 124]. Because phage display can be employed to generate peptide sequences for virtually any protease, activatable fluorescent probes can be designed for a wide library of targets [125].

In special cases, enzyme activity can be imaged by catalyzing the intracellular synthesis of fluorescent contrast agents. Although this approach is not generally applicable to a large family of enzymes, it has generated one particularly useful approach to optical metabolic imaging: the generation of protoporphyrin IX (PpIX) from 5-aminolevulinic acid (5-ALA). The steady-state concentration of PpIX formed from 5-ALA is higher in certain cancers, particularly of the brain, than in healthy tissue because of a higher ratio of the enzymes that promote PpIX formation relative to enzymes that degrade PpIX [126]. Consequently, 5-ALA can be added to cancer-bearing tissue to induce a high level of PpIX production, which in turn provides preferential fluorescence signal to demarcate a diseased region for optically guided resection. Clinical trials have demonstrated improved resection and increased patient survival when surgery was guided by PpIX fluorescence [127–129].

5.3.4 Local Chemical Environment

In addition to optical imaging of targeted metabolic processes, exogenous contrast agents can reveal general markers of metabolic state. Of particular importance are pH, oxygenation, and redox potential—the local environment's propensity to reduce or oxidize molecules [117, 130–133]. These parameters broadly impact chemical reactivity, especially for the innumerable molecules that can gain or lose hydrogen or oxygen atoms. Different cellular compartments can have dramatically different local chemical environments, yielding insight into their metabolic function and opportunities for selective imaging. Inflamed or cancerous tissues can also be chemically distinguished from healthy surrounding tissue by changes in redox potential and pH [132, 134, 135].

Given the breadth of chemicals sensitive to pH, oxygen concentration, and redox potential, many avenues to sensing local chemical environment exist. Despite the various approaches, virtually all optical contrast agents for chemical environment sensing operate by the same principle: a structural change occurs and can be externally calibrated, when a molecule is exposed to a specific set of chemical conditions. The structural change typically either activates or changes a fluorescent molecule (in terms of spectra, lifetime, intensity, etc.), often through quenching or dequenching processes. The resultant changes in optical readout yield an optical mechanism for sensing [136–138].

Activatable fluorescent probes are commonly employed for sensing pH and reactive oxygen species, although they are less common for quantification of molecular oxygen and redox potential (i.e., a direct measurement in millivolts) [136, 139–141]. The use of fluorescent pH sensors is ubiquitous, for example, in pH-measuring paper strips, and occurs as a result of the addition or removal of a hydrogen ion causing a spectral shift or intensity change in fluorescence [142]. Typically, this occurs in a single molecule, for example, by a ring-opening or ring-closing reaction, but it can also occur for polymeric nanoparticles that reversibly change from condensed, quenched structures to open fluorescent configurations [137]. Similar principles underlie the activation of fluorescence in response to reactive oxygen species, although the structural changes tend to be more significant on the molecular level, as in the oxidation of boronates by hydrogen peroxide [136]. In order for quantitative measurements to be made, a second reference fluorophore that is insensitive to the local chemical environment is often required as an internal standard for ratiometric measurements [98, 143].

The optical detection of molecular oxygen and redox potential often involves the use of nanoparticles coupled to molecules [98, 144]. In the case of molecular oxygen, a phosphorescent molecule coupled to a quantum dot (i.e., a semiconductor nanoparticle) can be calibrated to identify the partial pressure of oxygen, pO_2 [145]. For example, when the quantum dot is optically excited, it can transfer its energy to the phosphorescent molecule which subsequently emits light. Upon collisional interactions with oxygen, however, the phosphorescent molecule becomes quenched, and light is only emitted from the quantum dot [145, 146]. Thus, the quantum dot luminescence provides an internal standard for ratiometric imaging. Calibrating the luminescence ratio from the quantum dot-molecule conjugate to the partial pressure of oxygen enables in vivo measurements of pO_2 [144].

Redox potential can be accurately measured by means of surface-enhanced Raman scattering (SERS) nanoparticles [138]. Rather than an absorption-emission process, SERS utilizes the vibrational motions of molecules on the surface of nanoparticles, usually made of gold or silver, to impart detectable scattering signals that have been enhanced by surface plasmon effects from the metallic core [147, 148]. Because the vibrational motion of a molecule is unique to its structure, SERS spectra serve as molecular "fingerprints." Depending on the molecule, structural changes as small as the addition of a single hydrogen can be readily detected in SERS spectra by the appearance or disappearance of characteristic peaks [149, 150]. The ratio of peak heights in SERS spectra can then be calibrated to the chemical environment, including the electrical potential as measured by an external electrode. By monitoring the spectrum of a SERS nanoparticle sensitive to redox environment, optical measurements of local redox potential can be performed [138].

5.3.5 Cell Signaling

The communication of cells with their surroundings provides a showcase for the importance of optical metabolic imaging with exogenous contrast. Biochemical signaling involves networks of proteins rapidly relaying messages via intracellular and extracellular changes in chemical composition. Detection of these events often requires subcellular spatial resolution and real-time imaging of chemical gradients. Because most signal cascades are not intrinsically detectable, exogenous contrast is required to enable optical readout of changes in local chemical concentrations [151]. Accordingly, contrast agents sensitive to messenger species are particularly useful for imaging spikes in signaling activity [152].

Signaling ion gradients are imaged by exogenous probe molecules that generate an optical change upon binding an ion of interest [151–153]. The binding selectivity is achieved by designing unique chelators—molecules that entrap target species based upon their size, charge, and coordination chemistry—for each targeted ion [154]. The optical signal is generated as a result of the ion modifying the probe molecule's electronic structure. Typically, the ion binding induces fluorescence by preventing an internal quenching mechanism that inhibits fluorescence when the ion is not present [155, 156]. Alternative methods of investigation can detect subtler changes upon ion binding, albeit at the expense of more complex instrumentation. For example, changes to the fluorescence lifetime—the time between absorption and emission of a photon—can be detected upon ion binding using fluorescence lifetime imaging microscopy (FLIM) [96, 157]. While FLIM requires pulsed illumination sources and extremely short detector response times, the molecular contrast agents can have simpler designs because activated fluorescence is not required.

Imaging signaling molecules is more complicated than imaging small ions but can be accomplished by an analogous approach. While signaling ions like Ca^{2+} can be entrapped by small molecules, signaling molecules like adenosine triphosphate (ATP) are too large to be selectively bound by simple chelators. Instead, large molecules called aptamers must be tailor-made by combinatorial chemistry techniques to enable selective binding of the targeted molecule (e.g., ATP). Aptamers are comprised of specific peptide or nucleic acid sequences that change structure upon interacting with their target to form a stable complex. Methods like systematic evolution of ligands by exponential enrichment (SELEX) enable aptamer synthesis for virtually any target. Once the aptamer-target complex forms, a secondary exogenous compound binds to generate a fluorescent signal [158]. The fluorescence is only achieved if the aptamer, target, and secondary compound all bind together [159]. This approach has been established for a wide array of signaling molecules and metabolites including guanosine triphosphate, adenosine diphosphate, and *S*-adenosylmethionine [160].

Although the spatial resolution of conventional fluorescence is sufficient for in vitro metabolic studies, visible light scattering by tissues often necessitates modified imaging techniques for in vivo applications [161]. Two-photon imaging (TPI) enables the use of minimally scattered near-infrared excitation and suppresses background signal by requiring that two photons be absorbed for a single fluorescent event [162]. The high spatial resolution of TPI is ideal for in vivo imaging of cell signaling. After administrating a Ca^{2+}-activated fluorescent dye, signaling activity in neural tissue can be monitored by TPI of living mice [153, 163]. These studies have the added benefit of decreased photobleaching (i.e., light-induced destruction of contrast agents) relative to conventional fluorescence, because the contrast agents are not excited by out-of-focus light [162].

References

1. Ntziachristos V. Going deeper than microscopy: the optical imaging frontier in biology. Nat Methods. 2010;7:603–14.
2. Jacques SL, Pogue BW. Tutorial on diffuse light transport. J Biomed Opt. 2008;13(4):041302.
3. Culver JP, et al. Three-dimensional diffuse optical tomography in the parallel plane transmission geometry: evaluation of a hybrid frequency domain/continuous wave clinical system for breast imaging. Med Phys. 2003;30(2):235–47.
4. Jiang S, et al. Evaluation of breast tumor response to neoadjuvant chemotherapy with tomographic diffuse optical spectroscopy: case studies of tumor region-of-interest changes. Radiology. 2009;252(2):551–60.

5. Teng F, et al. A wearable optical device for continuous monitoring during neoadjuvant chemotherapy infusions. J Biomed Opt. 2016;22:14001.
6. Tromberg BJ, et al. Imaging in breast cancer: diffuse optics in breast cancer: detecting tumors in pre-menopausal women and monitoring neoadjuvant chemotherapy. Breast Cancer Res. 2005;7(6):279–85.
7. Stojanovic R, Karadaglic D. Design of an oximeter based on LED-LED configuration and FPGA technology. Sensors (Basel). 2013;13(1):574–86.
8. Muehlemann T, Haensse D, Wolf M. Wireless miniaturized in-vivo near infrared imaging. Opt Express. 2008;16(14):10323–30.
9. Pogue B, et al. Instrumentation and design of a frequency-domain diffuse optical tomography imager for breast cancer detection. Opt Express. 1997;1(13):391–403.
10. Yu Y, et al. Near-infrared spectral imaging of the female breast for quantitative oximetry in optical mammography. Appl Opt. 2009;48(10):D225–35.
11. Deng B, et al. Characterizing breast lesions through robust multimodal data fusion using independent diffuse optical and x-ray breast imaging. J Biomed Opt. 2015;20(8):80502.
12. Flexman ML, et al. Digital optical tomography system for dynamic breast imaging. J Biomed Opt. 2011;16(7):076014.
13. Carpenter CM, et al. Image-guided optical spectroscopy provides molecular-specific information in vivo: MRI-guided spectroscopy of breast cancer hemoglobin, water, and scatterer size. Opt Lett. 2007;32(8):933–5.
14. Zhu Q, et al. Noninvasive monitoring of breast cancer during neoadjuvant chemotherapy using optical tomography with ultrasound localization. Neoplasia. 2008;10(10):1028–40.
15. Pian Q, et al. Hyperspectral time-resolved wide-field fluorescence molecular tomography based on structured light and single-pixel detection. Opt Lett. 2015;40(3):431–4.
16. Cuccia DJ, et al. Quantitation and mapping of tissue optical properties using modulated imaging. J Biomed Opt. 2009;14(2):024012.
17. Durduran T, et al. Diffuse optics for tissue monitoring and tomography. Rep Prog Phys. 2010;73(7):076701.
18. Cerussi AE, et al. Frequent optical imaging during breast cancer neoadjuvant chemotherapy reveals dynamic tumor physiology in an individual patient. Acad Radiol. 2010;17(8):1031–9.
19. Shah N, et al. Noninvasive functional optical spectroscopy of human breast tissue. Proc Natl Acad Sci U S A. 2001;98(8):4420–5.
20. Jiang S, et al. Predicting breast tumor response to neoadjuvant chemotherapy with diffuse optical spectroscopic tomography prior to treatment. Clin Cancer Res. 2014;20(23):6006–15.
21. Zhou C, et al. Diffuse optical monitoring of blood flow and oxygenation in human breast cancer during early stages of neoadjuvant chemotherapy. J Biomed Opt. 2007;12(5):051903.
22. Falou O, et al. Diffuse optical spectroscopy evaluation of treatment response in women with locally advanced breast cancer receiving neoadjuvant chemotherapy. Transl Oncol. 2012;5(4):238–46.
23. Anderson PG, et al. Broadband optical mammography: chromophore concentration and hemoglobin saturation contrast in breast cancer. PLoS One. 2015;10(3):e0117322.
24. Pakalniskis MG, et al. Tumor angiogenesis change estimated by using diffuse optical spectroscopic tomography: demonstrated correlation in women undergoing neoadjuvant chemotherapy for invasive breast cancer? Radiology. 2011;259(2):365–74.
25. Cerussi A, et al. Predicting response to breast cancer neoadjuvant chemotherapy using diffuse optical spectroscopy. Proc Natl Acad Sci U S A. 2007;104(10):4014–9.
26. Rastogi P, et al. Preoperative chemotherapy: updates of National Surgical Adjuvant Breast and Bowel Project Protocols B-18 and B-27. J Clin Oncol. 2008;26(5):778–85.
27. Bevilacqua F, et al. Broadband absorption spectroscopy in turbid media by combined frequency-domain and steady-state methods. Appl Opt. 2000;39(34):6498–507.
28. Ueda S, et al. Baseline tumor oxygen saturation correlates with a pathologic complete response in breast cancer patients undergoing neoadjuvant chemotherapy. Cancer Res. 2012;72(17):4318–28.
29. Roblyer D, et al. Optical imaging of breast cancer oxyhemoglobin flare correlates with neoadjuvant chemotherapy response one day after starting treatment. Proc Natl Acad Sci U S A. 2011;108(35):14626–31.
30. Taga G, et al. Brain imaging in awake infants by near-infrared optical topography. Proc Natl Acad Sci U S A. 2003;100(19):10722–7.
31. Wilcox T, et al. Using near-infrared spectroscopy to assess neural activation during object processing in infants. J Biomed Opt. 2005;10(1):11010.
32. Devor A, et al. Frontiers in optical imaging of cerebral blood flow and metabolism. J Cereb Blood Flow Metab. 2012;32(7):1259–76.
33. Franceschini MA, et al. Diffuse optical imaging of the whole head. J Biomed Opt. 2006;11(5):054007.
34. Zeff BW, et al. Retinotopic mapping of adult human visual cortex with high-density diffuse optical tomography. Proc Natl Acad Sci U S A. 2007;104(29):12169–74.
35. Vishwanath K, et al. Using optical spectroscopy to longitudinally monitor physiological changes within solid tumors. Neoplasia. 2009;11(9):889–900.
36. Singh-Moon RP, et al. Spatial mapping of drug delivery to brain tissue using hyperspectral spatial frequency-domain imaging. J Biomed Opt. 2014;19(9):96003.
37. Lin AJ, et al. Spatial frequency domain imaging of intrinsic optical property contrast in a mouse

model of Alzheimer's disease. Ann Biomed Eng. 2011;39(4):1349–57.
38. Maslov K, Stoica G, Wang LV. In vivo dark-field reflection-mode photoacoustic microscopy. Opt Lett. 2005;15:625–7.
39. Zhang HF, et al. Functional photoacoustic microscopy for high-resolution and noninvasive in vivo imaging. Nat Biotechnol. 2006;24:848–51.
40. Zhang H, Maslov K, Sivaramakrishnan M, et al. Imaging of hemoglobin oxygen saturation variations in single vessels in vivo using photoacoustic microscopy. Appl Phys Lett. 2007;90:053901.
41. Chance B, et al. Optical and nuclear magnetic resonance studies of hypoxia in human tissue and tumors. Ann N Y Acad Sci. 1988;55:1–16.
42. Maslov K, et al. Optical-resolution photoacoustic microscopy for in vivo imaging of single capillaries. Opt Lett. 2008;33:929–31.
43. Hu S, et al. Functional transcranial brain imaging by optical-resolution photoacoustic microscopy. J Biomed Opt. 2009;14:040503.
44. Yao J, et al. High-speed label-free functional photoacoustic microscopy of mouse brain in action. Nat Methods. 2015;12:407–10.
45. Rumsey WL, Vanderkooi JM, Wilson DF. Imaging of phosphorescence: a novel method for measuring oxygen distribution in perfused tissue. Science. 1988;24:1649–51.
46. Yaseen MA, et al. Optical monitoring of oxygen tension in cortical microvessels with confocal microscopy. Opt Express. 2009;17:22341–50.
47. Estrada AD, et al. Microvascular oxygen quantification using two-photon microscopy. Opt Lett. 2008;33:1038–40.
48. Shonat RD, et al. Near-simultaneous hemoglobin saturation and oxygen tension maps in mouse brain using an AOTF microscope. Biophys J. 1997;73:1223–31.
49. Yaseen MA, et al. Microvascular oxygen tension and flow measurements in rodent cerebral cortex during baseline conditions and functional activation. J Cereb Blood Flow Metab. 2011;31:1051–63.
50. Vovenko E. Distribution of oxygen tension on the surface of arterioles, capillaries and venules of brain cortex and in tissue in normoxia: an experimental study on rats. Pflugers Arch. 1999;437:617–23.
51. Tomlins P, Wang R. Theory, developments and applications of optical coherence tomography. J Phys D Appl Phys. 2005;38:2519–35.
52. Wang RK, An L. Doppler optical micro-angiography for volumetric imaging of vascular perfusion *in vivo*. Opt Express. 2009;17:8926–40.
53. Faber DJ, et al. Light absorption of (oxy-)hemoglobin assessed by spectroscopic optical coherence tomography. Opt Lett. 2003;28:1436–8.
54. Faber DJ, et al. Toward assessment of blood oxygen saturation by spectroscopic optical coherence tomography. Opt Lett. 2005;30:1015–7.
55. Kagemann L, et al. Spectral oximetry assessed with high-speed ultra-high-resolution optical coherence tomography. J Biomed Opt. 2007;12:041212.
56. Yi J, Li X. Estimation of oxygen saturation from erythrocytes by high-resolution spectroscopic optical coherence tomography. Opt Lett. 2010;35:2094–6.
57. Yi J, et al. Visible-light optical coherence tomography for retinal oximetry. Opt Lett. 2013;38:1796–8.
58. Chong SP, et al. Quantitative microvascular hemoglobin mapping using visible light spectroscopic Optical Coherence Tomography. Biomed Opt Express. 2015;6:1429–50.
59. Chance B, Legallais V, Schoener B. Metabolically linked changes in fluorescence emission spectra of cortex of rat brain, kidney and adrenal gland. Nature. 1962;195:1073–5.
60. Chance B, Estabrook RW, Ghosh A. Damped sinusoidal oscillations of cytoplasmic reduced pyridine nucleotide in yeast cells. Proc Natl Acad Sci. 1964;51:1244–51.
61. Scholz R, Thurman R, Williamson JF, Chance B, Bucher T. Flavin and pyridine nucleotide oxidation-reduction changes in perfused rat liver. I. Anoxia and subcellular localization of fluorescent flavoproteins. J Biol Chem. 1969;244:2317–24.
62. Mayevsky A, Chance B. Repetitive patterns of metabolic changes during cortical spreading depression of the awake rat. Brain Res. 1974;65:529–33.
63. Harbig K, Chance B, Kovach AG, Reivich M. In vivo measurement of pyridine nucleotide fluorescence from cat brain cortex. J Appl Physiol. 1976;41:480–8.
64. Ji S, Chance B, Stuart BH, Nathan R. Two-dimensional analysis of the redox state of the rat cerebral cortex in vivo by NADH fluorescence photography. Brain Res. 1977;119:357–73.
65. Skala MC, et al. In vivo multiphoton microscopy of NADH and FAD redox states, fluorescence lifetimes, and cellular morphology in precancerous epithelia. Proc Natl Acad Sci U S A. 2007;104(49):19494–9.
66. Skala MC, et al. In vivo multiphoton fluorescence lifetime imaging of protein-bound and free NADH in normal and pre-cancerous epithelia. J Biomed Opt. 2007;12(2):024014.
67. Walsh AJ, Cook R, Manning HC, Hicks DJ, Lafontant A, Arteaga CL, Skala MC. Optical metabolic imaging identifies breast cancer glycolytic levels, sub-types, and early treatment response. Cancer Res. 2013;15(73):6164–74.
68. Shah AT, Demory Beckler M, Walsh AJ, Jones WP, Pohlmann PR, Skala MC. Optical metabolic imaging of treatment response in human head and neck squamous cell carcinoma. Plus ONE. 2014;9(3):e90746.
69. Walsh AJ, Cook R, Sanders ME, Aruisicchio L, Ciliberto G, Arteaga CL, Skala MC. Quantitative optical imaging of primary tumor organoid metabolism predicts drug response in breast cancer. Cancer Res. 2014;74(18):5184–94.

70. Walsh AJ, et al. Optical imaging of drug-induced metabolism changes in murine and human pancreatic cancer organoids reveals heterogeneous drug response. Pancreas. 2015;45:863–9.
71. Shah AT, et al. In Vivo autofluorescence imaging of tumor heterogeneity in response to treatment. Neoplasia. 2015;17(12):862–70.
72. Mayevsky A, Chance B. Intracellular oxidation-reduction state measured in situ by a multichannel fiber-optic surface fluorometer. Science. 1982;217:537–40.
73. Rice WL, Kaplan D, Georgakoudi I. Two-photon microscopy for non-invasive, quantitative monitoring of stem cell differentiation. Plus ONE. 2010;5:e10075.
74. Chance B, Schoener B, Oshino R, Itshak F, Nakase Y. Oxidation-reduction ratio studies of mitochondria in freeze-trapped samples: NADH and flavoprotein signals. J Biol Chem. 1979;254:4764–71.
75. Lee IY, Chance B. Activation of malate-linked reductions of NAD and flavoproteins in Ascaris muscle mitochondria by phosphate. Biochem Biophys Res Commun. 1968;32:547–33.
76. Georgakoudi I, Jacobson B, Muller MG, Sheets EE, Badizadegan K, et al. NAD(P)H and collagen as in vivo quantitative fluorescent biomarkers of epithelial precancerous changes. Cancer Res. 2002;62:682–7.
77. Levitt JM, ME ML-D, Munger K, Georgakoudi I. Automated biochemical, morphological, and organizational assessment of precancerous changes from endogenous two-photon fluorescence images. Plus ONE. 2011;6:e24765.
78. Lakowicz JR. Principles of fluorescence spectroscopy, vol. 13. 2nd ed. New York: Springer Science and Business Media; 1999. p. 698.
79. Sato K, et al. Hydrogen-bonding dynamics of free flavins in benzene and FAD in electron-transferring flavoprotein upon excitation. J Photochem Photobiol B Biol. 2003;70(2):67–73.
80. Muller F, Mayhew S, Massey V. The effect of temperature on the absorption spectra of free and protein-bound flavins. Biochemistry. 1973;12:4654–62.
81. Heikal AA. Intracellular coenzymes as natural biomarkers for metabolic activities and mitochondrial anomalies. Biomark Med. 2010;4(2):221–63.
82. Nelson DL, Lehninger AL, Cox MM. Lehninger principles of biochemistry. New York: Macmillan; 2008.
83. Chance B, T B. Localization and kinetics in oxygen delivery to tissue. Microvasc Res. 1959;8:276–82.
84. Chance B, Mayevsky A, Goodwin C, Mela L. Factors in oxygen delivery to tissue. Microvasc Res. 1974;8:276–82.
85. Chance B. Optical method. Annu Rev Biophys Biophys Chem. 1991;20:1–28.
86. Walsh AJ, et al. Optical metabolic imaging identifies glycolytic levels, subtypes, and early-treatment response in breast cancer. Cancer Res. 2013;73(20):6164–74.
87. Ramanujam N, et al. Low temperature fluorescence imaging of freeze-trapped human cervical tissues. Opt Express. 2001;8:335–43.
88. Bird DK, Yan L, Vrotsos KM, Eliceiri KW, Vaughan EM, et al. Metabolic mapping of MCF10A human breast cells via multiphoton fluorescence lifetime imaging of the coenzyme NADH. Cancer Res. 2005;65:8766–73.
89. Schneckenburger H, et al. Autofluorescence lifetime imaging of cultivated cells using a UV picosecond laser diode. J Fluoresc. 2004;14(5):649–54.
90. Mujat C, Greiner C, Baldwin A, Levitt JM, Tian F, et al. Endogenous optical biomarkers of normal and human papillomavirus immortalized epithelial cells. Int J Cancer. 2008;122:363–71.
91. Ostrander JH, McMahon C, Lem S, Millon SR, Borwn JQ, et al. Optical redox ratio differentiates breast cancer cell lines based on estrogen receptor status. Cancer Res. 2010;70:4759–66.
92. Mayevsky A. Mitochondrial function and energy metabolism in cancer cells: past overview and future perspectives. Mitochondrion. 2009;9(3):165–79.
93. Conklin MW, et al. Fluorescence lifetime imaging of endogenous fluorophores in histopathology sections reveals differences between normal and tumor epithelium in carcinoma in situ of the breast. Cell Biochem Biophys. 2009;53(3):145–57.
94. Centonze VE, White JG. Multiphoton excitation provides optical sections from deeper within scattering specimens than confocal imaging. Biophys J. 1998;75(4):2015–24.
95. Squirrell JM, et al. Long-term two-photon fluorescence imaging of mammalian embryos without compromising viability. Nat Biotechnol. 1999;17(8):763–7.
96. Becker W. Fluorescence lifetime imaging—techniques and applications. J Microsc. 2012;247(2):119–36.
97. Becker W. The bh TCSPC handbook. Berlin: Becker & Hickl; 2014.
98. Sondergaard RV, et al. Facing the Design Challenges of Particle-Based Nanosensors for Metabolite Quantification in Living Cells. Chem Rev. 2015;115(16):8344–78.
99. Drake CR, Miller DC, Jones EF. Activatable Optical Probes for the Detection of Enzymes. Curr Org Synth. 2011;8(4):498–520.
100. DeBerardinis RJ, et al. The biology of cancer: metabolic reprogramming fuels cell growth and proliferation. Cell Metab. 2008;7(1):11–20.
101. Plathow C, Weber WA. Tumor cell metabolism imaging. J Nucl Med. 2008;49:43S–63S.
102. Heiden MGV, Cantley LC, Thompson CB. Understanding the Warburg effect: the metabolic requirements of cell proliferation. Science. 2009;324(5930):1029–33.
103. Kondoh H, et al. A high glycolytic flux supports the proliferative potential of murine embryonic stem cells. Antioxid Redox Signal. 2007;9(3):293–9.
104. Gambhir SS. Molecular imaging of cancer with positron emission tomography. Nat Rev Cancer. 2002;2(9):683–93.
105. Rohren EM, Turkington TG, Coleman RE. Clinical applications of PET in oncology. Radiology. 2004;231(2):305–32.

106. Perani D, et al. Evidence of multiple memory-systems in the human brain—A F-18 FDG PET metabolic study. Brain. 1993;116:903–19.
107. Holcomb HH, et al. Functional sites of neuroleptic drug action in the human brain: PET/FDG studies with and without haloperidol. Am J Psychiatr. 1996;153(1):41–9.
108. Mosconi L. Brain glucose metabolism in the early and specific diagnosis of Alzheimer's disease—FDG-PET studies in MCI and AD. Eur J Nucl Med Mol Imaging. 2005;32(4):486–510.
109. Cheng Z, et al. Near-infrared fluorescent deoxyglucose analogue for tumor optical imaging in cell culture and living mice. Bioconjug Chem. 2006;17(3):662–9.
110. Yoshioka K, et al. A novel fluorescent derivative of glucose applicable to the assessment of glucose uptake activity of Escherichia coli. Biochim Et Biophy Acta-Gen Sub. 1996;1289(1):5–9.
111. Zou CH, Wang YJ, Shen ZF. 2-NBDG as a fluorescent indicator for direct glucose uptake measurement. J Biochem Biophys Methods. 2005;64(3):207–15.
112. Hu F, et al. Vibrational imaging of glucose uptake activity in live cells and tissues by stimulated raman scattering. Angew Chem Int Ed Eng. 2015;54(34):9821–5.
113. Hu FH, et al. Live-cell vibrational imaging of choline metabolites by stimulated Raman scattering coupled with isotope-based metabolic labeling. Analyst. 2014;139(10):2312–7.
114. Wei L, et al. Live-cell imaging of alkyne-tagged small biomolecules by stimulated Raman scattering. Nat Methods. 2014;11(4):410.
115. Yamakoshi H, et al. Alkyne-tag Raman imaging for visualization of mobile small molecules in live cells. J Am Chem Soc. 2012;134(51):20681–9.
116. Saar BG, et al. Video-rate molecular imaging in vivo with stimulated Raman scattering. Science. 2010;330(6009):1368–70.
117. Berg JT, Tymoczko JL, Stryer L. Biochemistry. 6th ed. San Francisco: Freeman, W. H. & Company; 2006.
118. Talvensaari-Mattila A, et al. Matrix metalloproteinase-2 immunoreactive protein—a marker of aggressiveness in breast carcinoma. Cancer. 1998;83(6):1153–62.
119. Weissleder R, et al. In vivo imaging of tumors with protease-activated near-infrared fluorescent probes. Nat Biotechnol. 1999;17(4):375–8.
120. Joyce JA, et al. Cathepsin cysteine proteases are effectors of invasive growth and angiogenesis during multistage tumorigenesis. Cancer Cell. 2004;5(5):443–53.
121. Ntziachristos V, et al. Fluorescence molecular tomography resolves protease activity in vivo. Nat Med. 2002;8(7):757–60.
122. Frangioni JV. In vivo near-infrared fluorescence imaging. Curr Opin Chem Biol. 2003;7(5):626–34.
123. Tung CH, et al. In vivo imaging of proteolytic enzyme activity using a novel molecular reporter. Cancer Res. 2000;60(17):4953–8.
124. Bremer C, Tung CH, Weissleder R. In vivo molecular target assessment of matrix metalloproteinase inhibition. Nat Med. 2001;7(6):743–8.
125. Kelly KA, et al. Detection of early prostate cancer using a hepsin-targeted imaging agent. Cancer Res. 2008;68(7):2286–91.
126. Hinnen P, et al. Biochemical basis of 5-aminolaevulinic acid induced protoporphyrin IX accumulation: a study in patients with (pre)malignant lesions of the oesophagus. Br J Cancer. 1998;78(5):679–82.
127. Stummer W, et al. Fluorescence-guided resection of glioblastoma multiforme by using 5-aminolevulinic acid-induced porphyrins: a prospective study in 52 consecutive patients. J Neurosurg. 2000;93(6):1003–13.
128. Denzinger S, et al. Clinically relevant reduction in risk of recurrence of superficial bladder cancer using 5-aminolevulinic acid-induced fluorescence diagnosis: 8-year results of prospective randomized study. Urology. 2007;69(4):675–9.
129. Stummer W, et al. Fluorescence-guided surgery with 5-aminolevulinic acid for resection of malignant glioma: a randomised controlled multicentre phase III trial. Lancet Oncol. 2006;7(5):392–401.
130. Gatenby RA, Gillies RJ. Why do cancers have high aerobic glycolysis? Nat Rev Cancer. 2004;4(11):891–9.
131. Roos A, Boron WF. Intracellular PH. Physiol Rev. 1981;61(2):296–434.
132. Hanahan D, Weinberg RA. Hallmarks of cancer: the next generation. Cell. 2011;144(5):646–74.
133. Vaupel P, Kallinowski F, Okunieff P. Blood-flow, oxygen and nutrient supply, and metabolic microenvironment of human-tumors—a review. Cancer Res. 1989;49(23):6449–65.
134. Aggarwal BB, Harikumar KB. Potential therapeutic effects of curcumin, the anti-inflammatory agent, against neurodegenerative, cardiovascular, pulmonary, metabolic, autoimmune and neoplastic diseases. Int J Biochem Cell Biol. 2009;41(1):40–59.
135. Rahman I, MacNee W. Oxidative stress and regulation of glutathione in lung inflammation. Eur Respir J. 2000;16(3):534–54.
136. Lippert AR, De Bittner GCV, Chang CJ. Boronate oxidation as a bioorthogonal reaction approach for studying the chemistry of hydrogen peroxide in living systems. Acc Chem Res. 2011;44(9):793–804.
137. Wang Y, et al. A nanoparticle-based strategy for the imaging of a broad range of tumours by nonlinear amplification of microenvironment signals. Nat Mater. 2014;13(2):204–12.
138. Jamieson LE, et al. Simultaneous intracellular redox potential and pH measurements in live cells using SERS nanosensors. Analyst. 2015;140(7):2330–5.
139. Geisow MJ, Hart PD, Young MR. Temporal changes of lysosome and phagosome PH during phagolysosome formation in macrophages—studies by fluorescence spectroscopy. J Cell Biol. 1981;89(3):645–52.
140. Urano Y, et al. Selective molecular imaging of viable cancer cells with pH-activatable fluorescence probes. Nat Med. 2009;15(1):104–9.

141. Gomes A, Fernandes E, Lima J. Fluorescence probes used for detection of reactive oxygen species. J Biochem Biophys Methods. 2005;65(2–3):45–80.
142. Martin MM, Lindqvist L. PH-dependence of fluorescein fluorescence. J Lumin. 1975;10(6):381–90.
143. Xu H, et al. A real-time ratiometric method for the determination of molecular oxygen inside living cells using sol-gel-based spherical optical nanosensors with applications to rat C6 glioma. Anal Chem. 2001;73(17):4124–33.
144. Silvi S, Credi A. Luminescent sensors based on quantum dot-molecule conjugates. Chem Soc Rev. 2015;44(13):4275–89.
145. Lemon CM, et al. Two-photon oxygen sensing with quantum dot-porphyrin conjugates. Inorg Chem. 2013;52(18):10394–406.
146. Dmitriev RI, Papkovsky DB. Optical probes and techniques for O2 measurement in live cells and tissue. Cell Mol Life Sci. 2012;69(12):2025–39.
147. Campion A, Kambhampati P. Surface-enhanced Raman scattering. Chem Soc Rev. 1998;27(4):241–50.
148. Lombardi JR, Birke RL. A unified view of surface-enhanced Raman scattering. Acc Chem Res. 2009;42(6):734–42.
149. Kneipp J, et al. Following the dynamics of pH in endosomes of live cells with SERS nanosensors. J Phys Chem C. 2010;114(16):7421–6.
150. Alvarez-Puebla RA, Liz-Marzan LM. SERS-based diagnosis and biodetection. Small. 2010;6(5):604–10.
151. Tsien RY. Fluorescence measurement and photochemical manipulation of cytosolic free calcium. Trends Neurosci. 1988;11(10):419–24.
152. Mao BQ, et al. Dynamics of spontaneous activity in neocortical slices. Neuron. 2001;32(5):883–98.
153. Stosiek C, et al. In vivo two-photon calcium imaging of neuronal networks. Proc Natl Acad Sci U S A. 2003;100(12):7319–24.
154. Grinvald A, et al. Optical imaging of neuronal-activity. Physiol Rev. 1988;68(4):1285–366.
155. Li XH, et al. Design strategies for water-soluble small molecular chromogenic and fluorogenic probes. Chem Rev. 2014;114(1):590–659.
156. Martinez-Manez R, Sancenon F. Fluorogenic and chromogenic chemosensors and reagents for anions. Chem Rev. 2003;103(11):4419–76.
157. Bastiaens PIH, Squire A. Fluorescence lifetime imaging microscopy: spatial resolution of biochemical processes in the cell. Trends Cell Biol. 1999;9(2):48–52.
158. Paige JS, Wu KY, Jaffrey SR. RNA mimics of green fluorescent protein. Science. 2011;333(6042):642–6.
159. Paige JS, et al. Fluorescence imaging of cellular metabolites with RNA. Science. 2012;335(6073):1194.
160. Strack RL, Song W, Jaffrey SR. Using Spinach-based sensors for fluorescence imaging of intracellular metabolites and proteins in living bacteria. Nat Protoc. 2014;9(1):146–55.
161. Helmchen F, et al. A miniature head-mounted two-photon microscope: high-resolution brain imaging in freely moving animals. Neuron. 2001;31(6):903–12.
162. Cahalan MD, et al. Two-photon tissue imaging: Seeing the immune system in a fresh light. Nat Rev Immunol. 2002;2(11):872–80.
163. Dombeck DA, et al. Imaging large-scale neural activity with cellular resolution in awake, mobile mice. Neuron. 2007;56(1):43–57.

Part III

Metabolic Diseases

Cancer Metabolism

6

Daniel R. Wahl and Sriram Venneti

6.1 Introduction

Altered cellular metabolism is one of the hallmarks of cancers. Otto Warburg, a German biochemist, observed that cancer cells take up and metabolized large amounts of glucose and ferment it to lactate even in the presence of oxygen. This unexpected observation that cancer cells convert glucose to lactate even in aerobic conditions led Warburg to hypothesize that cancer cells have defective mitochondria. We now know that mitochondria are not defective in cancer cells but that this process, called the Warburg effect, represents a form of metabolic adaptation in cancer cells.

In the era of precision medicine and next-generation sequencing, we have learned a lot about different genetic alterations in various cancers. It is essential to understand the biology of these tumors beyond genetic alterations in order to develop treatment strategies to effectively cure them. One avenue of research that shows a lot of promise is how metabolism is rewired in cancer cells. Metabolic pathways in cells represent core mechanisms that cells use to fuel their growth and survival. Cancer cells significantly alter their metabolism compared to normal tissues, making these pathways attractive therapeutic targets. Cancer cells also constantly adapt to harsh conditions such as diminished nutrient supply, hypoxia, and changes in microenvironment. Tumor cells reprogram their metabolism by altering nutrient uptake and metabolism to support their aberrant proliferation and survival. The recent years have seen the emergence of the concept that metabolic reprograming in cancers cells is not a passive process. Rather, oncogenes and inactivated tumor suppressors in cancer cells directly reprogram the metabolism of cancer cells [1, 2]. These metabolic pathways provide novel avenues to develop newer diagnostic and therapeutic targets.

6.1.1 The Warburg Effect Is a Hallmark of Cancer Cells

Glucose is a key fuel that cancer cells use to support their energy production and the synthesis of a vast array of metabolic intermediaries. Glucose can be metabolized via glycolysis into three-carbon pyruvate thereby generating ATP, NADH, and many intermediaries of metabolism. The functions of glycolysis are threefold: (1) to supply fuel in the form of pyruvate to mitochondria; (2) coupled with its anabolic branch, the phosphate pathway (PPP), to facilitate macromolecular synthesis; and (3) to generate reducing equivalents to maintain cellular

D.R. Wahl
Department of Radiation Oncology, University of Michigan Medical School, Ann Arbor, MI 48104, USA

S. Venneti (✉)
Department of Pathology, University of Michigan Medical School, Ann Arbor, MI 48104, USA
e-mail: svenneti@med.umich.edu

J.S. Lewis, K.R. Keshari (eds.), *Imaging and Metabolism*, DOI 10.1007/978-3-319-61401-4_6

redox balance and enable macromolecular synthesis. Glycolysis occurs in ten steps. The first five steps are called the "preparatory phase" where two molecules of ATP are consumed to generate the three-carbon glyceraldehyde-3-phosphate. The last five steps are referred to as the "payoff phase" where glyceraldehyde-3-phosphate is metabolized to the three-carbon pyruvate. The payoff phase yields (a) four molecules of ATP from ADP and phosphate and (b) two molecules of NADH derived from the reduction of NAD+. Overall, glycolysis yields, from one molecule of glucose, two molecules each of pyruvate, ATP, and NADH.

After its generation from glucose, pyruvate can (1) be converted to lactate by lactate dehydrogenase (LDH) and secreted from cells, (2) decarboxylated by pyruvate dehydrogenase (PDH) and enter the TCA cycle as acetyl-CoA, or (3) undergo carboxylation by pyruvate carboxylase (PC) and enter the TCA cycle as oxaloacetate to fuel anaplerosis. In aerobic conditions, pyruvate follows the second option and is oxidized to acetyl-coenzyme A, which enters the tricarboxylic acid (TCA) cycle to be completely oxidized to carbon dioxide through the process of oxidative phosphorylation. Glycolysis and oxidative phosphorylation together generate 38 molecules of ATP from one molecule of glucose.

Proliferative cells including cancer cells show increased metabolism of glucose-derived pyruvate to lactate even in the presence of oxygen. When pyruvate is fermented into lactate, there is lowered pyruvate entry into the mitochondrial and thus lowered oxidative phosphorylation yielding only two molecules of ATP form glucose. This is accomplished both by LDH overexpression and by inhibition of PDH, which is phosphorylated and inhibited by pyruvate dehydrogenase kinase (PDK), which is often overexpressed in cancers (Fig. 6.1) [3]. This phenomenon is not intuitive from the perspective of energy production as only two molecules of ATP are produced compared to 38 molecules of ATP generated by aerobic glycolysis coupled with oxidative. However, there are other advantages to the Warburg effect beyond energy production. For example, glycolytic intermediaries generated support macromolecular synthesis of DNA, RNA, proteins, and lipids. For example, 3-phosphoglycerate, a metabolite in the glycolytic pathway, can contribute carbons for the synthesis of purines and amino acids such as cysteine, glycine, and serine. Further, the rate of glycolysis may compensate for the low efficiency of ATP synthesis, as it may be preferable to produce ATP at a faster rate since the conversion of glucose to lactate is very rapid. The metabolism of pyruvate to lactate dehydrogenase generates NAD+. This NAD+ can be recycled to catalyze the generation of 1,3-bisphosphoglycerate from 3-phosphoglycerate in glycolysis. Further, lactate acidifies and alters the microenvironment to let tumors adapt to hypoxic environments and enable tumor invasion and evasion of immune responses [4–6]. Thus, the Warburg effect is an adaptation that enables tumors to survive and proliferate in hostile environments. More recent studies in animal models and human subjects suggest that some cancers oxidize glucosederived carbons in the mitochondria, which suggests the presence of multiple active glycolytic pathways in cancers rather than a "pure" Warburg effect. [7, 8].

6.1.2 Cancer-Associated Alterations in Glycolysis

Cancer cells regulate glycolysis in many ways including altering glycolytic enzymes and glucose transporters. Oncogenic alterations in pathways involving the PI3K/AKT pathway, MYC, and p53/Tigar can directly influence many glycolytic enzymes (Fig. 6.1).

For example, the enzyme hexokinase (HK) catalyzes the first committed step in glycolysis by phosphorylating glucose at the sixth carbon to yield glucose-6-phosphate. There are four different isoforms of hexokinase (HK1–4), but in many cancer cells, HK2 is the predominant isoform [9–11]. HK2 expression is expressed at higher levels in glioblastomas and in metastatic breast cancers [12, 13]. Genetic lowering of HK2 leads to decreased tumor proliferation in animal models of lung and breast cancer [9, 10]. In Kras-driven lung cancer cells, HK2 is also required for nucleotide synthesis via the pentose phosphate pathway, for mitochondrial oxidative phosphorylation of citrate, and for glutamine metabolism in the TCA cycle [10]. Thus HK2 is

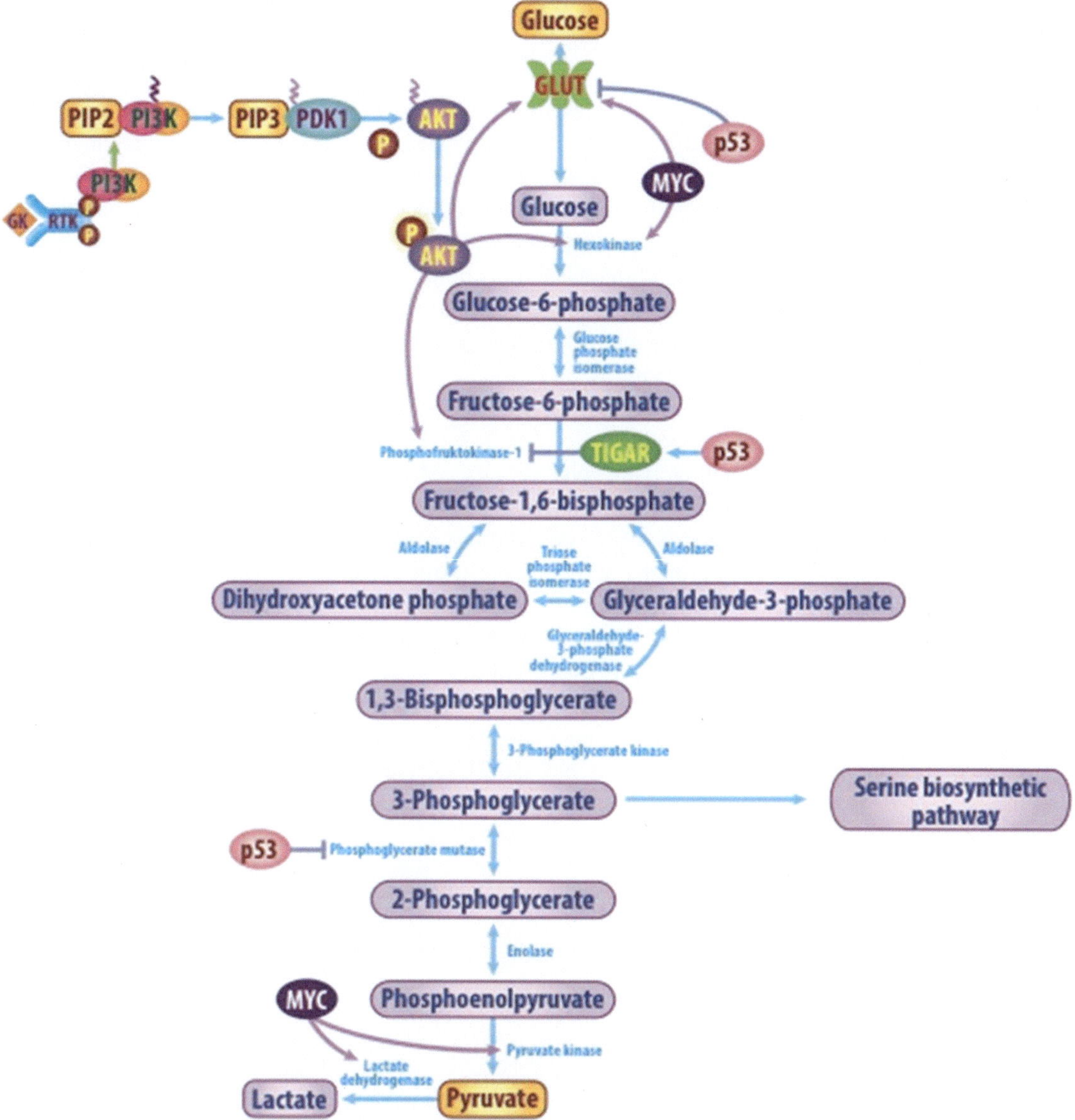

Fig. 6.1 Glycolytic reprograming in cancer cells. Many oncogenic pathways including those regulated by the PI3 kinase/AKT pathway, P53, and MYC can reprogram glycolysis in tumor cells by regulating transcription of glycolytic enzymes and glucose transporters

one of the critical enzymes that cancer cells use to regulate glycolysis.

Increased expression of glucose transporters and HK2 can be taken advantage of to image glucose uptake in cancer cells using positron emission tomography (PET) imaging with the glucose analog ^{18}F (2-[^{18}F]fluoro-2-deoxyglucose or ^{18}FDG). ^{18}FDG, like glucose, is transported into the cells by glucose transporters and phosphorylated by HK to 2-[^{18}F]fluoro-2-deoxyglucose-6-phosphate. This intermediate is unable to be further catabolized and becomes trapped in the cell, accumulating at a rate proportional to glucose utilization due to its inability to diffuse out of the cell and the slow rate of dephosphorylation. It is therefore a direct measure of glucose uptake and metabolism [14].

Pyruvate kinase catalyzes the final step in glycolysis by converting phosphoenolpyruvate into pyruvate and ATP [15] (Fig. 6.1). Pyruvate kinase is encoded by two genes: *PKLR*, which encodes the L (PKL) and R (PKR) isoforms of pyruvate kinase, and *PKM*, which encodes the M1 (PKM1) and M2 (PKM2) isoforms of pyruvate kinase. The expression of pyruvate kinase is tissue specific with PKL dominating in the liver; PKR in red blood cells; PKM1 in the brain, skeletal muscle, and heart; and PKM2 in numerous cell types including cancers and proliferating cells [15]. PKM1 and PKM2 differ in a single exon, but this difference leads to markedly different behaviors [16]. Unlike the constitutively active tetrameric PKM1, PKM2 can exist as an active tetramer or a relatively inactive dimer [17].

The activity of PKM2 is regulated both allosterically and by intracellular signaling pathways. The upstream glycolytic metabolite frutctose-1,6-bisphosphate is a major allosteric activator of PKM2 and promotes the formation of the active tetramer [18]. Numerous other small molecules and metabolites can also regulate PKM2. Similar to FBP, serine is an allosteric activator PKM2 that coordinates the fluxes of glucose toward catabolic or anabolic pathways [19]. PKM2 can thus be regulated as a rheostat in cancer cells and can be switched from active to inactive states [20]. Lower PKM2 activity promotes accumulation of glycolytic intermediaries that can feed into anabolic pathways [20]. For example, deletion of PKM2 causes the cells to arrest due to lowered nucleotide biosynthesis resulting in thymidine depletion and ineffective DNA synthesis [21]. This rheostat-like modulation of PKM2 activity by various factors may help cancer cells adapt to changing metabolic needs during tumor formation, progression, metastasis, and changes in the microenvironment [20].

6.1.3 Cancer-Associated Alterations in Amino Acid Metabolism

Amino acid metabolism is altered in many cancers. Amino acids including glutamine, glutamate, methionine, glycine, serine, cysteine, and aspartate can be metabolized to support many cellular functions including protein synthesis, nucleotide synthesis, redox modulation, and anaplerosis (the process by which TCA cycle substrates are replenished, Figs. 6.2 and 6.3).

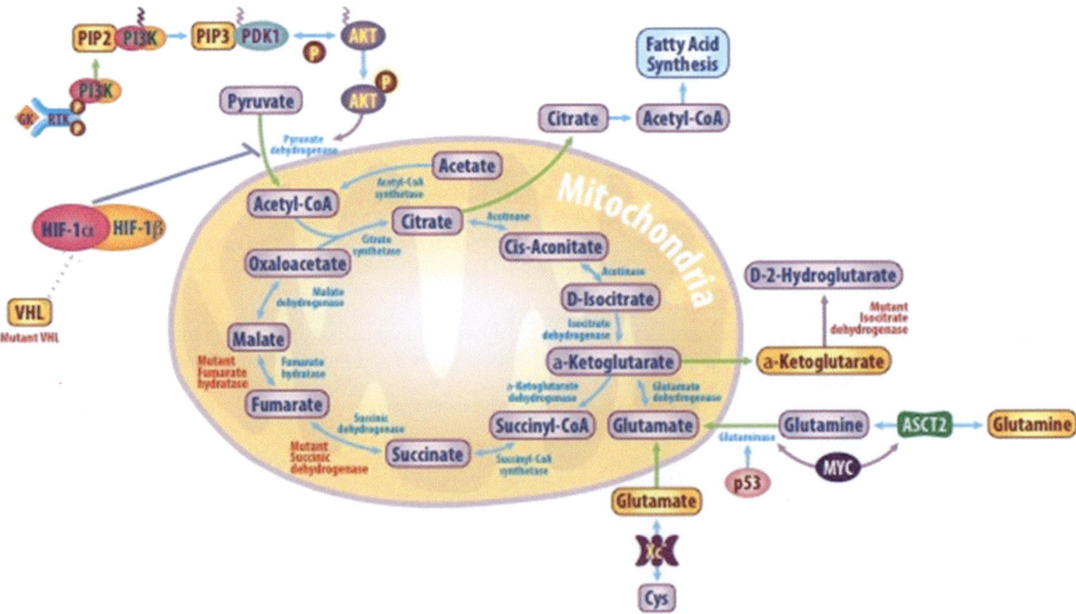

Fig. 6.2 The TCA cycle as a metabolic hub in cancer. TCA cycle-related enzymes such as fumarate hydratase, succinate dehydrogenase, and isocitrate dehydrogenase 1/2 are mutated in cancers such as renal cancers and gliomas, respectively. Additionally, oncogenic pathways involving VHL, PI3 kinase/AKT, and MYC can reprogram TCA cycle metabolism in many tumors

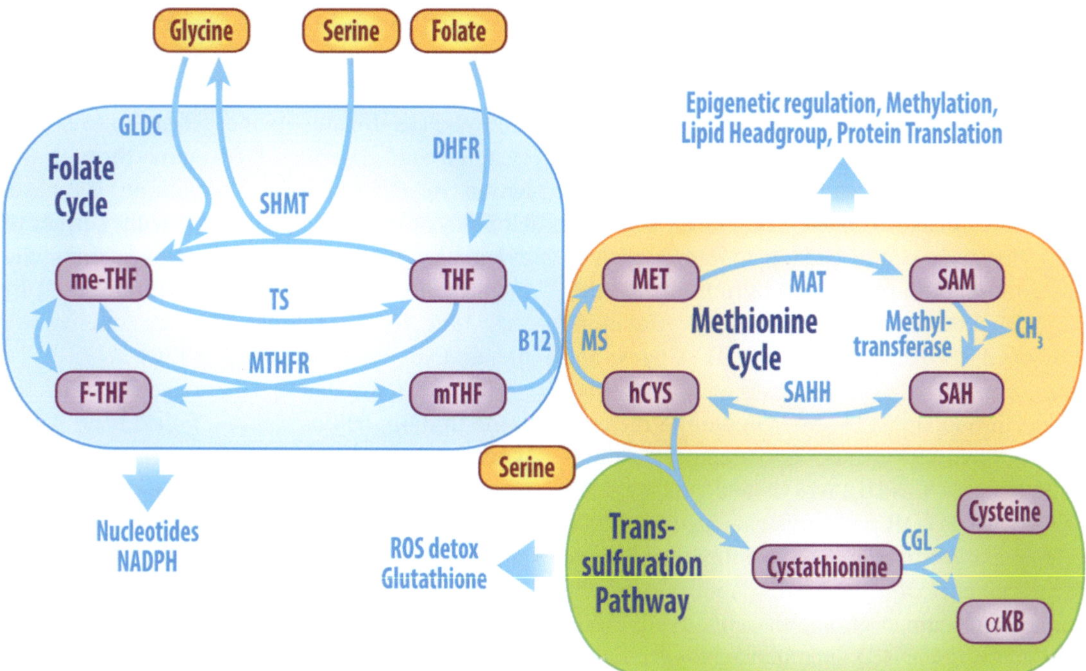

Fig. 6.3 Canonical cycles in one-carbon metabolism. Dietary folate enters the folate cycle and is converted to tetrahydrofolate (THF), by dihydrofolate reductase (DHFR). THF is converted to 5,10-methylene-THF (me-THF) by either serine hydroxymethyltransferase (SHMT), which is coupled to the conversion of serine to glycine, or glycine decarboxylase (GLDC), which catalyzes the conversion of glycine and THF to me-THF. Serine and glycine are derived from numerous sources including glycolytic intermediates. me-THF can be converted to either methyl-THF (mTHF) or 10-formyl-THF (F-THF). Methionine synthase (MS) and its cofactor vitamin B12 catalyze the demethylation of mTHF to regenerate THF and complete the folate cycle, whose major products include nucleotides and reducing potential in the form of NADPH. The methyl group from mTHF is added to homocysteine (hCYS) to form methionine (MET) and start the methionine cycle. Methionine adenosyltransferase (MAT) combines ATP and MET to form S-adenosylmethionine (SAM), which is the major cellular methyl donor. When it loses its methyl group, SAM is converted to S-adenosylhomocysteine (SAH), which is converted back to homocysteine by S-adenosylhomocysteine hydrolase (SAHH)-mediated deadenylation. The major outputs of the methionine cycle are methyl groups used to regulate numerous cellular processes as described in the text. In the transsulfuration pathway, hCYS condenses with serine to form cystathionine, which can be cleaved by cystathionine lyase (CGL) to form cysteine and α-ketobutyrate (αKB). Cysteine is then used to generate glutathione to help maintain cellular redox balance

Cancer cells via specific transporters can take up extracellular amino acids. Further, mutant Ras or c-Src in cancer cells enables uptake of extracellular proteins by a mechanism termed macropinocytosis mediated via remodeling of the actin cytoskeleton. Extracellular proteins thus taken up are broken down in the lysosome causing cells to recover free amino acids that can be shunted into various biosynthetic pathways including anaplerosis [22].

Glutamine is the most abundant amino acid in the plasma, and many cancers show altered glutamine metabolism. Proliferating cancer cells increase glutamine utilization as a source of nitrogen for de novo amino acid and nucleotide synthesis as well as a carbon source to replenish TCA cycle intermediates [23]. Glutamine is metabolized via a two-step process termed glutaminolysis. In the first step, glutamine is metabolized to glutamate by the enzyme glutaminase (GLS), which in turn is metabolized to ammonia and αKG by the enzyme glutamate dehydrogenase (GDH) (Fig. 6.2). There are two isoforms of GLS in mammals: GLS1, which primarily affects the entry of glutamine-derived carbons in the TCA cycle, and GLS2, which plays a larger role in regulating redox balance [24]. Glutamine metabolism can contribute to many cellular functions in cancer cells. For example, glutaminase and glutamate dehydrogenase generate ammonia from the γ and α nitrogens of glutamine, which can contribute to purine and pyrimidine synthesis [23]. Further, the carbons from glutamine contained in αKG can enter the TCA cycle and serve as a crucial contributor to anaplerosis and energy production [25–27]. Glutamine metabolism is rewired by many oncogenic alterations including RAS, VHL, MYC, and p53, and the PI3K/AKT/mTOR pathways can regulate glutamine metabolism (Fig. 6.2). Noninvasive in vivo measurement of glutamine uptake can be achieved in human glioma patients using radiolabeled 4-^{18}F-(2S,4R)-fluoroglutamine (^{18}F-FGln). ^{18}F-FGln uptake is increased in gliomas compared to normal brain enabling clear tumor to background delineation [28].

Glutamate along with cysteine and glycine can be used for the synthesis of glutathione. Glutathione is essential for the maintenance of redox balance in cells. NRF2 is a transcriptional factor that is a master regulator of redox balance and can control the expression of biosynthesis enzyme in the serine/glycine to support glutathione production [29]. Methionine, serine, and glycine contribute significantly to one-carbon metabolism as discussed below.

6.1.4 Cancer Cells Reprogram One-Carbon Metabolism

One-carbon metabolism broadly consists of the folate cycle, the methionine cycle, and the transsulfuration pathway and plays important roles in numerous biosynthetic pathways, maintaining redox balance and cellular methylation reactions [30] (Fig. 6.3). In the folate cycle, folate obtained from the diet is reduced through a series of reactions to form tetrahydrofolate (THF). THF is then converted to 5,10-methylene-THF (me-THF) through the action of the serine hydroxymethyltransferase enzymes [31] or the glycine cleavage system [32]. The folate cycle is coupled to the methionine cycle when methyl-THF donates its methyl group to homocysteine and generates methionine through the action of B^{12}-requiring methionine synthase. Homocysteine can also react with serine to eventually form glutathione, which links the methionine cycle to the transsulfuration pathway and forms a link between one-carbon metabolism and redox balance [30].

The substrates that fuel these interlinked cycles come from numerous sources. Folate is primarily derived from the diet. The serine that drives the formation of me-THF can either be derived from nutritional sources or from the metabolism of glucose, where the glycolytic intermediate 3-phosphoglycerate can be converted to serine by 3-phosphoglycerate dehydrogenase (PHGDG) and subsequent transamination [33]. Glycine can be imported into cells or be generated from numerous other carbon sources including threonine, choline, sarcosine, and others [30, 34].

These interconnected cycles produce numerous outputs that are required for cellular growth and proliferation. The nucleotides needed to form DNA and RNA require numerous substrates generated by one-carbon metabolism pathways. The formation of dUTP from dUMP requires the donation of a methyl group from methyl-THF. De novo purine synthesis requires carbons from glycine as well as the folate cycle intermediate 10-formyl-tetrahydrofolate to form the backbone of purine rings [35]. Lipids and their phosphatidylcholine head group also require methyl donation from S-adenosylmethionine (SAM), which is generated in the methionine cycle [36, 37] (Fig. 6.3). Several nodes of one-carbon metabolism are also important for the generation of reducing potential and the maintenance of redox balance. MTHFD1, an important enzyme in the folate cycle, was recently shown to be a major cellular producer of cellular reducing potential, and glutathione, the primary cellular antioxidant, is a major output of the transsulfuration pathway [38]. Finally, numerous cellular reactions and posttranslational modifications including histone, DNA, RNA, and amino acid methylation require methyl donation from SAM produced in one-carbon metabolism [39–41].

The importance of one-carbon metabolism to cancer was documented as early as the 1940s when Sidney Farber made his seminal discovery of anti-folates as the first chemotherapeutics. During the recent renaissance in cancer metabolism research, interest in these pathways has resurfaced. Studies in the 1980s showed that the entry of serine into one-carbon pathways increased as rat tumors progressed [42]. More recently, studies revealed that a significant fraction of cancers including many melanomas and triple negative breast cancers recurrently amplify PHGDH [43, 44]. Interestingly, the genomic regions harboring PHGDG amplifications contained no known oncogenes, suggesting that PHGDH itself may be a driver of these cancers. Indeed, PHGDG amplifications increased the shunting of glucose-derived carbon toward serine biosynthesis and one-carbon metabolism and were associated with a vulnerability to PHGDH inhibition.

Like PHGDH amplification, the actions of pyruvate kinase can facilitate the shunting of glucose-derived carbons into one-carbon metabolism. For example, FBP and serine can act to increase PKM2 activity when the pools of upstream glycolytic and one-carbon intermediate are replete and the absence of this allosteric stimulation slows PKM2 flux and increases flux through the pentose phosphate cycle and one-carbon metabolism when upstream metabolite pools fall [17]. Phosphorylated tyrosine residues can displace FBP from its allosteric pocket and thus inactivate PKM2, which suggests that oncogene-mediated signal transduction could help maintain PKM2 in an inactive form and facilitate flux through one-carbon pathways in many cancers [45].

The glycine cleavage pathway has also recently been implicated in the proliferation of cancer cells. A metabolomic study of the NCI-60 panel of cancer cell lines asked whether rates of proliferation correlated with the uptake or release of numerous metabolites [46]. While neither glucose uptake nor lactate production was correlated with proliferation, increased glycine uptake correlated tightly with increased proliferation. Further studies showed that this glycine was being metabolized by glycine dehydrogenase (GLDC) to enter the folate cycle via glycine cleavage (Fig. 6.3). GLDC may also be a driver of oncogenesis, as its overexpression is sufficient to drive tumorigenesis in xenograft models and its activity is especially high in subsets of tumor-initiating cells [47] . There are numerous other mechanisms by which enzymes in or related to one-carbon metabolism are related to oncogenesis and cancer progression and maintenance. Both ribonucleotide reductase and thymidylate synthase can function as oncogenes [48, 49], while other enzymes related to purine synthesis have recently been found to be tumor suppressors [50]. Together, these studies suggest that alterations in numerous steps of one-carbon metabolism can contribute to oncogenesis and further emphasize the opportunities that exist to therapeutically target different nodes in these pathways.

6.2 Oncogenic Reprogramming of Metabolism

One of the emerging paradigms in cancer metabolism is that oncogenes rewire metabolic pathways to drive tumor growth and adaptation to stress. Oncogenes can converge on central pathways via multiple mechanisms such as regulating transcription levels of nutrient transporters and metabolic enzymes, allosteric regulation of metabolic enzyme activity, and regulating epigenetics including histone and DNA modifications. These mechanisms vary depending on the cancer subtype, tissue origin, and tissue microenvironment. We examine these phenomena in the context of specific cancer subtypes below.

6.2.1 PI3K/AKT/mTOR Pathway Rewires Metabolism in Glioblastomas (GBMs)

Next-generation sequencing of GBMs in adults reveals that more than 90% of GBMs exhibit aberrant receptor tyrosine kinase/RAS/

phosphatidylinositol 3-kinase (RTK/RAS/PI3K) signaling mainly due to genetic alterations such as EGFR amplifications and PTEN deletions or alterations in downstream effectors of this pathway [51]. Growth factors such as EGF or PDGF bind their receptor tyrosine kinases to activate the PI3K cascade of intracellular signaling that closely regulates growth, metabolism, proliferation, and survival in cells. AKT and mTOR are central effectors of the PI3K pathway, while the lipid phosphatase PTEN is a negative regulator of this pathway. The PI3K/AKT/mTOR pathway is a central regulator of metabolism. Phosphorylated AKT (on Ser473) enhances glycolysis by increasing expression of glucose transporters and activating glycolytic enzymes such as HK2 and phosphofructokinase-1 (PFK-1) [52–54]. Similarly, AKT activation results in upregulating glutamine transporters [55] (Fig. 6.1).

The PI3K/AKT pathway directly influences the mammalian target of rapamycin (mTOR). mTOR is a master regulator of cellular homeostasis, nutrient sensing, and cellular metabolism [56]. mTOR is an atypical, PI3K family-related serine/threonine kinase that exists in two complexes termed mTOR complex 1 (mTORC1) and 2 (mTORC2) [56]. mTORC1 is an activator of anabolic growth and inhibitor of catabolism. Further, mTORC1 is a sensor for changes in growth factors, oxygen, and amino acid levels. Additionally, mTORC1 enhances protein synthesis by phosphorylating eukaryotic translation initiation factor 4E (eIF4E) binding protein 1 (4E-BP1) and S6 kinase 1 (S6K1) [57]. mTORC1 also promotes growth by suppressing autophagy. For example, ULK1, an essential factor required to initiate autophagy, can be negatively regulated by mTORC1 [58]. Activated mTORC1 reprograms glucose metabolism and glycolytic gene expression by regulating c-Myc activity in EGFRvIII-driven GBMs [59]. mTORC1 can also stimulate glutamine metabolism by enhancing the activity of GDH. This is achieved by repressing the transcription of SIRT4, an inhibitor of GDH [60]. The mTORC2 complex can also regulate many metabolic pathways. Activated mTORC2 can phosphorylate AKT and thus promote glucose uptake and metabolism [61]. Therefore, deregulation of the RTK/RAS/PI3K pathway is a central mediator of metabolic reprograming.

6.2.2 Isocitrate Dehydrogenase Is Mutated in Gliomas

The isocitrate dehydrogenases (IDHs) are a family of enzymes that catalyze the oxidative decarboxylation of isocitrate to α-ketoglutarate. In humans, there are three predominant isoforms that differ in subcellular localization, reversibility, and cofactor utilization. IDH1 is located in the cytosol and functions as a homodimer using $NADP^+$ as a substrate to catalyze the isocitrate to α-ketoglutarate reaction. IDH2 primarily localizes to the mitochondria and also functions as a homodimer using $NADP^+$ as a substrate. IDH3 functions as a heterotetramer composed of two α subunits, one β subunit, and one γ subunit. IDH3 localizes to the mitochondria and, unlike IDH1 and IDH2, uses NAD^+ rather than $NADP^+$ as a substrate thereby contributing to the TCA cycle and generation of NADH to fuel oxidative phosphorylation [62]. While the IDH1 and IDH2 reactions are reversible under physiologic conditions, the IDH3 reaction is thought to be irreversible [63].

The three IDH isoforms are regulated through distinct mechanisms. IDH3 is allosterically activated by citrate, calcium, and ADP, while it is inhibited by ATP, NADH, and NADPH. Together, these regulators couple the activity of IDH3 and the TCA cycle to energetic demand, which appears to be the dominant function of IDH3 [63–66]. Less is known about the regulation of IDH1 and IDH2. On a transcriptional level, IDH1 is regulated by the presence of sterols through the binding of SREBP-1a and REBP-2 to its promoter [67]. IDH1 transcription is also upregulated in response to exogenous signals such as prolactin and oxidative stress, although the precise transcription factors involved are not clear [68, 69]. These regulatory mechanisms underscore the view that a dominant function of IDH1 is to generate cytosolic NADPH that can be used for lipogenesis or ROS detoxification. While little has been reported on the transcriptional regulation of IDH2, recent studies suggest an important role for posttranslational control of IDH2 activity. IDH2 can be acetylated on lysine 413, which decreases its activity by more than 40-fold. SIRT3 is responsible for deacetylating this residue, thereby maintaining IDH2 activity, NADPH production, and the mitigation of oxidative stress [70]. Indeed, the generation of NADPH to maintain mitochondrial redox balance appears to the major function of IDH2 [71]. Under hypoxic conditions, IDH1 and IDH2 can reverse the direction of their typical flux and catalyze the reductive carboxylation of α-ketoglutarate to generate isocitrate [72, 73]. This reversed reaction allows the incorporation of glutamine-derived carbons into the acetyl-CoA pool, which then supports lipogenesis. These results reveal that IDH1 and IDH2 play critical albeit distinct roles in the lipogenesis necessary for proliferation under both normoxia (the generation of NADPH) and hypoxia (the incorporation of glutamine-derived carbons into lipids).

In the late 2000s, several groups performed sequencing efforts on low- and high-grade gliomas, which revealed a recurrent monoallelic mutation at Arg132 of IDH1 [74–76]. This mutation is found in the large majority of low-grade gliomas and secondary glioblastomas (GBMs), while those tumors lacking the IDH1 mutation often carry a mutation in the analogous codon (Arg172) of IDH2 [77, 78]. By contrast, primary GBMs and pediatric GBMs only rarely carried mutations of IDH1 or IDH2 [78, 79]. Similar efforts in other disease sites soon revealed both IDH1 and IDH2 mutations in many cancers including acute myeloid leukemia (AML, 5–20% mutational frequency) [80], myelodysplastic syndrome (MDS, 5–10% mutational frequency) [81], intrahepatic cholangiocarcinoma (up to 30% mutational frequency) [82, 83], and chondrosarcomas (approximately 50% mutational frequency) [84]. Many other cancers including lung and prostate cancer have been reported to contain mutations in IDH1 or IDH2, albeit at a much lower frequency [63].

While IDH mutations occur in many malignancies, there is variation between cancers with respect to the IDH isoform most commonly mutated, the amino acid that typically replaces arginine, and the prognostic importance of an IDH mutation. In gliomas, IDH1 is the dominant isoform affected, arginine is almost always replaced by a histidine (i.e., R132H), and the presence of an IDH mutation dramatically improves prognosis [78]. In AML, IDH1 and IDH2 mutations occur with similar frequencies with the most frequent substitutions being R132H and R132C in IDH1 or R140Q in IDH2 [85]. There is controversy regarding the prognostic importance of IDH mutations in AML as numerous reports have shown conflicting data [85–87]. In myelodysplastic syndrome, IDH1 and IDH2 mutations are relatively evenly mixed and are consistently associated with poor prognosis and increased likelihood of transformation to AML [81, 88]. In intrahepatic cholangiocarcinoma, most mutations occur in IDH1 and appear to have little prognostic importance [89–91].

The IDH1 and IDH2 mutations detailed above occur exclusively within the enzymatic active site. Initial studies revealed that cell lines engineered to overexpress mutant IDH1 or IDH2 had deficiencies in the ability to convert isocitrate to α-ketoglutarate, suggesting that these were loss of function mutations [78]. However, additional work soon revealed that mutations in both IDH1 and IDH2 encode for a gain of function in which the enzymes now convert α-ketoglutarate to (D)-2-hydroxyglutarate ((D)-2HG) while converting NADPH into $NADP^+$ [92, 93] (Fig. 6.4). This neomorphic enzymatic activity occurs because the mutated arginine residues (100 and 132 in IDH1 and 140 and 172 in IDH2) normally coordinate the binding of isocitrate carboxyl groups [94]. When these arginine residues are mutated, the binding affinity for isocitrate decreases while increasing the binding affinity for NADPH thereby severely limiting the rate of the oxidative decarboxylation of isocitrate (the canonical forward reaction of IDH1/IDH2) [92]. The reverse reaction can still partially occur in mutated IDH1/IDH2; however, the active site mutation results in the reduction of α-ketoglutarate to (D)-2HG, which is coupled to the oxidation of

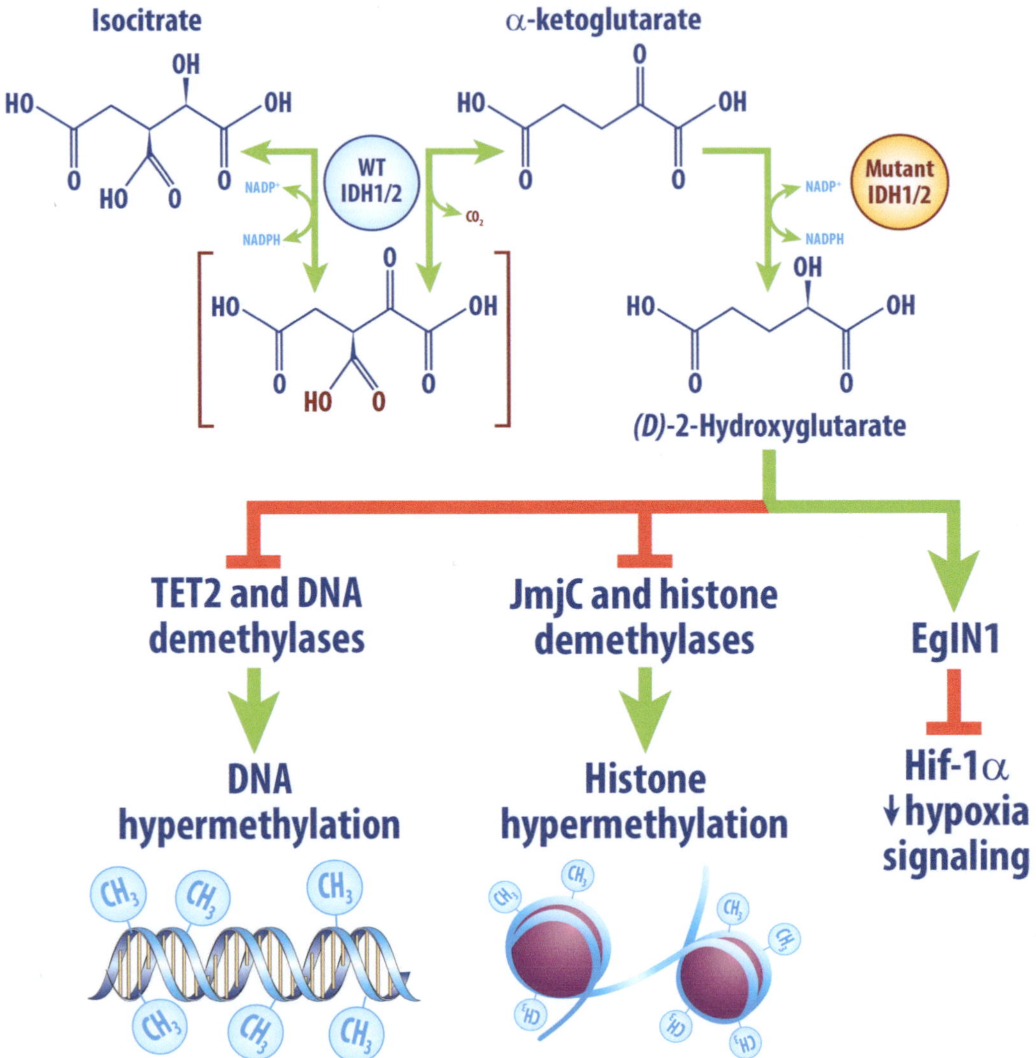

Fig. 6.4 Mutant Isocitrate dehydrogenase-mediated oncogenesis. Wild-type isocitrate dehydrogenase 1 and 2 (wtIDH1/2) catalyzes the reversible conversion of isocitrate and α-ketoglutarate. Mutant IDH1/IDH2 catalyzes the conversion of α-ketoglutarate to (D)-2-hydroxyglutarate, which inhibits TET2 and DNA demethylases, inhibits histone demethylases including the jumonji C (JmjC) family, and stimulates the EGLN prolyl hydroxylases. These discrete functions induce DNA hypermethylation and histone hypermethylation and decrease hypoxia signaling, which in turn induce oncogenesis

NADPH to NADP+. Additional carboxylation of (D)-2HG cannot occur and leads to a net reaction in which α-ketoglutarate and NADPH are consumed and (D)-2HG and NADP+ are produced. Because cells have limited ability to consume (D)-2HG, the IDH1/IDH2 mutations cause dramatic accumulations of (D)-2HG into the millimolar range [93, 95, 96].

The IDH1 mutation is an early event in gliomagenesis, suggesting that it might be a driver of oncogenesis [77, 97, 98]. Indeed, the forced expression of mutant IDH or treatment with cell-permeable (D)-2HG impairs cellular differentiation in numerous models including immortalized astrocytes, neuronal stem cells, erythroleukemia lines, liver progenitor cells, and chondrosarcoma models [63, 99–103]. Investigations into the tumorigenic effects of mutant IDH in vivo suggest that, on their own, these mutations are not sufficient to induce cancer. A brain-specific IDH1 R132H knock-in mouse was found to have more than a 100-fold increase in brain (D)-2HG levels, but the mice died from fatal cerebral hemorrhage shortly after birth, which precluded the investigation of oncogenesis [104]. A similar knock-in model of IDH1 R132H into hematopoietic stem cells caused impaired hematopoietic differentiation but no frank leukemia [104].

Rather being a sole oncogenic driver of malignant transformation, IDH mutations appear to function as an early genetic lesion that requires the acquisitions of additional lesions in order for cancer to form. This model has been best dissected in intrahepatic cholangiocarcinoma. Forced expression of the IDH2-R172K isoform in biliary cells caused the apparent migration of biliary cells away from bile ducts but did not induce tumor formation. However, when this model was crossed with a mouse that expressed an activating $Kras^{G12D}$ mutation, nearly all animals developed multifocal and metastatic intrahepatic cholangiocarcinoma in contrast to the complete absence of tumors in IDH2-R172K mice or the delayed development of hepatocellular carcinoma in the parental $Kras^{G12D}$ mice [103]. Further evidence for this multiple hit model comes from IDH1-mutated gliomas, where the development of low-grade or high-grade tumors seems to only occur when an early IDH1 mutation is followed by later alterations such as p53, TERT, and ATRX mutations, or deletion of chromosomal arms 1p and 19q [98, 105, 106].

The question then remains: What is the mechanistic basis by which IDH mutations contribute to oncogenesis? Because cell-permeable (D)-2HG recapitulates the transformative properties of IDH mutations [99, 107], (D)-2HG has been termed an "oncometabolite" and is thought to be responsible for the bulk of the ability of mutant IDH to induce oncogenesis. It appears that the ability of (D)-2HG to mediate oncogenesis is due to its structural similarity to αKG, which allows (D)-2HG to alter the activity of αKG-dependent dioxygenases, thereby altering DNA methylation, histone methylation, and hypoxia signaling [107] (Fig. 6.4).

In 2010, analysis performed by the Cancer Genome Atlas Research Network revealed that a subset of gliomas are characterized by widespread concerted DNA hypermethylation [108]. This glioma-specific CpG island methylator phenotype (G-CIMP) was highly enriched for the transcriptionally defined proneural GBM subtype [109], and approximately 80% of G-CIMP-positive tumors also carried an IDH1 mutation [108]. Furthermore, the forced expression of mutant IDH1 was sufficient to induce a hypermethylator phenotype similar to G-CIMP in immortalized astrocytes and other cell line models [100, 102, 110]. A similar association has been found in AML, where both IDH1 and IDH2 mutations are associated with global DNA hypermethylation [111]. In AML, IDH mutations are mutually exclusive with loss of function mutations in TET2, which catalyzes the αKG-dependent hydroxylation of 5-methylcytosine (5-mC) and is thought to be an important mediator of DNA demethylation [111]. (D)-2HG produced by mutant IDH inhibits TET2-mediated 5-mC hydroxylation in vitro and in several cellular systems [111, 112]. Furthermore, both IDH-mutated and TET2-mutated AML clinical samples displayed a similar DNA hypermethylation signature [111]. While inactivating TET2 mutations have not been described in gliomas, there do appear to be a subset of IDH wild-type grade II/III gliomas in which the TET2 promoter is hypermethylated, which presumably leads to TET2 silencing [113]. Together, these results suggest that some of the oncogenic potential of IDH mutations is due to their ability to inhibit enzymes such as TET2, which are involved in DNA demethylation, thereby inducing a hypermethylator phenotype, altered gene expression, and impaired differentiation.

In addition to DNA hypermethylation, IDH mutations may also promote oncogenesis by inducing histone hypermethylation and altered gene expression (Fig. 6.4). Jumonji C (JmjC) histone lysine demethylases comprise the largest family of histone demethylases and require αKG as a cofactor for their catalytic activity, in which the methyl group attached to lysine is hydroxylated and then lost as formaldehyde [114, 115]. Loss of function or decreased expression of JmjC demethylases is associated with oncogenesis in numerous cancers including AML, MDS, and glioma [107, 116]. The expression of mutant IDH causes histone hypermethylation in both cell lines and tumors as evidenced by increased trimethylation of histone marks including H3K9, H3K27, and H3K36 [102, 110, 112, 117, 118]. These effects appear to be due to the ability of (D)-2HG to compete with αKG and thereby inhibit JmjC demethylase activity [117, 119]. Together, DNA and histone hypermethylation affect the expression of many genes and are thought to contribute to suppressing cell differentiation and promoting oncogenesis.

(D)-2HG produced by mutant IDH affects several processes apart from DNA and histone methylation including collagen maturation, hypoxia signaling, and mitochondrial ATP production. Mice bearing a brain-specific IDH1 R132H knock-in die due to cerebral hemorrhage caused by abnormal collagen maturation. Proline hydroxylation is an important posttranslational modification that stabilizes collagen, and it appears that 2-HG may inhibit the αKG-dependent hydroxylation of collagen prolines much in the same way it inhibits other αKG-dependent hydroxylation reactions [104].

(D)-2HG also affects the proline hydroxylases that regulate hypoxia signaling. HIF-1α is the master transcriptional regulator of hypoxia signaling and is primarily regulated posttranscriptionally. Under normoxia, HIF-1α is hydroxylated by αKG- and oxygen-dependent prolyl hydroxylases including the EGLN family, which leads to HIF-1α degradation by the VHL complex. Under hypoxia, prolyl hydroxylase activity decreases leading to HIF-1α accumulation and the transcriptional activation of numerous hypoxia target genes. Initial studies suggested that the presence of IDH1 mutations in cell lines or human glioma samples was associated with increased levels of HIF-1α, presumably due to decreased αKG levels or (D)-2HG-mediated inhibition of prolyl hydroxylases [120]. This phenotype was recapitulated in the brain-specific IDH1 R132H knock-in mice, which also exhibit increased brain HIF-1α levels [104]. Several subsequent studies have presented evidence that (D)-2HG may activate rather than inhibit the EGLN hydroxylases responsible for hydroxylating HIF-1α and thereby decrease HIF-1α levels [101, 107]. Indeed, (D)-2HG serves as an EGLN cosubstrate in vitro, and the presence of mutant IDH1decreases HIF levels in immortalized astrocytes and promotes colony formation on soft agar [101]. Consistent with these findings, patient level data from the TCGA showed that the presence of an IDH1 mutation in astrocytomas was associated with decreased expression of HIF-responsive target genes [101]. These apparently conflicting data can be reconciled by the realization that EGLN hydroxylase activity is only one of many inputs that determine HIF stability. Indeed, detailed histopathologic analysis reveals that IDH1 mutant gliomas can focally increase HIF-1α levels in areas that correlate well with regions of hypoxia and necrosis [121].

Additional functions of the oncometabolite (D)-2HG continue to be discovered. Provocative recent studies in *C. elegans* reveal that (D)-2HG, like αKG, can inhibit the mitochondrial ATP synthase, inhibit mTOR signaling, and extend worm life span [122, 123]. These studies were extended to glioblastoma, where the presence of mutant IDH1 decreases oxygen consumption and hyperpolarizes the mitochondrial membrane potential, which is consistent with ATP synthase inhibition [122]. Together, these results suggest that IDH mutant tumors may be more dependent on glycolysis for ATP generation than their IDH wild-type counterparts and may be selectively vulnerable to therapeutic strategies that limit glucose availability.

6.2.3 MYC Is a Central Metabolic Regulator in Many Tumors

c-MYC (hereafter termed MYC) is a transcription factor that heterodimerizes with its partner MAX and induces a broad transcriptional program that regulates numerous pro-growth cellular programs [95].

MYC is a widely expressed member of the *myc* family, which also includes L-MYC and N-MYC, and its expression is tightly regulated in normal cells [124]. In the late 1970s and early 1980s, *MYC* was discovered as the cellular homolog of the retroviral oncogene *v-myc* [125, 126]. *MYC* was one of the first described oncogenes, and alterations in *MYC* including amplification and translocation characterize many types of human cancer [95, 127].

In normal cells, the *MYC* proto-oncogene is tightly regulated at the transcriptional and post-transcriptional levels, while the MYC protein is heavily regulated posttranslationally [124]. Together, these numerous regulatory mechanisms allow the activity of MYC to increase as a function of pro-growth signal transduction pathways so that MYC activity increases when a non-transformed cell needs to proliferate. Indeed, when fibroblasts are stimulated to proliferate by the addition of serum, MYC levels increase approximately 20-fold [128]. In cancers, the expression and activity of MYC often become growth factor independent, which allows MYC to help coordinate the constitutive proliferation characterized by transformed cells.

MYC is estimated to regulate around 15% of the protein-coding genes in mammalian cells [129, 130]. Given this broad transcriptional control, the importance of MYC in driving proliferation, and the role that altered metabolism plays in fueling proliferation, it is perhaps not surprising that MYC regulates numerous metabolic genes. Indeed, overexpression of MYC increases the expression of numerous genes involved in glycolysis and glutaminolysis and increases cellular utilization of both glucose and glutamine [23, 131–134] (Figs. 6.1, 6.2, and 6.5). MYC not only controls rates of carbon substrate uptake but also the intracellular metabolic pathways through which carbon substrates pass. For example, the absence of MYC forces proliferating fibroblasts to metabolize pyruvate through pyruvate carboxylase rather than pyruvate dehydrogenase due to transcriptional effects on the kinases that regulate pyruvate dehydrogenase [130]. These results suggest that proliferating cells without MYC may be more dependent on glucose for anaplerosis, while those with increased MYC signaling may instead be able to rely on glutamine.

MYC also facilitates increased flux through metabolic pathways that share intermediates with glycolysis. Indeed, MYC increases the entry of glucose-derived carbon into the pentose phosphate cycle and one-carbon folate metabolism to facilitate the synthesis of ribose sugars,

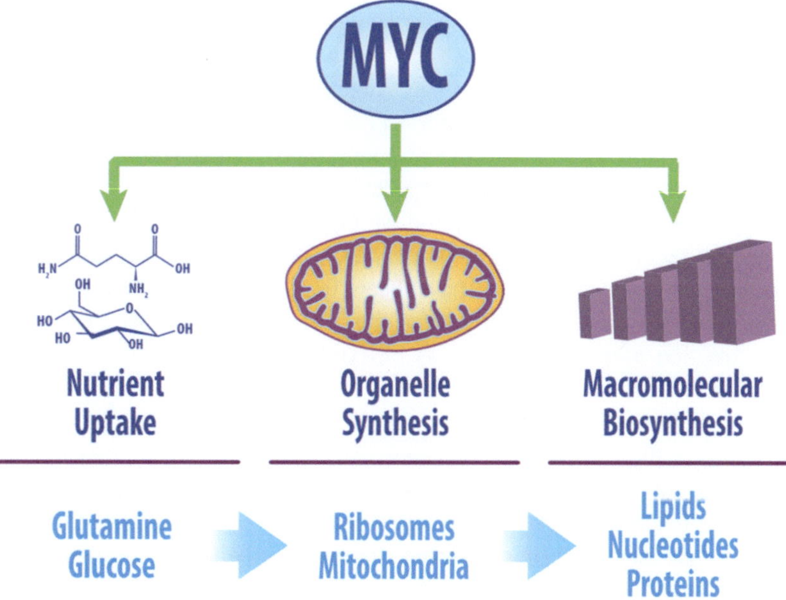

Fig. 6.5 MYC reprograms cellular metabolism. MYC induces a broad transcriptional program that increases nutrient uptake, synthesis of organelles, and anabolic enzyme expression. Together, these coordinated changes allow for the simultaneous increase in the raw materials, subcellular synthetic compartments, and key enzymes needed to synthesize the biomolecules required for proliferation

nucleotides, and amino acids as well as to generate NADPH, which fuels reductive biosynthesis [130]. MYC replete proliferating fibroblasts have increased levels of glucose, alanine, glycine, adenine, and ribose [130]. MYC also facilitates the synthesis of the lipids that proliferating cells require to duplicate their plasma membranes. As noted above, MYC stimulates the entry of glucose- and glutamine-derived carbons into the TCA cycle. One of the important anaplerotic roles of the TCA cycle is to form citrate, which is an important precursor of fatty acids and cholesterol. In addition to providing the carbon substrates for fatty acid synthesis, MYC also induces the expression of numerous enzymes involved in the production of fatty acids including ATP citrate lyase, acetyl-CoA carboxylase, fatty acid synthase, and stearoyl-CoA desaturase [135, 136]. The functional significance of these changes points toward an importance for MYC driving anabolic lipid synthesis. Indeed, when MYC-deficient fibroblasts proliferate, they oxidize fatty acids at a rate four- to five-fold higher than replete cells and incorporate less pyruvate-derived acetyl-CoA into lipids. Therefore, the transcriptional effects of MYC not only facilitate increased carbon uptake but also funnel this carbon toward the anabolic reactions necessary for cell division [136].

When a cell divides, it must replicate not only its simple biomolecules but also complex organelles. This process is promoted by MYC, which facilitates the biogenesis of many organelles such as ribosomes and mitochondria [124, 137] (Fig. 6.5). The ability of MYC to promote mitochondrial biogenesis appears to be related to its ability to increase the transcription of PGC-1β through direct binding to its promoter [129, 138], although other MYC targets have been implicated as well [139, 140]. Because of the important role that mitochondria play as biosynthetic hubs, the ability of MYC to promote mitochondrial biogenesis provides the machinery necessary to turn the increased carbon sources driven by MYC into the biomolecules necessary for cancer cells to proliferate. Hence, MYC not only supplies the raw materials (carbons) necessary for biosynthesis but also the workshops (mitochondria) where much of the biosynthesis occurs.

The global role of MYC in controlling cancer metabolism is well illustrated by the case of triple negative breast cancer (TNBC). TNBC is defined by the absence of estrogen receptors, progesterone receptors, or human epidermal growth factor receptor 2 (HER2) overexpression and exhibits worse clinical outcomes than hormone receptor-positive cancers. Transcriptional analysis of TNBC suggests that many of these cancers are characterized by overexpression of MYC [141–143]. ^{18}FDG PET imaging of patients with TNBC suggests that these cancers exhibit increased glycolysis compared to hormone receptor-positive breast cancers and that this increased glycolysis correlates with increased MYC transcript levels [141]. Furthermore, knockdown of MYC decreases glycolytic metabolism in TNBC through a mechanism involving thioredoxin-interacting protein, which suggests that there are additionally layers of MYC regulation of glycolysis beyond the simple transcriptional activation of glycolytic genes [144]. TNBC also display increased glutamine uptake compared to other subtypes of breast cancer [145]. While glutamine restriction slows the growth of most TNBC lines, knockdown of MYC does not slow glutamine utilization in triple negative breast cancer [144, 145]. These results suggest that there may be MYC-independent signals that can support glutamine metabolism in TNBC. In fact, there is increasing data that the role of MYC in dictating glutaminolysis may be context dependent. While MYC-driven liver tumors display high rates of glutaminolysis, MYC-driven lung tumors may be net producers of glutamine rather than consumers [146].

6.2.4 Renal Carcinomas Show Mutations in Metabolic Regulators

Renal cancers show profound metabolic alterations. The von Hippel-Lindau (VHL) factor is a tumor suppressor gene that is frequently mutated in a common subtype of renal cancers termed clear cell renal cell carcinomas [147]. VHL is a director regulator of the oxygen-sensing pathway, and renal cancers with VHL mutations show alterations in both glycolysis and TCA cycle metabolism. Of note, rare subsets of renal cancers show mutations in TCA cycle-related genes. Papillary type 2 renal cell carcinomas seen in hereditary leiomyomatosis and renal cell carcinoma syndrome are characterized by mutations in fumarate hydratase (Fig. 6.2). Succinate dehydrogenase mutations are noted in rare subsets of oncocytic renal cancers (Fig. 6.2) [148]. Both these mutations result in rewiring of many aspects of metabolism including glycolysis and the TCA cycle [149–151]. We examine some of these metabolic changes using VHL mutant cancers as an example.

VHL is a regulator of hypoxia-inducible factors (HIFs) in the oxygen-sensing pathway and is an E3 ubiquitin ligase that ubiquitinates HIF for degradation in the proteasome. HIFs form a heterodimer composed of HIF-1α and HIF-1β (Fig. 6.2). In normoxia, HIF-1α is bound by VHL and undergoes proteasomal degradation following hydroxylation by HIF prolyl hydroxylases. HIF prolyl hydroxylases such as EglN1 depend on oxygen as a cofactor for their enzyme activity. Thus, hypoxia causes lowered HIF prolyl hydroxylase activity resulting in stabilization of HIF-1α. Stable HIF-1α then binds with HIF1-β/ARNT and mediates the transcription of a number of genes that reprogram metabolism [152, 153].

HIF reprograms glucose metabolism to promote the Warburg effect by influencing glycolysis and the entry of glucose-derived carbons into the TCA cycle. HIF increases glycolytic flux by increasing glucose uptake and metabolism by upregulating glucose transporters and enzymes such as HK and PKM2 [154–156]. PKM2 can also interact with HIF-1α to enhance its binding to hypoxia response elements [156]. HIF activation promotes lactate formation by increasing LDHA expression and decreasing conversion of pyruvate to acetyl-CoA by upregulating PDK1 resulting in decreased activity of PDH (Fig. 6.2) [3, 154, 157]. Interestingly, this shunting of glucose carbons away from the TCA cycle results in reprograming of glutamine metabolism. HIF activation or VHL insufficiency (resulting in increased HIF activity) switches from oxidative decarboxylation to reductive carboxylation of glutamine to generate citrate and acetyl-CoA for lipid synthesis [158–162]. These data suggest that HIF activation is critical for metabolic adaptations that tumor cells undergo in hypoxic environments.

6.3 Therapeutic Targeting of Cancer Metabolism

The increasing understanding of altered metabolism in cancer has rekindled the idea that metabolic enzymes can be selective and efficacious therapeutic targets to treat cancer [163, 164]. This idea dates to the initial discovery by Sidney Farber in the 1940s that the anti-folate aminopterin could induce temporary remissions in childhood leukemia [165, 166]. This discovery was followed by the development of another anti-folate, methotrexate, which is notable both for its role in one of the first cures of a solid tumor with chemotherapy and its continued use in the clinic today [166]. Newer anti-folates continue to be introduced to the clinic in the modern era, and pemetrexed, which was approved by the FDA in 2004, is currently used to treat a number of malignancies including lung cancer [167].

The historical success of metabolically targeted therapies is not limited to targeting folate metabolism. Nucleoside analogs inhibit thymidylate synthase, ribonucleotide reductase, or DNA polymerase and have been used for decades to effectively treat numerous malignancies [165]. These agents, which include 5-fluorouracil, capecitabine, gemcitabine, fludarabine, and hydroxyurea, remain first-line therapies for many cancers today both on their own and in combination with radiation [168].

A third "historical" example of targeting cancer metabolism is the example of L-asparaginase. In the 1950s, investigators found that the administration of guinea pig serum could cause regression of lymphomas and this was later attributed to the presence of the enzyme L-asparaginase [169, 170]. Further studies revealed that subsets of transformed hematopoietic cells were incapable of synthesizing their own asparagine (i.e., were asparagine auxotrophs) and underwent cell death when exogenous asparaginase depleted the systemic asparagine pool [171]. Numerous clinical trials have demonstrated the efficacy of

L-asparaginase in hematologic malignancies over the past 40 years, and it remains a cornerstone of therapy for acute lymphoblastic leukemia today [172].

Because both cancerous and noncancerous cells express the same core metabolic machinery, it is often assumed that the utility of agents targeting aberrant cancer metabolism would be limited by untoward side effects caused by the inhibition of metabolic pathways in normal tissues. While normal tissue toxicities can be limiting for anti-folates, nucleoside analogs, and L-asparaginase [173, 174], the clinical benefit derived from these agents over the past 50 years emphasizes the presence of a therapeutic window that exists for targeting metabolic pathways in cancer. This therapeutic window cannot be entirely explained by the increased rates of proliferation in cancers and is likely also related to altered DNA damage repair machinery and cell cycle checkpoint aberrations that characterize many cancers [24]. This therapeutic window, combined with the historical successes of targeting cancer metabolism and the burgeoning knowledge being developed by the cancer metabolism field, has led to numerous new attempts to therapeutically target cancer metabolism.

6.3.1 Targeting Glucose Uptake and Glycolysis

The widespread phenotype of increased glycolysis in cancer has been exploited clinically for diagnostic and prognostic benefit with ^{18}FDG-PET imaging, which is now standardly used in many cancers [175]. Inhibition of increased glycolysis is now being explored clinically with strategies such agents such as 2-deoxyglucose (2DG) and dietary modifications such as the ketogenic diet.

2DG is a glucose analog that is imported to cells by glucose transporters and phosphorylated by hexokinase to produce 2-deoxyglucose-6-phosphate, which is a competitive inhibitor of the enzymes that metabolize glucose-derived glucose-6-phosphate. 2DG treatment is cytotoxic at sufficient (e.g., millimolar) concentrations and can potentiate the effects of numerous chemotherapeutics and radiation [176, 177]. The clinical utility of 2DG has been investigated as a single agent in patients with cancer as early as the late 1950s [178]. However, the NCI abandoned this approach due to untoward side effects including compensatory hyperglycemia, nausea, and vomiting, presumably due to the effects of 2DG on glycolysis in normal tissues. While these side effects could make long-term 2DG treatment intolerable, they were not life threatening. In the last two decades, several small studies from India have again investigated the clinical use of 2DG, this time as part of combination therapy. These studies showed the feasibility of combining oral administration of high-dose 2DG (sufficient to give rise to millimolar concentrations in patients) with radiation therapy for patients with gliomas. While life-threatening side effects were not seen, most patients developed hyperglycemia and mild-to-moderate nausea or vomiting, consistent with early trials from the NCI [179, 180]. As of 2009, a phase III trial of this strategy was underway in India, but no results have been published at this time [177]. These clinical experiences with 2DG suggest that metabolically targeted agents that may have little to no therapeutic window on their own could still have clinical utility when combined with anatomically targeted therapies such as radiation or molecularly targeted therapies.

An alternative to pharmacologically inhibiting glycolysis is to alter circulating metabolic substrate levels through dietary modifications. One such dietary program is the ketogenic diet in which fats comprise approximately 90% of calories and carbohydrates are limited to 5% or less (compared to 50% in a typical diet) [181]. Such a diet promotes the oxidation of fats in the liver leading to high levels of circulating ketones such as acetoacetate and β-hydroxybutyrate. Despite extremely low levels of ingested carbohydrates, the ketogenic diet only modestly lowers circulating glucose levels due to a compensatory increase in gluconeogenesis [182]. The ketogenic diet has been used to treat certain inborn errors of metabolism and intractable epilepsy [183]. Recently, there has been increased interest in utilizing the ketogenic diet to augment cancer therapy. Preclinical studies show that the ketogenic diet increases oxidative stress in xenograft models of lung cancer and sensitizes these tumors to both radiation and chemotherapy [184]. It is hypothesized that the presence of high circulating levels of ketones increases oxidative ATP production in cancer cells, which both increases mitochondrial ROS generation and limits antioxidant production by limiting pentose phosphate cycle flux. While scattered case reports and a small pilot study support the safety of the ketogenic diet in patients with cancer [185–187], this approach remains investigational. As of 2014, there were at least ten clinical trials investigating the use of the ketogenic diet for the treatment cancer either as monotherapy or in combination with chemotherapy or radiotherapy [181]. The results of these trials will help clarify whether the ketogenic diet could truly be useful to augment cancer therapy.

6.3.2 Inhibiting Glutamine Metabolism

There has been much investigation of the enzymes related to glutamine metabolism as potential therapeutic targets. Inhibitors of GLS1 have been developed, and these compounds slow the growth of many cancer cell lines in vitro and in xenograft models in vivo [188, 189]. Because glutamine is the source of most of the carbon that eventually forms (D)-2HG in IDH mutant tumors, glutaminase inhibitors are also efficacious in the treatment of models of IDH mutant cancer [190]. Clinical trials of glutaminase inhibitors are in progress, and preliminary results have been reported. In a phase I trial, CB-839, a glutaminase inhibitor produced by Calithera, was given to 35 patients with a variety of solid tumors. Active concentrations were achieved in tumors, and disease stability was achieved in 30% of patients with a tolerable safety profile [191]. CB-839 has also been investigated in hematologic malignancies in phase I studies. In 23 patients with multiple myeloma or non-Hodgkin's lymphoma, CB-839 was well tolerated, but preliminary results showed few clinically significant responses [192].

6.3.3 Mutant IDH Inhibitors

The combination of the oncogenic effects of mutant IDH and its cancer-specific expression have led to tremendous interest in inhibiting IDH enzymatic activity as a therapeutic strategy. Pharmacologic inhibitors of mutants IDH1 and IDH2 have been synthesized and show great promise in cell lines, animal models, and patients [63, 193–197]. Treatment of oligodendroglioma cell lines bearing 1p/19q co-deletions and IDH1 R132H mutations with IDH1 mutant-specific inhibitors significantly decreases (D)-2HG production. These inhibitors also slow subcutaneous glioma xenografts in animal models. IDH1 inhibition decreases the methylation of histone H3K9me3 and increases the expression of genes associated with glial differentiation, suggesting that its therapeutic effects arise from reversing (D)-2HG-mediated histone hypermethylation. Intriguingly, DNA methylation did not appreciably decrease after treatment [194]. Treatment of patient-derived AML cells with a mutant IDH2 inhibitor induces differentiation in vitro with early reversal of increased histone methylation but in contrast to glioma models showed a slower reversal of DNA hypermethylation [196, 197].

Given these promising preclinical data, clinical trials have commenced in patients with IDH1 and IDH2 mutant AML and solid tumors. While final results await publication, early abstract reports from these trials have been promising. In a phase I/II trial, an inhibitor of mutant IDH2 (AG-221) was administered to around 200 patients with IDH2-mutated advanced hematologic malignancies, many of which were heavily pretreated. AG-221 treatment was well tolerated and induced overall response rates of around 40% and complete response rates of around 20% [198]. In a similar phase I trial, 66 patients with IDH1-mutated advanced hematologic malignancies were treated with an inhibitor of mutant IDH1 (AG-120). Similar to the trials of IDH2 inhibition, AG-120 induced responses in 36% of patients and complete responses in nearly 20% of patients [87]. IDH inhibition has also been pursued clinically in solid malignancies including gliomas. While data are still maturing, initial reports suggest that

AG-120 is well tolerated, reduces (D)-2HG levels in both intracranial and extracranial malignancies, and leads to clinically meaningful responses in a variety of solid tumors [199]. While these clinical data are still immature, they raise the possibility that the inhibition of mutant IDH could become an important tool in the clinical management of patients with IDH-mutated malignancies. Importantly, the allelic frequency of mutated IDH did not significantly change during treatment, even in patients obtaining a complete response [198]. These data suggest that mutant IDH1 inhibitor agents act by inducing differentiation rather than cytotoxicity. This mechanism of action is consistent with in vitro results and suggests that these agents may require chronic administration, even in patients that achieve a complete response.

6.4 Targeting Pyruvate Dehydrogenase

Because of the important role that increased glycolytic metabolism and lactate production may play in cancer growth, therapeutic strategies have developed to increase the relative flux of pyruvate metabolism away from lactate and toward the mitochondria. Dichloroacetate (DCA) is a small molecule that inhibits PDK and therefore activates PDH and increases the mitochondrial metabolism of pyruvate [200]. DCA is conventionally used to treat the lactic acidosis that accompanies rare inborn errors of metabolism [201]. More recently, interest in DCA has been increasing as an anticancer agent. DCA treatment of cell lines and xenografts derived from multiple cancer types increases glucose oxidation, induces apoptosis, and slows proliferation [202]. DCA has also been used as a combination therapy in preclinical models where it sensitizes cervical cancer cell lines to cisplatin and glioblastoma cell lines to radiation [144, 203]. DCA is well tolerated by patients, and a small study published in 2010 showed encouraging results in five patients with glioblastoma treated with DCA [204]. At this time, several clinical trials investigating the clinical use of DCA in a variety of tumors are either accruing or will be reporting data soon.

6.5 Alternative Strategies to Modulate Cancer Metabolism

Several other metabolic strategies to treat cancer are currently being investigated in clinical trials. Vitamin C has been investigated over several decades as a potential cancer preventative agent, but to date little evidence supports this hypothesis [205, 206]. More recently, studies looking at the pharmacologic administration of vitamin C suggest that high doses of this compound may lead to ROS-mediated inactivation of GADPH and preferentially kill cancer cells with high rates of glycolysis [207]. Vitamin C may also be useful as combination therapy with ionizing radiation [208]. Strides are also being made to inhibit the monocarboxylate transporters (MCTs) responsible for lactate export as a therapeutic strategy. AZD3965 inhibits MCT1 and has anticancer activity in a number of preclinical cancers both on its own and as combination therapy [209–211]. Clinical trials of AZD3965 are ongoing. The requirement for high rates of fatty acid synthesis has also been investigated as a potential cancer treatment. Agents that inhibit fatty acid synthase such as TVB-3166 have shown promising in vitro activity and are currently being investigated in phase I clinical trials [212].

Metformin is a biguanide antidiabetic that is the standard of care initial pharmacologic treatment for type 2 (non-insulin-dependent) diabetes. Metformin acts by specifically inhibiting complex I of the mitochondrial respiratory chain, which perturbs the AMP/ATP energy balance in cells and leads to the LKB1-dependent phosphorylation of AMPK. These changes cause cells to switch from anabolic to catabolic metabolic programs, thereby inhibiting gluconeogenesis, increasing fatty acid oxidation, and increasing hepatic glucose uptake leading to the normalization of systemic glucose levels [213, 214].

In 2005, a retrospective case-control study suggested that diabetic patients taking metformin had an approximately 20% decreased risk of developing cancer compared to control patients with diabetes [215]. Since then, numerous additional retrospective studies have found an association between metformin use and decreased cancer incidence [216, 217]. Reanalysis of patient data from randomized trials involving metformin did not recapitulate these data; however, these retrospective analyses were post hoc and unplanned [218]. In addition to its potential preventative effects, metformin may also have direct anticancer activity. In cell culture and preclinical animal models, metformin decreases cancer cell proliferation across numerous cancer types [219]. The exact mechanism of action of the anticancer activity of metformin is debated but may involve lowering systemic glucose levels, decreased insulin signaling, or direct activation of AMPK in cancer cells [214]. The anticancer effects of metformin have been evaluated in patients in several contexts. In several studies in women with breast cancer, neoadjuvant metformin treatment caused decreased proliferation and increased apoptosis of cancer cells at the time of surgery [220–222]. Given the results of these observational studies and the promising results of these neoadjuvant randomized clinical trials, several randomized trials have opened to test whether metformin improves disease-free survival in breast cancer, ovarian cancer, and others [214].

6.6 Summary

Altered metabolism in cancer cells is an active phenomena that tumors use to sustain their uncontrolled proliferation. Many oncogenes can reprogram metabolism. Cancer cells display the Warburg effect that leads to generation of lactate from glucose carbons. This along with altered glucose uptake and metabolism sustains many biologic functions in cancer cells. Amino acid metabolism is also reprogrammed in cancer cells. Amino acids such as glutamine and glutamate support the TCA cycle and redox function and meet the nitrogen demand in cancer cells. Amino acids such as serine, glycine, and methionine are closely linked to one-carbon metabolism that contributes to redox, nucleotide synthesis, and methylation reactions in cells. Oncogenes driving the RTK/RAS/PI3K pathway directly regulate mTOR function to alter metabolism. IDH mutations produce the oncometabolite 2-HG that can influence histone and DNA methylation in cells. VHL mutations directly regulate the oxygen-sensing pathway including HIFs to reprogram metabolism. Many of these pathways serve as novel therapeutic targets for the development of more effective cancer therapies.

References

1. Vander Heiden MG, Cantley LC, Thompson CB. Understanding the Warburg effect: the metabolic requirements of cell proliferation. Science. 2009;324:1029–33.
2. Ward PS, Thompson CB. Metabolic reprogramming: a cancer hallmark even warburg did not anticipate. Cancer Cell. 2012;21:297–308.
3. Kim JW, Tchernyshyov I, Semenza GL, Dang CV. HIF-1-mediated expression of pyruvate dehydrogenase kinase: a metabolic switch required for cellular adaptation to hypoxia. Cell Metab. 2006;3:177–85.
4. Baumann F, et al. Lactate promotes glioma migration by TGF-beta2-dependent regulation of matrix metalloproteinase-2. Neuro-Oncology. 2009;11:368–80.
5. Colen CB, et al. Metabolic targeting of lactate efflux by malignant glioma inhibits invasiveness and induces necrosis: an in vivo study. Neoplasia. 2011;13:620–32.
6. Crane CA, et al. Immune evasion mediated by tumor-derived lactate dehydrogenase induction of NKG2D ligands on myeloid cells in glioblastoma patients. Proc Natl Acad Sci U S A. 2014;111:12823–8.
7. Marin-Valencia I, et al. Analysis of tumor metabolism reveals mitochondrial glucose oxidation in genetically diverse human glioblastomas in the mouse brain in vivo. Cell Metab. 2012;15:827–37.
8. Hensley CT, et al. Metabolic heterogeneity in human lung tumors. Cell. 2016;164:681–94.
9. Wolf A, Agnihotri S, Munoz D, Guha A. Developmental profile and regulation of the glycolytic enzyme hexokinase 2 in normal brain and glioblastoma multiforme. Neurobiol Dis. 2011;44:84–91.
10. Patra KC, et al. Hexokinase 2 is required for tumor initiation and maintenance and its systemic deletion is therapeutic in mouse models of cancer. Cancer Cell. 2013;24:213–28.
11. Rempel A, Mathupala SP, Griffin CA, Hawkins AL, Pedersen PL. Glucose catabolism in cancer cells: amplification of the gene encoding type II hexokinase. Cancer Res. 1996;56:2468–71.
12. Wolf A, et al. Hexokinase 2 is a key mediator of aerobic glycolysis and promotes tumor growth

in human glioblastoma multiforme. J Exp Med. 2011;208:313–26.
13. Palmieri D, et al. Analyses of resected human brain metastases of breast cancer reveal the association between up-regulation of hexokinase 2 and poor prognosis. Mol Cancer Res. 2009;7:1438–45.
14. Kelloff GJ. Progress and promise of FDG-PET imaging for cancer patient management and oncologic drug development. Clin Cancer Res. 2005;11:2785–808.
15. Wong N, Ojo D, Yan J, Tang D. PKM2 contributes to cancer metabolism. Cancer Lett. 2015;356:184–91.
16. Noguchi T, Inoue H, Tanaka T. The M1- and M2-type isozymes of rat pyruvate kinase are produced from the same gene by alternative RNA splicing. J Biol Chem. 1986;261:13807–12.
17. Israelsen WJ, Vander Heiden MG. Pyruvate kinase: function, regulation and role in cancer. Semin Cell Dev Biol. 2015;43:43–51.
18. Taylor CB, Bailey E. Activation of liver pyruvate kinase by fructose 1,6-diphosphate. Biochem J. 1967; 102:32c–33c.
19. Chaneton B, et al. Serine is a natural ligand and allosteric activator of pyruvate kinase M2. Nature. 2012;491:458–62.
20. Israelsen WJ, et al. PKM2 isoform-specific deletion reveals a differential requirement for pyruvate kinase in tumor cells. Cell. 2013;155:397–409.
21. Lunt SY, et al. Pyruvate kinase isoform expression alters nucleotide synthesis to impact cell proliferation. Mol Cell. 2015;57:95–107.
22. Commisso C, et al. Macropinocytosis of protein is an amino acid supply route in Ras-transformed cells. Nature. 2013;497:633–7.
23. DeBerardinis RJ, Cheng T. Q's next: the diverse functions of glutamine in metabolism, cell biology and cancer. Oncogene. 2010;29:313–24.
24. Vander Heiden MG, et al. Metabolic pathway alterations that support cell proliferation. Cold Spring Harb Symp Quant Biol. 2011;76:325–34.
25. DeBerardinis RJ, et al. Beyond aerobic glycolysis: transformed cells can engage in glutamine metabolism that exceeds the requirement for protein and nucleotide synthesis. Proc Natl Acad Sci U S A. 2007;104:19345–50.
26. Wise DR, Thompson CB. Glutamine addiction: a new therapeutic target in cancer. Trends Biochem Sci. 2010;35:427–33.
27. Daye D, Wellen KE. Metabolic reprogramming in cancer: unraveling the role of glutamine in tumorigenesis. Semin Cell Dev Biol. 2012.
28. Venneti S. et al. Glutamine-based PET imaging facilitates enhanced metabolic evaluation of gliomas in vivo. Sci Transl Med. 2015; 7:274ra17.
29. DeNicola GM, et al. NRF2 regulates serine biosynthesis in non-small cell lung cancer. Nat Genet. 2015;47:1475–81.
30. Locasale JW. Serine, glycine and one-carbon units: cancer metabolism in full circle. Nat Rev Cancer. 2013;13:572–83.
31. Schirch V, Szebenyi DM. Serine hydroxymethyltransferase revisited. Curr Opin Chem Biol. 2005;9:482–7.
32. Pai YJ, et al. Glycine decarboxylase deficiency causes neural tube defects and features of non-ketotic hyperglycinemia in mice. Nat Commun. 2015;6:6388.
33. Amelio I, Cutruzzolá F, Antonov A, Agostini M, Melino G. Serine and glycine metabolism in cancer. Trends Biochem Sci. 2014;39:191–8.
34. Wang J, et al. Dependence of mouse embryonic stem cells on threonine catabolism. Science. 2009;325:435–9.
35. Lane AN, Fan TW-M. Regulation of mammalian nucleotide metabolism and biosynthesis. Nucleic Acids Res. 2015.
36. Zatz M, Dudley PA, Kloog Y, Markey SP. Nonpolar lipid methylation. Biosynthesis of fatty acid methyl esters by rat lung membranes using S-adenosylmethionine. J Biol Chem. 1981;256:10028–32.
37. Hickman MJ, et al. Coordinated regulation of sulfur and phospholipid metabolism reflects the importance of methylation in the growth of yeast. Mol Biol Cell. 2011;22:4192–204.
38. Fan J, et al. Quantitative flux analysis reveals folate-dependent NADPH production. Nature. 2014;510:298–302.
39. Yang W, et al. PKM2 phosphorylates histone H3 and promotes Gene transcription and tumorigenesis. Cell. 2012;150:685–96.
40. Katada S, Imhof A, Sassone-Corsi P. Connecting threads: epigenetics and metabolism. Cell. 2012;148:24–8.
41. Teperino R, Schoonjans K, Auwerx J. Histone methyl transferases and demethylases; can they link metabolism and transcription? Cell Metab. 2010;12:321–7.
42. Snell K. Enzymes of serine metabolism in normal, developing and neoplastic rat tissues. Adv Enzym Regul. 1984;22:325–400.
43. Locasale JW, et al. Phosphoglycerate dehydrogenase diverts glycolytic flux and contributes to oncogenesis. Nat Genet. 2011;43:869–74.
44. Possemato R, et al. Functional genomics reveals serine synthesis is essential in PHGDH-amplified breast cancer. Nature. 2011;476:346–50.
45. Christofk HR, et al. The M2 splice isoform of pyruvate kinase is important for cancer metabolism and tumour growth. Nature. 2008;452:230–3.
46. Jain M, et al. Metabolite profiling identifies a key role for glycine in rapid cancer cell proliferation. Science. 2012;336:1040–4.
47. Zhang WC, et al. Glycine decarboxylase activity drives non-small cell lung cancer tumor-initiating cells and tumorigenesis. Cell. 2012;148:259–72.
48. Rahman L, et al. Thymidylate synthase as an oncogene: a novel role for an essential DNA synthesis enzyme. Cancer Cell. 2004;5:341–51.

49. Xu X, et al. Broad overexpression of ribonucleotide reductase genes in mice specifically induces lung neoplasms. Cancer Res. 2008;68:2652–60.
50. Bester AC, et al. Nucleotide deficiency promotes genomic instability in early stages of cancer development. Cell. 2011;145:435–46.
51. Brennan CW, et al. The somatic genomic landscape of glioblastoma. Cell. 2013;155:462–77.
52. Kohn AD, Summers SA, Birnbaum MJ, Roth RA. Expression of a constitutively active Akt Ser/Thr kinase in 3T3-L1 adipocytes stimulates glucose uptake and glucose transporter 4 translocation. J Biol Chem. 1996;271:31372–8.
53. Deprez J, Vertommen D, Alessi DR, Hue L, Rider MH. Phosphorylation and activation of heart 6-phosphofructo-2-kinase by protein kinase B and other protein kinases of the insulin signaling cascades. J Biol Chem. 1997;272:17269–75.
54. Gottlob K, et al. Inhibition of early apoptotic events by Akt/PKB is dependent on the first committed step of glycolysis and mitochondrial hexokinase. Genes Dev. 2001;15:1406–18.
55. Rosario FJ, Kanai Y, Powell TL, Jansson T. Mammalian target of rapamycin signalling modulates amino acid uptake by regulating transporter cell surface abundance in primary human trophoblast cells. J Physiol. 2013;591:609–25.
56. Laplante M, Sabatini DM. mTOR signaling in growth control and disease. Cell. 2012;149:274–93.
57. Ma XM, Blenis J. Molecular mechanisms of mTOR-mediated translational control. Nat Rev Mol Cell Biol. 2009;10:307–18.
58. Kim YC, Guan KL. mTOR: a pharmacologic target for autophagy regulation. J Clin Invest. 2015;125:25–32.
59. Babic I, et al. EGFR mutation-induced alternative splicing of max contributes to growth of glycolytic tumors in brain cancer. Cell Metab. 2013;17:1000–8.
60. Csibi A, et al. The mTORC1 pathway stimulates glutamine metabolism and cell proliferation by repressing SIRT4. Cell. 2013;153:840–54.
61. Zoncu R, Efeyan A, Sabatini DM. mTOR: from growth signal integration to cancer, diabetes and ageing. Nat Rev Mol Cell Biol. 2011;12:21–35.
62. Huh TL, Kim YO, Oh IU. Song, B.J. & Inazawa, J. Assignment of the human mitochondrial NAD+ −specific isocitrate dehydrogenase alpha subunit (IDH3A) gene to 15q25.1-->q25.2by in situ hybridization. Genomics. 1996;32:295–6.
63. Losman J-A, et al. (R)-2-Hydroxyglutarate is sufficient to promote Leukemogenesis and its effects are reversible. Science. 2013;339:1621–5.
64. Soundar S, Park JH, Huh TL, Colman RF. Evaluation by mutagenesis of the importance of 3 arginines in alpha, beta, and gamma subunits of human NAD-dependent isocitrate dehydrogenase. J Biol Chem. 2003;278:52146–53.
65. Cohen PF, Colman RF. Diphosphopyridine nucleotide dependent isocitrate dehydrogenase from pig heart. Characterization of the active substrate and modes of regulation. Biochemistry. 1972;11:1501–8.
66. Denton RM, Richards DA, Chin JG. Calcium ions and the regulation of NAD+−linked isocitrate dehydrogenase from the mitochondria of rat heart and other tissues. Biochem J. 1978;176:899–906.
67. Shechter I, Dai P, Huo L, Guan G. IDH1 gene transcription is sterol regulated and activated by SREBP-1a and SREBP-2 in human hepatoma HepG2 cells: evidence that IDH1 may regulate lipogenesis in hepatic cells. J Lipid Res. 2003;44:2169–80.
68. Liu W, Capuco AV, Romagnolo DF. Expression of cytosolic NADP+−dependent Isocitrate dehydrogenase in bovine mammary epithelium: modulation by regulators of differentiation and metabolic effectors. Exp Biol Med. 2006;231:599–610.
69. Jo SH, et al. Cellular defense against UVB-induced phototoxicity by cytosolic NADP(+)-dependent isocitrate dehydrogenase. Biochem Biophys Res Commun. 2002;292:542–9.
70. Yu W, Dittenhafer-Reed KE, Denu JM. SIRT3 protein deacetylates isocitrate dehydrogenase 2 (IDH2) and regulates mitochondrial redox status. J Biol Chem. 2012;287:14078–86.
71. Lee JH, Kim SY, Kil IS, Park JW. Regulation of ionizing radiation-induced apoptosis by mitochondrial NADP+−dependent isocitrate dehydrogenase. J Biol Chem. 2007;282:13385–94.
72. Metallo CM, et al. Reductive glutamine metabolism by IDH1 mediates lipogenesis under hypoxia. Nature. 2012;481:380–4.
73. Filipp FV, Scott DA, Ronai ZA, Osterman AL, Smith JW. Reverse TCA cycle flux through isocitrate dehydrogenases 1 and 2 is required for lipogenesis in hypoxic melanoma cells. Pigment Cell Melanoma Res. 2012;25:375–83.
74. Parsons DW, et al. An integrated genomic analysis of human glioblastoma multiforme. Science. 2008;321:1807–12.
75. Balss J, et al. Analysis of the IDH1 codon 132 mutation in brain tumors. Acta Neuropathol. 2008;116:597–602.
76. Bleeker FE, et al. IDH1 mutations at residue p.R132 (IDH1(R132)) occur frequently in high-grade gliomas but not in other solid tumors. Hum Mutat. 2009;30:7–11.
77. Hartmann C, et al. Type and frequency of IDH1 and IDH2 mutations are related to astrocytic and oligodendroglial differentiation and age: a study of 1,010 diffuse gliomas. Acta Neuropathol. 2009;118:469–74.
78. Yan H, et al. IDH1 and IDH2 mutations in gliomas. N Engl J Med. 2009;360:765–73.
79. Byeon SJ, et al. Distinct genetic alterations in pediatric glioblastomas. Childs Nerv Syst. 2012;28:1025–32.
80. Mardis ER, et al. Recurring mutations found by sequencing an acute myeloid leukemia genome. N Engl J Med. 2009;361:1058–66.

81. Thol F, et al. IDH1 mutations in patients with myelodysplastic syndromes are associated with an unfavorable prognosis. Haematologica. 2010;95:1668–74.
82. Borger DR, et al. Frequent mutation of isocitrate dehydrogenase (IDH)1 and IDH2 in cholangiocarcinoma identified through broad-based tumor genotyping. Oncologist. 2012;17:72–9.
83. Wang P, et al. Mutations in isocitrate dehydrogenase 1 and 2 occur frequently in intrahepatic cholangiocarcinomas and share hypermethylation targets with glioblastomas. Oncogene. 2013;32:3091–100.
84. Amary MF, et al. IDH1 and IDH2 mutations are frequent events in central chondrosarcoma and central and periosteal chondromas but not in other mesenchymal tumours. J Pathol. 2011;224:334–43.
85. Marcucci G, et al. IDH1 and IDH2 gene mutations identify novel molecular subsets within de novo cytogenetically normal acute myeloid leukemia: a cancer and leukemia group B study. J Clin Oncol. 2010;28:2348–55.
86. Abdel-Wahab O, Patel J, Levine RL. Clinical implications of novel mutations in epigenetic modifiers in AML. Hematol Oncol Clin North Am. 2011;25:1119–33.
87. DiNardo, C. et al. Molecular Profiling and Relationship with Clinical Response in Patients with IDH1 Mutation-Positive Hematologic Malignancies Receiving AG-120, a First-in-Class Potent Inhibitor of Mutant IDH1, in Addition to Data from the Completed Dose Escalation Portio…. Blood. 2015; 126:1306.
88. Patnaik MM, et al. Differential prognostic effect of IDH1 versus IDH2 mutations in myelodysplastic syndromes: a Mayo Clinic study of 277 patients. Leukemia. 2012;26:101–5.
89. Goyal L, et al. Prognosis and Clinicopathologic features of patients with advanced stage Isocitrate dehydrogenase (IDH) mutant and IDH wild-type intrahepatic Cholangiocarcinoma. Oncologist. 2015;20:1019–27.
90. Churi CR, et al. Mutation profiling in cholangiocarcinoma: prognostic and therapeutic implications. PLoS One. 2014;9:e115383.
91. Zhu AX, et al. Genomic profiling of intrahepatic cholangiocarcinoma: refining prognosis and identifying therapeutic targets. Ann Surg Oncol. 2014;21:3827–34.
92. Dang L, et al. Cancer-associated IDH1 mutations produce 2-hydroxyglutarate. Nature. 2009;462:739–44.
93. Ward PS, et al. The common feature of leukemia-associated IDH1 and IDH2 mutations is a neomorphic enzyme activity converting alpha-ketoglutarate to 2-hydroxyglutarate. Cancer Cell. 2010;17:225–34.
94. Xu X, et al. Structures of human cytosolic NADP-dependent isocitrate dehydrogenase reveal a novel self-regulatory mechanism of activity. J Biol Chem. 2004;279:33946–57.
95. Dang L, et al. Cancer-associated IDH1 mutations produce 2-hydroxyglutarate. Nature. 2010;465:966.
96. Gross S, et al. Cancer-associated metabolite 2-hydroxyglutarate accumulates in acute myelogenous leukemia with isocitrate dehydrogenase 1 and 2 mutations. J Exp Med. 2010;207:339–44.
97. Watanabe T, Nobusawa S, Kleihues P, Ohgaki H. IDH1 mutations are early events in the development of astrocytomas and oligodendrogliomas. Am J Pathol. 2009;174:1149–53.
98. Lai A, et al. Evidence for sequenced molecular evolution of IDH1 mutant glioblastoma from a distinct cell of origin. J Clin Oncol. 2011;29:4482–90.
99. Lu C, et al. IDH mutation impairs histone demethylation and results in a block to cell differentiation. Nature. 2012;483:474–8.
100. Lu C, et al. Induction of sarcomas by mutant IDH2. Genes Dev. 2013;27:1986–98.
101. Koivunen P, et al. Transformation by the (R)-enantiomer of 2-hydroxyglutarate linked to EGLN activation. Nature. 2012;483:484–8.
102. Turcan S, et al. IDH1 mutation is sufficient to establish the glioma hypermethylator phenotype. Nature. 2012;483:479–83.
103. Saha SK, et al. Mutant IDH inhibits HNF-4alpha to block hepatocyte differentiation and promote biliary cancer. Nature. 2014;513:110–4.
104. Sasaki M, et al. D-2-hydroxyglutarate produced by mutant IDH1 perturbs collagen maturation and basement membrane function. Genes Dev. 2012;26:2038–49.
105. Network TCGAR. Comprehensive, integrative genomic analysis of diffuse lower-grade gliomas. N Engl J Med. 2015;372:2481–98.
106. Eckel-Passow JE, et al. Glioma groups based on 1p/19q, IDH, and TERT promoter mutations in tumors. N Engl J Med. 2015;372:2499–508.
107. Losman J-A, Kaelin WG. What a difference a hydroxyl makes: mutant IDH, (R)-2-hydroxyglutarate, and cancer. Genes Dev. 2013;27:836–52.
108. Noushmehr H, et al. Identification of a CpG island methylator phenotype that defines a distinct subgroup of glioma. Cancer Cell. 2010;17:510–22.
109. Verhaak RG, et al. Integrated genomic analysis identifies clinically relevant subtypes of glioblastoma characterized by abnormalities in PDGFRA, IDH1, EGFR, and NF1. Cancer Cell. 2010;17:98–110.
110. Duncan CG, et al. A heterozygous IDH1R132H/WT mutation induces genome-wide alterations in DNA methylation. Genome Res. 2012.
111. Figueroa ME, et al. Leukemic IDH1 and IDH2 mutations result in a hypermethylation phenotype, disrupt TET2 function, and impair hematopoietic differentiation. Cancer Cell. 2010;18:553–67.
112. Xu W, et al. Oncometabolite 2-hydroxyglutarate is a competitive inhibitor of alpha-ketoglutarate-dependent dioxygenases. Cancer Cell. 2011;19:17–30.
113. Kim YH, et al. TET2 promoter methylation in low-grade diffuse gliomas lacking IDH1/2 mutations. J Clin Pathol. 2011;64:850–2.

114. Klose RJ, Kallin EM, Zhang Y. JmjC-domain-containing proteins and histone demethylation. Nat Rev Genet. 2006;7:715–27.
115. Chen Z, et al. Structural insights into histone demethylation by JMJD2 family members. Cell. 2006;125:691–702.
116. Hu Z, et al. A novel nuclear protein, 5qNCA (LOC51780) is a candidate for the myeloid leukemia tumor suppressor gene on chromosome 5 band q31. Oncogene. 2001;20:6946–54.
117. Lu C, Thompson CB. Metabolic regulation of epigenetics. Cell Metab. 2012;16:9–17.
118. Venneti S, et al. Histone 3 lysine 9 trimethylation is differentially associated with isocitrate dehydrogenase mutations in oligodendrogliomas and high-grade astrocytomas. J Neuropathol Exp Neurol. 2013;72:298–306.
119. Chowdhury R, et al. The oncometabolite 2-hydroxyglutarate inhibits histone lysine demethylases. EMBO Rep. 2011;12:463–9.
120. Zhao S, et al. Glioma-derived mutations in IDH1 dominantly inhibit IDH1 catalytic activity and induce HIF-1α. Science. 2009;324:261–5.
121. Williams SC, et al. R132H-mutation of isocitrate dehydrogenase-1 is not sufficient for HIF-1alpha upregulation in adult glioma. Acta Neuropathol. 2011;121:279–81.
122. Fu X, et al. 2-Hydroxyglutarate Inhibits ATP Synthase and mTOR Signaling. Cell Metab. 2015.
123. Chin RM, et al. The metabolite alpha-ketoglutarate extends lifespan by inhibiting ATP synthase and TOR. Nature. 2014;510:397–401.
124. Stine ZE, Walton ZE, Altman BJ, Hsieh AL, Dang CV, MYC, Metabolism, and cancer. Cancer Discov. 2015.
125. Duesberg PH, Vogt PK. Avian acute leukemia viruses MC29 and MH2 share specific RNA sequences: evidence for a second class of transforming genes. Proc Natl Acad Sci U S A. 1979;76:1633–7.
126. Hu SS, Lai MM, Vogt PK. Genome of avian myelocytomatosis virus MC29: analysis by heteroduplex mapping. Proc Natl Acad Sci U S A. 1979;76:1265–8.
127. Beroukhim R, et al. The landscape of somatic copy-number alteration across human cancers. Nature. 2010;463:899–905.
128. Dean M, et al. Regulation of c-myc transcription and mRNA abundance by serum growth factors and cell contact. J Biol Chem. 1986;261:9161–6.
129. Zeller KI, et al. Global mapping of c-Myc binding sites and target gene networks in human B cells. Proc Natl Acad Sci U S A. 2006;103:17834–9.
130. Morrish F, Isern N, Sadilek M. Jeffrey, M. & Hockenbery, D.M. C-Myc activates multiple metabolic networks to generate substrates for cell cycle entry. Oncogene. 2009;28:2485–91.
131. Kim JW, et al. Evaluation of myc E-box phylogenetic footprints in glycolytic genes by chromatin immunoprecipitation assays. Mol Cell Biol. 2004;24:5923–36.
132. Shim H, et al. C-Myc transactivation of LDH-A: implications for tumor metabolism and growth. Proc Natl Acad Sci U S A. 1997;94:6658–63.
133. Osthus RC, et al. Deregulation of glucose transporter 1 and glycolytic gene expression by c-Myc. J Biol Chem. 2000;275:21797–800.
134. Gao P, et al. C-Myc suppression of miR-23a/b enhances mitochondrial glutaminase expression and glutamine metabolism. Nature. 2009;458:762–5.
135. Morrish F, et al. Myc-dependent mitochondrial generation of acetyl-CoA contributes to fatty acid biosynthesis and histone acetylation during cell cycle entry. J Biol Chem. 2010;285:36267–74.
136. Edmunds LR, et al. C-Myc programs fatty acid metabolism and dictates acetyl-CoA abundance and fate. J Biol Chem. 2014;289:25382–92.
137. Li F, et al. Myc stimulates nuclearly encoded mitochondrial genes and mitochondrial biogenesis. Mol Cell Biol. 2005;25:6225–34.
138. Zhang H, et al. HIF-1 inhibits mitochondrial biogenesis and cellular respiration in VHL-deficient renal cell carcinoma by repression of C-MYC activity. Cancer Cell. 2007;11:407–20.
139. Kim J, Lee JH, Iyer VR. Global identification of Myc target genes reveals its direct role in mitochondrial biogenesis and its E-box usage in vivo. PLoS One. 2008;3:e1798.
140. Wonsey DR, Zeller KI, Dang CV. The c-Myc target gene PRDX3 is required for mitochondrial homeostasis and neoplastic transformation. Proc Natl Acad Sci U S A. 2002;99:6649–54.
141. Palaskas N, et al. 18F-fluorodeoxy-glucose positron emission tomography marks MYC-overexpressing human basal-like breast cancers. Cancer Res. 2011;71:5164–74.
142. Alles MC, et al. Meta-analysis and gene set enrichment relative to er status reveal elevated activity of MYC and E2F in the "basal" breast cancer subgroup. PLoS One. 2009;4:e4710.
143. Chandriani S, et al. A core MYC gene expression signature is prominent in basal-like breast cancer but only partially overlaps the core serum response. PLoS One. 2009;4:e6693.
144. Shen L, et al. Metabolic reprogramming in triple-negative breast cancer through Myc suppression of TXNIP. Proc Natl Acad Sci U S A. 2015;112:5425–30.
145. Timmerman, Luika A, et al. Glutamine sensitivity analysis identifies the xCT antiporter as a common triple-negative breast tumor therapeutic target. Cancer Cell. 2013; 24:450–65.
146. Yuneva MO, et al. The metabolic profile of tumors depends on both the responsible genetic lesion and tissue type. Cell Metab. 2012;15:157–70.
147. Gnarra JR, et al. Mutations of the VHL tumour suppressor gene in renal carcinoma. Nat Genet. 1994;7:85–90.
148. Williamson SR, et al. Succinate dehydrogenase-deficient renal cell carcinoma: detailed characterization of 11 tumors defining a unique subtype of renal cell carcinoma. Mod Pathol. 2015;28:80–94.

149. Linehan WM, Rouault TA. Molecular pathways: Fumarate hydratase-deficient kidney cancer-targeting the Warburg effect in cancer. Clin Cancer Res. 2013;19:3345–52.
150. Lussey-Lepoutre C, et al. Loss of succinate dehydrogenase activity results in dependency on pyruvate carboxylation for cellular anabolism. Nat Commun. 2015;6:8784.
151. Sullivan LB, et al. The proto-oncometabolite fumarate binds glutathione to amplify ROS-dependent signaling. Mol Cell. 2013;51:236–48.
152. Bertout JA, Patel SA, Simon MC. The impact of O2 availability on human cancer. Nat Rev Cancer. 2008;8:967–75.
153. Keith B, Johnson RS, Simon MC. HIF1alpha and HIF2alpha: sibling rivalry in hypoxic tumour growth and progression. Nat Rev Cancer. 2012;12:9–22.
154. Semenza GL, Roth PH, Fang HM, Wang GL. Transcriptional regulation of genes encoding glycolytic enzymes by hypoxia-inducible factor 1. J Biol Chem. 1994;269:23757–63.
155. Mathupala SP, Rempel A, Pedersen PL. Glucose catabolism in cancer cells: identification and characterization of a marked activation response of the type II hexokinase gene to hypoxic conditions. J Biol Chem. 2001;276:43407–12.
156. Luo W, et al. Pyruvate kinase M2 is a PHD3-stimulated coactivator for hypoxia-inducible factor 1. Cell. 2011;145:732–44.
157. Lum JJ, et al. The transcription factor HIF-1alpha plays a critical role in the growth factor-dependent regulation of both aerobic and anaerobic glycolysis. Genes Dev. 2007;21:1037–49.
158. Metallo CM, et al. Reductive glutamine metabolism by IDH1 mediates lipogenesis under hypoxia. Nature. 2011.
159. Wise DR, et al. Hypoxia promotes isocitrate dehydrogenase-dependent carboxylation of alpha-ketoglutarate to citrate to support cell growth and viability. Proc Nat Acad Sci U S A. 2011.
160. Mullen AR, et al. Reductive carboxylation supports growth in tumour cells with defective mitochondria. Nature. 2011.
161. Le A, et al. Glucose-independent glutamine metabolism via TCA cycling for proliferation and survival in B cells. Cell Metab. 2012;15:110–21.
162. Gameiro PA, et al. In vivo HIF-mediated reductive carboxylation is regulated by citrate levels and sensitizes VHL-deficient cells to glutamine deprivation. Cell Metab. 2013;17:372–85.
163. Galluzzi L, Kepp O, Vander Heiden MG, Kroemer G. Metabolic targets for cancer therapy. Nat Rev Drug Discov. 2013;12:829–46.
164. Vander Heiden MG. Targeting cancer metabolism: a therapeutic window opens. Nat Rev Drug Discov. 2011;10:671–84.
165. Chabner BA, Roberts TG Jr. Timeline: chemotherapy and the war on cancer. Nat Rev Cancer. 2005;5:65–72.
166. Farber S, Diamond LK. Temporary remissions in acute leukemia in children produced by folic acid antagonist, 4-aminopteroyl-glutamic acid. N Engl J Med. 1948;238:787–93.
167. Joerger M, Omlin A, Cerny T, Fruh M. The role of pemetrexed in advanced non small-cell lung cancer: special focus on pharmacology and mechanism of action. Curr Drug Targets. 2010;11:37–47.
168. Shewach DS, Lawrence TS. Antimetabolite radiosensitizers. J Clin Oncol. 2007;25:4043–50.
169. Kidd JG. Regression of transplanted lymphomas induced in vivo by means of normal guinea pig serum. I. Course of transplanted cancers of various kinds in mice and rats given guinea pig serum, horse serum, or rabbit serum. J Exp Med. 1953;98:565–82.
170. Muller HJ, Boos J. Use of L-asparaginase in childhood ALL. Crit Rev Oncol Hematol. 1998;28:97–113.
171. Broome JD. L-Asparaginase: discovery and development as a tumor-inhibitory agent. Cancer Treat Rep. 1981;65:111–4.
172. Fu CH, Sakamoto KM. PEG-asparaginase. Expert Opin Pharmacother. 2007;8:1977–84.
173. Earl M. Incidence and management of asparaginase-associated adverse events in patients with acute lymphoblastic leukemia. Clin Adv Hematol Oncol. 2009;7:600–6.
174. Wong A, Soo RA, Yong WP, Innocenti F. Clinical pharmacology and pharmacogenetics of gemcitabine. Drug Metab Rev. 2009;41:77–88.
175. Cohade C, Wahl RL. Applications of positron emission tomography/computed tomography image fusion in clinical positron emission tomography-clinical use, interpretation methods, diagnostic improvements. Semin Nucl Med. 2003;33:228–37.
176. Kaplan O, et al. Effects of 2-deoxyglucose on drug-sensitive and drug-resistant human breast cancer cells: toxicity and magnetic resonance spectroscopy studies of metabolism. Cancer Res. 1990;50:544–51.
177. Dwarakanath BS, et al. Clinical studies for improving radiotherapy with 2-deoxy-D-glucose: present status and future prospects. J Cancer Res Ther. 2009;5(Suppl 1):S21–6.
178. Landau BR, Laszlo J, Stengle J, Burk D. Certain metabolic and pharmacologic effects in cancer patients given infusions of 2-deoxy-D-glucose. J Natl Cancer Inst. 1958;21:485–94.
179. Mohanti BK, et al. Improving cancer radiotherapy with 2-deoxy-D-glucose: phase I/II clinical trials on human cerebral gliomas. Int J Radiat Oncol Biol Phys. 1996;35:103–11.
180. Singh D, et al. Optimizing cancer radiotherapy with 2-deoxy-d-glucose dose escalation studies in patients with glioblastoma multiforme. Strahlenther Onkol. 2005;181:507–14.
181. Allen BG, et al. Ketogenic diets as an adjuvant cancer therapy: history and potential mechanism. Redox Biol. 2014;2:963–70.

182. Valayannopoulos V, et al. Successful treatment of severe cardiomyopathy in glycogen storage disease type III with D,L-3-hydroxybutyrate, ketogenic and high-protein diet. Pediatr Res. 2011;70:638–41.
183. Neal EG, et al. The ketogenic diet for the treatment of childhood epilepsy: a randomised controlled trial. Lancet Neurol. 2008;7:500–6.
184. Allen BG, et al. Ketogenic diets enhance oxidative stress and radio-chemo-therapy responses in lung cancer xenografts. Clin Cancer Res. 2013;19:3905–13.
185. Nebeling LC, Miraldi F, Shurin SB, Lerner E. Effects of a ketogenic diet on tumor metabolism and nutritional status in pediatric oncology patients: two case reports. J Am Coll Nutr. 1995;14:202–8.
186. Zuccoli G, et al. Metabolic management of glioblastoma multiforme using standard therapy together with a restricted ketogenic diet: case report. Nutr Metab (Lond). 2010;7:33.
187. Schmidt M, Pfetzer N, Schwab M, Strauss I, Kammerer U. Effects of a ketogenic diet on the quality of life in 16 patients with advanced cancer: a pilot trial. Nutr Metab (Lond). 2011;8:54.
188. Gross MI, et al. Antitumor activity of the Glutaminase inhibitor CB-839 in triple-negative breast cancer. Mol Cancer Ther. 2014;13:890–901.
189. Xiang Y, et al. Targeted inhibition of tumor-specific glutaminase diminishes cell-autonomous tumorigenesis. J Clin Invest. 2015;125:2293–306.
190. Seltzer MJ, et al. Inhibition of glutaminase preferentially slows growth of glioma cells with mutant IDH1. Cancer Res. 2010;70:8981–7.
191. Harding JJ, et al. ASCO Annual Meeting Proceedings 2512. 2015.
192. Vogl DT, et al. Blood (Amer Soc Hematology 2021 L ST NW, SUITE 900, WASHINGTON, DC 20036 USA, 2015).
193. Popovici-Muller J, et al. Discovery of the first potent inhibitors of mutant IDH1 that lower tumor 2-HG in vivo. ACS Med Chem Lett. 2012;3:850–5.
194. Rohle D, et al. An inhibitor of mutant IDH1 delays growth and promotes differentiation of glioma cells. Science. 2013;340:626–30.
195. Chaturvedi A, et al. Mutant IDH1 promotes leukemogenesis in vivo and can be specifically targeted in human AML. Blood. 2013;122:2877–87.
196. Wang F, et al. Targeted inhibition of mutant IDH2 in leukemia cells induces cellular differentiation. Science. 2013;340:622–6.
197. Kernytsky A, et al. IDH2 mutation-induced histone and DNA hypermethylation is progressively reversed by small-molecule inhibition. Blood. 2015;125:296–303.
198. Stein EM, et al. AG-221, an oral, selective, first-in-class, potent inhibitor of the IDH2 mutant metabolic enzyme, induces durable remissions in a phase I study in patients with IDH2 mutation positive advanced hematologic malignancies. Blood. 2014;124:115.
199. Burris H, et al. Abstract PL04-05: the first reported results of AG-120, a first-in-class, potent inhibitor of the IDH1 mutant protein, in a phase I study of patients with advanced IDH1-mutant solid tumors, including gliomas. Mol Cancer Ther. 2015;14:PL04-05.
200. Michelakis ED, Webster L, Mackey JR. Dichloroacetate (DCA) as a potential metabolic-targeting therapy for cancer. Br J Cancer. 2008;99:989–94.
201. Kankotia S, Stacpoole PW. Dichloroacetate and cancer: new home for an orphan drug? Biochim Biophys Acta. 2014;1846:617–29.
202. Bonnet S, et al. A mitochondria-K+ channel axis is suppressed in cancer and its normalization promotes apoptosis and inhibits cancer growth. Cancer Cell. 2007;11:37–51.
203. Xie J, et al. Dichloroacetate shifts the metabolism from glycolysis to glucose oxidation and exhibits synergistic growth inhibition with cisplatin in HeLa cells. Int J Oncol. 2011;38:409–17.
204. Michelakis ED, et al. Metabolic modulation of glioblastoma with dichloroacetate. Sci Transl Med. 2010;2:31ra34.
205. Lee B, Oh S-W, Myung S-K. Efficacy of vitamin C supplements in prevention of cancer: a meta-analysis of randomized controlled trials. Korean J Family Med. 2015;36:278–85.
206. Coulter ID, et al. Antioxidants vitamin C and vitamin e for the prevention and treatment of cancer. J Gen Intern Med. 2006;21:735–44.
207. Yun J, et al. Vitamin C selectively kills KRAS and BRAF mutant colorectal cancer cells by targeting GAPDH. Science. 2015;350:1391–6.
208. Du J, et al. Pharmacological Ascorbate Radiosensitizes pancreatic cancer. Cancer Res. 2015;75:3314–26.
209. Blackhall F. O11.5Activity of the monocarboxylate transporter 1 inhibitor AZD3965 in small cell lung cancer. Annals of oncology 26. In: ii15; 2015.
210. Hong, Candice S, et al. MCT1 modulates cancer cell pyruvate export and growth of tumors that co-express MCT1 and MCT4. Cell Rep. 14:1590–601.
211. Bola BM, et al. Inhibition of monocarboxylate transporter-1 (MCT1) by AZD3965 enhances radiosensitivity by reducing lactate transport. Mol Cancer Ther. 2014;13:2805–16.
212. Brenner AJ, et al. ASCO Annual Meeting Proceedings TPS2615. 2015.
213. Stumvoll M, Nurjhan N, Perriello G, Dailey G, Gerich JE. Metabolic effects of metformin in non-insulin-dependent diabetes mellitus. N Engl J Med. 1995;333:550–4.
214. Morales DR, Morris AD. Metformin in cancer treatment and prevention. Annu Rev Med. 2015;66:17–29.
215. Evans JM, Donnelly LA, Emslie-Smith AM, Alessi DR, Morris AD. Metformin and reduced risk of cancer in diabetic patients. BMJ. 2005;330:1304–5.
216. Franciosi M, et al. Metformin therapy and risk of cancer in patients with type 2 diabetes: systematic review. PLoS One. 2013;8:e71583.

217. Thakkar B, Aronis KN, Vamvini MT, Shields K, Mantzoros CS. Metformin and sulfonylureas in relation to cancer risk in type II diabetes patients: a meta-analysis using primary data of published studies. Metabolism. 2013;62:922–34.
218. Home PD, et al. Experience of malignancies with oral glucose-lowering drugs in the randomised controlled ADOPT (a diabetes outcome progression trial) and RECORD (rosiglitazone evaluated for cardiovascular outcomes and regulation of glycaemia in diabetes) clinical trials. Diabetologia. 2010;53:1838–45.
219. Rizos CV, Elisaf MS. Metformin and cancer. Eur J Pharmacol. 2013;705:96–108.
220. Hadad S, et al. Evidence for biological effects of metformin in operable breast cancer: a pre-operative, window-of-opportunity, randomized trial. Breast Cancer Res Treat. 2011;128:783–94.
221. Niraula S, et al. Metformin in early breast cancer: a prospective window of opportunity neoadjuvant study. Breast Cancer Res Treat. 2012;135:821–30.
222. Bonanni B, et al. Dual effect of metformin on breast cancer proliferation in a randomized presurgical trial. J Clin Oncol. 2012;30:2593–600.

7 Inflammation and Immune Metabolism

Carmen Paus, Derk Draper, Mangala Srinivas, and Erik H.J.G. Aarntzen

7.1 Introduction

7.1.1 Biology and Function of Inflammation

Inflammation is a complex biological response of body tissues to harmful stimuli, with the intention to eliminate the cause of injury, protect from further damage, and initiate tissue repair. Inflammation is a rather generic term that covers a broad range of types of responses which, depending on the causal stimulus and subsequent actions, involve pathogenic cells, stromal cells, and cells of the innate and adaptive immune system, in varying composition (Figs. 7.1 and 7.2). However, common to all inflammatory conditions is the delicate balance between too little or too severe and inappropriate timing or duration, all of which can lead to progressive tissue destruction. For example, chronic inflammation may lead to a host of diseases, such as autoimmune diseases and even cancer [1]. Thus, inflammation is a highly dynamic and tightly regulated process that demands metabolic reprogramming of the involved cell types at various stages to respond with appropriate cell numbers and cell types. In this chapter, we will discuss how imaging can play a role in the assessment of inflammation and immune metabolism. We propose a simplified five-step model to indicate the potential targets for imaging in the ensuing immune response, while acknowledging that these simplified steps are iterative and overlapping in practice.

7.1.1.1 Step 1: Triggering Inflammatory Responses

Inflammatory responses can be triggered by physical stimuli (thermal wounds, trauma, ionizing radiation, foreign bodies), chemical stimuli (radical oxygen species, chemotherapeutic agents, tobacco smoke, toxins), or biological stimuli (pathogens like bacteria, viruses, and parasites or mutated cells with abnormal expression of antigens like in cancer or aberrant immune responses as in allergies). Although it seems trivial, the initial cause of inflammation influences subsequent responses. Chemical and physical injuries elicit danger-associated molecular patterns (DAMPs), such as high-mobility group box 1 (HMGB1) [2]. On the other hand, pathogens express pathogen-associated molecular patterns (PAMPs), like lipopolysaccharide (LPS), which elicits a different immunological response.

Carmen Paus and Derk Draper contributed equally to this work.

C. Paus • D. Draper • M. Srinivas
Department of Tumor Immunology, Radboud University Medical Centre, Nijmegen, The Netherlands

E.H.J.G. Aarntzen (✉)
Department of Radiology, Radboud University Medical Centre, Nijmegen, The Netherlands
e-mail: Erik.Aarntzen@radboudumc.nl

J.S. Lewis, K.R. Keshari (eds.), *Imaging and Metabolism*, DOI 10.1007/978-3-319-61401-4_7

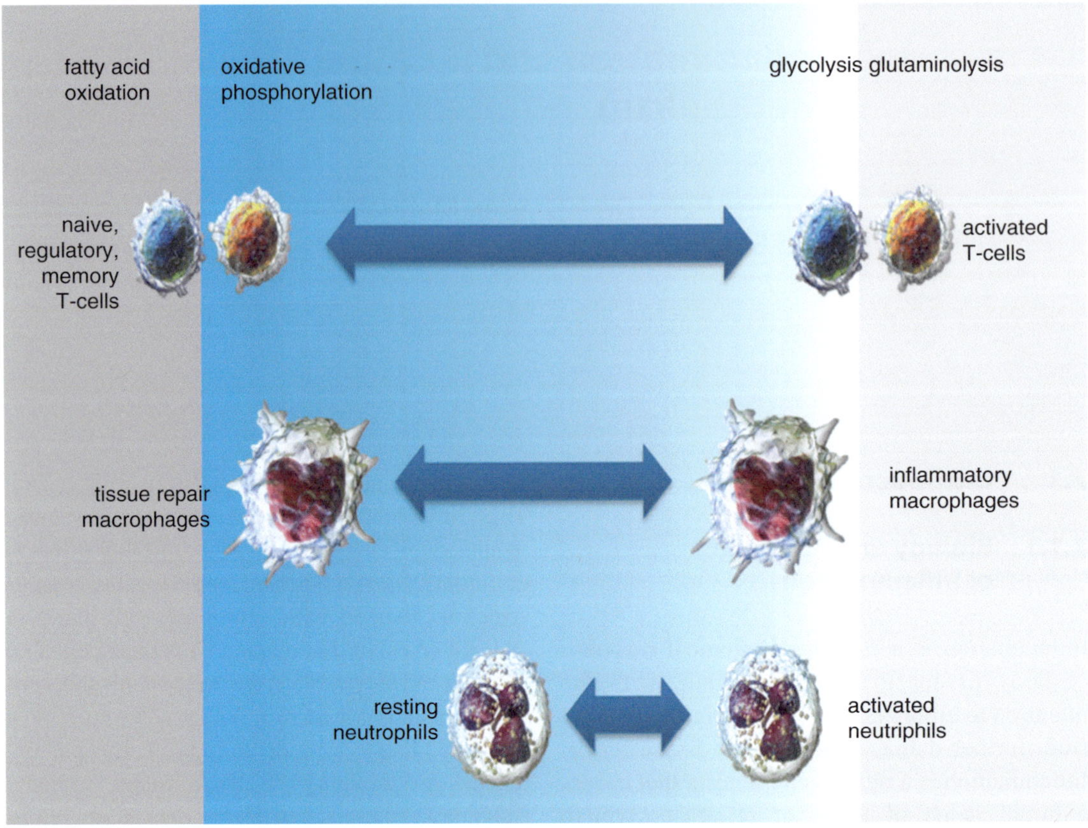

Fig. 7.1 Stepwise model of inflammation

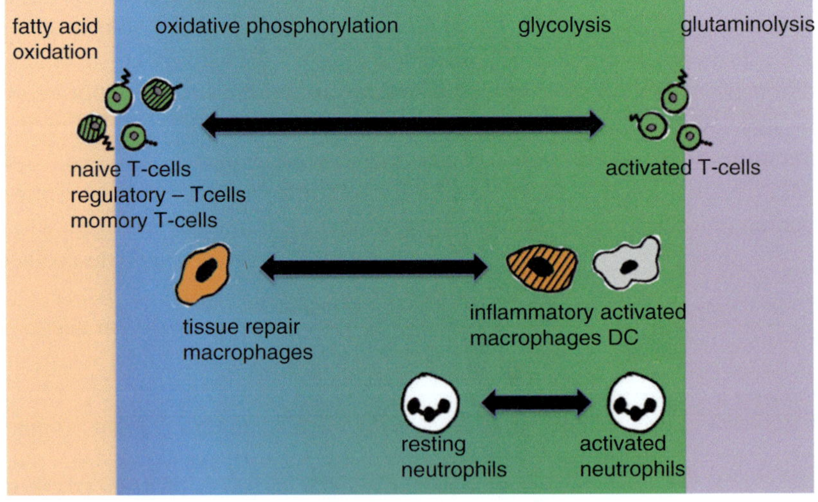

Fig. 7.2 Metabolic profiles of different immune cells

In general, DAMPs tend to induce milder inflammatory responses as compared to PAMPs and involve different subsets of immune cells, exemplified by the different responses to apoptosis and necrosis [2]. Cancer, on the other hand, tends to go relatively unnoticed, although these cells can express mutated or neo-antigens, overexpress self-antigens, or reexpress embryonic antigens.

7.1.1.2 Step 2: Activation of the Innate Immune System

Once pathogens have crossed the epithelial barriers, e.g., the skin, mucosal lining of the gastrointestinal tract, or respiratory system, they can enter tissues and start replication. At these target sites, cells of the innate immune system, such as neutrophils and tissue-resident macrophages (e.g., Kupffer cells, Langerhans cells, alveolar macrophages), are activated [3]. Although these cells lack the specificity of the adaptive immune system, they do distinguish self from nonself by expressing pattern recognition receptors that recognize classes of molecules present on pathogens. For example, Toll-like receptors (TLRs) recognize molecular patterns that are not found in normal vertebrates, e.g., TLR-4 recognizes lipopolysaccharide (LPS), a component of bacterial cell walls. Mannose receptors are expressed on macrophages to recognize certain sugar molecules present on most bacteria and some viruses. Scavenger receptors bind negatively charged cell wall components from gram-positive bacteria, such as lipoteichoic acid. The innate immune system, e.g., macrophages and neutrophils, has two important tasks: (1) rapid elimination of pathogens and (2) initiation of an inflammatory cascade. Ligation of most of the cell-surface receptors of innate immune cells leads to phagocytosis of the pathogen and subsequent killing in the intracellular milieu. Phagocytosis, e.g., surrounding the pathogen with cell membrane and subsequent internalization in a membrane-bound vesicle called phagosomes, is an active process that requires high levels of energy [4]. In addition, macrophages and neutrophils have membrane-bound granules, called lysosomes, that contain a variety of toxic products, such as nitric oxide (NO), oxygen radicals (generated during the "respiratory burst"), and hydrogen peroxide, which can be released to destroy pathogens. Rapidly, macrophages release lipid mediators, e.g., prostaglandins, leukotrienes, and platelet-activating factors. Next, tissue-resident macrophages and neutrophils release cytokines and chemokines, which contribute to local inflammation and facilitate the recruitment of other immune cells. For example, tumor necrosis factor α (TNFα) is an activator of endothelial cells, interleukin-8 (CXCL8) is involved in the recruitment of neutrophils to the site of infection, interleukin-12 (IL-12) activates natural killer (NK) cells, and interleukin-1β (IL-1β) and interleukin-6 (IL-6) induce systemic acute-phase responses in the liver. Antibody-antigen complexes and surface molecules on pathogens can induce the activation of other, non-eukaryotic, components of the immune system: the complement system and platelets. The complement system consists of plasma proteins that react to mark pathogens for phagocytosis, a process called opsonization, and help exaggerate immune responses. Platelets have long been regarded to be key players in hemostasis, but recent insights have revealed a potent role as immune modulator [5]. Owed to their broad repertoire of cell surface molecules and soluble mediators, platelets not only recognize pathogens but also assist leukocytes to tether and extravasate from the blood. Furthermore, specific neutrophil functions are induced by platelet activation. Thus, both systems help to limit the spread of pathogens.

7.1.1.3 Step 3: Recruitment of Immune Cells

The production of inflammatory cytokines leads to local changes that facilitate the recruitment of more immune cells, dilatation of local small blood vessels, and increased expression of adhesion molecules of endothelial cells [6]. These changes help neutrophils and inflammatory monocytes slow down and begin tethering, rolling, and extravasation into the inflamed tissue [7–10]. Driven by chemokines [11], these newly recruited neutrophils and inflammatory monocytes are guided to the focus of inflammation. The blood vessels also become more permeable, which allows proteins from the plasma and fluids to leak into the interstitial tissue. Altogether, these changes result in the classical signs of inflammation: heat (calor), pain (dolor), redness (rubor), and swelling (edema).

7.1.1.4 Step 4: Involvement of the Adaptive Immune System

The highly inflammatory environment and cytokines, mainly TNFα, also promote the immune stimulatory capacity of antigen-presenting cells. Although macrophages are mainly phagocytic, they can be activated to express co-stimulatory molecules and major histocompatibility complexes (MHC) containing antigens. B-cells bind specific soluble molecules derived from pathogens with cell-surface-bound immunoglobulins, which are internalized, processed, and displayed as antigen fragments in MHC complexes. Similarly, tissue-resident macrophages and recruited monocytes can undergo a phenotypic switch to become professional antigen-presenting cells, known as dendritic cells. Endowed by specific chemokine receptors, e.g., CCR7, these cells respond to chemokines like CCL21 and home to draining lymph nodes, bridging innate and adaptive immunity. Whereas macrophages are found throughout the lymph node, predominantly in the marginal sinuses, B-cells locate to follicles and dendritic cells enter the lymph node cortex in T-cell areas. Activated antigen-presenting cells induce local inflammation that slows down the passing cells of the adaptive immune system, T-cells and B-cells.

Naïve T-cells constantly circulate from the bloodstream and enter lymphoid tissue by crossing high endothelial venules (HEVs), sampling for their cognate antigen. Naïve T-cells that recognize their specific antigen, presented in MHC-peptide complexes in the proper context of co-stimulation and inflammatory cytokines, stop further migration and start differentiation and proliferation to generate large numbers of antigen-specific effector T-cells. This process continues in an autocrine fashion by the secretion of interleukin-2 (IL-2) and expression of IL-2-receptors by activated T-cells. The armament of the adaptive immune system includes $CD8^+$ cytotoxic T-cells, capable of killing virus-infected cells and mutated cancer cells, and $CD4^+$ helper T-cells (T_h-cells); grossly, T_{h1}-cells activate macrophages, and T_{h2}-cells activate B-cells as well as long-lived memory T-cell populations.

The clonally expanded effector T-cell populations egress from the lymph nodes into the circulation and provide a "second wave" of immune cell infiltration in inflamed tissues. These cells now trigger their effector functions, e.g., Fas ligand expression and release of granzymes and perforin, to induce killing of their target without the need for co-stimulation. Furthermore, effector T- and B-cells produce a wide array of cytokines that exaggerates the inflammatory cascade, resulting in iteration of the previous steps 2–4.

7.1.1.5 Step 5: Systemic Inflammatory Responses

Macrophage-derived pro-inflammatory cytokines, mainly TNFα, IL-6, and IL-1β, not only act on immune cells with professional antigen-presenting capacity but also systemically. The liver responds by producing acute-phase proteins, stimulating the activation of complement system, and fibrinogen. The hypothalamus, fat, and muscle tissue respond by mobilizing protein and energy to allow increased body temperature, and the bone marrow and endothelium mobilize loads of neutrophils. In case of a systemic infection, called sepsis, there is widespread leakage from blood vessels, leading to edema, decreased blood volume, collapse of vessels, and disseminated intravascular coagulation. Such multiple organ failure is potentially fatal.

7.1.2 Requirements to Image Inflammation

7.1.2.1 The Unique Features of Inflammation

The unique features of the inflammation pose challenges for in vivo imaging. The previous section illustrates that inflammation involves highly mobile immune cell subsets, which require the imaging field of view to not only include the complete area of inflammation but also draining lymph node regions and eventually other lymphoid organs such as the thymus, spleen, and bone marrow. Imaging modalities with limited field of view or penetration depth, such as ultrasound, fluorescence, and bioluminescence, are therefore less suitable. Next, the distinct steps that we have introduced actually represent a highly dynamic process that covers minutes to hours for the first steps but hours to days for the latter steps and in principal even lifelong imaging for immunological memory responses. This broad imaging time window also affects the choice for imaging method, as short-lived radiotracers and highly invasive techniques are less feasible for longitudinal monitoring. Moreover, the complexity of an ongoing immune response is enormous, involving many soluble factors and cell subsets, challenging the specificity of the imaging system, e.g., labeling specific subsets of cells or imaging a single receptor provide only fractional information. Lastly, inflammatory processes span a broad range of magnitudes; cancer-associated inflammation or parasitic infections go relatively silent, whereas gram-positive cocci result in fulminant and purulent inflammation that can rapidly end in sepsis and death. The sensitivity of the imaging system should allow coverage of the whole spectrum, rendering highly sensitive techniques such as PET more attractive than other techniques, although its use can be limited by exposure limits and costs (Table 7.1).

7.1.2.2 Choice of Target

Closely related to the imaging modality of choice is the question of choosing suitable targets for imaging inflammation.

Related to the first step in the inflammatory model, directly imaging the presence, numbers, and dynamics of pathogens would allow study of the interaction of pathogens with the immune system [12] and possibly guide the development of antibiotics. Several pathogens have been visualized using substrates for virus- or bacteria-specific enzymes [13, 14], radiolabeled antibiotics [15], pathogen-specific antibodies, and antibody fragments or via targeting bacterial products. However, most studies are performed in preclinical models [16] and are beyond the scope of this chapter.

During subsequent steps in inflammation, several studies have investigated radiolabeled cytokines and chemokines [reviewed in [17]] to image presence of cells expressing specific receptors, e.g., ^{99m}Tc-IL-2 to visualize activated lymphocytes [18] or ^{99m}Tc-CXCL8 to image neutrophil recruitment [19, 20]. Radiolabeled antibodies against cell-type-specific cell-surface molecules have also been designed, e.g., anti-CD4 and anti-CD3 antibodies [21] or anti-CD56 to target NK cells [22]. But also ^{111}In-labeled polyclonal IgG has been widely applied in the clinic [23]. Several disadvantages exist for an antibody-based approach; often the expression of cell-surface molecules is dynamic, molecules are internalized and sometimes reexpressed, and the expression is often not specific but part of physiological processes as well. Moreover, radiolabeled antibodies suffer from slow kinetics, often days to accumulate in tissues, whereas many inflammatory steps go much faster. High background in the liver, spleen, bone marrow, and blood circulation, due to unspecific uptake by phagocytic cells, is another drawback. Finally, high-affinity and high-specificity antibodies are seldom available for newly identified ligands.

Table 7.1 Characteristics of imaging modalities in relation to inflammation specific features

Inflammation specific feature	Related imaging requirement	Fluorescence	SPECT	PET	MR	MRS	CT	US
Highly mobile cells	Extended field of view	−−−	+++	+++	+++	+	+++	−
Highly dynamic processes	Imaging time window	−−−	−	−−	+	+	+	++
Many factors, many cell subsets	Specificity	+++	+++	+++	−	+	−−−	−−−
Wide range of magnitudes	Sensitivity	+++	++	+++	+	+	−−−	−−−
Ongoing process	Repeated imaging sessions	−−−	−−−	−−	−	−	−−−	+++

Endothelial activation is the next event in inflammation, and the upregulation of selectins, integrins, and adhesion molecules is targeted with various imaging techniques, including SPECT, PET, and MR imaging to visualize microparticles of iron oxide conjugated to antibodies. Related to the later steps in the inflammatory model, tissue characteristics are often used in clinical imaging modalities that include intravenous contrast, e.g., contrast-enhanced computed tomography (CT) using iodine contrast- or dynamic contrast-enhanced (DCE) magnetic resonance imaging (MRI) using gadolinium compounds. Enhanced perfusion and permeability are assessed by more rapid and more abundant passage of intravenous contrast than under physiological conditions. Although these imaging modalities have many favorable characteristics, the structural changes to the tissue follow functional changes in cell behavior and occur relatively late during the process. The lower sensitivity probably does not allow visualization of the small changes in tissue microstructure at earlier time points. Moreover, given the diverse nature of inflammatory responses, changes in tissue structure do not provide information on the type of inflammation.

Immune metabolism has a few characteristics that make it more attractive for imaging than other targets. In general, metabolism involves smaller molecules as substrate that rapidly diffuse over the cells and tissues and thus are less dependent on tissue structure and perfusion, and metabolic substrates are often abundantly present. Imaging metabolic processes would result in the most minimal perturbation of the system, other than labeling functional receptors or cells. Moreover, the sensitivity of imaging systems, including clinical systems, has greatly improved, enabling the measurement of relatively small amounts of substrate.

However, the challenge in imaging metabolic processes is to link metabolic features to functional processes. In the past decade, we have begun to understand that distinct cell function phenotypes require distinct metabolic profiles and, in turn, how the metabolic environment fuels, or even enforces, cell function [3, 24–26].

The next paragraphs describe current systems for imaging inflammation, focusing on the most dominant cell types, macrophages, neutrophils, and lymphocytes, using the stepwise model described above as reference.

7.2 Metabolism in Relation to Immune Cell Function

7.2.1 Lymphocytes

Lymphocytes are the main effectors of the adaptive immune system, mounting a specific attack against pathogens or diseased cells. This large and vital arm of the immune system consists of T- and B-cells, further divided in various functional subsets. With regard to the inflammatory model, lymphocytes are typically long-lived cells with a multiphasic life span including proliferation, differentiation, and recall, which coincide with specific bioenergetic profiles, as will be discussed in this paragraph.

Naïve lymphocytes continuously circulate throughout the vascular system, spleen, lymph nodes, and lymphatic system. They survey lymph nodes for an encounter with antigen-presenting cells presenting peptide-MHC complexes, cognate to their T-cell receptor (TCR) [27]. The time from their passage through the high endothelial venules (HEVs) to the cortical areas of lymph nodes is estimated between 20 min and 4 h, and then they slow down in T-cell areas of lymph nodes to better scrutinize their microenvironment for peptide-MHC complexes, egress from the lymph nodes, reenter the lymphatics, and return to the venous circulation in about 4–16 h [28]. Although T-cells are regarded as highly mobile cells, under steady-state conditions, only a few percent of naïve T-cells are present in the blood, and they spend the vast majority of their time in secondary lymph nodes, traveling micro-distances.

In this, rather quiescent, phase the metabolic demands of naïve T-cells is low. The basal rates of nutrient uptake and minimal levels of biosynthesis allow oxidative phosphorylation and mitochondrial fatty acid oxidation to prevail over glycolysis for generation of adenosine triphosphate (ATP) [29].

However, once activated in the secondary lymphoid tissue by antigen-presenting cells that present their cognate antigen in peptide-MHC complexes, naïve T-cells start to (1) proliferate and (2) differentiate into effector T-cells. This process known as clonal selection and expansion results in a highly specific immune response and enables the generation of long-lived memory cells. The proliferation rates are incredibly high, as most inflammatory conditions require manifold of antigen-specific effector T-cells.

While quiescent (naïve and memory) T-cells rely on oxidative phosphorylation for their ATP production, activated proliferating cells mainly switch to glycolysis. A critical substrate in activated T-cells is glucose whose uptake is facilitated by the increased localization of the glucose transporter Glut1 to the plasma membrane [30]. Glucose is broken down to pyruvate with a net production of two ATP molecules. Despite the availability of oxygen, activated lymphocytes convert pyruvate into lactate, which regenerates NAD^+ for use in glycolysis. This is known as the Warburg effect and is seen in many types of proliferating cells [29, 31]. ATP and glycolytic intermediates are used for the increase in biomass such as protein synthesis to execute their cytotoxic or helper effector functions and lipid synthesis to meet the increased need for organelle and cell membranes. Although the shift to glycolysis is a main event in effector T-cells, oxidative phosphorylation still occurs to produce reactive oxygen species (ROS) which is needed for activating T-cells [32], and also glutaminolysis is increased.

For the process of differentiation, the bioenergetic profiles are more diverse. Effector functions depend on the available nutrients available in the microenvironment [29, 33]. For example, the extent of the role of oxidative phosphorylation is also important in the differentiation of $CD4^+$ T-cells into regulatory T-cells or effector T-cells [34]. In $CD4^+$ T-cells, the glucose transporter Glut1 is crucial for the activation of $CD4^+$ T-cells and the differentiation into effector cells, whereas memory $CD4^+$ T-cells are not affected by the expression of Glut1 [35, 36]. In general, effector T-cells rely on aerobic glycolysis and oxidative phosphorylation, in contrast to memory T-cells and regulatory T-cells, which depend on oxidative phosphorylation, but do not exploit aerobic glycolysis.

After the pathogen is cleared and the cascade of inflammatory events runs dry, a retraction phase occurs that will leave a small population of memory T-cells [37] that differ from naïve T-cells in their capacity to respond rapidly upon restimulation. Thus, although they rely on oxidative phosphorylation again, their mitochondrial mass and respiratory capacity are increased compared to naïve T-cells.

B-cells share the main metabolic characteristics with T-cells; however, the role of metabolism in affecting the differentiation in either plasma or memory cells is not fully known.

7.2.2 Macrophages

Most tissues, especially epithelial linings that are constantly invaded by pathogens, contain tissue-resident mononuclear phagocytic cells, commonly known as macrophages: Kupffer cells in the liver, Langerhans cells in the skin, alveolar macrophages in the lungs, and lamina propria macrophages in the gut [38]. If the damage to these tissues, and subsequent release of DAMPs, reaches a certain threshold, macrophages are activated [39] and alarm other components of the immune system [9]. From the large pool of circulating monocytes, the subset of inflammatory monocytes, characterized by the low expression of CCR2 and high expression of CX3CR1, enter the tissue and differentiate in a plethora of phenotypes [10], with bioenergetic profiles according to the specific environmental stimuli. Two extremes of this spectrum are so-called pro-inflammatory (M1) macrophages, stimulated by TLR-4 triggering by LPS, and pro-tumorigenic (M2) macrophages, stimulated by interleukin-4 (IL-4) or interleukin-13 (IL-13), among others [40, 41]. Typical to (pro-inflammatory) macrophages are the wide range of effector functions, from phagocytosis and intracellular killing to production of chemo- and cytokines, present in the first steps of the inflammatory model. However, macrophages also play a role in later steps as they are essential in wound healing and tissue repair.

Thus, with respect to the inflammatory model, these cells are rather long-lived and constantly renewing their effector functions, such as cytolytic granules, in contrast to other cells in the first line of defense such as neutrophils. However, as opposed to other long-lived cells like lymphocytes, macrophages do not proliferate. Pro-inflammatory macrophages heavily depend on aerobic glycolysis, whereas macrophages with a tissue repair phenotype rely on oxidative phosphorylation. Due to their association with high-impact infections such as tuberculosis and with atherosclerotic plaque rupture, pro-inflammatory macrophages are most studied and will be discussed here.

Specific to macrophages is their role in iron homeostasis [3, 24]. Iron is an important growth factor for many pathogens, including bacteria and parasites, which have adapted systems to acquire as many free iron atoms as are available upon their invasion of host tissue. As bacteriostatic mechanism during inflammation, pro-inflammatory macrophages tend to retain both free and heme-bound iron intracellularly, to withhold its uptake by pathogens. Further mechanism to hinder iron uptake by pathogens is the decreased expression of ferroportin to reduce iron export and the secretion of lipocalin-2, which prevents iron uptake by bacteria [42]. Next to the first steps in the inflammation model, the acute phase of systemic inflammation (step 5) induces the liver to secrete iron-binding proteins, e.g., lactoferrin and hepcidin. This mechanism not only helps pro-inflammatory macrophages to sequester iron from local sites but also induce iron retention in phagocytic cells located in the liver (Kupffer cells) and spleen [43]. If these conditions endure, restricted iron availability affects the development of erythrocyte precursors, resulting in chronic inflammation-related anemia, a well-known clinical condition in patients with infections, cancer, and autoimmune diseases.

As inflammatory responses reside, damaged tissue should be repaired, and alternatively activated (M2) macrophages in this stage show distinct properties with regard to iron metabolism [44]. The increased expression of scavenger receptors (e.g., CD163) and folate receptor captures hemoglobin derived from hemolysis and hemoproteins such as peroxidases and myeloperoxidases derived from neutrophils, before its toxic effects do further harm to tissue. Next to increased uptake receptors, macrophages in the latter steps of inflammation increase their export of free (heme-derived) iron via ferroportin, to promote matrix remodeling and angiogenesis.

7.2.3 Neutrophils

Neutrophils are considered to be short-lived innate immune cells and are continuously circulating between the bone marrow, spleen, liver, and lung. In healthy individuals, they make up the majority of leukocytes. In the absence of neutrophils, i.e., neutropenia, recurrent infections are the result from overgrowth of bacteria and fungi.

After triggering the innate immune system, one of the very next steps is the recruitment of neutrophils to the inflammatory site. Similar to lymphocytes, this requires drastic changes in their migratory capacities, for example, in cytoskeleton, in order to efficiently migrate into interstitial tissue [7, 8]. Neutrophils play a key role in the direct elimination of invading pathogens. Their secretory vesicles and granules in the cytoplasm contain high loads of bactericidal proteins. The primary granules, known as azurophilic granules, contain the enzyme myeloperoxidase (MPO), the secondary granules contain lactoferrin, and the tertiary (i.e., gelatinase) granules contain matrix metalloproteinase-9 (MMP9). Next to degranulation, neutrophils can also engulf pathogens by phagocytosis and form phagosomes into which hydrolytic enzymes and reactive oxygen species (ROS) are released for intracellular killing. The generation of ROS requires high oxygen consumption, which is termed as the respiratory burst. A third mechanism by which neutrophils eliminate bacteria is the production of neutrophil extracellular traps (NETs) in which invasive bacteria are trapped and killed by extracellular fibers composed of DNA, histones, and granule contents [45]. The shift to glycolysis is essential for the formation of NETs.

In steady state, neutrophil relies on glycolysis, rather than oxidative phosphorylation as reflected by the low number of mitochondria. This dependency on glycolysis is even further increased once activated, similar to the differentiation of lymphocytes; the main reason for neutrophils to stick to aerobic glycolysis and the oxidative pentose phosphate pathway is their need to produce effector molecules, mainly microbicidal products like hydrogen peroxide. The increased need for glucose mainly occurs upon priming of neutrophils, but is not so much required for executing the effector functions itself, such as the respiratory burst or degranulation [46]. Indeed, in patients with bronchiectasis, there is an increase in neutrophils in the alveolar space, determined by imaging ^{111}In-labeled white blood cells (WBC) on a gamma camera, due to diffuse damage to the bronchial wall, but no increase in 2-deoxy-2-^{18}F-fluoro-D-glucose (^{18}F-FDG) uptake measured on PET/CT. On the other hand, in lobar pneumonia there is increased ^{18}F-FDG uptake in the lung without evident emigration of ^{111}In-labeled WBC in alveolar space [47]. This indicates that ^{18}F-FDG PET/CT might represent a biomarker for *early* inflammatory processes, reflecting neutrophil activation and priming. The strong correlation of increased ^{18}F-FDG uptake in the lung with both the number of neutrophils and their activation status supports this notion [48].

7.3 Targets for Imaging Immune Cell Metabolism

7.3.1 Imaging Cell-Surface Receptors and Transporters

7.3.1.1 Translocator Protein

The translocator protein, also known as peripheral benzodiazepine receptor (TSPO), is expressed on the outer membrane of mitochondria. Inflammatory macrophages are the main source of its expression in peripheral tissue, besides neutrophils and lymphocytes [49]. Activated glial cells and astrocytes are its major source in the central nervous system [50]; therefore, several proteins that bind this receptor have been investigated as tracer for atherosclerosis and neuroinflammation, respectively [51].

Examples. ^{18}F-FEDAA1106 suggest a higher specific binding to inflammatory sites as compared to ^{18}F-FDG [52], providing a marker to visualize pro-inflammatory macrophages in vulnerable atherosclerotic plaques. ^{11}C-PK11195 is regarded a method of visualizing the microglial component of neuroinflammation [53]. In tuberculosis, the mycobacterium is taken up by alveolar macrophages. The mycobacterium tuberculosis has developed certain mechanisms to evade the immune system and can eventually cause a granulomatous inflammation in which many infected macrophages are present. In some studies ^{125}I-DPA 713 for the use in SPECT has been compared to ^{18}F-FDG PET [54].

7.3.1.2 Iron-Binding Proteins

^{67}Ga is a trivalent metal with a half-life of 3.2 days; in blood (normal pH), it binds to the most abundant iron-binding protein, transferrin with high affinity. The increased permeability of capillaries in inflamed tissue causes ^{67}Ga-transferrin complexes to leak into the interstitial tissue. Due to increased anaerobic glycolysis, lactate concentrations in inflammation increase and result in a localized and gradual decline of pH. Low pH favors the dissociation of ^{67}Ga-transferrin, and free ^{67}Ga then binds to other iron-binding proteins produced by neutrophils and macrophages, such as lactoferrin and siderophores [55].

Example. ^{67}Ga-citrate, and more recently ^{68}Ga-citrate [56], has demonstrated high sensitivity for both acute and chronic infection as well as noninfectious inflammation [57]. For example, pulmonary tuberculosis infection nearly always showed increased ^{67}Ga accumulation to a higher extent as compared to non-tuberculosis pulmonary infections in non-HIV-infected patients. ^{67}Ga-uptake grade and ratio could thus be used to predict active pulmonary tuberculosis in acid-fast bacilli smear-positive patients [58]. However, its specificity is poor because of bowel excretion and accumulation in other acid environments such as cancer bone remodeling. In addition, the imaging window is up to 3 days after injection to allow for sufficient clearance from normal tissue.

7.3.1.3 Scavenger Receptor

Under physiological conditions, macrophages take up lipid complexes via scavenger receptors. Several studies have used such lipid complexes to target the presence of macrophages in atherosclerotic plaques in preclinical models. For example, scavenger receptor-targeted immunomicelles were tested in ApoE−/− and WT mice by using MRI, demonstrating a higher increase in signal intensity of atherosclerotic aortas in ApoE−/− mice after 24 h compared with untargeted micelles and no enhancement using gadolinium-DTPA. Colocalization with macrophages in plaques was confirmed with confocal laser scanning microscopy [59]. In another preclinical approach to target tumor-associated macrophages, high-density lipoproteins (HDL) have been complexed with ^{89}Zr for imaging with PET. These particles have been shown to specifically accumulate in tumor regions with increased presence of macrophages [60].

7.3.1.4 Folate Receptor

The folate receptor (FR) is a glycosylphosphatidylinositol-anchored protein that binds the vitamin folic acid with high affinity and internalizes it via endocytosis. In normal tissues and organs, FR-α expression is restricted to the luminal surface of polarized epithelia and thus does not have access to intravenously administered folic acid conjugates. However, FR-β is expressed on activated macrophages; its restricted expression makes this receptor an interesting target for both imaging and therapy of inflammation [61, 62]. In a preclinical lung inflammation model induced by *Escherichia coli* LPS, FR-β expression was markedly increased in lung macrophages after intratracheal LPS administration. In vivo molecular imaging with a fluorescent probe (cyanine 5 polyethylene glycol folate) showed that the fluorescence signal over the chest peaked at 48 h after administration and was reduced after depletion of macrophages. Flow cytometry identified the cells responsible for uptake of cyanine 5-conjugated folate as FRβ-positive interstitial macrophages and pulmonary monocytes, co-expression markers associated with a pro-inflammatory phenotype [63]. With similar intention, different murine models of inflammatory disease (rheumatoid arthritis, ulcerative colitis, pulmonary fibrosis, and atherosclerosis) were studied during treatment and evaluated with a folate receptor-targeted near-infrared dye. The dye accumulated at sites of inflammation in all four models and changes in uptake preceded changes in clinical symptoms in mice treated with all anti-inflammatory drugs examined [64]. Also in clinical settings, FR-β has been investigated as a target for activated macrophages, reviewed in [65]. A large number of radiolabeled folate conjugates with variable chemical structures have been developed over the last 25 years. Accumulation of radioactivity in healthy organs and tissues was always seen in the kidneys due to the expression of the FR in the proximal tubule cells, presumably due to nonspecific uptake of radiolabeled folate in the liver and the intestinal tract. To improve the target-to-background ratio, several chemical modifications of the folate conjugates are employed to modify their pharmacokinetic and pharmacodynamic properties, with increasing success [66].

7.3.1.5 Endocytosis

Directly related to their functional role during the initial phases of inflammation, tissue-resident macrophages and phagocytic cells differentiated from recruited inflammatory monocytes showed enhanced endocytic capacity. Although endocytosis, including actin-dependent macropinocytosis, is not entirely restricted to mononuclear phagocytic cells of the immune system, but also occurs in tumor cells, this mechanism is often exploited to visualize the presence of macrophages in inflammatory diseases. Nanoparticles, which can be modified in size, have been functionalized to enhance endocytosis-mediated specificity for certain cell types for imaging with MR, SPECT, PET, and fluorescence [67, 68]. Using advanced MR acquisition and registration techniques, it has been demonstrated in patients with type 1 diabetes that ferumoxytol nanoparticles, taken up by macrophages, allows visualization of pancreatic inflammation [69]. The most frequently studied nanoparticles are loaded with superparamagnetic iron oxide, potentially delivering a high load of iron to the phagocytic cells. The central role of macrophages in iron metabolism and the mutual relation of iron concentrations directly extracellularly and intracellularly with cell function [42, 44] suggest that those diagnostic nanoparticles can have an effect on macrophage function, although no systematic studies have been conducted so far.

7.3.2 Imaging Specific Metabolic Substrates

7.3.2.1 Glucose Metabolism

As a consequence to the increased glucose uptake in activated immune cells, ^{18}F-FDG PET is a common metabolic tracer to image inflammation [16]. ^{18}F-FDG is a glucose analogue, which is taken up in large amounts by Glut transporters in metabolic active cells. It is trapped in the cell as a result of phosphorylation by the enzyme hexokinase, allowing detection of active glucose metabolism using the high sensitivity of PET imaging.

^{18}F-FDG PET has been successfully applied in many inflammatory diseases like infections, atherosclerosis, and autoimmune diseases such as vasculitis [70]. In the appropriate clinical context, the diagnostic accuracy for ^{18}F-FDG to detect inflammatory activity is high. Physiological uptake ^{18}F-FDG in the myocardium, brain, liver, and bone marrow, however, makes it less sensitive for imaging inflammation at these sites. In patients with type 2 diabetes mellitus, the biodistribution of ^{18}F-FDG might be altered, with increased ^{18}F-FDG uptake in the larger and smaller intestines and decreased ^{18}F-FDG uptake in the myocardium, likely as a result of antidiabetic medication [71].

Example: bacterial infection. ^{18}F-FDG PET/CT is able to detect infectious foci with high diagnostic accuracy in patients with gram-positive bacteremia, resulting in lower mortality rates [20, 72]. In patients with *Staphylococcus aureus* bacteremia, relapse rates decreased significantly after inclusion of ^{18}F-FDG PET/CT in the diagnostic workup. Similar results were found for neutropenic patients [73].

Example: vasculitis. The diagnostic accuracy of ^{18}F-FDG PET/CT for patients with large vessel vasculitis is good; a recent meta-analysis shows a pooled sensitivity and specificity of 75.9% (95% CI 68.7–82.1) and 93.0% (95% CI 88.9–96.0), respectively. Especially for giant cell arteritis, the pooled sensitivity and specificity were 83.3% (95% CI 72.1–91.4) and 89.6% (95% CI 79.7–95.7) [74]. Although high glucose levels or diabetes mellitus is commonly regarded to impair the diagnostic accuracy of ^{18}F-FDG PET/CT in the diagnosis of inflammation, comparative analyses show that its influence is trivial [75].

Other glucose derivatives have been investigated in preclinical models to identify and localize infection-specific pathogens. For example, ^{18}F-FDG is used to produce 2-(^{18}F)-fluorodeoxysorbitol (^{18}F-FDS), a radioactive probe specific for *Enterobacteriaceae*. ^{18}F-FDS selectively accumulated in *Enterobacteriaceae*, but not in gram-positive bacteria or healthy mammalian or cancer cells in vitro. In mouse models increased accumulation of this tracer demonstrated to differentiate infection from sterile inflammation, and its signal intensity was proportional to the bacterial burden [76]. Mouse models indicate that 6-(^{18}F)-fluoromaltose is taken up by multiple strains of pathogenic bacteria, but not by mammalian cancer cell lines or inflamed tissue [77].

7.3.2.2 DNA Synthesis

An important feature that can be used to image activated lymphocytes is proliferation [4]. Thymidine has been labeled with radioactive ^{11}C, but due to several problems for clinical imaging, thymidine analogues which could be labeled with ^{18}F were developed [78].

The most promising tracer to detect proliferation by DNA synthesis has been 3′-deoxy-3′(^{18}F)-fluorothymidine (^{18}F-FLT) [79], which is increasingly used to monitor treatment responses in solid tumors [80]. ^{18}F-FLT is a thymidine analogue but is unlike thymidine in that it is not incorporated in the DNA. In the salvage pathway, thymidine is transported across the cell membrane and phosphorylated by thymidine kinase 1 (TK1) to thymidine monophosphate (TMP). Alternatively, TMP is formed by the conversion of deoxyuridine monophosphate (dUMP) by the enzyme thymidylate synthase (TS). This alternative de novo pathway is able to provide all the thymidine needed for DNA synthesis [81]. The activity of TK is directly related to DNA synthesis and therefore correlates with cell proliferation. ^{18}F-FLT is taken up by the salvage pathway and phosphorylated similarly to thymidine but is instead trapped in the cell.

Example. Rapidly proliferating cells in secondary lymphoid organs rely extensively on the salvage pathway, which suggests that ^{18}F-FLT PET is an effective modality for monitoring lymphocytes in the context of lymphoma [82, 83], as well as inflammation [84, 85]. In melanoma patients who underwent dendritic cell-based vaccinations, antigen-specific responses were measured by immune assays in peripheral blood as well as by ^{18}F-FDG and ^{18}F-FLT PET/CT scans; the signal intensity in vaccinated lymph nodes correlated with the magnitude of antigen-specific T-cell and B-cell responses for ^{18}F-FLT, but not with ^{18}F-FDG [84].

Deoxycytidine kinase (dCK) is a rate-limiting enzyme in the deoxyribonucleoside salvage pathway involved in the production and maintenance of a balanced pool of deoxyribonucleoside triphosphates (dNTPs) for DNA synthesis. The biodistribution and radiation dosimetry of three fluorinated dCK substrates, ^{18}F-D-FAC, ^{18}F-L-FAC, and ^{18}F-L-FMAC, have been evaluated in humans for PET imaging of dCK activity in vivo. The different probes have distinct affinities for nucleoside transporters, dCK, and catabolic enzymes such as cytidine deaminase (CDA). Dosimetry demonstrates that all three probes can be used safely to image the deoxyribonucleoside salvage pathway in humans. ^{18}F-D-FAC uptake is characteristic of activated lymphocytes, and biodistribution is predominantly seen in the spleen, thymus, and bone marrow. It has also been demonstrated to be sensitive to sites where immune activation takes place and has allowed visualization of lymphoid organs in a mouse model of antitumor immunity [86, 87]. Intriguingly, innate and adaptive immune cells from tissues of mice challenged with a retrovirus-induced sarcoma differentially accumulate ^{18}F-FDG and ^{18}F-D-FAC: ^{18}F-FDG accumulated to the highest levels in innate immune cells, while ^{18}F-D-FAC accumulated predominantly in CD8^{+} T-cells in a manner that correlated with the extent of proliferation. This study demonstrates that innate and adaptive cell types may differ in glycolytic and deoxycytidine salvage demands during an immune response which can be detected with specific PET probes [88].

7.3.2.3 Lipid Synthesis

Choline is a precursor for the biosynthesis of phospholipids and is present in cell and mitochondrial membranes. High levels of choline metabolites are found in proliferating tumor cells, suggesting that choline is a potential target for proliferation imaging. PET tracers ^{11}C-choline or ^{18}F-fluorocholine integrates in newly synthesized membranes upon injection. ^{1}H-MRS measurements of total choline also allow the assessment of membrane turnover.

Example: choline. To assess vulnerable atherosclerotic plaques, both ^{18}F-choline and ^{11}C-choline have been investigated in mouse models and shown to accumulate in macrophage-rich areas of aortic plaques, more specifically than ^{18}F-FDG [89, 90]. Similarly, in a pilot clinical study in five patients, ^{18}F-choline was demonstrated to correlate with structural vessel wall alterations. Positive ^{18}F-choline uptake was found in 14 lesions, more often in vessel walls with calcification, whereas 16 out of 17 ^{18}F-choline negative lesions were identified as completely calcified without additional structural vessel wall alteration. One of the major advantages of ^{18}F-choline compared to ^{18}F-FDG is the lower uptake in the myocardium, making it the favorable choice in imaging coronary obstructions. Although choline has demonstrated to accumulate in inflammatory sites [70], its exploitation as dedicated inflammation marker remains anecdotal in clinical settings [91].

7.3.2.4 Amino Acid Metabolism

Several tracers have been developed to image increased amino acid metabolism. Most tracers to detect increased amino acid metabolism have been used in preclinical and clinical tumor detection with PET but have also shown to be able to detect inflammation. The most frequently used radiolabeled amino acid is ^{11}C-methionine, as it contains sulfur; it is highly involved in protein synthesis. Uptake has been associated with an increased amino acid transport, and, despite the higher sensitivity for proliferating tumor cells, ^{11}C-methionine uptake is also significantly increased in inflammatory cells [92].

Example. Physiological high 18F-FDG accumulation in the cortical regions of the brain warrants the development of tracers that target other metabolic pathways. Preclinical studies revealed high uptake of methionine tracers in brain abscesses in particular [93, 94]. PET imaging before and after treatment in patients with brain abscess showed uptake of both tracers in the abscess before treatment. The region in the abscess with an increased uptake of ^{11}C-methionine corresponded closely to the enhanced area on both CT and MR images. After treatment the lesions became smaller on CT or MRI, and both ^{11}C-methionine and ^{18}F-FDG showed reduced uptake, suggesting that also ^{11}C-methionine imaging allows response monitoring of antibiotic treatment for brain abscesses.

The tracer trans-1-amino-3-(^{18}F)-fluorocyclobutanecarboxylic acid (^{18}F-FACBC) is a synthetic amino acid that is taken up by activated immune cells [95, 96]. In direct comparison with ^{18}F-FDG and ^{11}C-methionine in a rat model, ^{18}F-FACBC uptake ratios of stimulated versus non-stimulated T-cells increased threefold in the first minutes after incubation, for B-cells and macrophages the uptake ratio as compared to non-stimulated cells only slightly increased, while activated neutrophils showed an continuous increase over 60 min of incubation. However, the ratio of ^{14}C-FACBC uptake compared to tumor cells was less than the uptake of ^{18}F-FDG ratios. Thus the low ^{18}F-FACBC accumulation in granulocytes/macrophages may be advantageous in discriminating inflamed regions from tumors.

Glutamine is an essential precursor of proteins, amino sugars, nucleic acids, purines, and pyrimidines and abundantly present extracellularly. Its immediate metabolite glutamate is present extracellularly. Several PET probes have been developed to image glutaminolysis, e.g., ^{18}F-(2S,4S)-4-(3-fluoropropil)glutamine or 5-(^{11}C)-glutamine, mostly to image malignancies that are not dependent on glucose for the primary metabolism [97, 98], but studies specific on immune metabolism are lacking.

7.3.3 Imaging Enzyme Activity

7.3.3.1 Myeloperoxidase Activity

MPO activity is most abundant in the azurophilic granules of neutrophils but also seen in macrophages. During the respiratory burst, ROS are produced for direct killing of pathogens, which is associated with increased MPO activity. Monitoring ROS in living animals is challenging due to the rapid turnover of ROS and the limited sensitivity and specificity of ROS probes. Bioluminescent imaging studies in preclinical models of inflammation, including arthritis, dermatitis, and inflammatory tumors, have shown to correlate with MPO activity. In MPO knockout mice, no signal was seen which suggests specificity toward ROS converted by MPO and not to other oxidizing enzymes [99–101].

Another strategy to image MPO is the use of an MPO-activatable gadolinium-based contrast agent for MR imaging. Upon activation by MPO, the contrast agent binds to plasma proteins in the inflammatory site, resulting in delayed clearance from tissues and thus an enhanced image contrast. In mice with inflammation after stroke, the intensity of the MRI signal correlated to MPO levels as analyzed with biochemical assays, and specificity of the contrast agent toward MPO activity has been confirmed with MPO knockout mice [102].

7.3.3.2 Cyclooxygenase Activity

The enzyme cyclooxygenase (COX) is also known as prostaglandin H and produces prostaglandins out of conversion of arachidonic acid. This enzyme comes in three isoforms, and particularly the inducible isoform COX-2 plays an important role in inflammation and is the target of nonsteroidal anti-inflammatory drugs (NSAIDs). Several drugs that selectively inhibit COX-2, e.g., celecoxib and rofecoxib, have been radiolabeled to study enzyme activity in vivo in inflammation [103–105]. However, nonspecific binding and low sensitivity hamper successful implementation in larger studies.

7.3.3.3 Elastase and Matrix Metalloproteinase Activity

Imaging depth of bioluminescent imaging is limited, and therefore near-infrared (NIR) optical probe has been developed to target neutrophil-associated products with enhanced depth resolution. Optical imaging of probes targeting neutrophil elastase, an enzyme needed for destruction of bacteria, has been able to detect increased elastase activity, which correlated to the number of neutrophils at the inflammation site [106].

Similar associations with neutrophil burden were made with another NIR probe, specific for matrix metalloproteinase (MMP). These probes can be activated by MMP and were investigated in the heart after myocardial infarction in mice [107]. Confocal microscopy showed co-localization of neutrophils in the infarct zone with the NIR signal, which were confirmed by cytometric analysis. However, these techniques are restricted to preclinical models.

7.3.4 Imaging Metabolites

Magnetic resonance spectroscopy (MRS) is a noninvasive technique that has been used to detect the relative concentrations of metabolites in tissues. Like MR, MRS is based on nuclear magnetic resonance in which the hydrogen atom is often the main target due to its high sensitivity. Obtained MR spectra contain information of metabolite composition and have therefore been of clinical importance to study metabolic changes in disease [108].

MRS and serum analysis with ^{1}H-NMR have identified several biomarkers in patients with autoimmune diseases. In multiple sclerosis, MRS was capable of identifying increased metabolites compared to healthy controls, which are associated with increased glycolysis such as lactate, pyruvate, glucose, lipids, and several amino acids including glutamine [109]. Proliferating T-cells utilize tenfold more glutamine than any other amino acid, and this is necessary to regenerate oxaloacetic acid (OAA) which is consumed by biosynthesis [34]. Additionally, glutamine is an essential amine donor, required for biosynthesis of purine and amino acids in activated T-cells. Serum analysis with ^{1}H-NMR in rheumatoid arthritis identified a correlation between disease severity and the increase of several metabolites that are associated with upregulated biosynthetic pathways in inflammation [109].

7.4 Future Developments

The field of immune metabolism is rapidly evolving, driven by our increased understanding of the mutual relationship between bioenergetic profiles of immune cells and their contemporary functions. A few developments with high potential to influence the imaging approach of immune metabolism will be highlighted here.

7.4.1 Integrative Analysis of Multiscale Data

The past decades have revealed a manifold of individual receptors, enzymes, substrates, and metabolites that have a spatially and temporally restricted role in the inflammatory cascade. If the number of different pathogens and involved immune cells are considered, this adds to an enormously complex system that works together to balance pathogen clearance with tissue homeostasis. Recently, techniques have become available that integrate high-throughput data from various sources, including proteomics, transcriptomics, epigenomics, and genomics, providing a more comprehensive evaluation of the human immune response [110, 111].

Macrophages are to date the most well-studied immune cells, and such integrative analysis of metabolic and transcriptional data has demonstrated distinct modules that support specific functional polarization of macrophages [112]. Applying such transcriptional modules to human alveolar macrophages from smokers and patients with chronic obstructive pulmonary disease (COPD) has revealed an unexpected loss of inflammatory signatures in COPD patients [113]. As these developments go together with advanced image acquisition and analysis, e.g., texture feature analysis [114–116], there is no doubt that the next decade will allow a standardized and quantitative noninvasive assessment of metabolic profiles during inflammation.

7.4.2 Manipulation of Immune Cell Metabolism

As immune response requires major changes to metabolic processes in immune cells to determine their ability to divide, differentiate, and perform effector functions, immune cell metabolism is an attractive target therapy [25]. Mononuclear phagocytic cells, including tissue-resident macrophages and inflammatory monocytes, are the most plastic cells that orchestrate the immune response on site and have a large role in the local metabolic conditions [3, 24, 25]. Therefore, drugs that specifically target macrophages and their function are increasingly being introduced in the clinic [117]. Although this development is currently driven by the need to confer cancer-related inflammation and tumor-associated macrophages, translation to inflammation in infection and autoimmunity is near. In a similar fashion, metabolism supports many aspects of T-cell function. Recently, metabolic pathways can be manipulated in anticancer immunity, as well as in autoimmunity. Especially preventing T-cell dysfunction in hostile microenvironments might direct T-cell differentiation and function toward desired phenotypes in autoimmunity [118].

7.4.3 Hyperpolarized MR

An emerging imaging technique to measure metabolites is hyperpolarized MRI, which has two major advantages. First, using ^{13}C in its hyperpolarized state increases the signal drastically, up to 10^7 times. Second, it allows the use of several hyperpolarized probes simultaneously, thus the detection of multiple pathways at the same time. Furthermore, using hyperpolarized substrates, it is possible to measure its conversion in real time, whereas the other highly sensitive technique PET is not able to discriminate the parent from the formed metabolic product [119, 120].

7.4.4 Hybrid PET/MR Imaging

PET/MR imaging has many advantages over PET/CT, including a lower radiation exposure, higher soft tissue contrast, and better imaging of dynamic and moving processes. In inflammation imaging, dynamic contrast-enhanced (DCE) and diffusion-weighted (DW) imaging would add information on the tissue structure to the increased rate of glycolysis measured with ^{18}F-FDG PET. This can improve the diagnostic accuracy in body regions with high background ^{18}F-FDG accumulation, such as the bone marrow and spondylodiscitis, or with moving organs such as the intestines and inflammatory bowel diseases [121]. The complementary data from MR has recently been shown to enable accurate noninvasive imaging of tissue classes in tumor regions [122], illustrating that also inflammation imaging can benefit from hybrid imaging.

From the previous history of in vivo imaging, it is learned that imaging developments are boosted if there is a clinical relevance in other medical disciplines. As our understanding of immune metabolism has made big leaps forward in the recent years and therapeutic options for manipulation of immune metabolism are only just being explored, the future of imaging immune metabolism in inflammation looks bright.

Acknowledgments This work was supported by a European Research Council (ERC) Grant ERC-2104-StG-336454-CoNQUeST and Dutch Cancer Society grant KUN2015-8106.

References

1. Mantovani A, Allavena P, Sica A, Balkwill F. Cancer-relatedinflammation.Nature.2008;454(7203):436–44.
2. Green DR, Ferguson T, Zitvogel L, Kroemer G. Immunogenic and tolerogenic cell death. Nat Rev Immunol. 2009;9(5):353–63.
3. Chawla A, Nguyen KD, Goh YP. Macrophage-mediated inflammation in metabolic disease. Nat Rev Immunol. 2011;11(11):738–49.
4. Gordon S. Phagocytosis: an Immunobiologic process. Immunity. 2016;44(3):463–75.
5. Jenne CN, Kubes P. Platelets in inflammation and infection. Platelets. 2015;26(4):286–92.
6. Pober JS, Sessa WC. Evolving functions of endothelial cells in inflammation. Nat Rev Immunol. 2007;7(10):803–15.
7. Friedl P, Weigelin B. Interstitial leukocyte migration and immune function. Nat Immunol. 2008;9(9):960–9.
8. Weninger W, Biro M, Jain R. Leukocyte migration in the interstitial space of non-lymphoid organs. Nat Rev Immunol. 2014;14(4):232–46.
9. Abtin A, Jain R, Mitchell AJ, Roediger B, Brzoska AJ, Tikoo S, et al. Perivascular macrophages mediate neutrophil recruitment during bacterial skin infection. Nat Immunol. 2014;15(1):45–53.
10. Shi C, Pamer EG. Monocyte recruitment during infection and inflammation. Nat Rev Immunol. 2011;11(11):762–74.
11. Bachmann MF, Kopf M, Marsland BJ. Chemokines: more than just road signs. Nat Rev Immunol. 2006;6(2):159–64.
12. Coombes JL, Robey EA. Dynamic imaging of host-pathogen interactions in vivo. Nat Rev Immunol. 2010;10(5):353–64.
13. Diaz LA Jr, Foss CA, Thornton K, Nimmagadda S, Endres CJ, Uzuner O, et al. Imaging of musculoskeletal bacterial infections by [124I]FIAU-PET/CT. PLoS One. 2007;2(10):e1007.
14. Pullambhatla M, Tessier J, Beck G, Jedynak B, Wurthner JU, Pomper MG. [(125)I]FIAU imaging in a preclinical model of lung infection: quantification of bacterial load. Am J Nucl Med Mol Imaging. 2012;2(3):260–70.
15. Ferro-Flores G, Ocampo-Garcia BE, Melendez-Alafort L. Development of specific radiopharmaceuticals for infection imaging by targeting infectious micro-organisms. Curr Pharm Des. 2012;18(8):1098–106.
16. Dorward DAD. Imaging inflammation: molecular strategies to visualize key components of the inflammatory cascade, from initiation to resolution. Pharmacol Ther. 2012;135(2):182–99.
17. Malviya G, Signore A, Lagana B, Dierckx RA. Radiolabelled peptides and monoclonal antibodies for therapy decision making in inflammatory diseases. Curr Pharm Des. 2008;14(24):2401–14.
18. Annovazzi A, Biancone L, Caviglia R, Chianelli M, Capriotti G, Mather SJ, et al. 99mTc-interleukin-2 and (99m)Tc-HMPAO granulocyte scintigraphy in patients with inactive Crohn's disease. Eur J Nucl Med Mol Imaging. 2003;30(3):374–82.
19. Rennen HJ, Bleeker-Rovers CP, van Eerd JE, Frielink C, Oyen WJ, Corstens FH, et al. 99mTc-labeled interleukin-8 for scintigraphic detection of pulmonary infections. Chest. 2004;126(6):1954–61.
20. Vos FJ, Bleeker-Rovers CP, Sturm PD, Krabbe PF, van Dijk AP, Cuijpers ML, et al. 18F-FDG PET/CT for detection of metastatic infection in gram-positive bacteremia. J Nucl Med. 2010;51(8):1234–40.
21. Malviya G, Galli F, Sonni I, Signore A. Imaging T-lymphocytes in inflammatory diseases: a nuclear medicine approach. Q J Nucl Med Mol Imaging. 2014;58(3):237–57.
22. Galli F, Histed S, Aras O. NK cell imaging by in vitro and in vivo labelling approaches. Q J Nucl Med Mol Imaging. 2014;58(3):276–83.
23. de Kleijn EM, Oyen WJ, Corstens FH, van der Meer JW. Utility of indium-111-labeled polyclonal immunoglobulin G scintigraphy in fever of unknown origin. The Netherlands FUO imaging group. J Nucl Med. 1997;38(3):484–9.
24. Biswas SK, Mantovani A. Orchestration of metabolism by macrophages. Cell Metab. 2012;15(4):432–7.
25. Norata GD, Caligiuri G, Chavakis T, Matarese G, Netea MG, Nicoletti A, et al. The cellular and molecular basis of translational immunometabolism. Immunity. 2015;43(3):421–34.
26. Biswas SK. Metabolic reprogramming of immune cells in cancer progression. Immunity. 2015;43(3):435–49.
27. Germain RN, Miller MJ, Dustin ML, Nussenzweig MC. Dynamic imaging of the immune system: progress, pitfalls and promise. Nat Rev Immunol. 2006;6(7):497–507.
28. Lee M, Mandl JN, Germain RN, Yates AJ. The race for the prize: T-cell trafficking strategies for optimal surveillance. Blood. 2012;120(7):1432–8.
29. Pearce Erika LE. Metabolic pathways in immune cell activation and quiescence. Immunity. 2013;38(4):633–43.
30. Frauwirth KA, Thompson CB. Regulation of T lymphocyte metabolism. J Immunol. 2004;172(8):4661–5.
31. Palmer CS, Ostrowski M, Balderson B, Christian N, Crowe SM. Glucose metabolism regulates T cell activation, differentiation, and functions. Front Immunol. 2015;6:1.
32. Sena Laura AL. Mitochondria are required for antigen-specific T cell activation through reactive oxygen species signaling. Immunity. 2013;38(2):225–36.
33. Fox CJ, Hammerman PS, Thompson CB. Fuel feeds function: energy metabolism and the T-cell response. Nat Rev Immunol. 2005;5(11):844–52.

34. Pearce Erika LE. Fueling immunity: insights into metabolism and lymphocyte function. Science. 2013;342(6155).
35. Maekawa Y, Ishifune C, Tsukumo S, Hozumi K, Yagita H, Yasutomo K. Notch controls the survival of memory CD4+ T cells by regulating glucose uptake. Nat Med. 2015;21(1):55–61.
36. Macintyre AN, Gerriets VA, Nichols AG, Michalek RD, Rudolph MC, Deoliveira D, et al. The glucose transporter Glut1 is selectively essential for CD4 T cell activation and effector function. Cell Metab. 2014;20(1):61–72.
37. Lanzavecchia A, Sallusto F. Understanding the generation and function of memory T cell subsets. Curr Opin Immunol. 2005;17(3):326–32.
38. Ginhoux F, Schultze JL, Murray PJ, Ochando J, Biswas SK. New insights into the multidimensional concept of macrophage ontogeny, activation and function. Nat Immunol. 2015;17(1):34–40.
39. Zhang X, Mosser DM. Macrophage activation by endogenous danger signals. J Pathol. 2008;214(2):161–78.
40. Mosser DM, Edwards JP. Exploring the full spectrum of macrophage activation. Nat Rev Immunol. 2008;8(12):958–69.
41. Murray PJ, Wynn TA. Obstacles and opportunities for understanding macrophage polarization. J Leukoc Biol. 2011;89(4):557–63.
42. Cairo G, Recalcati S, Mantovani A, Locati M. Iron trafficking and metabolism in macrophages: contribution to the polarized phenotype. Trends Immunol. 2011;32(6):241–7.
43. Recalcati S, Locati M, Cairo G. Systemic and cellular consequences of macrophage control of iron metabolism. Semin Immunol. 2012;24(6):393–8.
44. Recalcati S, Locati M, Gammella E, Invernizzi P, Cairo G. Iron levels in polarized macrophages: regulation of immunity and autoimmunity. Autoimmun Rev. 2012;11(12):883–9.
45. Brinkmann VV. Neutrophil extracellular traps kill bacteria. Science. 2004;303(5663):1532–5.
46. Jones HA, Cadwallader KA, White JF, Uddin M, Peters AM, Chilvers ER. Dissociation between respiratory burst activity and deoxyglucose uptake in human neutrophil granulocytes: implications for interpretation of (18)F-FDG PET images. J Nucl Med. 2002;43(5):652–7.
47. Jones HA, Sriskandan S, Peters AM, Pride NB, Krausz T, Boobis AR, et al. Dissociation of neutrophil emigration and metabolic activity in lobar pneumonia and bronchiectasis. Eur Respir J. 1997;10(4):795–803.
48. Chen DL, Rosenbluth DB, Mintun MA, Schuster DP. FDG-PET imaging of pulmonary inflammation in healthy volunteers after airway instillation of endotoxin. J Appl Physiol. 2006;100(5):1602–9.
49. Campanella M, Turkheimer FE. TSPO: functions and applications of a mitochondrial stress response pathway. Biochem Soc Trans. 2015;43(4):593–4.
50. Janczar K, Su Z, Raccagni I, Anfosso A, Kelly C, Durrenberger PF, et al. The 18-kDa mitochondrial translocator protein in gliomas: from the bench to bedside. Biochem Soc Trans. 2015;43(4):579–85.
51. Cerami C, Perani D. Imaging neuroinflammation in ischemic stroke and in the atherosclerotic vascular disease. Curr Vasc Pharmacol. 2015;13(2):218–22.
52. Cuhlmann S, Gsell W, Van der Heiden K, Habib J, Tremoleda JL, Khalil M, et al. In vivo mapping of vascular inflammation using the translocator protein tracer 18F-FEDAA1106. Mol Imaging. 2014;13
53. Varley J, Brooks DJ, Edison P. Imaging neuroinflammation in Alzheimer's disease and other dementias: recent advances and future directions. Alzheimers Dement. 2015;11(9):1110–20.
54. Ordonez AA, Pokkali S, DeMarco VP, Klunk M, Mease RC, Foss CA, et al. Radioiodinated DPA-713 imaging correlates with bactericidal activity of tuberculosis treatments in mice. Antimicrob Agents Chemother. 2015;59(1):642–9.
55. Vallabhajosula SR, Harwig JF, Wolf W. The mechanism of tumor localization of gallium-67 citrate: role of transferrin binding and effect of tumor pH. Int J Nucl Med Biol. 1981;8(4):363–70.
56. Nanni C, Errani C, Boriani L, Fantini L, Ambrosini V, Boschi S, et al. 68Ga-citrate PET/CT for evaluat ing patients with infections of the bone: preliminary results. J Nucl Med. 2010;51(12):1932–6.
57. Weiner R, Hoffer PB, Thakur ML. Lactoferrin: its role as a Ga-67-binding protein in polymorphonuclear leukocytes. J Nucl Med. 1981;22(1):32–7.
58. Yeh JJ, Huang YC, Teng WB, Huang YF, Chuang YW, Hsu CC. The role of gallium-67 scintigraphy in comparing inflammatory activity between tuberculous and nontuberculous mycobacterial pulmonary diseases. Nucl Med Commun. 2011;32(5):392–401.
59. Amirbekian V, Lipinski MJ, Briley-Saebo KC, Amirbekian S, Aguinaldo JG, Weinreb DB, et al. Detecting and assessing macrophages in vivo to evaluate atherosclerosis noninvasively using molecular MRI. Proc Natl Acad Sci U S A. 2007;104(3):961–6.
60. Perez-Medina C, Tang J, Abdel-Atti D, Hogstad B, Merad M, Fisher EA, et al. PET imaging of tumor-associated macrophages with 89Zr-labeled high-density lipoprotein nanoparticles. J Nucl Med. 2015;56(8):1272–7.
61. Paulos CM, Turk MJ, Breur GJ, Low PS. Folate receptor-mediated targeting of therapeutic and imaging agents to activated macrophages in rheumatoid arthritis. Adv Drug Deliv Rev. 2004;56(8):1205–17.
62. Muller C. Folate based radiopharmaceuticals for imaging and therapy of cancer and inflammation. Curr Pharm Des. 2012;18(8):1058–83.
63. Han W, Zaynagetdinov R, Yull FE, Polosukhin VV, Gleaves LA, Tanjore H, et al. Molecular imaging of folate receptor beta-positive macrophages during acute lung inflammation. Am J Respir Cell Mol Biol. 2015;53(1):50–9.
64. Kelderhouse LE, Mahalingam S, Low PS. Predicting response to therapy for autoimmune and inflammatory diseases using a Folate receptor-

targeted near-infrared fluorescent imaging agent. Mol Imaging Biol. 2016;18(2):201–8.

65. Van De Wiele C, Sathekge M, Maes A. Targeting monocytes and macrophages by means of SPECT and PET. Q J Nucl Med Mol Imaging. 2014;58(3):269–75.
66. Siwowska K, Muller C. Preclinical development of small-molecular-weight folate-based radioconjugates: a pharmacological perspective. Q J Nucl Med Mol Imaging. 2015;59(3):269–86.
67. Weissleder R, Nahrendorf M, Pittet MJ. Imaging macrophages with nanoparticles. Nat Mater. 2014;13(2):125–38.
68. Sharifi S, Seyednejad H, Laurent S, Atyabi F, Saei AA, Mahmoudi M. Superparamagnetic iron oxide nanoparticles for in vivo molecular and cellular imaging. Contrast Media Mol Imaging. 2015;10(5):329–55.
69. Gaglia JL, Harisinghani M, Aganj I, Wojtkiewicz GR, Hedgire S, Benoist C, et al. Noninvasive mapping of pancreatic inflammation in recent-onset type-1 diabetes patients. Proc Natl Acad Sci U S A. 2015;112(7):2139–44.
70. Wu CC. PET imaging of inflammation biomarkers. Theranostics. 2013;3(7):448–66.
71. Ozguven MA, Karacalioglu AO, Ince S, Emer MO. Altered biodistribution of FDG in patients with type-2 diabetes mellitus. Ann Nucl Med. 2014;28(6):505–11.
72. Vos FJ, Kullberg BJ, Sturm PD, Krabbe PF, van Dijk AP, Wanten GJ, et al. Metastatic infectious disease and clinical outcome in Staphylococcus aureus and streptococcus species bacteremia. Medicine (Baltimore). 2012;91(2):86–94.
73. Vos FJ, Bleeker-Rovers CP, Oyen WJ. The use of FDG-PET/CT in patients with febrile neutropenia. Semin Nucl Med. 2013;43(5):340–8.
74. Lee YH, Choi SJ, Ji JD, Song GG. Diagnostic accuracy of 18F-FDG PET or PET/CT for large vessel vasculitis: a meta-analysis. Z Rheumatol. 2015;
75. Rabkin Z, Israel O, Keidar Z. Do hyperglycemia and diabetes affect the incidence of false-negative 18F-FDG PET/CT studies in patients evaluated for infection or inflammation and cancer? A Comparative analysis. J Nucl Med. 2010;51(7):1015–20.
76. Weinstein EA, Ordonez AA, DeMarco VP, Murawski AM, Pokkali S, MacDonald EM, et al. Imaging Enterobacteriaceae infection in vivo with 18F-fluorodeoxysorbitol positron emission tomography. Sci Transl Med. 2014;6(259):259ra146.
77. Gowrishankar G, Namavari M, Jouannot EB, Hoehne A, Reeves R, Hardy J, et al. Investigation of 6-[(1)(8)F]-fluoromaltose as a novel PET tracer for imaging bacterial infection. PLoS One. 2014;9(9):e107951.
78. Shields AF, Grierson JR, Dohmen BM, Machulla HJ, Stayanoff JC, Lawhorn-Crews JM, et al. Imaging proliferation in vivo with [F-18]FLT and positron emission tomography. Nat Med. 1998;4(11):1334–6.
79. Laing RE, Nair-Gill E, Witte ON, Radu CG. Visualizing cancer and immune cell function with metabolic positron emission tomography. Curr Opin Genet Dev. 2010;20(1):100–5.
80. Bollineni VR, Kramer GM, Jansma EP, Liu Y, Oyen WJ. A systematic review on [(18)F]FLT-PET uptake as a measure of treatment response in cancer patients. Eur J Cancer. 2016;55:81–97.
81. Bading James RJ. Imaging of cell proliferation: status and prospects. J Nucl Med. 49.
82. Schoder H, Zelenetz A, Hamlin P, Gavane S, Horwitz S, Matasar M, et al. Prospective study of FLT PET for early interim response assessment in advanced stage B-cell lymphoma. J Nucl Med. 2015;
83. Lee H, Kim SK, Kim YI, Kim TS, Kang SH, Park WS, et al. Early determination of prognosis by interim 3′-deoxy-3′-18F-fluorothymidine PET in patients with non-Hodgkin lymphoma. J Nucl Med. 2014;55(2):216–22.
84. Aarntzen EH, Srinivas M, De Wilt JH, Jacobs JF, Lesterhuis WJ, Windhorst AD, et al. Early identification of antigen-specific immune responses in vivo by [18F]-labeled 3′-fluoro-3′-deoxy-thymidine ([18F]FLT) PET imaging. Proc Natl Acad Sci U S A. 2011;108(45):18396–9.
85. Troost EG, Vogel WV, Merkx MA, Slootweg PJ, Marres HA, Peeters WJ, et al. 18F-FLT PET does not discriminate between reactive and metastatic lymph nodes in primary head and neck cancer patients. J Nucl Med. 2007;48(5):726–35.
86. Radu Caius GC. Molecular imaging of lymphoid organs and immune activation by positron emission tomography with a new [18F]-labeled 2′-deoxycytidine analog. Nat Med. 14(7):783–8.
87. Brewer S, Nair-Gill E, Wei B, Chen L, Li X, Riedinger M, Campbell DO, Wiltzius S, Satyamurthy N, Phelps ME, Radu C, Witte ON, Braun J. Uptake of [18F]1-(2′-deoxy-2′-arabinofuranosyl) cytosine indicates intestinal inflammation in mice. Gastroenterology. 2010;138(4):1266–75.
88. Nair-Gill E, Wiltzius SM, Wei XX, Cheng D, Riedinger M, Radu CG, et al. PET probes for distinct metabolic pathways have different cell specificities during immune responses in mice. J Clin Invest. 2010;120(6):2005–15.
89. Matter CM, Wyss MT, Meier P, Spath N, von Lukowicz T, Lohmann C, et al. 18F-choline images murine atherosclerotic plaques ex vivo. Arterioscler Thromb Vasc Biol. 2006;26(3):584–9.
90. Laitinen IE, Luoto P, Nagren K, Marjamaki PM, Silvola JM, Hellberg S, et al. Uptake of 11C-choline in mouse atherosclerotic plaques. J Nucl Med. 2010;51(5):798–802.
91. Le C, van de Weijer EP, Pos FJ, Vogel WV. Active inflammation in 18F-methylcholine PET/CT. Eur J Nucl Med Mol Imaging. 2010;37(3):654–5.
92. Huang TT. A comparative uptake study of multiplexed PET tracers in mice with turpentine-induced inflammation. Molecules. 2012;17(12):13948–59.
93. van Waarde Aren A. Proliferation markers for the differential diagnosis of tumor and inflammation. Curr Pharm Des. 2008;14(31):3326–39.
94. Tsuyuguchi Naohiro N. Evaluation of treatment effects in brain abscess with positron emission tomography:

comparison of fluorine-18-fluorodeoxyglucose and carbon-11-methionine. Ann Nucl Med. 17(1):47–51.
95. Kanagawa Masaru M. Comparison of trans-1-amino-3-[18F]fluorocyclobutanecarboxylic acid (anti-[18F]FACBC) accumulation in lymph node prostate cancer metastasis and lymphadenitis in rats. Nucl Med Biol. 41(7):545–51.
96. Oka Shuntaro S. Differences in transport mechanisms of trans-1-amino-3-[18F]fluorocyclobutanecarboxylic acid in inflammation, prostate cancer, and glioma cells: comparison with L-[methyl-11C] methionine and 2-deoxy-2-[18F]fluoro-D-glucose. Mol Imag Biol. 16(3):322–9.
97. Qu W, Oya S, Lieberman BP, Ploessl K, Wang L, Wise DR, et al. Preparation and characterization of L-[5-11C]-glutamine for metabolic imaging of tumors. J Nucl Med. 2012;53(1):98–105.
98. Qu W, Zha Z, Lieberman BP, Mancuso A, Stetz M, Rizzi R, et al. Facile synthesis [5-(13)C-4-(2)H(2)]-L-glutamine for hyperpolarized MRS imaging of cancer cell metabolism. Acad Radiol. 2011;18(8):932–9.
99. Kielland A, Blom T, Nandakumar KS, Holmdahl R, Blomhoff R, Carlsen H. In vivo imaging of reactive oxygen and nitrogen species in inflammation using the luminescent probe L-012. Free Radic Biol Med. 2009;47(6):760–6.
100. Imada I, Sato EF, Miyamoto M, Ichimori Y, Minamiyama Y, Konaka R, et al. Analysis of reactive oxygen species generated by neutrophils using a chemiluminescence probe L-012. Anal Biochem. 1999;271(1):53–8.
101. Daiber A, August M, Baldus S, Wendt M, Oelze M, Sydow K, et al. Measurement of NAD(P)H oxidase-derived superoxide with the luminol analogue L-012. Free Radic Biol Med. 2004;36(1):101–11.
102. Breckwoldt Michael OM. Tracking the inflammatory response in stroke in vivo by sensing the enzyme myeloperoxidase. Proc Natl Acad Sci. 2008;105(47):18584–9.
103. McCarthy TJ, Sheriff AU, Graneto MJ, Talley JJ, Welch MJ. Radiosynthesis, in vitro validation, and in vivo evaluation of 18F-labeled COX-1 and COX-2 inhibitors. J Nucl Med. 2002;43(1):117–24.
104. de Vries EF, Doorduin J, Dierckx RA, van Waarde A. Evaluation of [(11)C]rofecoxib as PET tracer for cyclooxygenase 2 overexpression in rat models of inflammation. Nucl Med Biol. 2008;35(1):35–42.
105. Gao M, Wang M, Miller KD, Zheng QH. Synthesis and preliminary in vitro biological evaluation of new carbon-11-labeled celecoxib derivatives as candidate PET tracers for imaging of COX-2 expression in cancer. Eur J Med Chem. 2011;46(9):4760–7.
106. Kossodo S, Zhang J, Groves K, Cuneo GJ, Handy E, Morin J, et al. Noninvasive in vivo quantification of neutrophil elastase activity in acute experimental mouse lung injury. Int J Mol Imaging. 2011;2011:581406.
107. Chen J, Tung CH, Allport JR, Chen S, Weissleder R, Huang PL. Near-infrared fluorescent imaging of matrix metalloproteinase activity after myocardial infarction. Circulation. 2005;111(14):1800–5.
108. van der Graaf Marinette M. In vivo magnetic resonance spectroscopy: basic methodology and clinical applications. Eur Biophys J. 39(4):527–40.
109. Kang JJ. Application of metabolomics in autoimmune diseases: insight into biomarkers and pathology. J Neuroimmunol. 2015;279:25–32.
110. Kidd BA, Wroblewska A, Boland MR, Agudo J, Merad M, Tatonetti NP, et al. Mapping the effects of drugs on the immune system. Nat Biotechnol. 2016;34(1):47–54.
111. Burel JG, Apte SH, Doolan DL. Systems approaches towards molecular profiling of human immunity. Trends Immunol. 2016;37(1):53–67.
112. Jha AK, Huang SC, Sergushichev A, Lampropoulou V, Ivanova Y, Loginicheva E, et al. Network integration of parallel metabolic and transcriptional data reveals metabolic modules that regulate macrophage polarization. Immunity. 2015;42(3):419–30.
113. Xue J, Schmidt SV, Sander J, Draffehn A, Krebs W, Quester I, et al. Transcriptome-based network analysis reveals a spectrum model of human macrophage activation. Immunity. 2014;40(2):274–88.
114. Aerts HJ, Velazquez ER, Leijenaar RT, Parmar C, Grossmann P, Carvalho S, et al. Decoding tumour phenotype by noninvasive imaging using a quantitative radiomics approach. Nat Commun. 2014;5:4006.
115. Gillies RJ, Kinahan PE, Hricak H. Radiomics: images are more than pictures. They Are Data Radiology. 2016;278(2):563–77.
116. Lambin P, Rios-Velazquez E, Leijenaar R, Carvalho S, van Stiphout RG, Granton P, et al. Radiomics: extracting more information from medical images using advanced feature analysis. Eur J Cancer. 2012;48(4):441–6.
117. Mantovani A, Vecchi A, Allavena P. Pharmacological modulation of monocytes and macrophages. Curr Opin Pharmacol. 2014;17:38–44.
118. O'Sullivan D, Pearce EL. Targeting T cell metabolism for therapy. Trends Immunol. 2015;36(2):71–80.
119. Colombo Serra S, Karlsson M, Giovenzana GB, Cavallotti C, Tedoldi F, Aime S. Hyperpolarized (13) C-labelled anhydrides as DNP precursors of metabolic MRI agents. Contrast Media Mol Imaging. 2012;7(5):469–77.
120. Viale A, Reineri F, Dastru W, Aime S. Hyperpolarized (13)C-pyruvate magnetic resonance imaging in cancer diagnostics. Expert Opin Med Diagn. 2012;6(4):335–45.
121. Glaudemans Andor WJMA. Pitfalls and limitations of radionuclide and hybrid imaging in infection and inflammation. Semin Nucl Med. 2015;45(6):500–12.
122. Divine MR, Katiyar P, Kohlhofer U, Quintanilla-Martinez L, Pichler BJ, Disselhorst JA. A population-based Gaussian mixture model incorporating 18F-FDG PET and diffusion-weighted MRI quantifies tumor tissue classes. J Nucl Med. 2016;57(3):473–9.

Imaging in Diabetes

8

Liang Zhang and Greg M. Thurber

8.1 Introduction

Diabetes refers to a group of metabolic disorders where insulin insensitivity and/or a lack of insulin production results in elevated blood glucose levels. These broadly include type 1 diabetes (previously known as "juvenile-onset" diabetes), type 2 diabetes (previously "adult onset"), and additional less prevalent variants (e.g., monogenic diabetes). Unregulated blood glucose levels have a negative impact on multiple organ systems and consequently pose a risk for stroke, heart disease, kidney failure, blindness, high blood pressure, and other chronic conditions that impair the quality of life. Currently, there are over 400 million cases of diabetes worldwide and the rate continues to rise [1]. Patients with diabetes must rely on medications and lifestyle changes to maintain glucose homeostasis. Aside from the morbidity, the financial burden of the disease constitutes approximately 10% of all healthcare costs in developed countries [2]. No cure currently exists and present strategies to prevent disease complications place a significant strain on healthcare systems. Therefore, it is important to understand the disease pathophysiology for the medical community and patients. The ability to image and follow disease progression would play a crucial role in understanding disease etiology and allow accurate monitoring during clinical trials for potential clinical translation of treatments. Ultimately, improved treatments, transplants, and understanding of basic and clinical pathophysiology of the disease may lead to a permanent cure.

8.1.1 Physiology of the Pancreas/Islets

Despite the multi-organ involvement of the disease, the pancreas is a critical organ due to its central role in regulating blood sugar levels and metabolism. Located behind the stomach in humans, the pancreas is part of both the endocrine and digestive systems. Macroscopically, it consists of three regions—the head, body, and tail (Fig. 8.1a). Distinct tissues within the organ carry out the functions for each organ system. The exocrine pancreas primarily serves the digestive system and forms ~99% of the organ mass [2]. It is formed by acini, with each acinus consisting of secretory epithelial cells. The lumen at the center of each layer mediates the drainage of cellular secretions into a series of connected ducts. The ducts join to form the pancreatic

L. Zhang
Department of Chemical Engineering, University of Michigan, Ann Arbor, MI 48109, USA
e-mail: liangzha@umich.edu

G.M. Thurber (✉)
Department of Chemical Engineering, University of Michigan, Ann Arbor, MI 48109, USA

Department of Biomedical Engineering, University of Michigan, 2800 Plymouth Rd, Ann Arbor, MI 48109, USA
e-mail: gthurber@umich.edu

J.S. Lewis, K.R. Keshari (eds.), *Imaging and Metabolism*, DOI 10.1007/978-3-319-61401-4_8

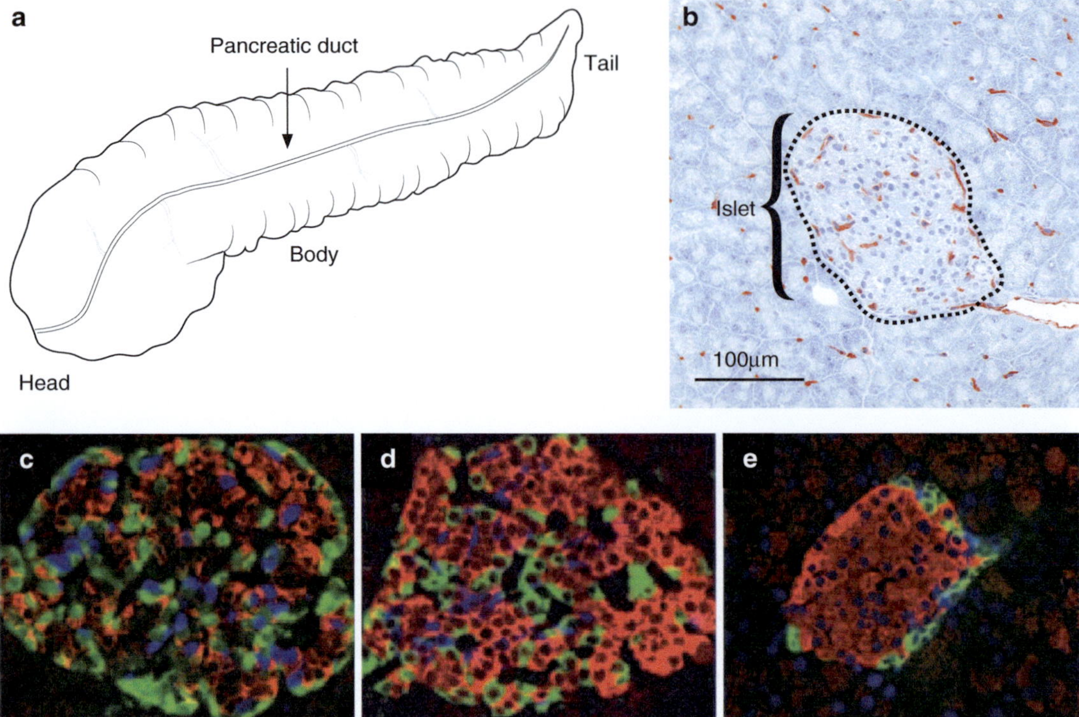

Fig. 8.1 Structure of the pancreas. (**a**) Schematic of the pancreas with head, body, and tail portions labeled. The pancreatic duct runs along the organ and empties into the duodenum (not shown). (**b**) Histology slide of a mouse islet with the blood vessels (CD31) stained in brown (hematoxylin counterstain). Adapted from Keliher et al., 2012. Notice the extensive vessels on the islet surface and within. A human (**c**), monkey (**d**), and mouse (**e**) islet of Langerhans stained for beta cells (insulin, *red*), alpha cells (glucagon, *green*), and delta cells (somatostatin, *blue*). The proportion of beta cells in humans is lower (~60%) than mice (~80%). Adapted from Cabrera et al., *Proc. Natl Acad. Sci.* USA 103 (7), 2334-2339; © (2006) National Academy of Sciences USA

duct, which empties into the duodenum. These secretions aid in digestion and include enzymes such as trypsin, chymotrypsin, elastase, ribonuclease, amylase, lipase, and others. The endocrine pancreas forms approximately 1% of the pancreas mass and carries out several functions through multiple distinct cell types. These functions include the secretion of insulin, glucagon, somatostatin, peptide YY, neuropeptide Y, and pancreatic polypeptide (PP) directly into the blood for tight glucose regulation (endocrine function). Although the pancreas is mostly exocrine tissue by mass, the organ's role in diabetes research is closely associated with the functionality of endocrine pancreas.

The endocrine pancreas is comprised of distinct microstructures known as islets of Langerhans. These individual clusters of cells range from 40–300 microns in diameter and account for 1–2% of pancreatic tissue (varying between species), although they receive 10–20% of arterial flow, a disproportionately higher amount compared to exocrine tissue [3]. They also have a higher density of vessels, with surface area measurements of 505 cm^2/cm^3 for the islets versus 182 cm^2/cm^3 for the exocrine tissue [4, 5] (Fig. 8.1b). Cell types within each islet include alpha, beta, delta, and PP cells with differences in cytoarchitecture across species (Fig. 8.1c–e). These cells secrete glucagon (alpha cells), insulin (beta cells), somatostatin (delta cells), and pancreatic polypeptide (PP) with beta cells responsible for the central role of secreting insulin and lowering blood glucose. Although the ratios of different cell types vary between the head, body, and tail of the pancreas, the beta cells are the most prevalent cell type (70–80% in mice) with the remaining fraction comprised of alpha, delta, and PP cells [6]. Incretins form another signaling axis in the regulation of metabolism. These peptides are secreted by the epithelial cells in the intestines and induce beta cell production of insulin. Two common incretin peptides include glucagon-like peptide-1 (GLP-1) and gastric inhibitory peptide (GIP).

8.1.2 Disease Background

The most common types of diabetes are type 1 diabetes mellitus and type 2 diabetes mellitus. Type 1 diabetes is an autoimmune disorder characterized by T-cell destruction of the insulin-producing beta cells in the pancreas. The drastic reduction in beta cell functionality results in hyperglycemia and requires patients to depend on lifelong insulin treatments to lower blood glucose levels for survival. Because the destruction occurs in adolescents and the early stages are largely asymptomatic, there is much to learn about disease progression. Though disease etiology is complex and the pathogenesis poorly understood, the examination of patient islet tissue from biopsies reveals the presence of insulitis in most patients (>50%). Much of this knowledge relies on histopathology from the 1960s, and there is limited availability from prediabetic patients due to the difficulty of obtaining samples from individuals at risk to develop the disease [7]. From these early studies and more recent data, disease progression is divided into two phases, the initial occult phase followed by overt diabetes. The occult phase, marked by insulitis, involves the aggressive infiltration of leukocytes (Fig. 8.2). The transition to overt diabetes occurs once the majority of beta cells (60–80%) are destroyed and the remaining beta cell mass can no longer adequately control blood sugar levels. Healthy fasting blood glucose levels should be less than 100 mg/dL, and levels between 100 and 125 mg/dL are considered prediabetes, while levels over 125 mg/dL indicate diabetes.

The much more prevalent type 2 diabetes is reaching epidemic levels given the worldwide increase in obesity [8]. Accounting for 90–95% of all cases, type 2 diabetes is a complex heterogeneous metabolic disorder responsible for simultaneous dysfunctions in multiple organs. Disease etiology is complex with physical inactivity and genetic predisposition as the two critical causes for disease onset [9]. Onset of hyperglycemia is caused by multiple defects in glucose homeostasis including increased liver glucose production, decreased insulin secretion in islets, and insulin insensitivity. Although screening and diagnosis of the disease is readily available and established, no cure currently exists. The majority of cases can be prevented by lifestyle changes such as routine exercise and dietary modifications, but most patients will eventually require medication. Numerous effective and FDA-approved medications exist to alleviate symptoms, and research into new agents continues. Metformin is an oral pill often used as first-line therapy to lower hepatic glucose production. Sulfonylureas can be used to increase insulin secretion, and glitazones are insulin sensitizers. Glucagon-like peptide-1 (GLP-1) agonists (e.g., exenatide, liraglutide, dulaglutide) are incretin mimetics that can control blood sugar and promote weight loss. These agents must be injected, but research into slower clearing agents has reduced the frequency of dosing. Oral formulations of these peptides are actively being researched. Rather than supplying exogenous incretins, DPP-4 inhibitors, such as sitagliptin and saxagliptin, slow the degradation rate of GLP-1. They have the advantage of oral administration but do not promote weight loss. The newest class of diabetes drugs is sodium-glucose co-transporter 2 (SGLT-2) inhibitors. Glucose is readily filtered from the blood by the kidneys, but these transporters facilitate reabsorption to avoid loss of glucose in the urine. By inhibiting this transporter, blood glucose levels are reduced. These agents promote modest weight loss without a risk of low blood sugar, but the most common side effects include vaginal yeast and urinary tract infections. Finally, in some cases exogenous insulin is indicated [10].

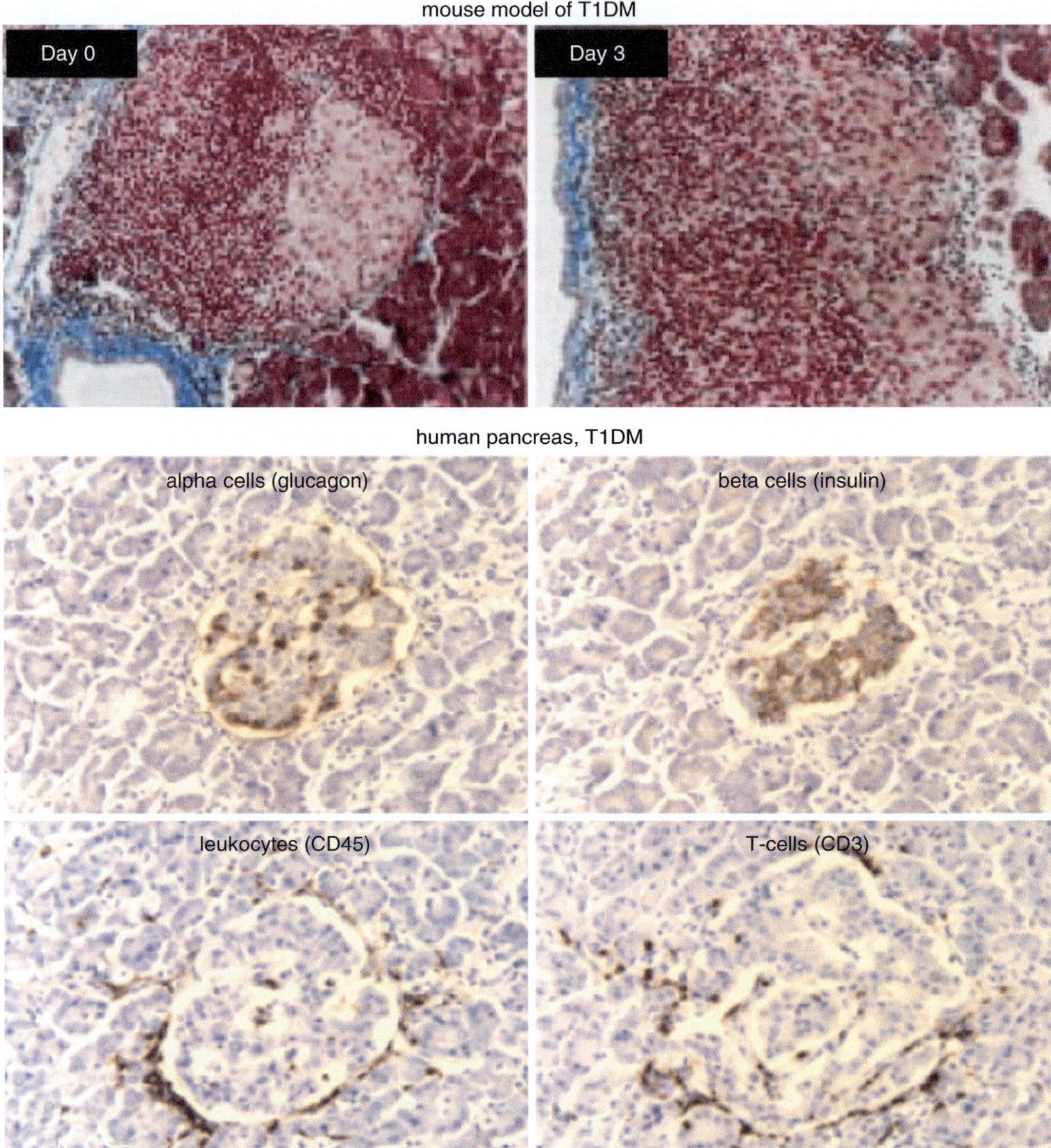

Fig. 8.2 *Top panel*: induced mouse model of type 1 diabetes. Cyclophosphamide is used to synchronize the transition from the insulitis stage (*left*) to the diabetes (*right*). Adapted from Schmutz et al., 1999. Representative samples from day 0 and 3 indicate beta cell death. Bottom panel: immunostaining indicates lymphocyte infiltration of endocrine islet in a patient with type 1 diabetes. Adapted from Willcox et al., 2009

8.1.3 Role of Imaging in Diabetes

Attempts to cure diabetes have primarily focused on restoring or preserving beta cell function within the pancreas. This has proven challenging as no clinical procedure currently exists to quantify the beta cell mass (BCM) noninvasively in patients. Instead, biochemical tests using blood samples are used to estimate beta cell mass functionality, but these methods are insensitive to the early phase of the disease when the pancreas has excess capacity to control blood sugar levels [11].

An imaging technique with the resolution and sensitivity to quantify the BCM would greatly benefit the diabetes community but has so far remained out of reach. For type 2 diabetes, understanding the role that BCM plays in the disease could open up new avenues for treatment. Imaging could play an even more significant role in type 1 diabetes by increasing insight into the early stages of immune attack and monitoring immunomodulatory therapy, transplant, and other treatment strategies. Accurately quantifying the beta cell mass during clinical trials would provide invaluable information on disease etiology and treatment efficacy, but the low fraction of beta cells in the pancreas is challenging to monitor.

Particularly for type 1 diabetes, extensive research has been conducted on islet transplantation, since this treatment has the potential for curative results. One of the most successful and well-studied methods is the Edmonton Protocol where islets from multiple donors are infused in the portal vein of the liver [12]. To date, long-term cures from transplantation are rare [13] due to several causes. The transplanted islets are susceptible to the same type of immune rejection as any organ transplant (and patients must maintain lifelong immunosuppressive therapy) and must also counter the autoimmune attack responsible for the initial loss of the islets. Additionally, the microvasculature must connect with the islets, since many are beyond the size where oxygen can efficiently diffuse from the surface to cells in the center [14]. Finally, the local microenvironment in the transplant site may impact long-term efficacy [6]. The ability to track transplanted islets would improve transplantation technique and postsurgical monitoring [15].

8.2 Imaging Modalities in Diabetes

A significant effort has been placed on developing imaging agents for the pancreas due to its central role in diabetes. The focus of this chapter is primarily on methods to quantify the BCM given the importance in diagnosis and treatment monitoring of type 1 diabetes and potential implications in type 2 diabetes. However, several studies and reviews of molecular and metabolic imaging strategies for tissues outside of the pancreas are also presented to show the breadth of imaging applications in these diseases.

Detecting changes in BCM and early stages of the immune attack in vivo hold high clinical relevance, but no current combination of imaging agent and modality is ideal (Table 8.1). At present, several imaging modalities are used in diabetes research each with their complementary strengths and weaknesses. These include magnetic

Table 8.1 Imaging modalities used in diabetes

Modality	Applications	Targets (examples and notes)	Pros/cons
MRI	Islet transplantation, insulitis	Inflammatory cells (nanoparticle uptake)	No ionizing radiation (safe), high resolution, limited molecular probe sensitivity (e.g., hyperpolarized probes only)
PET	BCM quantification, insulitis, islet transplantation	GLP-1R, VMAT2	Highest sensitivity (pM), limited spatial resolution
SPECT	BCM quantification, insulitis, islet transplantation	GLP-1R, VMAT2	High sensitivity (pM), limited spatial resolution
Fluorescence	Probe design, animal model imaging	GLP-1R (nM sensitivity), antibody probes	Highest resolution, convenient for in vitro work, poor translatability
US	Organ volume	Microbubbles (no current diabetes applications)	Inexpensive, no ionizing radiation (safe), limited contrast
CT	Organ volume, whole-pancreas transplantation	mM sensitivity (no current diabetes applications)	High resolution, limited contrast, ionizing radiation

resonance imaging (MRI), positron emission tomography (PET), single photon emission computed tomography (SPECT), fluorescence imaging, bioluminescence imaging, ultrasound (US), and X-ray computed tomography (CT). With the exception of bioluminescence, the remaining modalities have seen or have potential for clinical translation (albeit limited for fluorescence). Trade-offs such as spatial resolution, specificity, and the use or lack of non-ionizing radiation are considered in the following sections. Although it is a valuable research tool, bioluminescent techniques will not be discussed due to low imaging depth and difficulty of clinical translation. Each of the above imaging modalities will be described in turn, but, first, some of the unique considerations when imaging the endocrine pancreas, particularly for molecular imaging of beta cells in type 1 diabetes, will be discussed to provide context for the reported studies.

8.3 Imaging Limitations and Design Considerations for Pancreatic Imaging

Quantitative analysis of molecular imaging of islets reveals several challenges to BCM quantification [16]. The two biggest obstacles are the small size of individual islets (40–300 μm) and the incredibly low volume fraction of islets in the pancreas. The small islet size relative to the resolution of current imaging modalities results in significant partial volume effects. Because an islet only occupies a fraction of a voxel in an image, any contrast, be it intrinsic or from exogenous imaging agents, is "diluted" over the entire voxel volume. Voxel dimensions for PET and SPECT imaging are on the order of 1 cm^3 under ideal imaging conditions, which can be difficult to replicate in a clinical setting. Recent literature indicates that quantification of radiotracers in structures lower than 3 cm in diameter will be subject to such partial volume effects and will require correction factors for accurate quantification [17]. Voxel sizes for US, CT, and MRI are smaller (~1 mm^3), but these modalities suffer from a much lower sensitivity for exogenous contrast agents and are still well above the size of individual islets. Optical imaging has both high resolution and adequate sensitivity, but the lower depth of imaging limits this to invasive procedures [18].

The partial volume effects alone would not be a problem if the volume fraction were relatively large. For example, if islets occupied 50% of the tissue volume, this would only lower the measured contrast ~two-fold. Although islet volume fractions vary between species and disease states, and the low absolute value and distribution of islets in the pancreas can make it challenging to estimate [19–21], most measurements indicate 1–2% of the total pancreas mass is occupied by islets. This results in a 50- to 100-fold reduction in islet contrast due to the partial volume effect, which places severe limitations on probe selection and design.

Given the small size and low volume fraction discussed above, the intrinsic contrast between islets and the surrounding exocrine pancreas is insufficient for beta cell mass measurements using US, MRI, or CT. Therefore, exogenous contrast agents have been used to monitor various aspects of diabetes, particularly type 1. These can be divided into targeted and nontargeted exogenous contrast agents.

The type of contrast agent is generally dictated by the sensitivity of the imaging modality. For molecular contrast, meaning a specific binding interaction between the contrast agent and a target, the sensitivity must be high. Some of the most highly expressed disease-related targets, such as cell surface receptors overexpressed on cancer cells, have ~ 1 million receptors per cell [22]. Using a cell density of 5×10^8 cells/mL, if the targeting has no method for amplification (e.g., continuous internalization and recycling, a catalytic mechanism to trap probe, etc.), the maximum concentration of target would be ~800 nM. Even if a highly expressed target was completely saturated, this is far from the millimolar concentrations needed for CT contrast agents and well below the micromolar concentrations typically needed for MRI contrast. This also does not account for partial volume effects. Microbubbles are available for US contrast, but targeting is limited to blood vessels. This leaves PET, SPECT (both with picomolar sensitivity), and fluorescence (nanomolar sensitivity) for targeted molecular imaging. Nontargeted exogenous contrast agents in MRI, US, and CT must rely on changes in local physiology such as blood flow (small molecule contrast agents) or blood volume/permeability (for macromolecular contrast agents) [23]. An important exception is iron oxide nanoparticles for MRI contrast. These nanoparticles can be detected at lower concentrations than the common chelated gadolinium MRI contrast agents. Nanoparticles extravasate in areas of increased vascular permeability and are taken up by local macrophages, particularly in inflammatory environments. Efforts to target nanoparticles to specific receptors, however, have generally not worked due to poor washout of the nanoparticles from tissue (resulting in the enhanced permeation and retention, EPR, effect) [24]. Therefore, they target specific cells but not through the typical molecular binding of most targeted contrast agents.

Focusing on molecular imaging agents, which can be designed to provide signal specifically from the islets, PET, SPECT, and fluorescence are three modalities that have the necessary sensitivity. Despite this sensitivity, the selectivity for islets is challenging given their small volume fraction. Sweet et al. analyzed the targeting requirements for such a probe with estimates on the required selectivity and affinity that highlight the formidable challenges in probe development. In addition to the low volume fraction and partial volume effects, they also considered the challenge of measuring a loss in signal over time before the critical functional islet mass threshold is reached and a patient exhibits overt diabetes. For imaging probes that can reach intracellular targets, the probes must be 1000-fold more specific for beta cells than exocrine cells. Even cell surface targeting probes that completely lack binding to exocrine cells require extremely high affinity and rapid clearance to lower the signal from the extracellular space [16]. Despite these stringent requirements, there are probes that are close to meeting these criteria, although further work is required. For two of the probes, vesicular monoamine transporter 2 (VMAT2)- and glucagon-like peptide-1 (GLP-1) receptor-targeted agents, discussion on the presence of receptor expression in the exocrine pancreas is particularly salient in light of these strict requirements. Overall, an effective clinical agent will require a combination of a high expressing target, a high-fidelity probe with strong binding affinity, little to no interactions/uptake in off-target exocrine tissue, and fast systemic clearance.

In spite of the challenges, progress has been made in using several modalities to image various aspects of diabetes.

8.3.1 MRI

MRI offers relatively high spatial resolution in a noninvasive manner free from ionizing radiation. Many clinical instruments are capable of imaging with voxel dimensions of 1 mm × 1 mm × 1 mm, but submillimeter resolution is possible with higher field strengths [18]. High soft tissue contrast and potential for use with imaging probes make this a useful tool in diabetes imaging. The modality also allows for prolonged visualization of the region of interest compared to radionuclides. To date, MRI has been used to image transplanted islets as well as to study insulitis in animal models. The high resolution and lack of ionizing radiation makes MRI an attractive option for diabetes imaging, particularly in pediatric populations, but the inability to distinguish between exocrine and endocrine pancreas without contrast agents limits the modality to particles reacted ex vivo such as islet transplantation, particles taken up in vivo for imaging insulitis, and gadolinium contrast agents to measure changes in tissue physiology in the clinic.

There are multiple studies using MRI to study the efficacy of islet transplantation as a means of replacing the BCM for patients with type 1 diabetes. During islet transplantation surgery, significant cellular losses may occur due to multiple reasons including autoimmune rejection, mechanical stress on the cells, glucose toxicity, and damage incurred within the islets such as microvascular damage during the isolation process [6]. To study ways of minimizing islet failure during transplantation, cells are first labeled with a contrast agent prior to surgery. In mouse models, Turvey and colleagues were able to purify islets, load the cells with superparamagnetic iron oxide (SPIO) nanoparticles, and then visualize the particles in diabetic and healthy mice on T2-weighted MR images [25]. Distinguishing between functional and nonfunctional islets proved challenging although further studies by Kriz et al. suggested it may be possible to detect decreases in islet mass [26].

Insulitis is marked by multiple microvascular changes including increases in vessel permeability to small molecules, volumetric flow rate of blood to endocrine tissue, and the islet vascular volume [6]. These changes can be readily investigated using MRI contrast agents. Medarova et al. were able to detect vascular changes using a streptozotocin-induced mouse model of type 1 diabetes [27]. T1-weighted MR images revealed increased accumulation of the gadolinium-based contrast agent compared to healthy mice. Another example includes MR imaging using $CD8^+$ lymphocytes, where cells first internalize dextran-coated SPIO nanoparticles in vitro, resulting in intracellular accumulation. The readministered cells were used to track the immune response in animal models of type 1 diabetes using NOD mice and detected decreases in the parenchymal pancreas in NOD mice when compared to control animals [28, 29].

Gaglia et al. were able to visualize islet inflammation caused by microvascular changes through MR imaging of dextran-coated magnetic nanoparticles (MNP) taken up by monocytes/macrophages in the clinic [30, 31]. An earlier study using ferumoxtran as a negative T2 contrast agent was able to elucidate differences in delta T2 between patients with type 1 diabetes and healthy controls. The change in T2 signal is associated with macrophage uptake of the MNPs. Heterogeneity in MNP accumulation was also detected, and these heterogeneities are supported from past pancreatic histology from cadavers. A more extensive study using FDA-approved ferumoxytol and imaging advances such as higher field strength, optimized pulse sequences, and improved visualization tools measured increased levels of pancreatic inflammation in patients with type 1 diabetes and detected pronounced heterogeneities in pancreatic tissue (Fig. 8.3).

8.3.2 PET/SPECT

Significant progress has been made toward a noninvasive monitoring technique using targeted nuclear probes. PET and SPECT are modalities that offer some of the highest sensitivity (picomolar detection) with trade-offs in resolution compared to CT and MRI. Recent efforts to pair PET and SPECT with CT or MRI have helped address this shortcoming by overlaying a high-resolution anatomical image with the molecular PET/SPECT data. PET has a higher sensitivity than SPECT due to the coincidence detection rather than using a less efficient collimator for image formation. However, PET isotopes can be challenging to synthesize, and many have short decay half-lives. The high sensitivity of these nuclear imaging techniques allows for multiple approaches in diabetes research including the use of radiolabeled ligands to target beta cells specifically for BCM quantification and imaging insulitis to understand disease histopathology.

8.3.2.1 Targeted Molecular Imaging

Targeting cell receptors provides a robust method for labeling abnormal cells as well as monitoring disease progression and evaluating therapeutic response. A detectable label, which is typically chemically conjugated to the targeting moiety, allows researchers to track the targeting ligand in the tissue of interest. Two of the most promising biomarkers for targeted molecular imaging include vesicular monoamine transporter 2 (VMAT2) and glucagon-like peptide-1 receptor (GLP-1R) [2]. Neither ligand is perfect, and the search for alternative imaging probes continues [32, 33]. However, both of these targets and associated imaging agents (dihydrotetrabenazine (DTBZ) and exendin derivatives, respectively) have demonstrated potential in proof-of-principle

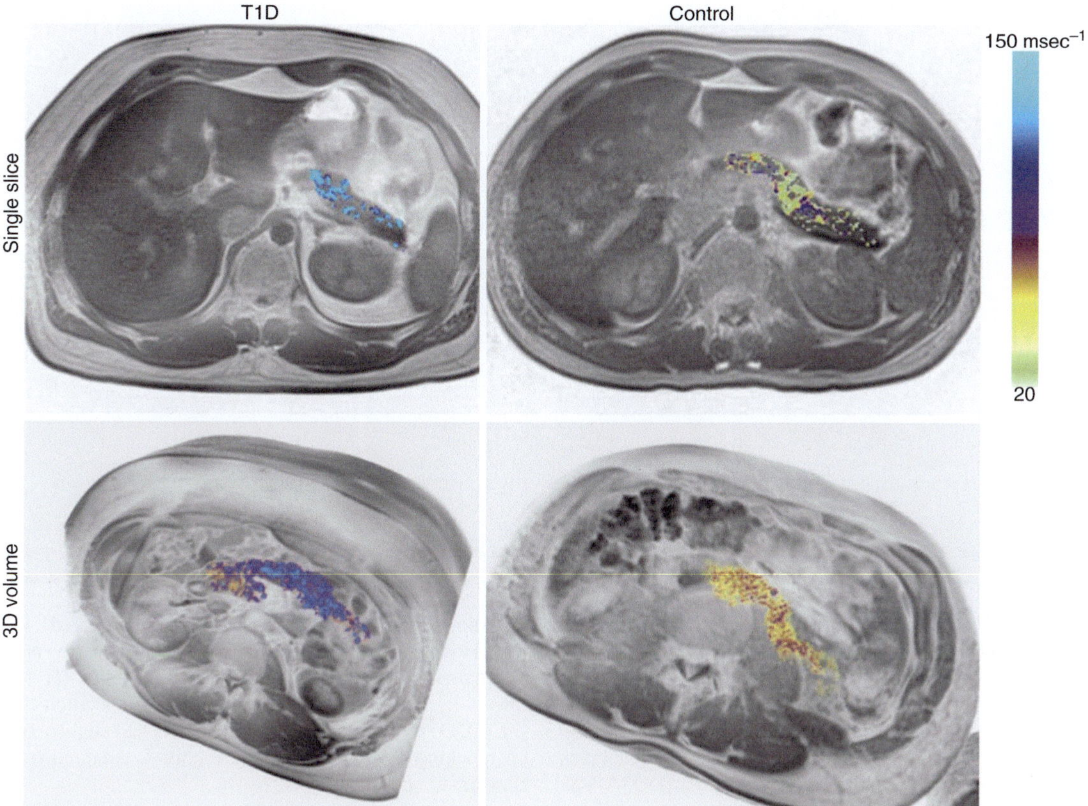

Fig. 8.3 MRI imaging of insulitis. The iron replacement therapy agent ferumoxytol accumulates in macrophages. The increase in $\Delta R2^*$ is higher in the pancreas of recent-onset type 1 diabetic patients (*left*) than the controls (*right*), shown for a slice (*top*) or 3D reconstruction (*bottom*). The data indicate heterogeneous nanoparticle distribution, consistent with insulitis models in animal models. Adapted from Gaglia et al., 2015

studies in the clinic and will be discussed in more detail. Antibody-targeted imaging and metabolic tracers are also mentioned as alternatives.

Vesicular monoamine transporters regulate the uptake of cytoplasmic monoamines to the secretory granules in neuroendocrine cells. Although VMAT2 was first used in the 1990s as a target for PET brain imaging in Parkinson's disease, more recent immunohistochemical staining revealed VMAT2 expression in the islets of Langerhans, making it an attractive target for beta cell imaging as well (Fig. 8.4). DTBZ is a strong binder for VMAT2, with subnanomolar K_d values and greater than 10,000-fold selectivity over VMAT1 (also expressed in the endocrine pancreas), and holds promise given that DTBZ is a clinically approved PET tracer. [^{11}C]-DTBZ has been traditionally used for neural imaging of VMAT2 with high specificity, and Freeby et al. were able to estimate rat BCM in models of spontaneous type 1 diabetes using this probe [34]. The probe also detected decreases in BCM in STZ-induced diabetic rats, although accumulation was not detectable in baboons. Variable expression across species makes interpretation challenging, and rodent studies may show the targeting of pancreatic nerve tissue rather than islets themselves [35].

The short half-life of C-11 (20 min) can lead to some challenges, so researchers have created F-18 derivatives (110 min half-life) with high affinity [36]. In vivo imaging of pancreatic BCM in type 1 diabetic patients compared to healthy controls with these agents has yielded promising results, but challenges remain. Using the VMAT2 radiotracer [^{18}F]-fluoropropyl-dihydrotetrabenazine (^{18}F-FP-(+)-DTBZ), Normandin et al. and Freeby et al. have

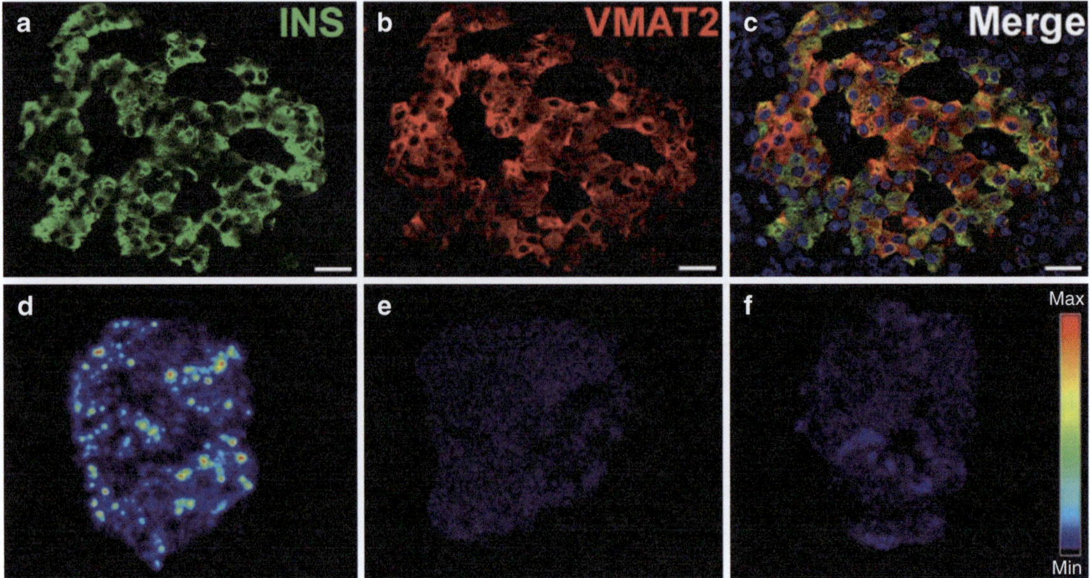

Fig. 8.4 VMAT2 and GLP-1R-targeted PET agents. Immunofluorescent staining of a healthy human islet; insulin (**a**), VMAT2 (**b**), and DAPI (*blue*, **c**). Merged image indicates most insulin-expressing cells also express VMAT2 (**c**). Scale bars are 30 um, adapted from Saisho et al., 2008. Ex vivo autoradiography of whole pancreas sections from healthy rats injected with [^{64}Cu]DO3A-VS-exendin-4. Punctate spots are islets of Langerhans (**d**). Rat with blocking injection of cold exendin-4 (**e**) and the non-internalizing antagonist exendin-(9-39) amide (**f**) followed by radiolabeled exendin indicate specificity of [^{64}Cu]DO3A-VS-exendin-4 for beta cells and slightly better blocking with internalizing exendin-4. Adapted from Bandara et al., 2015

measured significant differences in pancreatic standardized uptake and binding potential in healthy volunteers and patients [37, 38]. Higher-than-expected uptake of the radiotracer was measured in the body and tail of patient pancreata despite the near-complete loss of functionality. Nonspecific uptake of the radiotracer and possible exocrine expression of VMAT2 are possible explanations for the higher signal, although estimates for exocrine expression by Freeby et al. suggest a low contribution to overall measurements (<10%). Nonspecific contributions were estimated using the negative enantiomer and showed that uptake in pancreata accounted for at most 15% of the total signal [2]. The measured reduction in binding potential in patients compared to healthy controls (26% reduction) and the decreases in binding capacity (63% reduction) suggest VMAT2-targeted tracers hold clinical promise. However, since multiple groups have obtained findings that indicate patients with long-standing diabetes, where the BCM should be negligible, show pancreatic accumulation of labeled DTBZ (e.g., Goland et al. [39]), further investigation is required. Improvements in accuracy and decreases in off-target signal are needed for efficient clinical translation including accounting for VMAT2 expression in PP cells [17]. Expression differences in common lab species make this a challenging endeavor [35].

Glucagon-like peptide-1 receptor (GLP-1R) is a member of family B1 of G protein-coupled receptors. Activation of the receptor plays an important role in glucose homeostasis where the natural ligand GLP-1 helps stimulate insulin secretion in pancreatic beta cells [40]. Therefore, this receptor is a target of several clinically approved treatments for type 2 diabetes [41]. GLP-1R is highly expressed in islets, making GLP-1 and its analogues strong candidates for beta cell imaging (Fig. 8.4). The high expression, along with high vascularization of tissue within the islets, has led to the development of multiple GLP-1 analogues for beta cell targeting. Native GLP-1 is rapidly degraded by dipeptidyl peptidase 4 (DPP-4) resulting in a <2 min half-life in the blood [42]. To avoid high lysosomal breakdown of GLP-1, Gao et al. incorporated a lactam bridge along the peptide backbone, leading to higher binding affinity as well [43]. Perhaps even more promising is the exendin-4 peptide, originally isolated from *Heloderma suspectum*, more commonly known as the Gila monster. Multiple bioactive compounds were isolated from the venom of this foot-long lizard, one of only two poisonous lizards, including exendin-4 [44]. This peptide displays remarkable in vivo stability. Wild-type exendin-4 shares 53% homology to GLP-1 and binds to GLP-1R with subnanomolar affinity [45]. The peptide is currently approved for treatment of type 2 diabetes, and the interaction between the ligand and GLP-1R is well characterized. Gotthardt visualized GLP-1R positive tissues through SPECT imaging using [^{111}In]-DTPA-Lys^{40}-exendin-4 through in vivo imaging and biodistribution measurements in rats and mice [46]. Mukai demonstrated successful blocking of GLP-1R using pre-administration of excess nonradioactive exendin followed by subsequent delivery of truncated exendin in the form of [^{125}I]-Bolton-Hunter exendin-(9-39) [47]. The development of [^{18}F]-exendin-(9-39) by Toyoda et al. showed promising uptake in the pancreas at 30 min with receptor specificity confirmed by similar blocking experiments [48]. However, intracellular trapping of the agonist form (wild-type exendin-4) may improve retention compared to the non-internalized exendin-(9-39) antagonist. More recently, Brom et al. demonstrated pronounced differences in pancreas uptake with ^{111}In-labeled exendin in five patients with type 1 diabetes [49]. Quantitative PCR results from human tissue also suggested a favorable expression of GLP-1R in the islets compared to exocrine pancreas, indicating low off-target signal in patients. Similar to VMAT2 imaging, challenges remain. Karlsson and colleagues point out that the Brom et al. results may not account for the shrinking pancreas size, which may confound measurements in healthy versus diseased pancreata [32].

Despite the promising clinical results, a significant obstacle facing GLP-1 imaging is low GLP-1 receptor expression in non-beta cells. Although a diffuse signal was reported for human exocrine pancreas slides labeled with radioactive GLP-1 [50], recent studies have presented a clearer picture of the localization of this expression in humans and animal models [51, 52]. Zhang et al. used quantitative flow cytometry and biodistribution measurements to estimate the expression on beta cells and non-beta cells and found ~55,000 GLP-1 receptors per beta cell in a transgenic MIP-GFP mouse model [53]. Based on the specific uptake (%ID/g difference between blocked and unblocked mice) and a 1% beta cell fraction, the beta cell targeting only accounted for 50% of the specific signal. The other half appeared to be diffusely spread throughout the mouse pancreas. A lower expression in the exocrine pancreas (~850 GLP-1 receptors per cell [53]) could explain this non-beta cell-specific labeling and is consistent with other studies showing exocrine expression.

The low beta cell fraction in the pancreas makes the specificity of the target crucial to the success of a probe, and GLP-1R faces similar challenges as VMAT2 in this regard. Willekens argues that the uptake of exendin in mouse models indicates binding to a receptor other than GLP-1R [54]. This is based on their findings of (1) a similarly high transcription ratio between endocrine and exocrine tissue in mice and rats but (2) a much lower in vivo uptake between these two tissues. The comparable transcript levels indicate that expression may be similar in the exocrine pancreas between these species, but this is challenging to verify at the protein (translational) level due to the poor specificity of GLP-1R mouse antibodies [55]. Functional expression of GLP1-R has been reported in mouse acinar cells [56], and slightly higher translation in mouse exocrine pancreas (resulting in higher target expression) could be the culprit for the low (5:1) uptake between endocrine and exocrine pancreas in mice versus 50:1 for rats. The 20 pmol dose of radiolabeled exendin may saturate the exocrine pancreas, while the endocrine pancreas is strongly labeled but well below saturation due to higher expression. Higher doses, such as 200 pmol to 2 nmol used in fluorescence imaging, saturate both endocrine and exocrine tissue, resulting in higher endocrine to exocrine ratios.

Understanding the differences between mouse and rat pancreas (and other species such as pig and nonhuman primate [51, 57]) is crucial for preclinical studies, but ultimately the human pancreas is most important for clinical translation. Animal studies are critical for understanding the disease, but they can sometimes be misleading, such as variable density of beta cells in islets (Fig. 8.1d–f) [58] and differences in prevalence as a result of gender differences and unpredictability of disease onset in non-obese diabetic (NOD) mice [59–61]. Other animal models such as BioBreeding (BB) rats are lymphopenic and display a near absence of $CD4^+$ and $CD8^+$ T cells, deviating from type 1 diabetes in humans [62]. For targeted molecular imaging for diabetes research, differences between animals and humans can significantly impact results as well. Given the challenges in imaging beta cell mass, even small changes in receptor expression or beta cell number can influence imaging outcomes in preclinical models. Willekens et al. state that the rat pancreas is similar to humans given the low levels of In-111 exendin seen in some type 1 diabetic patients. Brom et al. show very low nonspecific uptake in humans, which appears promising. Alternatively, the variability seen in pancreas uptake could be impacted not just by variability in patient BCM but also variable exocrine pancreas expression, pancreas size, and potentially nonspecific uptake due to inflammation [49]. There are several studies indicating GLP-1R expression in the human exocrine pancreas with radiolabeled GLP-1 [50] and extensively validated antibodies [51, 52]. Whether this off-target expression is sufficient to interfere with beta cell quantification is currently unclear.

Although In-111 is not an ideal radioisotope for imaging (SPECT tracer versus PET, beta and Auger electron emissions, a longer half-life than needed), it is important to note that In-111 exendin does have some of the best imaging agent targeting properties for a cell surface receptor (Fig. 8.5). The low plasma protein interactions result in extremely low nonspecific interactions as seen by the high blocking efficiency when delivered with high doses of cold exendin [46, 49]. Tc-99m and Ga-68 can suffer

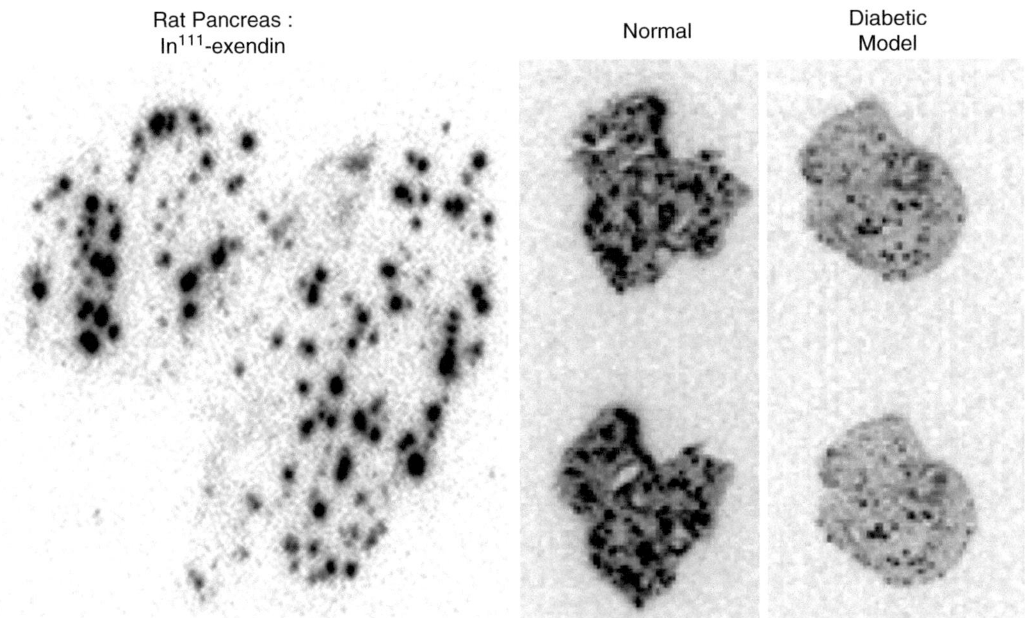

Fig. 8.5 SPECT Imaging of GLP-1R. Pancreatic sections from brown Norway rats showing accumulation of [111In]-exendin in the islets of Langerhans (*left*). Adapted from Willekens et al., 2016. Same model system in normal rats versus lower uptake in type 1 diabetes model (Alloxan-treated rat, 60 mg/kg). Adapted from Brom et al., 2014

from nonspecific interactions that decrease endocrine pancreas uptake and/or increase nonspecific signal [63]. Cu-64-labeled peptides appear to have better pharmacokinetics than technetium and gadolinium [64], but the islet uptake is slightly lower and the blocked pancreas (nonspecific) uptake slightly higher than In-111 [65]. Whether the higher sensitivity of PET outweighs these effects remains to be determined. In-111 is also a residualizing isotope, which is important for rapidly internalized agonists, such as exendin-4, that are trapped within the cell to avoid washout of probes that occurs even with seemingly high single-digit nanomolar affinity [5, 24]. This is in contrast to isotopes such as iodine and F-18 that can wash out of the target cells upon internalization and degradation (depending on the linker and associated chemistry [66]).

Antibodies specific to beta cell surface proteins that bind with high affinity have also been investigated as probes for BCM imaging and quantification. Several monoclonal antibodies (mAbs) have been reported that bind specifically to beta cells [67, 68]. These large (~150 kDa) proteins recognize specific epitopes through their variable regions, and their slow clearance results in efficient targeting. IC2, a rat IgM monoclonal antibody, is known to bind to sulfatide expressed on the beta cell surface in the insulin granula [69]. Results of the study using [^{111}In]-DTPA-IC2 were promising and demonstrated high uptake and specificity as well as high correlation between antibody accumulation in the pancreas and BCM between diabetic and healthy animals. However, several limitations exist for radiolabeled antibodies in the clinic, particularly the high background activity due to slow systemic clearance. Hampe and colleagues used fragments of K14D10 IgG to demonstrate that antibody fragments are able to clear systemic circulation quickly and bind to beta cells with high affinity [70]. However, analysis of the pharmacokinetics of protein imaging agents indicates the most efficient uptake occurs for either very low molecular weight probes (< 3 kDa) [5] or monoclonal antibodies [24], with low molecular weight probes providing more efficient background clearance than the latter.

Serotonin synthesis is localized in islets, and measurements of biosynthesis activity can be used to potentially quantify beta cells. One strategy uses a radiolabeled serotonin precursor hydroxy-tryptophan (HTP). Serotonin synthesis in healthy pancreata will result in the accumulation of radiolabeled precursor, whereas pancreas from patients with type 1 diabetes will lack the molecular machinery required for synthesis [71]. Although both exocrine and endocrine cells take up HTP, the precursor molecule is quickly trafficked out of the cell unless it is metabolized. Eriksson and colleagues demonstrated accumulation of [^{11}C]5-HTP in the pancreas of healthy volunteers, noticeably in the tail and body regions where islets are more abundant. Compensating for loss of pancreas volume in patients, there was an observable decrease in tracer accumulation in diabetic pancreata (0.0028%ID/g vs. 0.0046%ID/g for patients and volunteers, respectively) between 40 and 60 min post-administration [33]. Because all neuroendocrine tissue undergoes serotonin biosynthesis, the tracer is not specific to beta cells, indicating that the near-total beta cell loss found in patients with long-standing type 1 diabetes will result in only partial signal loss. Despite these challenges, [^{11}C]5-HTP has potential for use in islet transplantation and regenerative therapies.

Highly specific ligands to markers unique to beta cells are a challenge to develop. One of the reasons the debate over the significance of low-level expression in non-beta cell tissue for several imaging probes continues is due to the challenging circumstances from the small islet size and partial volume effects. For example, in cancer imaging, a few thousand EGFR receptors per cell in healthy tissue would not be a major concern when imaging a tumor with a million EGFR receptors per cell. However, the 1% mass fraction of islets makes even low expression extremely pertinent. Also important is the nonspecific uptake of probe in healthy tissue, particularly for residualizing radioisotopes that will be trapped in background tissue even once the plasma and interstitial probe has cleared. Even subtle changes to the molecule, such as the radiolabel, can impart large changes in protein interaction and nonspecific uptake rates. These considerations, and differences between animal species used for preclinical testing and humans, remain an important consideration for all probes, including VMAT2 and GLP-1R.

8.3.2.2 Nuclear Imaging of Insulitis

To date, noninvasive PET methods for imaging insulitis include labeled lymphocytes and labeled peptide and protein ligands specifically targeting lymphocytes. The labeling of lymphocytes is performed ex vivo and cells are readministered intravenously post-labeling. Ideally, the systemic circulating lymphocytes will migrate to the inflamed pancreatic tissue due to cytokine and chemokine signaling. Results from readministered lymphocytes showed poor pancreas targeting in patients, and animal work indicated uptake in the pancreas for both the control and test groups. As a result, the technique using labeled lymphocytes does not appear to be specific. A promising alternative for insulitis imaging involves radiolabeling interleukin-2 (IL-2) with SPECT tracers. In short, uptake of [^{123}I]-IL-2 resulting from lymphocyte invasion in the pancreas of non-obese diabetic (NOD) mice was quantifiable. Promising in vitro and in vivo results including high specificity and retention prompted administration of radiolabeled IL-2 in humans. Patients with a high risk of type 1 diabetes were also dosed and showed clear pancreatic uptake as well [72]. Additional SPECT tracers have been used including Tc-99m with similar qualitative results. However, additional improvements are needed for accurate quantification. A more detailed discussion can be found in Signore et al. [6].

8.3.3 Fluorescence

Fluorescence imaging uses visible or near-infrared light to detect a dye with high spatial resolution (< 1 μm) and sensitivity (nM range). The excitation wavelength photon excites the dye, and a longer wavelength photon is emitted. Near-infrared fluorescent dyes are often used due to reduced background (autofluorescence) and higher tissue-penetrating properties of the light. Similar to radiolabeled ligands for PET/SPECT, a fluorophore is attached to a targeting ligand to generate the probe. Commonly, a commercially available dye is chemically conjugated to the targeting ligand using common chemistries (ester-amine reactions, maleimide-sulfhydryl linkages, azide-alkyne click chemistry or copper-free click reactions, etc.) to create the imaging probe, which is then administered to a patient or animal to label specific antigens. Although near-infrared light can travel through several centimeters of tissue [73], the tissue is highly scattering. Even a large difference in contrast between the target and background can be lost as the signal "blurs" under increasing tissue depth. Due to the scattering and absorption associated with fluorescence imaging, it is not possible to develop a fluorescent probe that will allow for noninvasive real-time monitoring of BCM, where MRI or PET/SPECT may be more appropriate. However, the high resolution and ease of handling of fluorescent materials compared to radionuclides—including the ability to resolve subcellular structure and trafficking—make it an invaluable tool for research use in imaging agent design. Some pertinent parameters that can be measured using fluorescent molecular imaging include receptor expression quantification, binding affinity, internalization rate measurements, plasma protein interactions, and imaging agent stability.

With the availability of reactive fluorophores and fluorescent proteins, including near-infrared (NIR) probes with higher penetration depths, there is increased use of fluorescent microscopy for determining localization of biomolecules under normal and diseased conditions. Hara et al. stably generated transgenic mice with the specific expression of green fluorescent protein (GFP) in the insulin-producing beta cells [74]. The tool has improved flow cytometry analysis and quantification of BCM ex vivo, although low imaging depth and poor optical properties of GFP preclude this method's use for in vivo quantification. Given the low absorption of near-infrared light by hemoglobin, NIR probes are quickly gaining popularity for labeling targeting ligands. For example, Reiner et al. chemically conjugated an NIR fluorophore via copper-catalyzed click chemistry to exendin-4 to generate a highly specific beta cell binder and demonstrate the loss in signal following streptozotocin treatment of mice [75].

8.3.3.1 Fluorescence Imaging for Molecular Probe Design

The high resolution and real-time imaging of fluorescent probes make them excellent tools for insight into molecular probe design. For example, the rapid internalization and intracellular trapping of exendin derivatives visualized through live cell imaging provides insight into the necessary affinity for these imaging agents (Fig. 8.6). Distinct from the original analysis performed by Sweet et al. [16], the fast internalization rate results in effectively irreversible binding, so the requirement for binding affinity for internalized and residualizing probes (those trapped within cells following internalization) is not as strict as originally postulated. (In Sweet et al. it is assumed no internalization occurs and binding is at equilibrium.) Internalization and trapping using residualizing isotopes and/or linkers is an effective method to lower the required binding affinity and reduce washout of probe [5]. Notably, the slowly internalized exendin antagonist (exendin-9-39) is not an appropriate imaging agent, likely because it is not rapidly internalized and therefore it is subject to the strict affinity requirements for low molecular weight probes [24].

In addition to cellular trafficking, fluorescent derivatives can provide insight into absolute expression of imaging targets. Flow cytometry analysis of digested pancreas from mice that were administered fluorescent exendin-4 has provided absolute measurements of the accessible GLP-1 receptor expression in vivo. Absolute expression levels can be difficult to measure, but they can assist researchers in determining the optimal dose, blocking doses, and required affinity. Fluorescent derivatives for VMAT2 targeting are more challenging to develop given its intracellular location. However, the recent report of a fluorescent

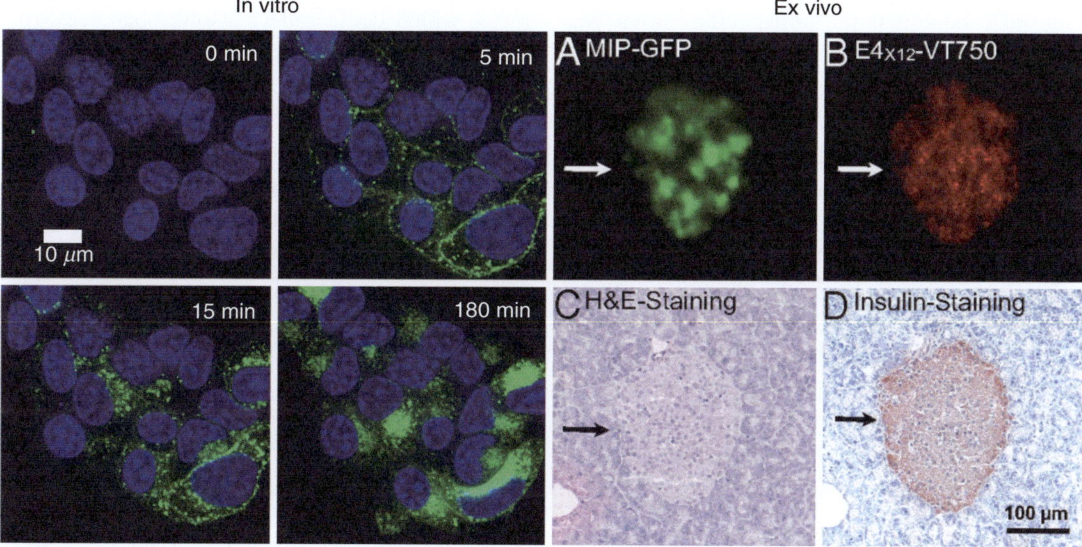

Fig. 8.6 *Left panel*: GLP-1R-positive NIT-1 cells are allowed to internalize fluorescent exendin conjugated with Alexa Fluor 488 at 37 C. Nuclei are stained blue with Hoechst 33342. Live cell imaging helps illustrate the rapid internalization kinetics of the ligand-receptor interaction. Adapted from Zhang et al., 2015. *Right panel*: exendin-4 conjugated with VT750 injected in MIPGFP mice to demonstrate probe and GFP colocalization. H&E and insulin staining of the same islet demonstrate successful targeting. Adapted from Reiner et al., 2011

derivative may aid in the understanding of VMAT2 targeting in the context of diabetes [76]. For these targets and others, a subsaturating dose is typically ideal to achieve maximum contrast between binding of probe in the target versus background tissues. This is balanced against a need for sufficient signal depending on the imaging modality. (For example, fluorescent doses are often higher than radiolabeled doses for animal imaging.)

Given the extremely small fraction of islets in pancreatic tissue, nonspecific targeting and uptake, even in low quantities, can result in drastic overestimates for BCM. Fluorescently labeled ligands have been used to correlate nonspecific in vivo uptake with plasma protein binding and nonspecific in vitro cellular uptake [5]. This may enable rapid in vitro screening for molecules with low nonspecific uptake in vivo. Fluorescently labeled exendin-4 derivatives were used to show that probes with increased plasma protein binding also had higher nonspecific cellular uptake rates, which can contribute to background signal. Even if the bound exendin was internalized and trapped within beta cells, a long washout period before imaging would provide little benefit if the nonspecific signal was also internalized. The longer washout would reduce extracellular probe that could intravasate into the blood and clear systemically, but the internalized probe would leak out of the beta cells and other cells at approximately the same rate. It is important to be cognizant of the impact of fluorophore conjugation on imaging agent properties similar to how chelators impact radiolabeled probes (along with the targeting ligand itself). The lipophilicity of a fluorophore can significantly impact clearance rates and the degree of off-target interactions. A parallel exists in radioimaging where additional chelator hydrophilicity may reduce sticking [77, 78]. This may be one reason why the In-111-labeled exendin was able to show large differences in the clinic [49]. Chelated In-111 is known to have very low interactions with plasma proteins, and In-111 has shown excellent specificity by having very low uptake in blocked controls in animal models [79].

8.3.4 Ultrasonography and Computed Tomography

Abdominal ultrasonography (US) and computed tomography (CT) are common techniques used for traditional pancreatic imaging. Due its noninvasive nature, lack of ionizing radiation, and abundance in the clinic, US is one of the most frequent diagnostic tools. Although organ functionality and anatomical structures can be visualized, US is rarely used to detect the structural changes that occur during type 1 diabetes, and the modality faces numerous challenges for quantifying and visualizing islets [6]. Computed tomography (CT) is an imaging technique used to visualize the anatomy of the pancreas due to differences in X-ray attenuation between tissues. Within the pancreas, however, both exocrine tissue and the islets share a similar density, making it difficult to differentiate between the two with available CT scanners. Though not suited for islet visualization, CT has been used to monitor tissue modifications during pancreas transplantation [80]. These methods have also been used to measure the size of the pancreas. The lower organ weight seen in some studies may complicate the interpretation of loss in beta cell mass, which could reflect a lower pancreas volume. Though not as common as type 1 and type 2 diabetes, monogenic diabetes mellitus displays multiple characteristics that are detectable with traditional US and CT imaging including increased US reflectivity and reduced X-ray attenuation on CT [81]. Therefore, these modalities play an important secondary role in pancreas imaging.

8.3.5 Multimodal Imaging

The trade-offs of different imaging modalities for detection and treatment of type 1 diabetes including islet transplantation therapy and beta cell quantification suggest there may not be one ideal modality for this purpose, mirroring conclusions found in other diseases such as cancer. Because of these non-overlapping weaknesses, multimodal imaging, which combines methods such as PET/MRI, has gained use for clinical diagnostics. For example, PET images can provide functional information, whereas

MRI provides the complementary high-resolution anatomical images [82]. Medarova et al. have detailed a method of islet transplantation that allows for facile monitoring post-surgery using both MR imaging and optical imaging in mice [83]. The MN-NIRF (superparamagnetic iron oxide nanoparticles conjugated with a near-infrared probe) particles label islets with fluorescent imaging to corroborate MRI results. Combinations of fluorescence and PET have been used to target *N*-glycoprotein with a monoclonal antibody specific for transmembrane protein 27 (TMEM27) and achieved measurable uptake in insulinoma xenografts in mouse models [84]. The expansion of multimodal imaging will likely expand given the intrinsic drawbacks of each individual modality.

8.4 Molecular Imaging Outside the Pancreas in Diabetes

Molecular and metabolic imaging outside of the pancreas is primarily focused on quantifying changes in metabolism and insulin resistance in organs such as the liver and skeletal muscle given the importance in type 2 diabetes. Additional studies have focused on pathological effects in organs such as the kidney and heart, which are common in the disease. Even with the important pathological role of insulin resistance, the failure of beta cells is considered the main culprit in the conversion to diabetes [85]. Although most diabetes research involves visualizing the pancreas, imaging other organs has increased our understanding of the pathogenesis of the disease, and examples of such studies are outlined below.

The most common techniques for examining metabolic changes associated with diabetes use radiolabeled metabolites for PET and SPECT imaging, magnetic resonance spectroscopy, and more recently, hyperpolarized MRI. Radiolabeled agents for metabolic studies include ^{18}F-fluorodeoxyglucose (FDG) for quantifying glucose metabolism, [^{11}C]-palmitate and [^{123}I]-BMIPP (beta-methyl-p-iodophenyl-pentadecanoic acid) for measuring fatty acid utilization with PET and SPECT, respectively, and [^{11}C]-glutamate and [^{11}C]-methionine for amino acid metabolism [86, 87]. For example, impaired glucose transport and phosphorylation in response to insulin using PET have been demonstrated in skeletal muscle, the most important tissue for insulin resistance, and results suggest there are deficiencies in glucose phosphorylation in the pathogenesis of type 2 diabetes [88]. This is consistent with magnetic resonance spectroscopy studies [89], and similar results have been shown for the liver [90]. [^{11}C]-palmitate has shown the reduced conversion of fatty acids into triglycerides in muscle for obese patients, a major risk factor in type 2 diabetes. Brehm and colleagues measured reductions in insulin-stimulated ATP synthase flux due to increases in lipid availability for patients with insulin sensitivity. These fatty acids are important regulators of glucose metabolism, further impacting insulin-mediated glucose utilization [91]. Other studies have focused on the pathological effects of diabetes in different organ systems. Recently, a hyperpolarized redox sensor, [^{13}C]-dehydroascorbate (DHA), has been used to show reduced redox capacity prior to the onset of nephropathy in a diabetic mouse model [92]. Particular emphasis has been placed on imaging the heart due to the increased risk of cardiovascular disease in diabetic patients. Blood flow imaging (^{201}Tl, ^{99m}Tc tetrofosmin, ^{99m}Tc-sestamibi) and glucose metabolism (FDG) have been used to detect mismatch between perfusion and viable tissue after myocardial infarction [86], which is more prevalent in diabetics. Specifically for diabetes, studies on metabolism include magnetic resonance spectroscopy, which has shown increased triglyceride content in the heart [93]. Molecular imaging will continue to develop in these areas to improve our understanding of the multi-organ pathological impact of the disease.

8.5 Conclusions and Future Directions

Molecular imaging in diabetes has primarily focused on the endocrine pancreas given its central role in controlling glucose metabolism. The small size and low volume fraction of islets of

Langerhans in the pancreas place considerable limitations on current imaging modalities. To date, a robust and widely adopted approach for quantifying beta cell mass remains elusive. This is a major limitation for researchers in the field when studying disease onset, progression, and treatment options. The use of highly specific targeting ligands to bind defined biomarkers on beta cells in PET and SPECT imaging is making progress toward the goal of clinical quantification of beta cell mass. The high resolution and ease of use of fluorescence imaging make this an increasingly valuable tool for aiding in the design of improved imaging agents. In addition to quantifying beta cell mass through imaging, the early stages of type 1 diabetes characterized by insulitis and the multi-organ effects of metabolism in type 2 diabetes have also been investigated as well using multiple modalities including MRI, PET, SPECT, fluorescence imaging, and bioluminescence. Each modality has a unique set of strengths and drawbacks, and each plays a crucial imaging role in studying the disease. The noninvasive nature of MRI and PET/SPECT and sensitivity to molecular markers (e.g., molecular resonance spectroscopy and hyperpolarized MRI contrast agents and radioactive PET and SPECT tracers) make these key modalities for clinical translation.

One of the biggest challenges for the future of this field remains the development of a robust imaging method for beta cell mass. What new approaches could help facilitate the development of such a probe (or adaptation of current probes to yield more reliable results)? Absolute quantification of target expression (across species and in humans), delivery rates (blood flow, vascular surface area, etc.) under various disease states, and probe properties (plasma clearance, cellular uptake and retention, binding affinity, etc.) can greatly facilitate the development of improved agents and interpretation of experimental results. For example, knowing the absolute number of GLP-1 receptors on endocrine versus exocrine cells rather than relative expression can facilitate strategies for improving specificity. Some of the basic principles of targeting specificity can be incorporated into screening methods [33] provided the in vitro expression profiles capture the in vivo situation. At the same time, it is important to revisit the assumptions of earlier analyses, since new probes may act by different mechanisms. For example, GLP-1R agonists and tryptophan precursors act by cellular trafficking and residualization rather than a simple binding interaction, thereby sidestepping some of the affinity limitations outlined in earlier analyses. Fortunately, a plethora of models exist to describe the pharmacokinetics of these types of agents (including FDG) that can be used to scale the results to animal and possibly human studies [23, 94].

In silico simulations of molecular distribution continue to improve and may be adapted for pharmacokinetic simulations of imaging agents. For the purpose of the discussion here, simulations differ from models in that simulations require little to no experimental data to predict in vivo outcomes. In contrast, models often use extensive experimental data and are fit to the results. For intracellular targets, simulations of first-in-animal and first-in-man drug distribution could be adapted (with suitable adjustments for targeting in tissues) to describe specific and nonspecific distribution of small molecule probes [95]. Similarly, non-steady state simulations of probe distribution [5, 96] can aid in the design of extracellular targeted agents. The use of in silico techniques can help guide experiments with current probes as well. As mentioned previously, recent evidence indicates that GLP-1R is expressed at very low levels in the exocrine pancreas in several species, including humans. Based on estimates of GLP-1R expression in mice and quantitative blocked and unblocked biodistribution, the expression is ~850 receptors per cell. However, this lower expression is significant versus endocrine uptake in the whole pancreas due to the low volume fraction of beta cells. If this low-level expression in the exocrine pancreas could be blocked specifically without completely blocking the beta cell receptor expression, the beta cell specificity of a subsequent radiolabeled agent would be greatly improved. The low molecular weight of exendin is close to optimal for an extracellular target in fenestrated tissue such as the pancreas, but it is still limited by permeability (the permeability surface area product or PS/V) and not blood flow. Assuming the fenestrated permeability is similar between the endocrine and exocrine pancreas, the relative uptake is determined by the surface area. Estimates of S/V (cm^2/cm^3) for endocrine and exocrine pancreas are 505 and 182, respectively [4, 97]. Although delivery to the exocrine pancreas is expected to be about threefold lower, the amount of probe required to block these receptors is >tenfold lower than what would completely block islet uptake. Therefore it is theoretically possible to block this low exocrine signal without blocking the beta cell receptors using a low dose of unlabeled peptide, and in silico simulations can be used to identify the appropriate scheme. (In contrast, the close association between nontarget cells expressing VMAT2 and reversible binding of DTBZ versus the "irreversible" internalization of GLP-1R make blocking less feasible for VMAT2.) "Cold dosing," using nonradioactive probes, has extensive precedent in the literature including the use with radiolabeled antibodies [98, 99] and in antibody-drug conjugate delivery [100]. It is important to clarify here that "low dose" refers to a dose that does not saturate the islets but does saturate the lower expression within exocrine tissue. Therefore, it may be much higher than the trace amounts of radioactive probe injected. A potential complication would be nausea and emesis seen with large doses of exendin, although these symptoms may be controlled for a single imaging session or an antagonist could be used. This may provide one avenue to improve specificity.

Another concern for agents delivered to sites of inflamed tissue includes accounting for changes in local transport properties due to the inflammation itself. For example, many probes will have a higher effective permeability in the inflamed tissue during insulitis, potentially increasing local probe uptake. A structurally similar nonbinding probe could be used to quantify the impact of inflammation on imaging agent concentration in the inflamed local environment. This could be critical if some of the significant interindividual variability seen in clinical trials is due to differences in delivery and not just differences in beta cell mass [101]. SPECT offers the possibility of gating on two gamma ray energies, providing "two-color" imaging, and adaptations for use with PET are being explored [102]. This could be employed for binding and nonbinding controls [94] to normalize results to differences in probe delivery from inflammation. Recently, Mathijs and colleagues used this dual isotope approach for delineating the pancreas relative to surrounding organs, such as the kidneys, in mouse imaging [103].

In conclusion, there are key challenges that must be overcome to develop an imaging agent for the clinic moving forward. One, there must be improvements in the specificity of PET and SPECT beta cell targeting probes as they represent the most advanced and well-characterized approaches for BCM assessment in humans. The promising results in the clinic for both VMAT2 and GLP-1R targets still show overlap between healthy controls and type 1 diabetics, which is short of the desired goal of quantifying a graded loss in beta cell mass. Two, the clinical application must be clearly defined for different imaging modalities. For example, given the radiation concern in pediatric populations, can a composite score of MRI-measured inflammation, autoantibody titer, and other clinical data (e.g., functional tests) provide enough information for measuring patient response to treatment? Each of these methods has drawbacks individually, but progress in several areas may allow reasonable measurements of clinical response. One could envision PET/SPECT imaging playing a critical role in clinical trials for developing new treatments, while MRI methods would be used for clinical practice to avoid the safety risk associated with ionizing radiation. Lastly, there is a need for more emphasis in imaging agent design. Due to the complexity of imaging beta cells, a clinically reliable probe needs to display ideal pharmacokinetic properties including high target uptake, low systemic concentrations during imaging, very low nonspecific sticking to proteins, and next to zero off-target uptake for maximum contrast. Given the expense of developing new probes and imaging techniques, particularly those requiring large animals, in vitro and in silico experiments can help guide the rational design of probes, efficiently set up animal experiments, and help interpret the results to maximize the information gained from animal imaging. These probes can facilitate our understanding of diabetes, open up opportunities for new drug targets, and monitor progress in clinical trials to improve the outcome for this increasingly prevalent and costly disease.

References

1. Scully T. Diabetes in numbers. Nature. 2012;485:S2–3.
2. Laurent D, et al. Pancreatic beta-cell imaging in humans: fiction or option? Diabetes Obes Metab. 2016;18:6–15.
3. Carlsson PO, Berne C, Jansson L. Angiotensin II and the endocrine pancreas: effects on islet blood flow and insulin secretion in rats. Diabetologia. 1998;41:127–33.
4. Keliher EJ, Reiner T, Thurber GM, Upadhyay R, Weissleder R. Efficient18F-labeling of synthetic Exendin-4 analogues for imaging Beta cells. ChemistryOpen. 2012;1:177–83.
5. Zhang L, Bhatnagar S, Deschenes E, Thurber GM. Mechanistic and quantitative insight into cell surface targeted molecular imaging agent design. Sci Rep. 2016;6
6. Di Gialleonardo V, et al. Imaging of beta-cell mass and Insulitis in insulin-Dependent (type 1) diabetes mellitus. Endocr Rev. 2012;33:892–919.
7. Foulis AK, Liddle CN, Farquharson MA, Richmond JA, Weir RS. The histopathology of the pancreas in type-1 (insulin-Dependent) diabetes-mellitus - a 25-year review of deaths in patients under 20 years of age in the United-Kingdom. Diabetologia. 1986;29:267–74.
8. Olokoba AB, Obateru OA, Olokoba LB. Type 2 diabetes mellitus: a review of current trends. Oman Med J. 2012;27:269–73.
9. Kahn CR. Banting lecture. Insulin action, diabetogenes, and the cause of type II diabetes. Diabetes. 1994;43:1066–84.
10. Defronzo RA. Banting lecture. From the triumvirate to the ominous octet: a new paradigm for the treatment of type 2 diabetes mellitus. Diabetes. 2009;58:773–95.
11. Ichise M, Harris PE. Imaging of beta-cell mass and function. J Nucl Med. 2010;51:1001–4.
12. Shapiro AMJ, et al. Islet transplantation in seven patients with type 1 diabetes mellitus using a glucocorticoid-free immunosuppressive regimen. N Engl J Med. 2000;343:230–8.
13. Brennan DC, et al. Long-term follow-up of the Edmonton protocol of islet transplantation in the United States. Am J Transpl. 2016;16:509–17.
14. Carlsson PO, Palm F, Andersson A, Liss P. Markedly decreased oxygen tension in transplanted rat pancreatic islets irrespective of the implantation site. Diabetes. 2001;50:489–95.
15. Pattou F, Kerr-Conte J, Wild D. GLP-1-receptor scanning for imaging of human beta cells transplanted in muscle. N Engl J Med. 2010;363:1289–90.
16. Sweet IR, Cook DL, Lernmark A, Greenbaum CJ, Krohn KA. Non-invasive imaging of beta cell mass: a quantitative analysis. Diabetes Technol Ther. 2004;6:652–9.
17. Blomberg BA, Codreanu I, Cheng G, Werner TJ, Alavi A. Beta-cell imaging: call for evidence-based and scientific approach. Mol Imaging Biol. 2013;15:123–30.
18. Frangioni JV. New technologies for human cancer imaging. J Clin Oncol. 2008;26:4012–21.
19. Bock T, Svenstrup K, Pakkenberg B, Buschard K. Unbiased estimation of total beta-cell number and mean beta-cell volume in rodent pancreas. APMIS. 1999;107:791–9.
20. Herbach N, Bergmayr M, Goke B, Wolf E, Wanke R. Postnatal development of numbers and mean sizes of pancreatic islets and beta-cells in healthy mice and GIPR(dn) transgenic diabetic mice. PLoS One. 2011;6:e22814.
21. Nir T, Melton DA, Dor Y. Recovery from diabetes in mice by beta cell regeneration. J Clin Invest. 2007;117:2553–61.
22. Engfeldt T, et al. Imaging of HER2-expressing tumours using a synthetic Affibody molecule containing the Tc-99m-chelating mercaptoacetyl-glycyl-glycyl-glycyl (MAG3) sequence. Eur J Nucl Med Mol Imaging. 2007;34:722–33.
23. Tofts PS, et al. Estimating kinetic parameters from dynamic contrast-enhanced T(1)-weighted MRI of a diffusable tracer: standardized quantities and symbols. J Magn Reson Imaging. 1999;10:223–32.
24. Schmidt MM, Wittrup KD. A modeling analysis of the effects of molecular size and binding affinity on tumor targeting. Mol Cancer Ther. 2009;8:2861–71.
25. Turvey SE, et al. Noninvasive imaging of pancreatic inflammation and its reversal in type 1 diabetes. J Clin Investig. 2005;115:2454–61.
26. Kriz J, et al. Magnetic resonance imaging of pancreatic islets in tolerance and rejection. Transplantation. 2005;80:1596–603.
27. Medarova Z, et al. Noninvasive magnetic resonance imaging of microvascular changes in type 1 diabetes. Diabetes. 2007;56:2677–82.
28. Dodd CH, et al. Normal T-cell response and in vivo magnetic resonance imaging of T cells loaded with HIV transactivator-peptide-derived superparamagnetic nanoparticles. J Immunol Methods. 2001;256:89–105.
29. Moore A, et al. MRI of insulitis in autoimmune diabetes. Magn Reson Med. 2002;47:751–8.
30. Gaglia JL, et al. Noninvasive mapping of pancreatic inflammation in recent-onset type-1 diabetes patients. Proc Natl Acad Sci U S A. 2015;112:2139–44.
31. Gaglia JL, et al. Noninvasive imaging of pancreatic islet inflammation in type 1A diabetes patients. J Clin Invest. 2011;121:442–5.

32. Karlsson F, Antonodimitrakis PC, Eriksson O. Systematic screening of imaging biomarkers for the islets of Langerhans, among clinically available positron emission tomography tracers. Nucl Med Biol. 2015;42:762–9.
33. Eriksson O, et al. Positron emission tomography ligand [C-11]5-Hydroxy-tryptophan can be used as a surrogate marker for the human endocrine pancreas. Diabetes. 2014;63:3428–37.
34. Freeby M, et al. VMAT2 quantitation by PET as a biomarker for beta-cell mass in health and disease. Diabetes Obes Metab. 2008;10:98–108.
35. Schafer MK, et al. Species-specific vesicular monoamine transporter 2 (VMAT2) expression in mammalian pancreatic beta cells: implications for optimising radioligand-based human beta cell mass (BCM) imaging in animal models. Diabetologia. 2013;56:1047–56.
36. Goswami R, et al. Fluoroalkyl derivatives of dihydrotetrabenazine as positron emission tomography imaging agents targeting vesicular monoamine transporters. Nucl Med Biol. 2006;33:685–94.
37. Freeby MJ, et al. Cross-sectional and test-retest characterization of PET with [F-18]FP-(+)-DTBZ for beta cell mass estimates in diabetes. Mol Imaging Biol. 2016;18:292–301.
38. Normandin MD, et al. Vivo imaging of endogenous pancreatic beta-cell mass in healthy and type 1 diabetic subjects using F-18-Fluoropropyl-Dihydrotetrabenazine and PET. J Nucl Med. 2012;53:908–16.
39. Goland R, et al. C-11-Dihydrotetrabenazine PET of the pancreas in subjects with long-standing type 1 diabetes and in healthy controls. J Nucl Med. 2009;50:382–9.
40. Runge S, Thogersen H, Madsen K, Lau J, Rudolph R. Crystal structure of the ligand-bound glucagon-like peptide-1 receptor extracellular domain. J Biol Chem. 2008;283:11340–7.
41. Fosgerau K, Hoffmann T. Peptide therapeutics: current status and future directions. Drug Discov Today. 2015;20:122–8.
42. Wu Z, Kandeel F. Radionuclide probes for molecular imaging of pancreatic beta-cells. Adv Drug Deliv Rev. 2010;62:1125–38.
43. Gao H, et al. PET of Insulinoma using 18F-FBEM-EM3106B, a new GLP-1 analogue. Mol Pharm. 2011;8(5):1775–82.
44. Furman BL. The development of Byetta (exenatide) from the venom of the Gila Monster as an anti-diabetic agent. Toxicon. 2012;59:464–71.
45. Eng J, Kleinman WA, Singh L, Singh G, Raufman JP. Isolation and characterization of Exendin-4, an Exendin-3 analog, from Heloderma-Suspectum venom - further evidence for an extending receptor on dispersed Acini from Guinea-pig pancreas. J Biol Chem. 1992;267:7402–5.
46. Gotthardt M, et al. A new technique for in vivo imaging of specific GLP-1 binding sites: first results in small rodents. Regul Pept. 2006;137:162–7.
47. Mukai E, et al. GLP-1 receptor antagonist as a potential probe for pancreatic beta-cell imaging. Biochem Biophys Res Commun. 2009;389:523–6.
48. Toyoda K, et al. Non-invasive PET imaging of pancreatic islets targeting glucagon-like peptide-1 receptors. Diabetes. 2010;59:A431.
49. Brom M, et al. Non-invasive quantification of the beta cell mass by SPECT with in-111-labelled exendin. Diabetologia. 2014;57:950–9.
50. Korner M, Stockli M, Waser B, Reubi JC. GLP-1 receptor expression in human tumors and human normal tissues: potential for in vivo targeting. J Nucl Med. 2007;48:736–43.
51. Pyke C, et al. GLP-1 receptor localization in monkey and human tissue: novel distribution revealed with extensively validated monoclonal antibody. Endocrinology. 2014;155:1280–90.
52. Waser B, Blank A, Karamitopoulou E, Perren A, Reubi JC. Glucagon-like-peptide-1 receptor expression in normal and diseased human thyroid and pancreas. Mod Pathol. 2015;28:391–402.
53. Zhang L, Thurber GM. Quantitative impact of plasma clearance and down-regulation on GLP-1 receptor molecular imaging. Mol Imaging Biol. 2016;18:79–89.
54. Willekens SM, et al. Strain differences determine the suitability of animal models for noninvasive in vivo Beta cell mass determination with radiolabeled Exendin. Mol Imaging Biol. 2016;18:705–14.
55. Pyke C, Knudsen LB. The glucagon-like peptide-1 receptor-or not? Endocrinology. 2013;154:4–8.
56. Hou Y, Ernst SA, Heidenreich K, Williams JA. Glucagon-like peptide-1 receptor is present in pancreatic acinar cells and regulates amylase secretion through cAMP. Am J Physiol Gastrointest Liver Physiol. 2016;310:G26–33.
57. Nalin L, et al. Positron emission tomography imaging of the glucagon-like peptide-1 receptor in healthy and streptozotocin-induced diabetic pigs. Eur J Nucl Med Mol Imaging. 2014;41:1800–10.
58. Cabrera O, et al. The unique cytoarchitecture of human pancreatic islets has implications for islet cell function. Proc Natl Acad Sci U S A. 2006;103:2334–9.
59. Hanafusa T, et al. The NOD mouse. Diabetes Res Clin Pract. 1994;24 Suppl:S307–11.
60. Pozzilli P, Signore A, Williams AJ, Beales PE. NOD mouse colonies around the world-recent facts and figures. Immunol Today. 1993;14:193–6.
61. King AJF. The use of animal models in diabetes research. Br J Pharmacol. 2012;166:877–94.
62. Mordes JP, Bortell R, Blankenhorn EP, Rossini AA, Greiner DL. Rat models of type 1 diabetes: genetics, environment, and autoimmunity. ILAR J. 2004;45:278–91.
63. Brom M, Oyen WJ, Joosten L, Gotthardt M, Boerman OC. 68Ga-labelled exendin-3, a new agent for the detection of insulinomas with PET. Eur J Nucl Med Mol Imaging. 2010;37:1345–55.
64. Mikkola K, et al. 64Cu- and 68Ga-labelled [Nle(14),Lys(40)(Ahx-NODAGA)NH2]-exendin-4

for pancreatic beta cell imaging in rats. Mol Imaging Biol. 2014;16:255–63.
65. Bandara N, et al. Evaluation of cu-64 and Ga-68 radiolabeled glucagon-like peptide-1 receptor agonists as PET tracers for pancreatic beta cell imaging. Mol Imaging Biol. 2016;18:90–8.
66. Schoffelen R, et al. Pretargeted immuno-positron emission tomography imaging of carcinoembryonic antigen-expressing tumors with a bispecific antibody and a 68Ga- and 18F-labeled hapten peptide in mice with human tumor xenografts. Mol Cancer Ther. 2010;9:1019–27.
67. Buschard K, Brogren CH, Ropke C, Rygaard J. Antigen expression of the pancreatic beta-cells is dependent on their functional-state, as shown by a specific, Bb rat monoclonal autoantibody Ic2. APMIS. 1988;96:342–6.
68. Konidaris C, Simonson W, Michelsen B, Papadopoulos GK. Specific monoclonal antibodies against the surface of rat islet beta cells. Cell Biol Int. 2002;26:817–28.
69. Moore A, Bonner-Weir S, Weissleder R. Noninvasive in vivo measurement of beta-cell mass in mouse model of diabetes. Diabetes. 2001;50:2231–6.
70. Hampe CS, Wallen AR, Schlosser M, Ziegler M, Sweet IR. Quantitative evaluation of a monoclonal antibody and its fragment as potential markers for pancreatic beta cell mass. Exp Clin Endocrinol Diabetes. 2005;113:381–7.
71. Wilson ME, Scheel D, German MS. Gene expression cascades in pancreatic development. Mech Dev. 2003;120:65–80.
72. Signore A, et al. In vivo imaging of insulitis in autoimmune diabetes. J Endocrinol Investig. 1999;22:151–8.
73. Weissleder R, Ntziachristos V. Shedding light onto live molecular targets. Nat Med. 2003;9:123–8.
74. Hara M, et al. Imaging pancreatic beta-cells in the intact pancreas. Am J Physiol Endocrinol Metab. 2006;290:E1041–7.
75. Reiner T, et al. Accurate measurement of pancreatic islet beta-cell mass using a second-generation fluorescent exendin-4 analog. Proc Natl Acad Sci U S A. 2011;108:12815–20.
76. Hu G, et al. New fluorescent substrate enables quantitative and high-throughput examination of vesicular monoamine transporter 2 (VMAT2). ACS Chem Biol. 2013;8:1947–54.
77. Maresca KP, et al. Novel polar single amino acid chelates for technetium-99m tricarbonyl-based radiopharmaceuticals with enhanced renal clearance: application to octreotide. Bioconjug Chem. 2010;21:1032–42.
78. Ray Banerjee S, et al. Effect of chelators on the pharmacokinetics of (99m)Tc-labeled imaging agents for the prostate-specific membrane antigen (PSMA). J Med Chem. 2013;56:6108–21.
79. Schmitt A, et al. Differences in biodistribution between 99mTc-depreotide, 111In-DTPA-octreotide, and 177Lu-DOTA-Tyr3-octreotate in a small cell lung cancer animal model. Cancer Biother Radiopharm. 2005;20:231–6.
80. Neri E, et al. Multirow CT in the follow-up of pancreas transplantation. Transplant Proc. 2004;36:597–600.
81. Haldorsen IS, Raeder H, Vesterhus M, Molven A, Njolstad PR. The role of pancreatic imaging in monogenic diabetes mellitus. Nat Rev Endocrinol. 2012;8:148–59.
82. Lee DE, et al. Multifunctional nanoparticles for multimodal imaging and theragnosis. Chem Soc Rev. 2012;41:2656–72.
83. Medarova Z, Evgenov NV, Dai G, Bonner-Weir S, Moore A. In vivo multimodal imaging of transplanted pancreatic islets. Nat Protoc. 2006;1:429–35.
84. Vats D, et al. Multimodal imaging of pancreatic beta cells in vivo by targeting transmembrane protein 27 (TMEM27). Diabetologia. 2012;55:2407–16.
85. Iozzo P. Metabolic imaging in obesity: underlying mechanisms and consequences in the whole body. Ann N Y Acad Sci. 2015;1353:21–40.
86. Osterholt M, Sen S, Dilsizian V, Taegtmeyer H. Targeted metabolic imaging to improve the management of heart disease. JACC Cardiovasc Imaging. 2012;5:214–26.
87. Morooka M, et al. 11C-methionine PET of acute myocardial infarction. J Nucl Med. 2009;50:1283–7.
88. Williams KV, Price JC, Kelley DE. Interactions of impaired glucose transport and phosphorylation in skeletal muscle insulin resistance: a dose-response assessment using positron emission tomography. Diabetes. 2001;50:2069–79.
89. Krssak M, et al. Intramyocellular lipid concentrations are correlated with insulin sensitivity in humans: a 1H NMR spectroscopy study. Diabetologia. 1999;42:113–6.
90. Borra R, et al. Inverse association between liver fat content and hepatic glucose uptake in patients with type 2 diabetes mellitus. Metab Clin Exp. 2008;57:1445–51.
91. Brehm A, et al. Increased lipid availability impairs insulin-stimulated ATP synthesis in human skeletal muscle. Diabetes. 2006;55:136–40.
92. Keshari KR, et al. Noninvasive in vivo imaging of diabetes-induced renal oxidative stress and response to therapy using hyperpolarized 13C dehydroascorbate magnetic resonance. Diabetes. 2015;64:344–52.
93. McGavock JM, et al. Cardiac steatosis in diabetes mellitus: a 1H-magnetic resonance spectroscopy study. Circulation. 2007;116:1170–5.
94. Tichauer KM, Wang Y, Pogue BW, Liu JT. Quantitative in vivo cell-surface receptor imaging in oncology: kinetic modeling and paired-agent principles from nuclear medicine and optical imaging. Phys Med Biol. 2015;60:R239–69.
95. Poulin P, et al. Prediction of drug distribution in subcutaneous xenografts of human tumor cell lines and healthy tissues in mouse: application of the tissue

composition-based model to antineoplastic drugs. J Pharm Sci. 2015;104:1508–21.
96. Thurber GM, Weissleder R. A systems approach for tumor pharmacokinetics. PLoS One. 2011;6:e24696.
97. Sweiry JH, Mann GE. Pancreatic microvascular permeability in Cerulein-induced acute-pancreatitis. Am J Phys. 1991;261:G685–92.
98. Hernandez M, Knox S. Radiobiology of radioimmunotherapy: targeting CD20 B-cell antigen in non-Hodgkin's lymphoma. Int J Radiat Oncol Biol Phys. 2004;59:1274–87.
99. Kaminski MS, et al. Radioimmunotherapy of B-cell lymphoma with I-131 anti-B1 (anti-Cd20) antibody. N Engl J Med. 1993;329:459–65.
100. Boswell CA, et al. Differential effects of predosing on tumor and tissue uptake of an 111In-labeled anti-TENB2 antibody-drug conjugate. J Nucl Med. 2012;53:1454–61.
101. Saisho Y, et al. Beta-cell mass and turnover in humans effects of obesity and aging. Diabetes Care. 2013;36:111–7.
102. Di Bella EVR, Kadrmas DJ, Christian PE. Feasibility of dual-isotope coincidence/single-photon imaging of the myocardium. J Nucl Med. 2001;42:944–50.
103. Mathijs I, et al. A standardized method for in vivo mouse pancreas imaging and semiquantitative beta cell mass measurement by dual isotope SPECT. Mol Imaging Biol. 2015;17:58–66.

9 Brain Disorders

Vesselin Z. Miloushev and Ronald G. Blasberg

9.1 Introduction and Scope

Brain metabolism is in itself a broad topic. Metabolism as a concept is an approach to understand the behavior of biological systems. It comprises the transient and steady-state chemical reactions and cellular machinery necessary to maintain homeostasis and dynamically respond to changing physiological environment on cellular, tissue, and organism levels. These processes permit basic cellular functions and have important consequences for pathological processes. Disorders in multiple enzymatic steps affect normal brain function and development. Manifestation of metabolic disorders in the brain is primarily due to the relatively high and constant metabolic demands. Brain metabolism is complex not only on a cellular level but also on a tissue level, with complex metabolic interactions between neurons and glia, and metabolic differences in based on brain anatomy [1].

This chapter highlights imaging approaches to disorders of brain metabolism, based on current technology and understanding of the underlying cellular/tissue biology. The subsequent core of this chapter introduces brain metabolic disorders accompanied by summaries of relevant imaging approaches, noting several more concise reviews of this subject [2, 3]. This chapter is far from comprehensive in cataloguing the multitude of observed, and the many more theoretically possible, metabolic disturbances which have phenotypes in the central nervous system. Rather, we concentrate on the most commonly described and representative disorders, to provide an overview of this expansive discipline.

We begin by providing a historical context for metabolic imaging of the brain followed by a brief survey of modern approaches. Subsequently, several categories of well-known metabolic disorders with brain "phenotypes" are discussed in further detail. The categories are disorders of central energy metabolism, urea cycle disorders, peroxisome biosynthesis disorders, cholesterol biosynthesis disorders, amino acid disorders, organic acidosis disorders, and lysosomal storage disorders. Finally, we explore the several prevalent multifactorial disorders including Alzheimer's disease, Parkinson's disease, depression, and diabetes, highlighting the metabolic perspective of disease and breadth of this topic.

9.2 History

The origins of brain imaging date back to the early 1900s, when a neurosurgeon (Walter Dandy) injected air into ventricles of the brain and later into the subarachnoid space via lumbar spinal puncture, to obtain contrast images of the

V.Z. Miloushev (✉) • R.G. Blasberg
Memorial Sloan Kettering Cancer Center,
1275 York Ave, New York, NY 10065, USA
e-mail: miloushv@mskcc.org

J.S. Lewis, K.R. Keshari (eds.), *Imaging and Metabolism*, DOI 10.1007/978-3-319-61401-4_9

ventricles and subarachnoid space on plain X-ray film. The procedure, known as ventriculography or pneumoencephalography, was initially used in patients suspected of having hydrocephalus and later in patients suspected of having a brain tumor. In 1927, cerebral angiography using an iodinated contrast agent was used to visualize normal and abnormal blood vessels of the brain with great detail. Radionuclide-based imaging, based on the radiotracer principle, was first described by George de Hevesy in 1935, using ^{32}P to study phosphorus metabolism, which led to radionuclide-based imaging (scintigraphy), with the Anger gamma camera in 1957. Three-dimensional X-ray imaging of the brain using computerized axial tomography (CAT or CT scanning) was introduced in the early 1970s, yielding more detailed anatomic images of the brain for both diagnostic and research applications. This advance was shortly followed by three-dimensional radionuclide imaging of the brain in the early 1980s with single-photon emission computed tomography (SPECT) and positron emission tomography (PET). Now, PET-CT hybrid tomographs are widely available. With respect radiopharmaceuticals, ^{18}F-fluorodeoxyglucose (FDG) was the first radiotracer for metabolic/molecular imaging of the brain using PET. It was approved by the FDA for clinical use in 2000, after a 20-year research/investigative/regulatory sojourn. Magnetic resonance imaging (MRI or MR) was developed concurrently with PET and provides much greater anatomical detail of different brain structures, compared to CT. During the 1980s, many technical refinements were introduced and diagnostic MR applications rose to its current predominance. Functional magnetic resonance imaging (fMRI) became a reality when it was shown that blood flow changes measured by PET could also be imaged by MRI (BOLD technique). Since the 1990s, fMRI has come to dominate several physiological measures that were initially obtained with PET (such as brain activation mapping) due to the lack of radiation exposure and low invasiveness of MRI. "Molecular imaging" of the brain and diseases of the brain are currently performed by both MR and PET using now standard techniques.

9.3 Description of Modern Imaging Approaches

Magnetic resonance imaging of the brain uses local differences in the concentration and relaxation properties of water proton nuclear spins to delineate anatomic structures. Currently, available clinical systems operate at 1.5–3.0 T, readily achieving resolution on the order of 1–2 mm. Abnormalities in volume and signal of anatomic structures can be readily detected. The so-called contrast enhancement results from breakdown or the absence of the blood-brain barrier; it is typically achieved by intravenous injection of inert gadolinium chelates, which shorten the T_1 relaxation time constant, increasing steady-state signal in short recycle delay sequences (T_1-weighting). The possible causes of underlying abnormalities can be inferred from the imaging pattern and clinical scenario, anchoring the rationale for the field of neuroradiology. While considered sensitive in broad terms, such *anatomical* MRI is not necessarily specific. For example, varied leukodystrophies have overlapping imaging features requiring additional information for diagnosis [4, 5]. Further, abnormalities detected by standard MRI often indicate damage or significant departure from normal metabolism in the underlying brain, but detection of subtle or physiological changes requires additional techniques.

Several so-called *advanced* MRI methods are targeted to specific physiological properties. The most commonly recognized subspecialty modality is functional MRI (fMRI). Neural activation can be inferred using the blood oxygenation-level dependent (BOLD) effect with paradigm-driven fMRI or paradigm-free approaches (resting-state fMRI). This technique can localize functional units in the brain. It has been applied to many clinical scenarios to gauge altered brain connectivity and function.

Magnetic resonance spectroscopic imaging (MRSI) typically of proton (^{1}H) nuclei, and others including phosphorus (^{31}P) and carbon (^{13}C), measures the resonant frequency or relative *chemical shift* of underlying nuclear spins. The nuclear chemical shift is sensitive to chemical structure and can be used to identify molecules, given some a priori knowledge of the set of possibilities. The primary limitation is low signal to noise. Spectral complexity is a secondary problem, unless multidimensional and less sensitive techniques are used. Notwithstanding, ^{1}H MRSI at clinically prevalent field strengths (1.5–3.0 T) and feasible scan times can detect molecules in the mM range of concentration, primarily limited to choline/phosphocholine (Cho), creatine (Cr), N-acetyl-aspartate (NAA), and lactate (Lac). The so-called *high-field* MRSI (7 T and above) can detect static pools of at least 20 different metabolites [6]. Given current limitations, however, the power of the MRI spectroscopy is to include/discount certain diagnoses, although in the context of additional information [7].

Hyperpolarization MRI (HP-MRI) techniques, such as dissolution dynamic nuclear polarization, are under active development with the aim of improving concentration limits (nM to uM range, approaching the sensitivity of PET) and sampling real-time metabolism [8]. Many challenges remain; however, HP-MRI has the potential for widespread clinical applications since it inherently images nontoxic endogenous metabolites, is fast and repeatable, and uses no ionizing radiation.

Diffusion tensor imaging/diffusion spectrum imaging (DTI/DSI) exploits the anisotropic and anomalous diffusion environment of white matter tracts to characterize their integrity and direction. The most common and simplest approach models diffusion as a Gaussian elliptical tensor, extracting the voxel-based orientations (eigenvectors) and amplitudes (eigenvalues) of diffusion in three dimensions; mean diffusivity (MD, average of eigenvalues) or equivalently apparent diffusion coefficient (ADC) and fractional anisotropy (similar to normalized standard deviation of eigenvalues) are commonly reported. This technique can infer the location of known white matter tracts. In addition to signal-to-noise limitations, disruption of the anisotropic environment, for example, due to "edema"—a term probably encompassing several pathophysiologies, affecting compaction of the white matter tracts—can prevent accurate delineation or assessment of integrity.

MRI perfusion imaging uses inert contrast agents and spin labeling techniques to quantify kinetic parameters related to mass/volume transfer from the vasculature to additional compartments. Typical parameters include the permeability of the vasculature (K_{trans}, or K_{12}) and plasma volume of (V_p).

An emerging class of MRI contrast agents exploits dynamic molecular properties for sensing the cellular/extracellular microenvironment or detection of low-concentration metabolites. Mechanistically, these probes rely on modulation of the chemical shift, for example, due to differences in pH, redox potential, or chemical exchange (i.e., chemical exchange saturation transfer – CEST) [9, 10]. Recent achievements include imaging of endogenous glucose and glutamate [11, 12].

Several photon emission methods have been developed under the realm of nuclear medicine to image brain metabolism, ligand localization, and perfusion. Typically detection of the emitted photons is coupled with anatomic localization, using computed tomography (SPECT/CT, PET/CT) or MRI (PET/MR). These methods currently achieve metabolic localization within resolution on the order of 5 mm, but provide invaluable metabolic information. Molecular imaging using PET and SPECT is largely based on the ability of specific radiopharmaceuticals to monitor specific molecular events. The most widely used positron emitter ^{18}fluorodeoxyglucose (^{18}FDG) images glucose utilization in normal brain structures, as well as specific brain lesions as discussed below. The accumulation of ^{18}FDG monitors the activity of the enzyme hexokinase, which reflects the rate of glucose utilization and glycolysis. For the past four decades, the radiochemistry and nuclear medicine disciplines have continued to generate an increasing number of radioligands/radiopharmaceuticals for molecular-targeted imaging. Recently, new MRI-PET hybrid methods have become available providing the combination of high anatomical spatial resolution (MRI), NMR spectroscopy, and PET imaging.

A notable development in functional/metabolic/molecular imaging is integration with informatics/data science and multiple "omics," concentrated on statistical correlations of imaging with other "big data." For quantitative imaging, referencing brain images to a standard image, a process called "statistical parametric mapping" (SPM) has provided invaluable insights in pathophysiologic correlates to changes in brain morphology and connectivity [13]. The future of metabolic imaging of the central nervous system has multifaceted potential in not only integrating the multiple viable techniques but the almost certain development of new methods.

9.4 Categories of Metabolic Disorders

9.4.1 Central Energy Metabolism

Defects in the primary energy metabolism are associated with perturbations of glycolysis and subsequent oxidative phosphorylation. Glycolysis is sequence of chemical reactions that sequentially convert glucose to pyruvate. Subsequently pyruvate can have canonical reductive or oxidative metabolic fates. Pyruvate can be directly reduced to lactate, by the enzyme lactate dehydrogenase, coupled to the oxidation of the electron acceptor nicotinamide adenine dinucleotide (NADH to NAD+). The reductive fate of pyruvate is less energetically efficient, but is critical for biomass generation, and hence upregulated in cancer and precancer states.

Alternatively, pyruvate can be transported to the mitochondrial matrix and oxidized to acetyl coenzyme-A (acetyl-CoA), by the pyruvate dehydrogenase complex. Acetyl-CoA is also the convergence of fatty acid and protein metabolism with oxidative phosphorylation. Acetyl-CoA can enter the chemical pools of the so-called tricarboxylic acid (TCA) cycle, citric acid cycle, or Krebs cycle. The TCA is a circular sequence of chemical reactions energetically coupled to reduction of electron acceptors (NAD+ to NADH), and the electron transport chain complexes, to ultimately generating adenosine triphosphate (ATP). Within the TCA, the succinate dehydrogenase complex catalyzes the oxidation of succinate to fumarate and is structurally coupled to reduction of flavin adenine dinucleotide (FAD) and the electron transport chain.

The clinically observed perturbations of central energy metabolism cluster in the pyruvate dehydrogenase complex, succinate dehydrogenase complex, pyruvate carboxylase, molecular transporters, and multiple defects in the electron transport chain. Specific mutations of genes encoded by nuclear and mitochondrial DNA are known, in addition to mitochondrial DNA deletions syndromes. Several syndromes can be caused by mutations in different genes, and several are associated with deletions in mitochondrial DNA.

Leigh's syndrome can be caused by mutations in multiple genes and is the most common mitochondrial disorder in the pediatric population [14]. Clinical presentation is variable but with characteristic presentation in infancy, after a period of normal development. Presentation in adults has been reported, although rare. Imaging hallmarks are bilateral necrotic lesions in the basal ganglia and leukoencephalopathy, (Fig. 9.1).

Compromise of the pyruvate dehydrogenase complex or pyruvate mitochondrial import factors cause clinically variable manifestations [16]. Clinical manifestations include neonatal lactic acidosis as well as delayed presentation in later infancy and early childhood. Fetal and neonatal MRI demonstrates ventriculomegaly [17] with subsequent findings of periventricular white matter abnormality (PVL, aka "leukomalacia") and disorders of cortical development such as polymicrogyria [18–20]. Progressive injury can present with necrotic lesions in the basal ganglia and brain stem, overlapping with presentation of Leigh's syndrome [18]. Additional associations between PDH and epilepsy [21] and inflammatory pain [20] underscore the multiple clinical manifestations.

Compromise of the succinate dehydrogenase complex (complex II) also has a variable clinical presentation. Mutations occur in both structural and catalytic components of complex and are exclusively encoded in the nucleus [22]. Clinical manifestations include multifocal brain abnormalities in the white matter and basal ganglia,

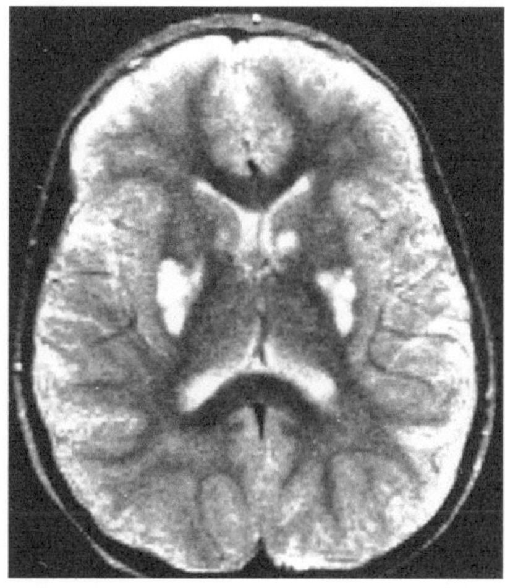
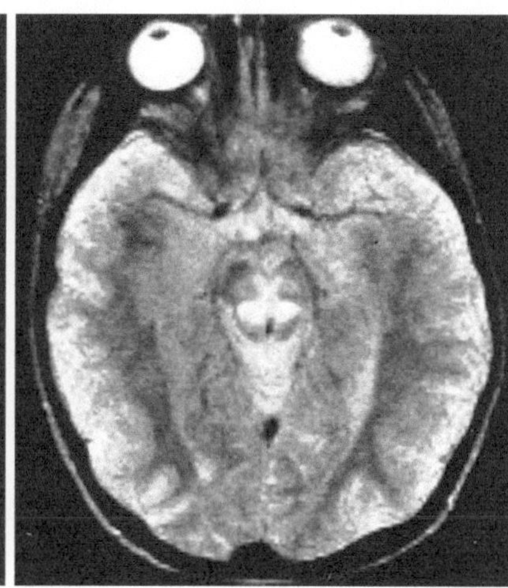

Fig. 9.1 Leigh's disease. The canonical defect in central energy metabolism is characterized by necrotic basal ganglionic and brain stem lesions. The images are reprinted from one of the first publications to describe the abnormality on MRI, with permission [15]

with multisystem involvement including myopathy and cardiomyopathy [23]. Beyond metabolic dysfunction, mutations in succinate dehydrogenase are seen in cancer predisposition to pheochromocytoma and paraganglioma, renal cell carcinomas, and gastrointestinal stromal tumors [24, 25].

The mitochondrial encephalopathy, lactic acidosis, and stroke-like episodes (MELAS) syndrome is causable by mutations in several genes, the most common of which is a leucine transfer RNA gene [26]. Clinical characteristics include leukoencephalopathy, stroke, and stroke-like episodes, as well as seizures. The mitochondrial encephalopathy with ragged-red fibers (MERRF) syndrome is causable by mutations in several genes. Characteristically, patients demonstrate leukoencephalopathy, myoclonic epilepsy, and myopathy; muscle biopsy demonstrates characteristic ragged-red fibers. The mitochondrial neurogastrointestinal encephalopathy (MNGIE) syndrome is caused by a defect in thymidine phosphorylase (TYMP), causing accumulation of pyrimidine; associated mitochondrial DNA deletions are probably resultant. Further, there is evidence that the pathologic correlate of white matter abnormalities is nevertheless thought to be axonal swelling due to pyrimidine accumulation rather than white matter damage [27].

Lactic acidosis is a common theme for defects of cell energy metabolism, when oxidative phosphorylation is compromised. Lactate can be detected by ^{1}H MRSI and is general considered an indicator of a *mitochondrial defect* when used for screening purposes. Increased lactate metabolite has been reported in pyruvate dehydrogenase deficiency [28, 29], MELAS syndrome [30], Leigh's syndrome [31], and succinate dehydrogenase complex deficiency. Nonspecific brain "damage" also manifests as decreased NAA, and this has been described in multiple disorders, including MERRF [32]. Notably, in the case of succinate dehydrogenase complex deficiency, ^{1}H MRSI can also directly detect increased pools of the un-metabolized substrate succinate [33].

9.4.2 Urea Cycle Disorders

The urea cycle is the enzymatic pathway that converts the ammonia to urea [34]. This conversion normally takes place in cytoplasmic and mitochondrial compartments of hepatocytes. In the mitochondrion, bicarbonate and ammonia are condensed to form carbamoyl phosphate. Subsequently, carbonyl phosphate and ornithine are converted to citrulline by ornithine transcarbamylase. In the cytoplasm, aspartate and citrulline are combined to form argininosuccinate by argininosuccinate synthase and broken into fumarate and arginine by argininosuccinate lyase. The conversion of arginine to ornithine is catalyzed by arginase-1, releasing urea [34].

The majority of disorders result in hyperammonemia, which may be marked in the infantile

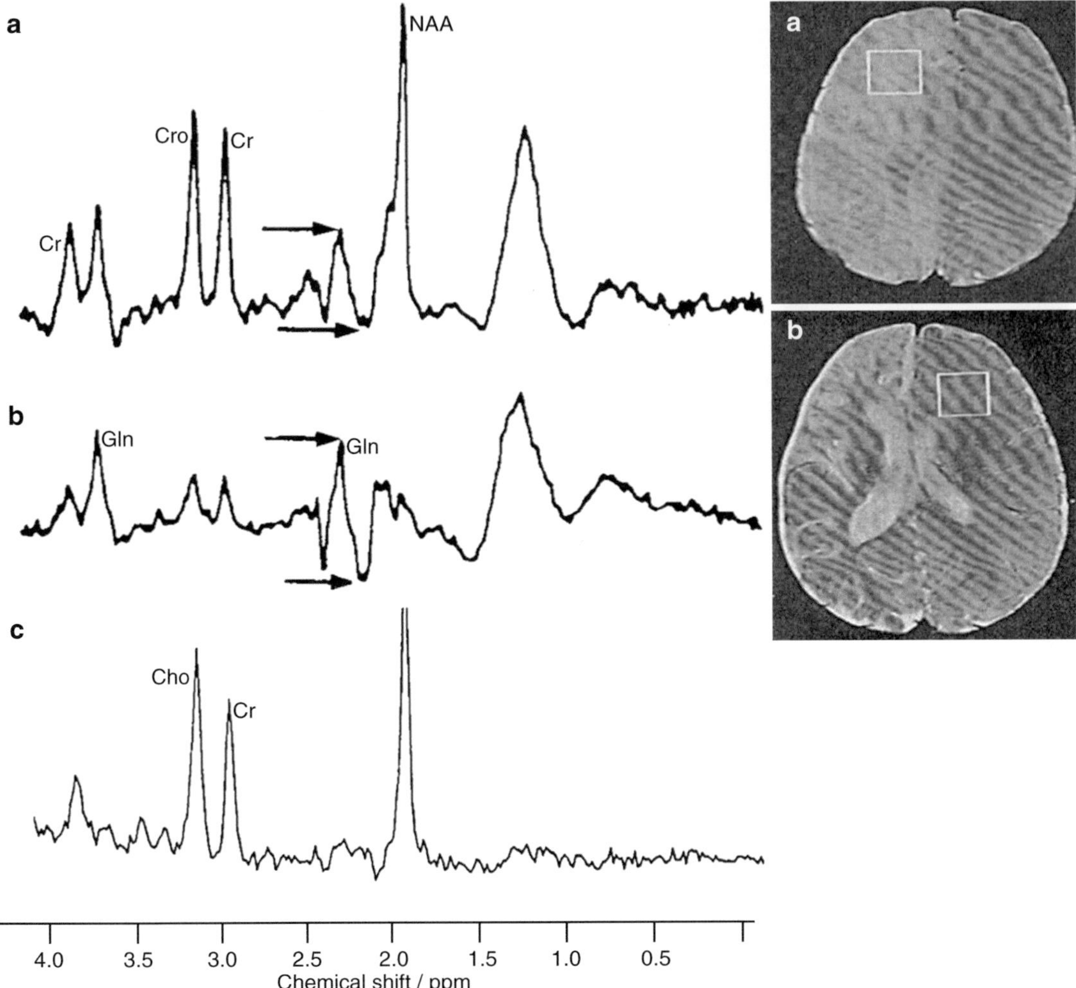

Fig. 9.2 Ornithine carbamoyl transferase deficiency. Spectra (**a**, **b**) corresponding to MRI abnormality demonstrate increased glutamine resonances. A normal reference spectrum (**c**) does not demonstrate the prominent glutamine resonance. The figure is adapted from one of the initial descriptions, with permission [35]

stages, episodic, or delayed into adulthood. In the central nervous system, urea cycle disorders result in increased glutamatergic transmission [34]. Many of the urea cycle disorders are characterized by increased glutamine levels, detectable by ^{1}H MRSI [2, 35] (Fig. 9.2). Anatomic ^{1}H MRI demonstrates differential sensitivity of astrocytes, which have increased T2-weighted signal, possibly due to direct toxicity of ammonia or glutamine levels. For example, the most common urea cycle disorder is ornithine transcarbamylase (OTC) deficiency and preferentially affects the insular and cingulate cortex. The notable exception to the urea cycle disorders is arginase-1 deficiency. In this case, hyperammonemia is delayed or episodic, and the disorder is characterized by congenital argininemia.

9.4.3 Cholesterol Synthesis Disorders

The brain is cholesterol rich due to myelin components that insulate axons [36]. Cholesterol biosynthesis is a multistep process, initiated by reaction of two molecules of acetyl-CoA, with the rate-limiting step being the subsequent formation of mevalonate by HMG-CoA reductase [37]. Despite cholesterol biosynthesis being a multistep process, only eight metabolic disorders are known. The most common is Smith-Lemli-Opitz syndrome (SLOS) [38]. Affected individuals demonstrate mental retardation and some dysmorphic features. The behavioral profile is characteristic with pervasive autism spectrum disorder [39, 40]. While dietary supplementation can ameliorate systemic effects, it does not rescue the central nervous system, since the brain relies on its own cholesterol synthesis. Anatomic MRI demonstrates midline brain malformations, most commonly affecting the septum pellucidum and corpus callosum [41]. MRSI of the cerebral white matter demonstrates elevations in lipid precursors and choline, correlating with severity [42].

9.4.4 Amino Acid Metabolism Disorders

Disorders of amino acid metabolism are due to enzymatic defects that either prevent the synthesis of critical metabolites or result in accumulation of precursors to toxic levels. Several well-known disorders fit into this category including phenylketonuria (PKU), maple syrup urine disease (MSUD), Canavan disease, and less well-known disorders such as nonketotic hyperglycinemia and Smith-Magenis syndrome. Clinical manifestations are varied as are the multitude of disorders, which fit into this broad category.

Phenylketonuria results from a defect in phenylalanine hydroxylase. Resulting accumulation of phenylalanine competes with tyrosine, a neurotransmitter precursor. Characteristic clinical manifestations include a "musty" odor, gait disturbance, epilepsy, seizures, and mental retardation [43, 44]. There are case reports of associated dementia and parkinsonism [45]. Brain abnormalities include periventricular white matter abnormality [46] and decreased cortical and basal ganglia volume in the absence of treatment [47, 48]. ^{1}H MRSI can directly detect increased phenylalanine metabolite [49], and ^{31}P MRSI demonstrates decreased levels of inorganic phosphate and phospholipids [50]. DTI demonstrates decreased mean diffusivity with normal fractional anisotropy [51]. Functional MRI demonstrates decreased prefrontal cortex function [52]. On ^{18}FDG-PET there is increased activity in frontal lobes and the anterior cingulate, with decreased parietal and cerebellar metabolism; changes in Broca's area can also be seen after treatment [53].

Maple syrup urine disease is a disorder caused by mutations in branched-chain alpha-keto acid dehydrogenase, in four component genes. The branched-chain amino acids are valine, leucine, and isoleucine, keto acids of which are excreted in the urine. Characteristic clinical manifestations are a "maple syrup" odor to the urine and varying degrees of mental and physical retardation [54]. There are four different clinical syndromes that correlate neurological disturbances with differences in enzymatic activity [55]: classic severe, intermediate, intermittent, and thiamine responsive [54]. Anatomic MRI demonstrates diffuse white matter abnormalities [56, 57] (Fig. 9.3). DTI demonstrates decreased mean diffusivity and fractional anisotropy in internal capsule [57]. MRSI demonstrates significant methyl peaks at 0.9 ppm due to branched-chain amino acids [58].

Canavan disease is caused by a defect in aminoacyclase 2, leading to increased levels of N-acetyl aspartate (NAA). Progressive clinical manifestations in early infancy are due to dysmyelination [59]. Anatomic MRI demonstrates diffuse white matter involvement with preferential involvement of the subcortical U-fibers [4, 60]. ^{1}H MRSI characteristically demonstrates increased NAA.

Nonketotic hyperglycinemia and the Smith-Magenis syndrome are both disorders of glycine metabolism. Nonketotic hyperglycinemia is defect in the four-protein components of the *glycine cleavage system* that breaks glycine down into carbon dioxide and ammonia, with coupled reduction of NAD to NADH and methyl transfer of tetrahydrofolate to methylenetetrahydrofolate [61]. Several clinical manifestations have been described, the most common being a severe neonatal phenotype [62]. Anatomic MRI and DTI demonstrate progressive white matter changes related to myelin vacuolization and subsequent

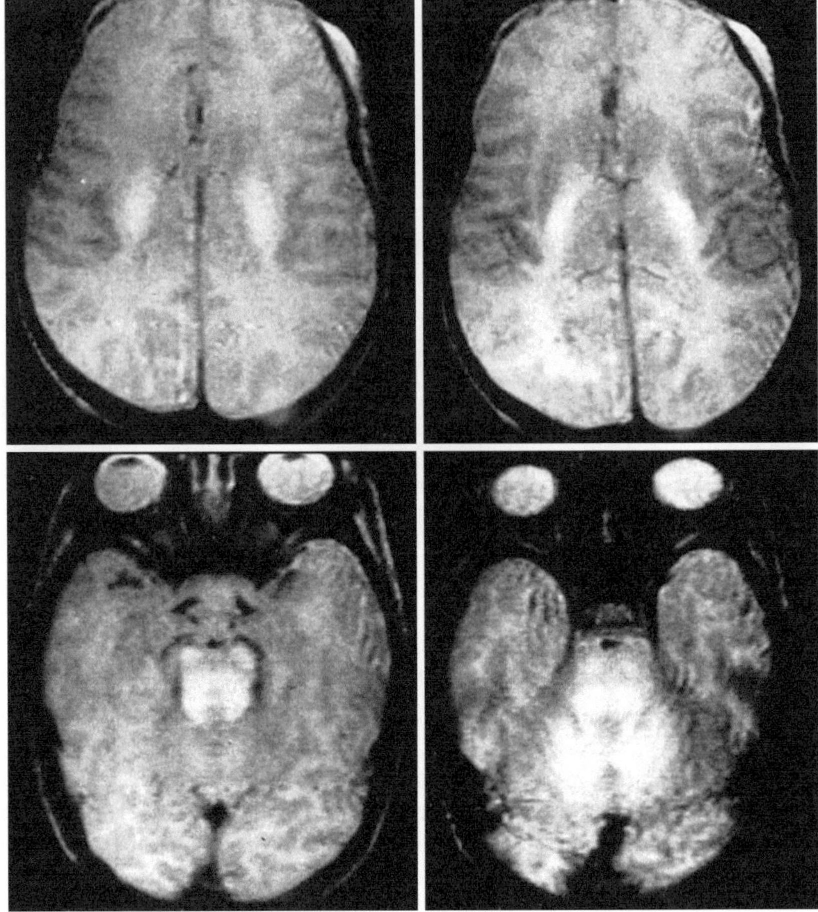

Fig. 9.3 Maple syrup urine disease. Images demonstrate involvement of the corticospinal tracts, brain stem, and cerebellum. The figure is adapted from one of the initial descriptions, with permission [56]

axonal loss [63]. The Smith-Magenis syndrome results from microdeletion of chromosome 17p, encoding the cytosolic serine hydroxymethyltransferase enzyme that catalyzes the reversible conversion of serine and tetrahydrofolate to glycine. Resulting low glycine levels alter NMDA signaling [64]. A variety of clinical manifestations have been described [65]. Anatomic abnormalities detectable by MRI include midline malformation and subependymal gray matter heterotopias [66].

9.4.5 Organic Acidosis Disorders

The organic acidosis disorders are a varied group of disorders in multiple pathways. Branched-chain acidoses include the well-known isovaleric acidemia, propionic acidemia, and methylmalonic acidemia.

Isovaleric acidemia results from accumulation of isovaleric acid, a product of leucine metabolism, due to inactivity of isovaleryl-CoA dehydrogenase activity. Clinical manifestations include severe neonatal ketoacidosis and episodic forms in later life [67]. Ring-like lesions in the basal ganglia are described in case reports [68].

Metabolism of odd-chain fatty acids, cholesterol side chains, and several amino acids (methionine, threonine, valine, isoleucine) generates propionic acid. Defects in propionyl-CoA carboxylase result in accumulation of propionic acid, and the disorder is associated with elevated glycine levels. Clinical manifestations include episodic vomiting, lethargy, encephalopathy, and immune deficiencies [69]. ^{1}H MRSI demonstrates increased glutamine, decreased NAA and myoinositol [70] in addition to high lactate levels [71].

The biotin-dependent reaction generates methylmalonyl-CoA from propionyl-CoA. Defects in methylmalonyl-CoA mutase prevent the conversion into succinyl-CoA and entry into the TCA cycle. Resulting methylmalonic acidemia (MMA) is heterogenous group of disorders with varied clinical manifestations [72]. It is associated with multiple brain abnormalities, including white matter abnormalities, cerebellar atrophy, and basal ganglia calcifications [73]. Basal ganglionic infarcts preferentially involve the globus pallidus externa [74]. DTI demonstrates decreased FA of cerebral white matter, indicative of white matter damage [75]. At least in case reports, ^{1}H MRSI can demonstrate normalization of lactate and NAA with treatment [76], in patients with MMA.

9.4.6 Peroxisome Disorders

The peroxisome is a membrane-bound organelle that compartmentalizes beta oxidation of very long-chain and branched-chain fatty acids and reduces the resultant hydrogen peroxide. Peroxisome disorders are group of disorders of peroxisome biogenesis and enzymatic defects. The two well-known disorders are the Zellweger syndrome and adrenoleukodystrophy (ALD).

The Zellweger syndrome is a spectrum of disorders, which include Refsum disease and neonatal ALD, which are characterized by the absence of peroxisomes, due to mutations in multiple PEX genes. Patients demonstrate plasma elevations of very long-chain fatty acids. Clinical MRI demonstrates an abnormal gyration pattern with malformations of cortical development, delayed myelination and progressive leukoencephalopathy and atrophy [77]. ^{1}H MRSI demonstrates nonspecific decrease in NAA correlating with disease severity in addition to lipids and lactate metabolites [78, 79].

Adrenoleukodystrophy results from mutations in the peroxisome membrane transporter ABCD1 gene, a member of the ATP-binding cassette D superfamily. The mutations result in defects in fatty acid oxidation and accumulation of very long-chain fatty acids. Classically, MRI demonstrates posterior white matter abnormalities and *leading-edge* enhancement. The adult-onset variant demonstrates abnormalities in the brain stem and cerebellum (Fig. 9.4). ^{1}H MRSI demonstrates nonspecific decrease in NAA [80]. ^{18}FDG-PET demonstrates increased glucose metabolism in frontal lobes and reduced glucose metabolism in cerebellum and temporal lobe areas [81].

9.4.7 Lysosomal Storage Disorders

The lysosome is a cellular organelle compartment responsible for a variety of hydrolytic reactions. Defects in lysosomal function are termed lysosomal storage diseases, because of accumulation of precursors within the lysosome. As expected, multiple disorders are combined in this group.

The sphingolipidoses are lysosomal storage disorders with altered sphingomyelin metabolism. Well-known disorders include Gaucher disease, Krabbe's disease, Fabry's disease, Niemann-Pick disease, Tay-Sachs disease, and metachromatic leukodystrophy. Of these, the most common lysosomal storage disease is Gaucher disease, which results from defects in beta-glucocerebrosidase and accumulation of glucosylceramide. Type 1 (non-neuronopathic) disease usually has mild neurological involvement, with decreased olfaction and cognition. Type 2 (acute neuronopathic) and type 3 (subacute neuronopathic) have more significant neurological compromise [83]. In type 1 disease, abnormalities are usually mild. ^{1}H MRSI shows relatively mild, considered subclinical, elevations in choline [84]. High-field MRSI has recently been shown to detect changes in glutathione metabolism in type 1 disease [85]. DTI demonstrates decreased FA in middle cerebral peduncles in type 1 disease [86]. Type 2–3 diffusion imaging demonstrates decreased MD in multiple regions [87].

Metachromatic leukodystrophy results from deficiency in arylsulfatase A, resulting in precursor elevation of sulfatides, which are important components of myelin. Clinically, the juvenile form is associated with neurological compromise, while the adult syndrome is associated with psychiatric disturbances. Anatomical MRI shows diffuse white matter involvement, sparing of the subcortical U-fibers and a "tigroid" pattern [4, 88].

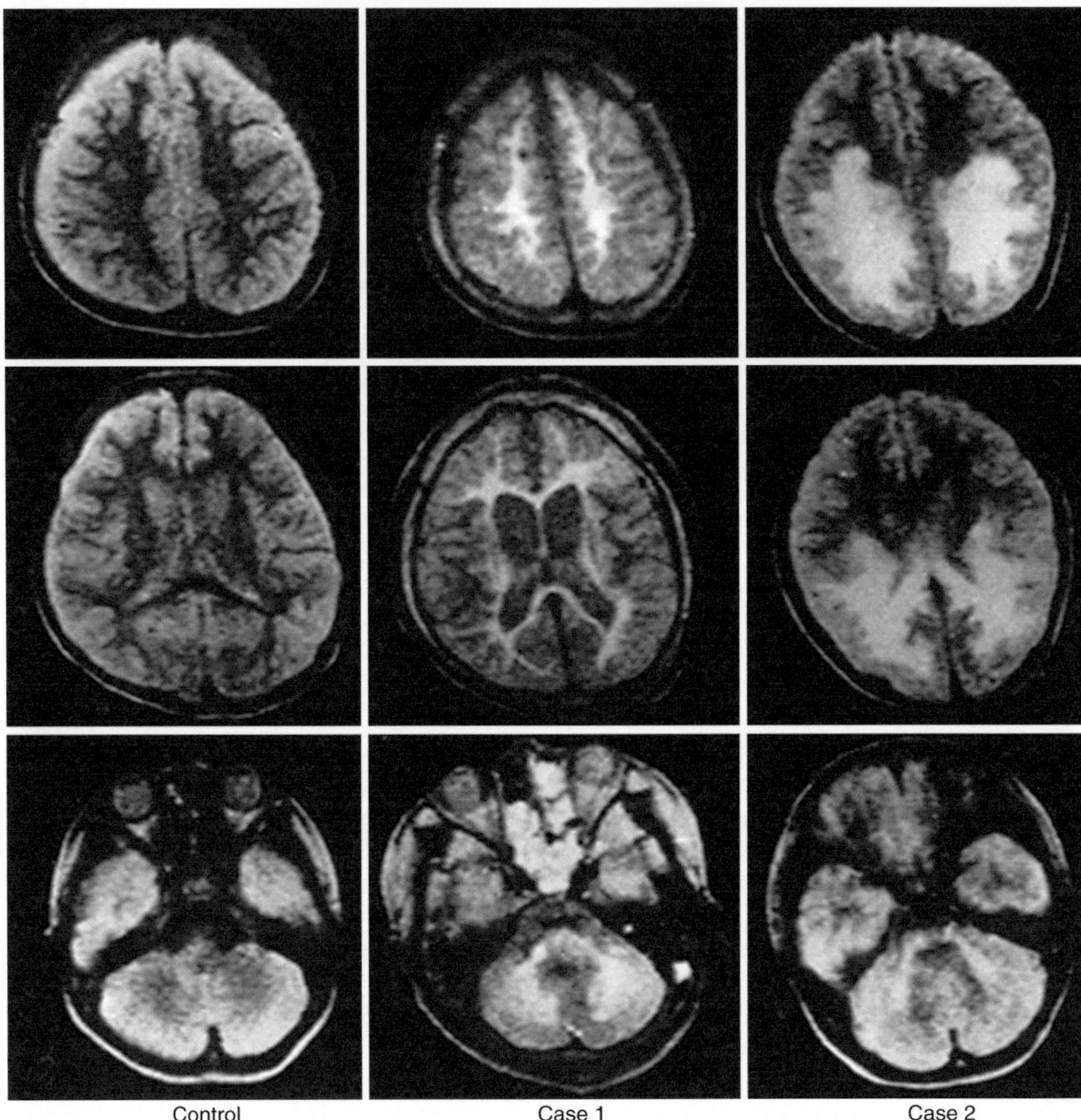

Fig. 9.4 Adrenoleukodystrophy. Images demonstrate the posterior predominant white matter involvement and involvement of the brain stem and cerebellum. The figure is reprinted from one of the initial descriptions, with permission [82]

^{1}H MRSI demonstrates decreased NAA, with elevations in lactate and myoinositol, indicative of white matter damage [89, 90].

Fabry's disease results from a deficiency in alpha-galactosidase A, resulting in accumulation of glycosphingolipids. Clinical manifestations in the central nervous system are primarily due to cerebrovascular disease, including transient ischemic attacks, stroke, and hemorrhage. Anatomic MRI shows expected correlates of ischemia with cortical and white matter involvement [91]. White matter lesions apparently occur preferentially in ^{18}F-FDG hypometabolic and hyperperfused regions [92]. However, MRI remains the preferred imaging modality, with limited long-term utility of FDG imaging [93]. ^{1}H MRSI demonstrates nonspecific diffusely decreased NAA, indicative of neuronal damage [94].

Niemann-Pick disease results from a deficiency in sphingomyelinase, resulting in accumulation of gangliosides and cholesterol with disrupted cholesterol intracellular trafficking [95]. Clinical manifestations of the disorder are very heterogeneous with several described forms, including the severe infantile (type A), visceral (type B), and juvenile (type C) forms [96]. On anatomic MRI, type A disease may show delayed myelination and frontal atrophy [97]. Type C disease may mimic multiple sclerosis and is characterized by atrophy of multiple brain structures and structural white matter abnormalities detected by DTI [98, 99]. ^{1}H MRSI demonstrates nonspecific findings of decrease in NAA and elevation in choline, in multiple structures [94].

Krabbe's globoid cell dystrophy is due to a defect in galactosylceramidase with resultant elevation in psychosine. Clinical manifestations begin at infancy, characterized by irritability, stiffness, and seizures. MRI demonstrates increased signal in posterior periventricular white matter, corticospinal tract, and corpus callosum [100]. Distinctively, this leukodystrophy is characterized by enhancement of multiple cranial nerves and optic nerve enlargement [101]. ^{1}H MRSI demonstrates increased lactate [102] and increased choline [103].

The well-known ganglioside lysosomal storage disorders are Tay-Sachs and Sandhoff disease. Tay-Sachs results from mutations in hexosaminidase A, while Sandhoff disease results from mutations in hexosaminidase B. Clinical manifestations of Tay-Sachs, essentially indistinguishable from Sandhoff disease, begin in infancy and demonstrate neurocognitive delay, followed by paralysis, dementia, and blindness, with death in the second or third year of life [104]. Clinical MRI early in the disease shows signal abnormalities in the deep gray nuclei with cortical and cerebral white matter abnormalities in the later stages, with cerebral atrophy [105, 106]. ^{1}H MRSI demonstrates increased choline and myoinositol with decreased NAA [107]. ^{18}FDG-PET demonstrates decreased metabolism in the cerebellum, temporal, and occipital lobes [106].

The mucopolysaccaridoses are lysosomal storage disorders that result in accumulation of glycosaminoglycans. Seven separate syndromes are described, including the eponymous Hurler, Hunter, Sanfilippo, and Morquio syndromes. Hurler syndrome results from defects in hydrolase-α-L-iduronidase [108]. Hunter syndrome is caused by defects in iduronate 2-sulfatase [109]. The Sanfilippo syndrome is causable by four separate enzyme deficiencies, resulting in accumulation in heparin sulfate. The Morquio syndrome is causable by mutations in galactosamine-6-sulfate sulfatase and beta galactosidase enzymes, resulting in accumulation of keratin sulfate. Characteristic MRI findings in the mucopolysaccaridoses include enlarged perivascular spaces, white matter lesions, ventriculomegaly, and atrophy, in addition to spinal canal stenosis as a result of the osseous abnormalities (Fig. 9.5) [110]. For Hurler and Hunter syndromes, ^{1}H MRSI demonstrates probable accumulation of mucopolysaccharides [111]. For Hurler syndrome, DTI demonstrates decreased FA thought to be due to decreased myelination [112].

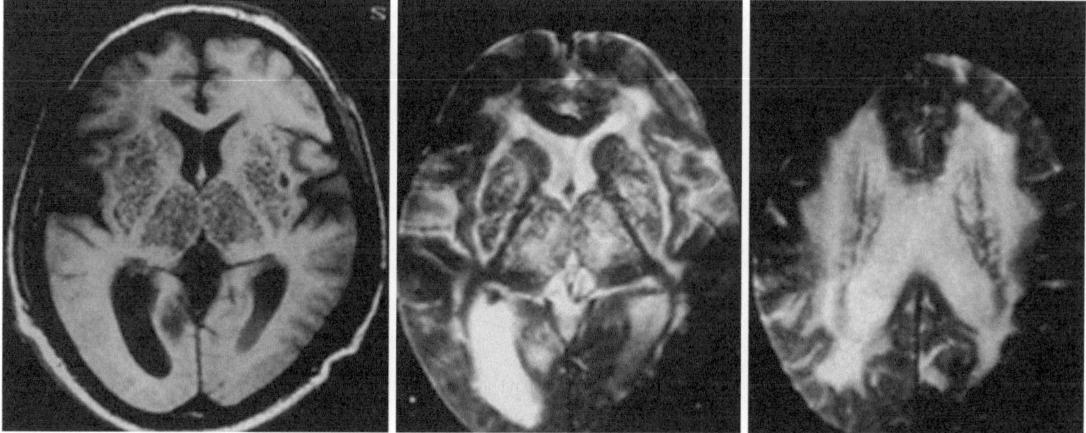

Fig. 9.5 Hunter's mucopolysaccharidosis II. The images show diffuse white matter changes and prominent perivascular spaces in the deep gray nuclei. The figure is adapted from one of the initial descriptions, with permission [113]

9.5 Multifactorial Disorders and Neurodegenerative Diseases

9.5.1 Alzheimer's Disease

Alzheimer's disease (AD) is the most prevalent form of dementia and is predicted to increase in prevalence as the population ages. In the prodromal/preclinical stages, it is often referred to as mild cognitive impairment (MCI), although not all patients with MCI progress to AD. AD is considered a medial temporal lobe dementia, initially effecting short-term memory formation. As the disease progresses, patients display language deficits, disorientation, and behavioral changes. The pathophysiological hallmarks are senile plaques (extracellular plaques composed of amyloid-ß protein) and neurofibrillary tangles (intracellular inclusions composed of hyperphosphorylated tau protein). Other dementias (e.g., dementia with Lewy bodies (DLB), frontotemporal dementia (FTD), mild cognitive impairment (MCI)) have been similarly imaged [114].

The diagnosis of Alzheimer's disease is currently made on the basis of clinical, neuropsychological, and neuroimaging assessments. Structural neuroimaging (CT and MRI) is based on nonspecific features, primarily on brain atrophy, which is a late feature in the progression of the disease. Involvement of the medial temporal lobes is detectable by structural MRI [115]. Volumes of the hippocampal formation and entorhinal cortex have strong inverse correlations with disease severity. Later stages of the disease display more generalized volume loss. More recently, three-dimensional (3D) volume imaging of specific brain structures (such the size of the hippocampus) by MRI (and to a lesser extent by CT) has been used as parameters of the disease and its progression.

FDG-PET was one of the first molecular imaging strategies to provide a more functional assessment of Alzheimer's disease and helped distinguish Alzheimer's disease from other forms of dementia. It was recognized very early in the initial FDG imaging studies that there was a characteristic hypometabolism of the parietotemporal, frontal, and cingulate cortex in Alzheimer's disease and that the extent of hypometabolism was correlated with the severity of the dementia [116]. Glucose hypometabolism in Alzheimer disease is considered to reflect a combination of neuronal cell loss and decreased synaptic activity [117]. Clinical studies have shown that FDG-PET has a sensitivity of 94% and a specificity of 73% and predicted a progressive course with a 91% sensitivity and a nonprogressive course with a 75% specificity [118].

Several extensive and excellent reviews of FDG-PET imaging in dementia were recently published [119, 120], which include excellent descriptions and images of other dementias, including (a) normal aging, (b) mild cognitive impairment (MCI, prodromal AD), (c) dementia with Lewy bodies, (d) frontotemporal dementia, (e) semantic dementia, and (f) corticobasal degeneration. An example of FDG-PET imaging in AD is shown in Fig. 9.6.

Direct imaging of amyloid beta-formation is possible with Pittsburgh compound B (PiB) [121, 122] (Fig. 9.7) and several PET tracers, including ^{18}F-florbetapir and ^{18}F-florbetaben [123]. The presence and density of beta-amyloid correlated closely in individuals who had florbetapir-PET imaging within 99 days before death and then upon autopsy [124]. Patients with mild cognitive impairment, or older healthy controls, showed significantly lower mean cortical florbetapir uptake values [125]. Differentiating mild cognitive impairment from Alzheimer's disease is also possible with a tau-specific ligand ^{18}F-FDDNP, which correlates with disease severity. Highly selective tau-specific ligands are under active development [126]. The amyloid imaging agents, as well as FDG-PET, have been used to detect persons at risk for Alzheimer disease even before the onset of symptoms [127].

The pattern of progression and involvement is congruent with BOLD-fMRI findings, initially demonstrating decreased activation in the medial temporal lobe [128]. In the frontal lobes, however, BOLD-fMRI demonstrates increased activity in frontal regions in AD at-risk individuals, suggesting preclinical reorganization of brain activity [129].

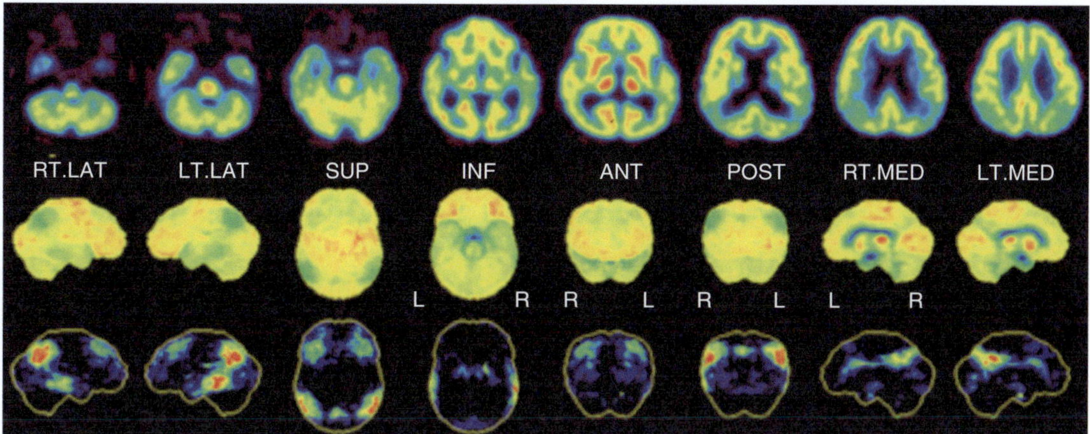

Fig. 9.6 FDG-PET images of a patient with AD dementia. Standard transaxial FDG-PET images (*upper row*), 3D-SSP images (*middle row*), and 3D-SSP Z score (hypometabolism) images (*bottom row*). Typical AD-like glucose hypometabolism is observed in the parietotemporal association area, posterior cingulate, precuneus, and frontal association area. The figure is adapted from a review article with permission [120]

Based on the *Cochrane Database Systematic Review*, a meta-analysis noted considerable variability of specificity values and lack of defined thresholds for determining test positivity in the ^{18}F-FDG-PET studies included in the analysis [130]. It was concluded that current evidence does not support the routine use of ^{18}F-FDG-PET scans in clinical practice for the evaluation of patients with MCI. Despite the good sensitivity achieved in many of the studies included in the meta-analysis that indicates a potential value for ^{11}C-PIB-PET imaging in MCI, the variability in performance and interpretation of the studies, existence of "outliers," and the lack of defined thresholds for determination of test positivity, ^{11}C-PIB-PET imaging was also not recommended for routine use in the clinical assessment of MCI [131]. Nevertheless, both imaging tests demonstrate characteristic anatomical patterns of functional abnormality in moderate-to-severe Alzheimer's Disease.

9.5.2 Parkinson's Disease

Parkinson's disease (PD) is the most frequent neurodegenerative movement disorder characterized clinically by rigidity, akinesia, resting tremor, postural instability, and often early presenting nonmotor deficits due to progressive degeneration of the dopaminergic nigrostriatal system, responsible for the core motor symptoms. Two forms of PD are described: (a) "familial" or early-onset PD involving a mutated gene and (b) "idiopathic/ sporadic" or late-onset PD (>85% of all patients). PD affects ~1.5% of people over 65 years and 2.5% over 80. PD involves degeneration of dopaminergic neurons in the substantia nigra resulting in a resting tremor, rigidity, and bradykinesia. A broader category of "Parkinsonian syndromes" includes a number of toxicity syndromes (Wilson disease, manganese and carbon monoxide poisoning, and chronic exposure to certain neuroleptic drugs), as well as other neurodegenerative syndromes such as multisystem atrophy (MSA) and progressive supranuclear palsy (PSP). Clinical differentiation of idiopathic Parkinson disease from causes such as multisystem atrophy may be difficult when patients do not respond to L-dopa therapy.

Presynaptic imaging studies of the dopamine (DA) system and its functionality can be studied using PET by measuring: (a) aromatic amino acid decarboxylase (AADC) activity with ^{18}F-DOPA; (b) dopamine transporter (DAT) activity with ^{11}C-nomifensine, ^{11}C-RT132, ^{11}C-CFT, ^{18}F-CFT PET [132] and with ^{123}I ioflupanc (FP-CIT) SPECT (DaT-Scan) [133]; and (c) vesicular monoamine transporter (VMAT2) density with ^{11}C-dihydrotetrabenazine (DTBZ)

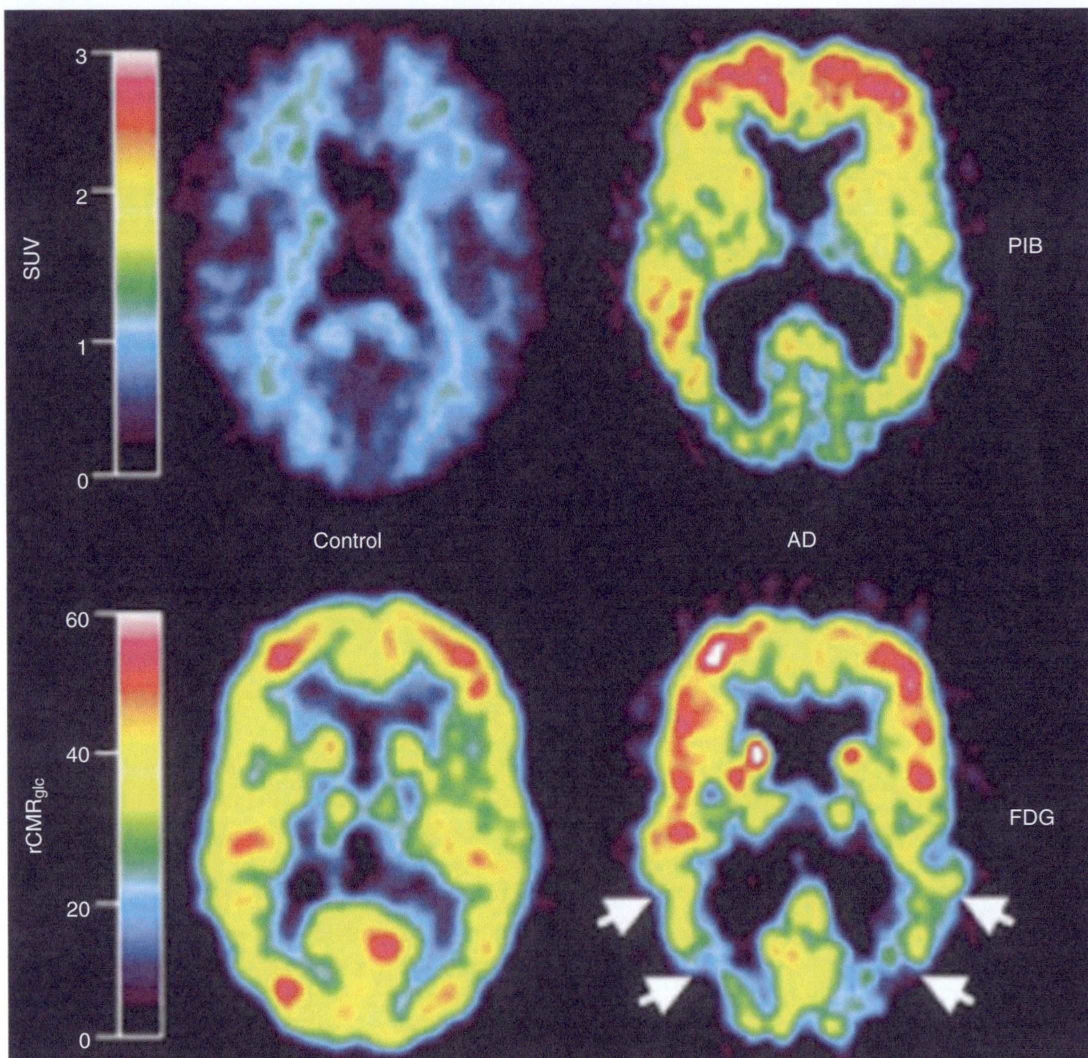

Fig. 9.7 PIB standardized uptake value (SUV) images demonstrate a marked difference between PIB retention in Alzheimer's disease (AD) patients and healthy control (HC) subjects. PET images of a 67-year-old HC subject (*left*) and a 79-year-old AD patient (AD6; MMSE _ 21; *right*). (*top*) SUV PIB images summed over 40–60 min; (*bottom*) ^{18}FDG rCMRglc images μmol/min/100 ml). The left column shows lack of PIB retention in the entire gray matter of the HC subject (*top left*) and normal ^{18}FDG uptake (*bottom left*). Nonspecific PIB retention is seen in the white matter (top left). The right column shows high PIB retention in the frontal and temporoparietal cortices of the AD patient (*top right*) and a typical pattern of ^{18}FDG hypometabolism present in the temporoparietal cortex (*arrows*; *bottom right*) along with reserved metabolic rate in the frontal cortex. PIB and ^{18}FDG scans were obtained within 3 days of each other. The figure is adapted from [121] with permission

[134], which provide a measure of presynaptic DA terminal function [135].

^{18}F-DOPA-PET has been used extensively to assess AADC activity in the DA terminals [136], since AADC converts L-DOPA to DA (which accumulates in the neuron). Thus, ^{18}F-DOPA-PET can be used as a measure of DA terminal functionality. Measurements of ^{18}F-DOPA uptake in the striatum of patients with PD will be influenced by the number of remaining dopaminergic cells. In addition, ^{18}F-DOPA uptake/binding correlates inversely with motor disability in PD (as measured by the Unified Parkinson's Disease Rating Scale [UPDRS]) [137]. Clinical progression has been studied with ^{18}F-DOPA-PET, and it has been shown that ^{18}F-DOPA uptake in the putamen is more correlated with disease progression than uptake in the caudate, which suggests that neuronal loss is slower in the caudate than in the putamen [137].

To compare changes and drug effects on D1 and D2 receptors in PD, a two-scan PET approach involving ^{11}C-SCH23390 to assess striatal D1 receptors and ^{11}C-raclopride to assess striatal D2 receptors has been used. Studies suggest there is abnormal binding of D2 and not D1 receptors in early PD [138]. In advanced PD cases, improvement in clinical function following oral L-DOPA administration was significantly correlated with reductions in ^{11}C-raclopride binding, suggesting an effect of increased DA on the striatal D2 receptors [139].

Non-dopaminergic imaging has also been performed in PD, including (a) imaging the cholinergic system with ^{11}C-PMP, ^{11}C-MP4A, and ^{11}C-NMPB, (b) imaging of the serotonergic system with ^{11}C-WAY100635, ^{11}C-DASB, and ^{11}C-McN5652, as well as (c) imaging the noradrenergic and opioid systems and activation of microglial in PD.

9.5.3 Differential Diagnosis of PD Based on Imaging

Since clinical features of PD may resemble other disorders, neuroimaging can often help with obtaining a correct diagnosis. As noted above, the broader category of "Parkinsonian syndromes" is often confused with PD during the early stages of disease. Corticobasal ganglionic degeneration (CGD), dementia with Lewy bodies (DLB), and Alzheimer's disease (AD) also share common clinical features with PD. It has been clearly shown that ^{18}F-DOPA and dopamine transporter PET imaging accurately reflect disturbances in monoamine (dopamine) metabolism in the striatum of patients with idiopathic PD and can be useful in situations where clinical uncertainty exists for patients with Parkinson-like movement disorders.

For example, drug-induced parkinsonism (DIP) is the most common of the secondary "Parkinsonian syndromes" [140], initially described as a complication of antipsychotic agents, but later recognized as possible side effects from antiemetics, cholinomimetics, antidepressants, anti-vertigo medications, calcium channel antagonists, antiarrhythmics, and antiepileptic drugs [141].^{18}F-DOPA (AADC activity) and dopamine transporter (DAT) PET and SPECT imaging have been used to differentiate between post-neuroleptic Parkinson-like symptoms from idiopathic PD. Neuroleptic-induced PD patients display intact DA terminals, normal ^{18}F-DOPA striatal PET scans, and normal dopamine transporter (DAT) scans; they do not respond to L-DOPA therapy and show no progression on follow-up, but may show improvement following cessation of the offending neuroleptic drug [142].

In another example, one study showed that volumetric analysis of MRI data and functional imaging of local metabolism (^{18}F-FDG-PET) and of postsynaptic D2 receptor density (^{11}C-raclopride PET) provides a clear distinction between PD and multiple system atrophy (MSA), consistent with the degeneration of striatal nuclei in MSA [143] (Fig. 9.8).

9.5.4 Diabetes

Type 2 diabetes mellitus (T2DM) and prediabetic insulin resistance (IR) are known to be associated with cognitive dysfunction and dementia later in life, including the development of Alzheimer's disease (AD) [144]. MRI and PET neuroimaging have contributed to a better understanding of the underlying brain processes involved in this association, as well as the relationships with other disease processes—such as hypertension, hypertensive cerebral vasculopathy (white matter lacunes and micro-hemorrhages), carotid artery atherosclerosis, and obesity. Brain imaging shows that changes associated with T2DM develop slowly over the course of many years. Both anatomical (structural MRI) and metabolic (functional PET) changes have been described comparing age-matched cohorts (nondiabetics with normal plasma glucose profiles, IR prediabetics, and T2DM). In addition, functional MRI

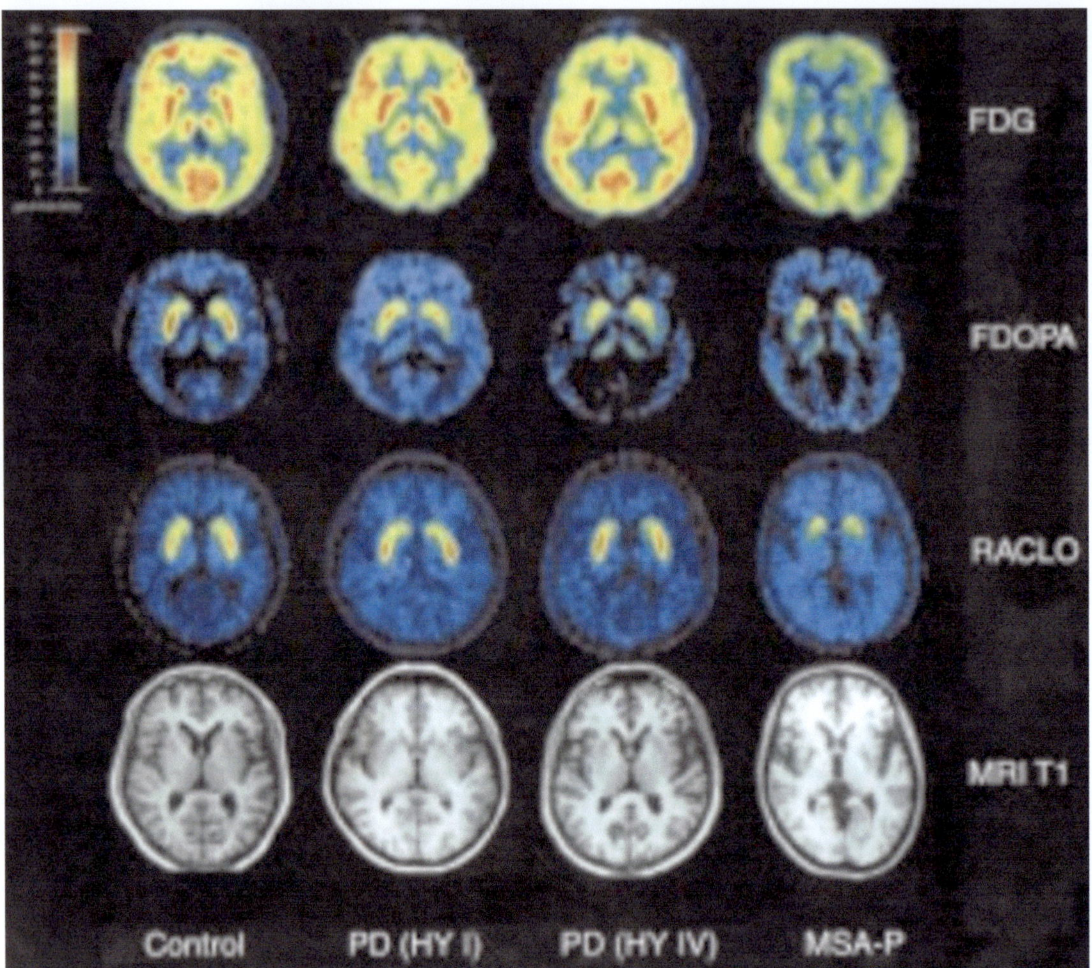

Fig. 9.8 Transaxial slices of FDG-PET, F-DOPA-PET, and RACLO-PET as well as T1-weighted MRI (from *top* to *bottom*) of a healthy control subject (control), two patients with idiopathic Parkinson's disease (early-stage PD HY I and advanced-stage PD HY IV), and a patient with striatonigral variant of multiple system atrophy (MSA-P) (from left to right). Note the marked decrease of putaminal volume (MRI), glucose consumption (FDG), and dopamine D2 receptor binding (RACLO) in MSA-P, which cannot be found in PD and controls. Reduction of putaminal F-DOPA influx constants are similarly visible in PD and MSA-P with an intranuclear gradient of radiotracer binding toward lower activity within the posterior part of the putamen. The figure is adapted from [143] with permission

(fMRI), diffusion tensor imaging, and magnetic resonance spectroscopy are current technologies being used to study the effects of IR prediabetes and T2DM on brain function [145].

Patients with T2DM develop slightly more global brain atrophy compared with normal aging, and these changes increase gradually over time. T2DM and IR prediabetics have more amygdala atrophy on MRI compared to normal subjects; T2DM also have greater hippocampal atrophy compared to normals. These changes were found to be independent of vascular pathology (although others state that the association with white matter hyperintensities and microbleeds is less clear). The longer the duration of T2DM, the greater the loss of brain volume, particularly in gray matter, which has been observed in serial MRI studies. In this T2DM cohort of patients, there was no association with small vessel ischemic disease [146].

A recent study investigated the causal risk factors for developing AD in three cohorts (IR and

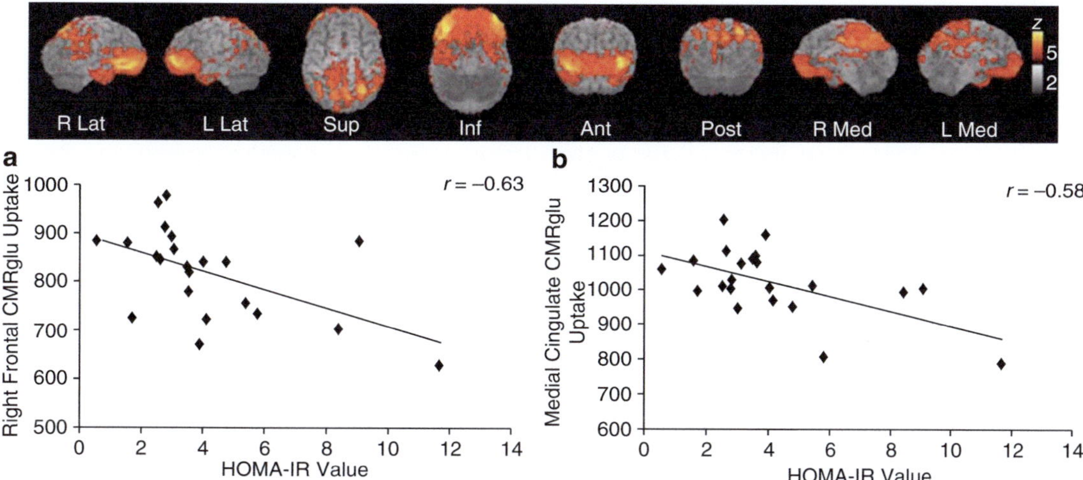

Fig. 9.9 *Upper Panel.* Brain regions in which a lower cerebral glucose metabolic rate was associated with greater insulin resistance as indexed by the homeostasis model assessment of insulin resistance. Regions in which the strongest negative associations were observed are represented in *yellow*. The vertical bar shows image color vs Z score scale. Image views are labeled as follows: *R* right, *L* left, *Lat* lateral, *Sup* superior, *Inf* inferior, *Ant* anterior, *Post* posterior, *Med* medial. *Lower Panel.* Scatterplots for cerebral glucose metabolic rate (CMRglu) and homeostasis model assessment of insulin resistance (HOMA-IR) values in frontal (**a**) and cingulate (**b**) cortices for adults with prediabetes or type 2 diabetes. The figure is adapted from [147] with permission

T2DM and normal age-matched controls) [147]. Cerebral glucose metabolic rate (CMRglu) was measured by ^{18}FDG-PET, and an assessment IR (HOMA-IR) was calculated using fasting glucose and insulin values obtained during an oral glucose tolerance test. HOMA-IR values were correlated with CMRglu values obtained during the resting scan. Greater insulin resistance was associated with an AD-like pattern of reduced CMRglu in frontal, parietotemporal, and cingulate regions in adults with PD/T2DM (Fig. 9.9). Resting CMRglu values were also subtracted from CMRglu values obtained during the memory encoding activation scan to examine task-related patterns of CMRglu. There was a different activation pattern in the IR/T2DM cohort compared to controls during the memory encoding task—a more diffuse and extensive activation pattern, associated with fewer recalled items on a delayed memory test.

As has been suggested in the literature, several questions remain: (1) Is the association between insulin resistance and AD causal? and (2) Are the mechanisms cerebrovascular or neurodegenerative (amyloid driven) [148]? Although there is a strong association between amyloid imaging and AD (less with MCI), it is not 100% predictive of AD. Nevertheless, the mechanistic link between IR/T2DM and AD would have been strengthened had the same cohorts in the Baker et al. study [147] undergone an amyloid imaging study as well. Maybe more important would be the clinical follow-up of these same patients, including sequential cognitive studies to assess for the development MCI or AD.

9.5.5 Depression

Depression is a complex neuropsychological disorder that has been sub-characterized as (a) major depressive disorder (MDD), (b) mono- and bipolar depressive disorder, and other less common subcategories. Major depressive episodes occur in both MDD and bipolar disorder, but bipolar disorder has distinct neuroimaging characteristics that distinguish it from MDD [149, 150]. The complex symptomatology is thought to be due to an imbalance of the neurotransmitter serotonin thought to be central to pathology. The precursor to serotonin is 5-hydroxytryptophan. The tryptophan-shuttle hypothesis ascribes the pathogenesis to shuttling of tryptophan from brain to the liver due increased cortisol [151].

Neuroimaging of cerebral blood flow (BF) identified the first physiological characteristic of depression, identifying increased BF in the *left* amygdala in unipolar depressives with familial pure depressive disease relative to healthy controls [152], which was confirmed in a later FDG-PET study and extended to bipolar disorder as well [153]. MDD is characterized by reduced FDG metabolism of the dorsolateral prefrontal cortex ("hypofrontality") and increased metabolism in limbic regions, such as the amygdala and insula, and in the subcallosal cingulate cortex [154].

Based on current "network models" of major depressive disorder, neuroimaging studies of MDD are now more focused on studying "aberrant function" within these intrinsically connected networks. Although there is not complete consistency, these studies point to identifying brain regions/structures contributing to specific networks that may be involved in specific types of mental activity. Coupling network models to neuroimaging technology as potential biomarkers has been a focus of research over the past decade. FDG-PET has been used to (a) characterize resting-state metabolic signatures and (b) measure the density of neurotransmitter receptors or transporters. MRI has been used to measure (a) the volume of specific brain structures (e.g., hippocampus), (b) functional metabolic activity patterns (fMRI) in response to specific challenges or tasks, or (c) white matter integrity and density (diffusion tensor imaging). fMRI patterns reflect states of brain metabolic activity. Enhanced (or diminished) metabolic activity of specific brain structures/regions is accompanied by corresponding changes in blood flow which can be detected by fMRI without exposure to radiation and with greater anatomical resolution. Both FDG-PET and fMRI images can also be examined in coordinated temporal patterns of activity across multiple regions (functional connectivity) [155].

Neuroimaging studies dating back to the late 1990s have suggested that pretreatment brain imaging of activity patterns can predict treatment efficacy [156] (Fig. 9.10). A potentially transformational development in the treatment of MDD is the application of neuroimaging to predict the best therapy for depression. Since only ~40% of patients treated for MDD achieve remission with initial treatment, the potential of a "treatment predictive" biological marker was tested in a small study (65 patients) [157]. This study showed that FDG-PET imaging of insula metabolism (relative to whole-brain mean metabolism) in MDD could predict treatment response. A good response to

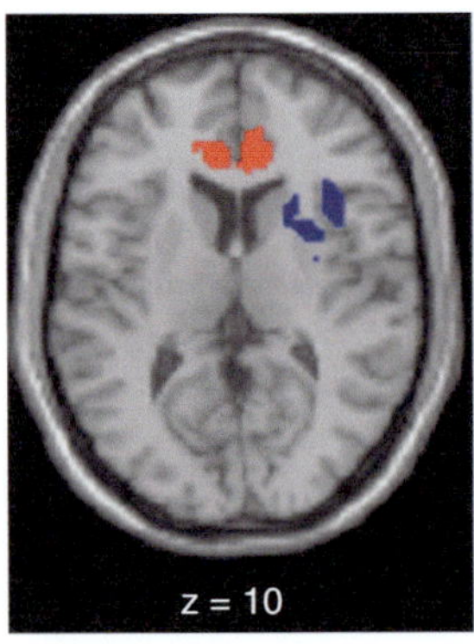

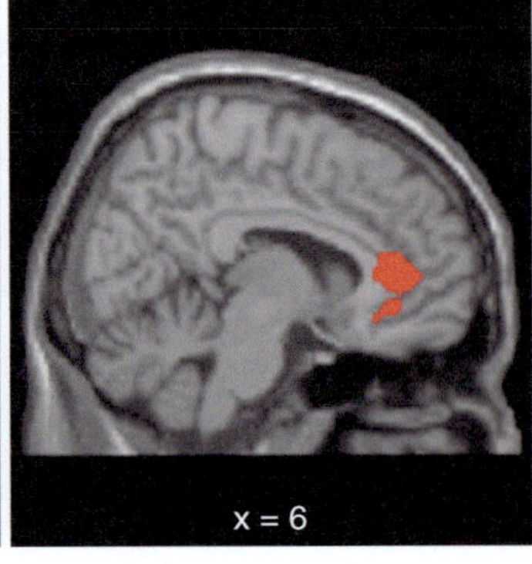

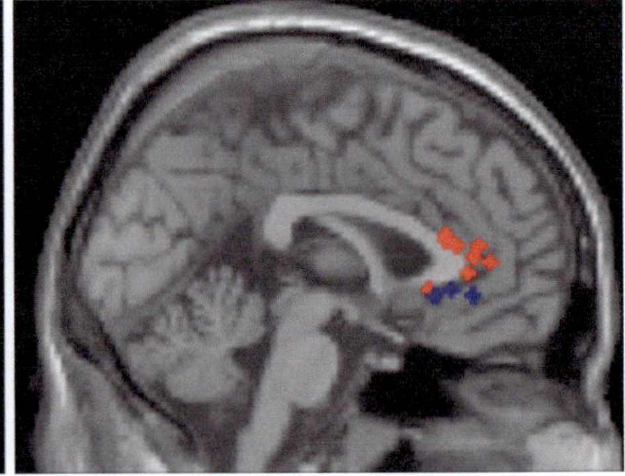

Fig. 9.10 Composite of a meta-analysis of functional predictors of treatment response in depression. Increased activation in anterior cingulate is predictive of positive response to treatment (in *red*), while increased activation in the right amygdala, striatum, and insula increases the likelihood of poor response (in *blue*). Results are $P < 0.05$ (with FDR multiple comparisons correction) (**a**). Analysis from an individual study findings in the anterior cingulate; areas of increased activation that were associated with a positive response to treatment are represented by red crosses, while the opposite finding of increased activation associated with a poor response are represented by *blue* crosses. The figure is adapted from [156] with permission

cognitive behavior therapy and a poor response to escitalopram were associated with "low" insula FDG metabolism, while insula "hypermetabolism" was associated with a good response to escitalopram and poor response to cognitive behavior therapy [157].

9.6 Concluding Remarks

This chapter has surveyed modern imaging approaches to brain metabolism and metabolic disorders. Having explored separate categories of canonical brain metabolic disorders and multifactorial disorders, we hope that the reader will come away with an understanding of the breadth of this topic and the utility of neuroimaging. This expansive field builds on discoveries in basic and clinical science, and is inherently linked to technical advances being made in neuroimaging.

References

1. Turner DA, Adamson DC. Neuronal-astrocyte metabolic interactions: understanding the transition into abnormal astrocytoma metabolism. J Neuropathol Exp Neurol. 2011;70:167–76.
2. Gropman AL. Patterns of brain injury in inborn errors of metabolism. Semin Pediatr Neurol. 2012;19:203–10.
3. Yoon HJ, Kim JH, Jeon TY, Yoo S-Y, Eo H. Devastating metabolic brain disorders of newborns and young infants. Radiographics. 2014;34:1257–72.
4. Cheon J-E, Kim I-O, Hwang YS, Kim KJ, Wang K-C, Cho B-K, Chi JG, Kim CJ, Kim WS, Yeon KM. Leukodystrophy in children: a pictorial review of MR imaging features. Radiographics. 2002;22:461–76.
5. Ibrahim M, Parmar HA, Hoefling N, Srinivasan A. Inborn errors of metabolism: combining clinical and radiologic clues to solve the mystery. Am J Roentgenol. 2014;203:W315–27.
6. Tkac I, Oz G, Adriany G, Ugurbil K, Gruetter R. In vivo ^{1}H NMR spectroscopy of the human brain at high magnetic fields: metabolite quantification at 4T vs. 7T. Magn Reson Med. 2009;62:868–79.
7. Kingsley PB, Shah TC, Woldenberg R. Identification of diffuse and focal brain lesions by clinical magnetic resonance spectroscopy. NMR Biomed. 2006;19:435–62.
8. Miloushev VZ, Keshari KR, Holodny AI. Hyperpolarization MRI: preclinical models and potential applications in neuroradiology. Top Magn Reson Imaging. 2016;25:31–7.
9. Sherry AD, Woods M. Chemical exchange saturation transfer contrast agents for magnetic resonance imaging. Annu Rev Biomed Eng. 2008;10:391–411.
10. Jasanoff A. MRI contrast agents for functional molecular imaging of brain activity. Curr Opin Neurobiol. 2007;17:593–600.
11. Nasrallah FA, Pages G, Kuchel PW, Golay X, Chuang KH. Imaging brain deoxyglucose uptake and metabolism by glucoCEST MRI. J Cereb Blood Flow Metab. 2013;33:1270–8.
12. Cai K, Haris M, Singh A, Kogan F, Greenberg JH, Hariharan H, Detre JA, Reddy R. Magnetic resonance imaging of glutamate. Nat Med. 2012;18:302–6.
13. Statistical Parametric Mapping. The analysis of functional brain images. 1st ed. New York: Academic; 2006.
14. Lake NJ, Compton AG, Rahman S, Thorburn DR. Leigh syndrome: one disorder, more than 75 monogenic causes. Ann Neurol. 2016;79:190–203.
15. Davis PC, Hoffman JC, Braun IF, Ahmann P, Krawiecki N. MR of Leigh's disease (subacute necrotizing encephalomyelopathy). Am J Neuroradiol. 1987;8:71–5.
16. Sperl W, Fleuren L, Freisinger P, Haack TB, Ribes A, Feichtinger RG, Rodenburg RJ, Zimmermann FA, Koch J, Rivera I, Prokisch H, Smeitink JA, Mayr JA. The spectrum of pyruvate oxidation defects in the diagnosis of mitochondrial disorders. J Inherit Metab Dis. 2015;38:391–403.
17. Natarajan N, Tully HM, Chapman T. Prenatal presentation of pyruvate dehydrogenase complex deficiency. Pediatr Radiol. 2016;46:1354–7.
18. Brown G. Pyruvate dehydrogenase deficiency and the brain. Dev Med Child Neurol. 2012;54:395–6.
19. Sharma R, Sharrard MJ, Connolly DJ, Mordekar SR. Unilateral periventricular leukomalacia in association with pyruvate dehydrogenase deficiency. Dev Med Child Neurol. 2012;54:469–71.
20. Jha MK, Song GJ, Lee MG, Jeoung NH, Go Y, Harris RA, Park DH, Kook H, Lee IK, Suk K. Metabolic connection of inflammatory pain: pivotal role of a pyruvate dehydrogenase kinase-pyruvate dehydrogenase-lactic acid Axis. J Neurosci. 2015;35:14353–69.
21. Prasad C, Rupar T, Prasad AN. Pyruvate dehydrogenase deficiency and epilepsy. Brain and Development. 2011;33:856–65.
22. Jain-Ghai S, Cameron JM, Al Maawali A, Blaser S, MacKay N, Robinson B, Raiman J, Complex II. Deficiency-a case report and review of the literature. Am J Med Genet A. 2013;161a:285–94.
23. O. Online Mendelian Inheritance in Man, Complex II, in, Johns Hopkins University, Baltimore, MD, 2016.
24. Hoekstra AS, Bayley JP. The role of complex II in disease. Biochim Biophys Acta. 2013;1827:543–51.

25. Baysal BE, Maher ER. 15 YEARS OF PARAGANGLIOMA: genetics and mechanism of pheochromocytoma-paraganglioma syndromes characterized by germline SDHB and SDHD mutations. Endocr Relat Cancer. 2015;22:T71–82.
26. O. Online Mendelian Inheritance in Man, MELAS, in, Johns Hopkins University, Baltimore, MD, 2016.
27. Haraguchi M, Tsujimoto H, Fukushima M, Higuchi I, Kuribayashi H, Utsumi H, Nakayama A, Hashizume Y, Hirato J, Yoshida H, Hara H, Hamano S, Kawaguchi H, Furukawa T, Miyazono K, Ishikawa F, Toyoshima H, Kaname T, Komatsu M, Chen ZS, Gotanda T, Tachiwada T, Sumizawa T, Miyadera K, Osame M, Yoshida H, Noda T, Yamada Y, Akiyama S. Targeted deletion of both thymidine phosphorylase and uridine phosphorylase and consequent disorders in mice. Mol Cell Biol. 2002;22:5212–21.
28. Shevell MI, Matthews PM, Scriver CR, Brown RM, Otero LJ, Legris M, Brown GK, Arnold DL. Cerebral dysgenesis and lactic acidemia: an MRI/MRS phenotype associated with pyruvate dehydrogenase deficiency. Pediatr Neurol. 1994;11:224–9.
29. Cross JH, Connelly A, Gadian DG, Kendall BE, Brown GK, Brown RM, Leonard JV. Clinical diversity of pyruvate dehydrogenase deficiency. Pediatr Neurol. 1994;10:276–83.
30. Wilichowski E, Pouwels PJ, Frahm J, Hanefeld F. Quantitative proton magnetic resonance spectroscopy of cerebral metabolic disturbances in patients with MELAS. Neuropediatrics. 1999;30:256–63.
31. Krageloh-Mann I, Grodd W, Schoning M, Marquard K, Nagele T, Ruitenbeek W. Proton spectroscopy in five patients with Leigh's disease and mitochondrial enzyme deficiency. Dev Med Child Neurol. 1993;35:769–76.
32. Chuang CS, Lo MC, Lee KW, Liu CS. Magnetic resonance spectroscopy study in basal ganglia of patients with myoclonic epilepsy with ragged-red fibers. Neurol India. 2007;55:385–7.
33. Helman G, Caldovic L, Whitehead MT, Simons C, Brockmann K, Edvardson S, Bai R, Moroni I, Taylor JM, Haren KV, Taft RJ, Vanderver A, van der Knaap MS. Magnetic resonance imaging spectrum of succinate dehydrogenase-related infantile leukoencephalopathy. Ann Neurol. 2016;79:379–86.
34. Natesan V, Mani R, Arumugam R. Clinical aspects of urea cycle dysfunction and altered brain energy metabolism on modulation of glutamate receptors and transporters in acute and chronic hyperammonemia. Biomed Pharmacother. 2016;81:192–202.
35. Connelly A, Cross JH, Gadian DG, Hunter JV, Kirkham FJ, Leonard JV. Magnetic resonance spectroscopy shows increased brain glutamine in ornithine carbamoyl transferase deficiency. Pediatr Res. 1993;33:77–81.
36. Zhang J, Liu Q. Cholesterol metabolism and homeostasis in the brain. Protein Cell. 2015;6:254–64.
37. Cerqueira NMFSA, Oliveira EF, Gesto DS, Santos-Martins D, Moreira C, Moorthy HN, Ramos MJ, Fernandes PA. Cholesterol biosynthesis: a mechanistic overview. Biochemistry. 2016;55:5483–506.
38. Herman GE. Disorders of cholesterol biosynthesis: prototypic metabolic malformation syndromes. Hum Mol Genet, 12 Spec. 2003;1:R75–88.
39. Tierney E, Nwokoro NA, Porter FD, Freund LS, Ghuman JK, Kelley RI. Behavior phenotype in the RSH/Smith-Lemli-Opitz syndrome. Am J Med Genet. 2001;98:191–200.
40. Sikora DM, Pettit-Kekel K, Penfield J, Merkens LS, Steiner RD. The near universal presence of autism spectrum disorders in children with Smith-Lemli-Opitz syndrome. Am J Med Genet A. 2006;140:1511–8.
41. Lee RW, Conley SK, Gropman A, Porter FD, Baker EH. Brain magnetic resonance imaging findings in Smith-Lemli-Opitz syndrome. Am J Med Genet A. 2013;161a:2407–19.
42. Caruso PA, Poussaint TY, Tzika AA, Zurakowski D, Astrakas LG, Elias ER, Bay C, Irons MB. MRI and ^{1}H MRS findings in Smith-Lemli-Opitz syndrome. Neuroradiology. 2004;46:3–14.
43. Paine RS. The variability in manifestations of untreated patients with phenylketonuria (phenylpyruvic aciduria). Pediatrics. 1957;20:290–302.
44. O. Online Mendelian Inheritance in Man, Phenylketonuria, in, Johns Hopkins University, Baltimore, MD, 2016.
45. Tufekcioglu Z, Cakar A, Bilgic B, Hanagasi H, Gurvit H, Emre M. Adult-onset phenylketonuria with rapidly progressive dementia and parkinsonism. Neurocase. 2016;22:273–5.
46. Anderson PJ, Leuzzi V. White matter pathology in phenylketonuria. Mol Genet Metab. 2010;99(Suppl 1):S3–9.
47. Bodner KE, Aldridge K, Moffitt AJ, Peck D, White DA, Christ SE. A volumetric study of basal ganglia structures in individuals with early-treated phenylketonuria. Mol Genet Metab. 2012;107:302–7.
48. Christ SE, Price MH, Bodner KE, Saville C, Moffitt AJ, Peck D. Morphometric analysis of gray matter integrity in individuals with early-treated phenylketonuria. Mol Genet Metab. 2016;118:3–8.
49. E.J. Novotny, Jr., M.J. Avison, N. Herschkowitz, O.A. Petroff, J.W. Prichard, M.R. Seashore, D.L. Rothman, In vivo measurement of phenylalanine in human brain by proton nuclear magnetic resonance spectroscopy, Pediatr Res, 37 (1995) 244–249.
50. Pietz J, Rupp A, Ebinger F, Rating D, Mayatepek E, Boesch C, Kreis R. Cerebral energy metabolism in phenylketonuria: findings by quantitative in vivo 31P MR spectroscopy. Pediatr Res. 2003;53:654–62.
51. Horder J, Lavender T, Mendez MA, O'Gorman R, Daly E, Craig MC, Lythgoe DJ, Barker GJ, Murphy DG. Reduced subcortical glutamate/glutamine in adults with autism spectrum disorders: a [(1)H]MRS study. Transl Psychiatry. 2013;3:e279.
52. Christ SE, Moffitt AJ, Peck D. Disruption of prefrontal function and connectivity in individuals with

phenylketonuria. Mol Genet Metab. 2010;99(Suppl 1):S33–40.

53. Ficicioglu C, Dubroff JG, Thomas N, Gallagher PR, Burfield J, Hussa C, Randall R, Zhuang H. A pilot study of Fluorodeoxyglucose positron emission tomography findings in patients with phenylketonuria before and during Sapropterin supplementation. J Clin Neurol. 2013;9:151–6.
54. O. Online Mendelian Inheritance in Man, MSUD, in, Johns Hopkins University, Baltimore, MD, 2016.
55. Indo Y, Akaboshi I, Nobukuni Y, Endo F, Matsuda I. Maple syrup urine disease: a possible biochemical basis for the clinical heterogeneity. Hum Genet. 1988;80:6–10.
56. Brismar J, Aqeel A, Brismar G, Coates R, Gascon G, Ozand P. Maple syrup urine disease: findings on CT and MR scans of the brain in 10 infants. AJNR Am J Neuroradiol. 1990;11:1219–28.
57. Cavalleri F, Berardi A, Burlina AB, Ferrari F, Mavilla L. Diffusion-weighted MRI of maple syrup urine disease encephalopathy. Neuroradiology. 2002;44:499–502.
58. Sato T, Muroya K, Hanakawa J, Asakura Y, Aida N, Tomiyasu M, Tajima G, Hasegawa T, Adachi M. Neonatal case of classic maple syrup urine disease: usefulness of (1) H-MRS in early diagnosis. Pediatr Int. 2014;56:112–5.
59. O. Online Mendelian Inheritance in Man, Canavan Disease, in, Johns Hopkins University, Baltimore, MD, 2016.
60. Brismar J, Brismar G, Gascon G, Ozand P. Canavan disease: CT and MR imaging of the brain. AJNR Am J Neuroradiol. 1990;11:805–10.
61. Hiraga K, Kochi H, Hayasaka K, Kikuchi G, Nyhan WL. Defective glycine cleavage system in nonketotic hyperglycinemia. Occurrence of a less active glycine decarboxylase and an abnormal aminomethyl carrier protein. J Clin Invest. 1981;68:525–34.
62. O. Online Mendelian Inheritance in Man, Nonketotic Hyperglycinemia, in, Johns Hopkins University, Baltimore, MD, 2016.
63. Mourmans J, Majoie CB, Barth PG, Duran M, Akkerman EM, Poll-The BT. Sequential MR imaging changes in Nonketotic Hyperglycinemia. Am J Neuroradiol. 2006;27:208–11.
64. Elsea SH, Juyal RC, Jiralerspong S, Finucane BM, Pandolfo M, Greenberg F, Baldini A, Stover P, Patel PI. Haploinsufficiency of cytosolic serine hydroxymethyltransferase in the Smith-Magenis syndrome. Am J Hum Genet. 1995;57:1342–50.
65. O. Online Mendelian Inheritance in Man, Smith-Magenis, in, Johns Hopkins University, Baltimore, MD, 2016.
66. Capra V, Biancheri R, Morana G, Striano P, Novara F, Ferrero GB, Boeri L, Celle ME, Mancardi MM, Zuffardi O, Parrini E, Guerrini R. Periventricular nodular heterotopia in Smith-Magenis syndrome. Am J Med Genet A. 2014;164a:3142–7.
67. O. Online Mendelian Inheritance in Man, Isovaleric Acidemia, in, Johns Hopkins University, Baltimore, MD, 2016.
68. Wani NA, Qureshi UA, Jehangir M, Ahmad K, Hussain Z. Atypical MR lenticular signal change in infantile isovaleric acidemia. Indian J Radiol Imaging. 2016;26:131–4.
69. O. Online Mendelian Inheritance in Man, Propionic Acidemia, in, Johns Hopkins University, Baltimore, MD, 2016.
70. Bergman AJ, Van der Knaap MS, Smeitink JA, Duran M, Dorland L, Valk J, Poll-The BT. Magnetic resonance imaging and spectroscopy of the brain in propionic acidemia: clinical and biochemical considerations. Pediatr Res. 1996;40:404–9.
71. Chemelli AP, Schocke M, Sperl W, Trieb T, Aichner F, Felber S. Magnetic resonance spectroscopy (MRS) in five patients with treated propionic acidemia. J Magn Reson Imaging. 2000;11:596–600.
72. O. Online Mendelian Inheritance in Man, Methylmalonic Acidemia, in, Johns Hopkins University, Baltimore, MD, 2016.
73. Radmanesh A, Zaman T, Ghanaati H, Molaei S, Robertson RL, Zamani AA. Methylmalonic acidemia: brain imaging findings in 52 children and a review of the literature. Pediatr Radiol. 2008;38:1054–61.
74. Baker EH, Sloan JL, Hauser NS, Gropman AL, Adams DR, Toro C, Manoli I, Venditti CP. MRI characteristics of globus pallidus infarcts in isolated methylmalonic acidemia. AJNR Am J Neuroradiol. 2015;36:194–201.
75. Gao Y, Guan WY, Wang J, Zhang YZ, Li YH, Han LS. Fractional anisotropy for assessment of white matter tracts injury in methylmalonic acidemia. Chin Med J. 2009;122:945–9.
76. Takeuchi M, Harada M, Matsuzaki K, Hisaoka S, Nishitani H, Mori K. Magnetic resonance imaging and spectroscopy in a patient with treated methylmalonic acidemia. J Comput Assist Tomogr. 2003;27:547–51.
77. Weller S, Rosewich H, Gartner J. Cerebral MRI as a valuable diagnostic tool in Zellweger spectrum patients. J Inherit Metab Dis. 2008;31:270–80.
78. Rosewich H, Dechent P, Krause C, Ohlenbusch A, Brockmann K, Gartner J. Diagnostic and prognostic value of in vivo proton MR spectroscopy for Zellweger syndrome spectrum patients. J Inherit Metab Dis. 2016;
79. Groenendaal F, Bianchi MC, Battini R, Tosetti M, Boldrini A, de Vries LS, Cioni G. Proton magnetic resonance spectroscopy (^{1}H-MRS) of the cerebrum in two young infants with Zellweger syndrome. Neuropediatrics. 2001;32:23–7.
80. Eichler FS, Barker PB, Cox C, Edwin D, Ulug AM, Moser HW, Raymond GV. Proton MR spectroscopic imaging predicts lesion progression on MRI in X-linked adrenoleukodystrophy. Neurology. 2002;58:901–7.

81. Salsano E, Marotta G, Manfredi V, Giovagnoli AR, Farina L, Savoiardo M, Pareyson D, Benti R, Uziel G. Brain fluorodeoxyglucose PET in adrenoleukodystrophy. Neurology. 2014;83:981–9.
82. Nishio H, Kodama S, Tsubota T, Takumi T, Takahashi T, Yokoyama S, Matsuo T. Adrenoleukodystrophy without adrenal insufficiency and its magnetic resonance imaging. J Neurol. 1985;232:265–70.
83. O. Online Mendelian Inheritance in Man, Gaucher Disease Type I, in, Johns Hopkins University, Baltimore, MD, 2016.
84. Mercimek-Mahmutoglu S, Gruber S, Rolfs A, Stadlbauer A, Woeber C, Kurnik P, Voigtlaender T, Moser E, Stoeckler-Ipsiroglu S. Neurological and brain MRS findings in patients with Gaucher disease type 1. Mol Genet Metab. 2007;91:390–5.
85. Holmay MJ, Terpstra M, Coles LD, Mishra U, Ahlskog M, Oz G, Cloyd JC, Tuite PJ. N-Acetylcysteine boosts brain and blood glutathione in Gaucher and Parkinson diseases. Clin Neuropharmacol. 2013;36:103–6.
86. Davies EH, Seunarine KK, Banks T, Clark CA, Vellodi A. Brain white matter abnormalities in paediatric Gaucher type I and type III using diffusion tensor imaging. J Inherit Metab Dis. 2011;34:549–53.
87. Abdel Razek AA, Abd El-Gaber N, Abdalla A, Fathy A, Azab A, Rahman AA. Apparent diffusion coefficient Vale of the brain in patients with Gaucher's disease type II and type III. Neuroradiology. 2009;51:773–9.
88. Reider-Grosswasser I, Bornstein N. CT and MRI in late-onset metachromatic leukodystrophy. Acta Neurol Scand. 1987;75:64–9.
89. Kruse B, Hanefeld F, Christen HJ, Bruhn H, Michaelis T, Hanicke W, Frahm J. Alterations of brain metabolites in metachromatic leukodystrophy as detected by localized proton magnetic resonance spectroscopy in vivo. J Neurol. 1993;241:68–74.
90. Assadi M, Wang DJ, Velazquez-Rodriquez Y, Leone P. Multi-voxel ^{1}H-MRS in metachromatic Leukodystrophy. J Cent Nerv Syst Dis. 2013;5:25–30.
91. Menzies DG, Campbell IW, Kean DM. Magnetic resonance imaging in Fabry's disease. J Neurol Neurosurg Psychiatry. 1988;51:1240–1.
92. Moore DF, Altarescu G, Barker WC, Patronas NJ, Herscovitch P, Schiffmann R. White matter lesions in Fabry disease occur in 'prior' selectively hypometabolic and hyperperfused brain regions. Brain Res Bull. 2003;62:231–40.
93. Korsholm K, Feldt-Rasmussen U, Granqvist H, Hojgaard L, Bollinger B, Rasmussen AK, Law I. Positron emission tomography and magnetic resonance imaging of the brain in Fabry disease: a Nationwide, long-time, prospective follow-up. PLoS One. 2015;10:e0143940.
94. Tedeschi G, Bonavita S, Banerjee TK, Virta A, Schiffmann R. Diffuse central neuronal involvement in Fabry disease: a proton MRS imaging study. Neurology. 1999;52:1663–7.
95. Vance JE. Lipid imbalance in the neurological disorder, Niemann-pick C disease. FEBS Lett. 2006;580:5518–24.
96. O. Online Mendelian Inheritance in Man, Niemann Pick Disease, in, Johns Hopkins University, Baltimore, MD, 2016.
97. D'Amico A, Sibilio M, Caranci F, Bartiromo F, Taurisano R, Balivo F, Melis D, Parenti G, Cirillo S, Elefante R, Brunetti A. Type a niemann-pick disease. Description of three cases with delayed myelination, Neuroradiol J. 2008;21:309–15.
98. Grau AJ, Brandt T, Weisbrod M, Niethammer R, Forsting M, Cantz M, Vanier MT, Harzer K. Adult Niemann-pick disease type C mimicking features of multiple sclerosis. J Neurol Neurosurg Psychiatry. 1997;63:552.
99. Masingue M, Adanyeguh I, Nadjar Y, Sedel F, Galanaud D, Mochel F. Evolution of structural neuroimaging biomarkers in a series of adult patients with Niemann-pick type C under treatment. Orphanet J Rare Dis. 2017;12:22.
100. Demaerel P, Wilms G, Verdru P, Carton H, Baert AL. MR findings in globoid cell leucodystrophy. Neuroradiology. 1990;32:520–2.
101. Jones BV, Barron TF, Towfighi J. Optic nerve enlargement in Krabbe's disease. AJNR Am J Neuroradiol. 1999;20:1228–31.
102. Kang PB, Hunter JV, Kaye EM. Lactic acid elevation in extramitochondrial childhood neurodegenerative diseases. J Child Neurol. 2001;16:657–60.
103. Zarifi MK, Tzika AA, Astrakas LG, Poussaint TY, Anthony DC, Darras BT. Magnetic resonance spectroscopy and magnetic resonance imaging findings in Krabbe's disease. J Child Neurol. 2001;16:522–6.
104. O. Online Mendelian Inheritance in Man, Tay-Sachs Disease, in, Johns Hopkins University, Baltimore, MD, 2016.
105. Mugikura S, Takahashi S, Higano S, Kurihara N, Kon K, Sakamoto K. MR findings in Tay-Sachs disease. J Comput Assist Tomogr. 1996;20:551–5.
106. Jamrozik Z, Lugowska A, Golebiowski M, Krolicki L, Maczewska J, Kuzma-Kozakiewicz M. Late onset GM2 gangliosidosis mimicking spinal muscular atrophy. Gene. 2013;527:679–82.
107. Aydin K, Bakir B, Tatli B, Terzibasioglu E, Ozmen M. Proton MR spectroscopy in three children with Tay-Sachs disease. Pediatr Radiol. 2005;35:1081–5.
108. Wraith JE, Jones S. Mucopolysaccharidosis type I. Pediatr Endocrinol Rev. 2014;12(Suppl 1):102–6.
109. Kosuga M, Mashima R, Hirakiyama A, Fuji N, Kumagai T, Seo JH, Nikaido M, Saito S, Ohno K, Sakuraba H, Okuyama T. Molecular diagnosis of 65 families with mucopolysaccharidosis type II (Hunter syndrome) characterized by 16 novel mutations in the IDS gene: genetic, pathological, and structural studies on iduronate-2-sulfatase. Mol Genet Metab. 2016;118:190–7.

110. Reichert R, Campos LG, Vairo F, de Souza CF, Perez JA, Duarte JA, Leiria FA, Anes M, Vedolin LM. Neuroimaging findings in patients with Mucopolysaccharidosis: what you really need to know. Radiographics. 2016;36:1448–62.
111. Takahashi Y, Sukegawa K, Aoki M, Ito A, Suzuki K, Sakaguchi H, Watanabe M, Isogai K, Mizuno S, Hoshi H, Kuwata K, Tomatsu S, Kato S, Ito T, Kondo N, Orii T. Evaluation of accumulated mucopolysaccharides in the brain of patients with mucopolysaccharidoses by (1)H-magnetic resonance spectroscopy before and after bone marrow transplantation. Pediatr Res. 2001;49:349–55.
112. Shapiro E, Guler OE, Rudser K, Delaney K, Bjoraker K, Whitley C, Tolar J, Orchard P, Provenzale J, Thomas KM. An exploratory study of brain function and structure in mucopolysaccharidosis type I: long term observations following hematopoietic cell transplantation (HCT). Mol Genet Metab. 2012;107:116–21.
113. Shimoda-Matsubayashi S, Kuru Y, Sumie H, Ito T, Hattori N, Okuma Y, Mizuno Y. MRI findings in the mild type of mucopolysaccharidosis II (Hunter's syndrome). Neuroradiology. 1990;32:328–30.
114. Quigley H, Colloby SJ, O'Brien JT. PET imaging of brain amyloid in dementia: a review. Int J Geriatr Psychiatry. 2011;26:991–9.
115. Morys J, Bobek-Billewicz B, Dziewiatkowski J, Bidzan L, Ussorowska D, Narklewicz O. Changes in the volume of temporal lobe structures related to Alzheimer's type dementia. Folia Neuropathol. 2002;40:47–56.
116. Salmon E. Functional brain imaging applications to differential diagnosis in the dementias. Curr Opin Neurol. 2002;15:439–44.
117. Mazziotta JC, Frackowiak RS, Phelps ME. The use of positron emission tomography in the clinical assessment of dementia. Semin Nucl Med. 1992;22:233–46.
118. Salmon E, Gregoire MC, Delfiore G, Lemaire C, Degueldre C, Franck G, Comar D. Combined study of cerebral glucose metabolism and [11C]methionine accumulation in probable Alzheimer's disease using positron emission tomography. J Cereb Blood Flow Metab. 1996;16:399–408.
119. Bohnen NI, Djang DS, Herholz K, Anzai Y, Minoshima S. Effectiveness and safety of ^{18}F-FDG PET in the evaluation of dementia: a review of the recent literature. J Nucl Med. 2012;53:59–71.
120. Kato T, Inui Y, Nakamura A, Ito K. Brain fluorodeoxyglucose (FDG) PET in dementia. Ageing Res Rev. 2016;30:73–84.
121. Klunk WE, Engler H, Nordberg A, Wang Y, Blomqvist G, Holt DP, Bergstrom M, Savitcheva I, Huang GF, Estrada S, Ausen B, Debnath ML, Barletta J, Price JC, Sandell J, Lopresti BJ, Wall A, Koivisto P, Antoni G, Mathis CA, Langstrom B. Imaging brain amyloid in Alzheimer's disease with Pittsburgh compound-B. Ann Neurol. 2004;55:306–19.
122. Fagan AM, Mintun MA, Mach RH, Lee SY, Dence CS, Shah AR, LaRossa GN, Spinner ML, Klunk WE, Mathis CA, DeKosky ST, Morris JC, Holtzman DM. Inverse relation between in vivo amyloid imaging load and cerebrospinal fluid Abeta42 in humans. Ann Neurol. 2006;59:512–9.
123. Ewers M, Sperling RA, Klunk WE, Weiner MW, Hampel H. Neuroimaging markers for the prediction and early diagnosis of Alzheimer's disease dementia. Trends Neurosci. 2011;34:430–42.
124. Clark CM, Schneider JA, Bedell BJ, Beach TG, Bilker WB, Mintun MA, Pontecorvo MJ, Hefti F, Carpenter AP, Flitter ML, Krautkramer MJ, Kung HF, Coleman RE, Doraiswamy PM, Fleisher AS, Sabbagh MN, Sadowsky CH, Reiman EP, Zehntner SP, Skovronsky DM. Use of florbetapir-PET for imaging beta-amyloid pathology. JAMA. 2011;305:275–83.
125. Fleisher AS, Chen K, Liu X, Roontiva A, Thiyyagura P, Ayutyanont N, Joshi AD, Clark CM, Mintun MA, Pontecorvo MJ, Doraiswamy PM, Johnson KA, Skovronsky DM, Reiman EM. Using positron emission tomography and florbetapir F18 to image cortical amyloid in patients with mild cognitive impairment or dementia due to Alzheimer disease. Arch Neurol. 2011;68:1404–11.
126. Dani M, Brooks DJ, Edison P. Tau imaging in neurodegenerative diseases. Eur J Nucl Med Mol Imaging. 2016;43:1139–50.
127. Silverman DH, Small GW, Chang CY, Lu CS, Kung De Aburto MA, Chen W, Czernin J, Rapoport SI, Pietrini P, Alexander GE, Schapiro MB, Jagust WJ, Hoffman JM, Welsh-Bohmer KA, Alavi A, Clark CM, Salmon E, de Leon MJ, Mielke R, Cummings JL, Kowell AP, Gambhir SS, Hoh CK, Phelps ME. Positron emission tomography in evaluation of dementia: regional brain metabolism and long-term outcome. JAMA. 2001;286:2120–7.
128. Sperling R. Potential of functional MRI as a biomarker in early Alzheimer's disease. Neurobiol Aging. 2011;32(Suppl 1):S37–43.
129. Bondi MW, Houston WS, Eyler LT, Brown GG. fMRI evidence of compensatory mechanisms in older adults at genetic risk for Alzheimer disease. Neurology. 2005;64:501–8.
130. Smailagic N, Vacante M, Hyde C, Martin S, Ukoumunne O, Sachpekidis C. (1)(8)F-FDG PET for the early diagnosis of Alzheimer's disease dementia and other dementias in people with mild cognitive impairment (MCI). Cochrane Database Syst Rev. 2015;1:Cd010632.
131. Zhang S, Smailagic N, Hyde C, Noel-Storr AH, Takwoingi Y, McShane R, Feng J. (11)C-PIB-PET for the early diagnosis of Alzheimer's disease dementia and other dementias in people with mild cognitive impairment (MCI). Cochrane Database Syst Rev. 2014;1:Cd010386.
132. Leenders KL, Salmon EP, Tyrrell P, Perani D, Brooks DJ, Sager H, Jones T, Marsden CD, Frackowiak

RS. The nigrostriatal dopaminergic system assessed in vivo by positron emission tomography in healthy volunteer subjects and patients with Parkinson's disease. Arch Neurol. 1990;47:1290–8.
133. Sixel-Doring F, Liepe K, Mollenhauer B, Trautmann E, Trenkwalder C. The role of 123I-FP-CIT-SPECT in the differential diagnosis of Parkinson and tremor syndromes: a critical assessment of 125 cases. J Neurol. 2011;258:2147–54.
134. de la Fuente-Fernandez R, Sossi V, McCormick S, Schulzer M, Ruth TJ, Stoessl AJ. Visualizing vesicular dopamine dynamics in Parkinson's disease. Synapse. 2009;63:713–6.
135. Marie RM, Barre L, Rioux P, Allain P, Lechevalier B, Baron JC. PET imaging of neocortical monoaminergic terminals in Parkinson's disease. J Neural Transm Park Dis Dement Sect. 1995;9:55–71.
136. Garnett ES, Firnau G, Nahmias C. Dopamine visualized in the basal ganglia of living man. Nature. 1983;305:137–8.
137. Broussolle E, Dentresangle C, Landais P, Garcia-Larrea L, Pollak P, Croisile B, Hibert O, Bonnefoi F, Galy G, Froment JC, Comar D. The relation of putamen and caudate nucleus ^{18}F-Dopa uptake to motor and cognitive performances in Parkinson's disease. J Neurol Sci. 1999;166:141–51.
138. Cropley VL, Fujita M, Bara-Jimenez W, Brown AK, Zhang XY, Sangare J, Herscovitch P, Pike VW, Hallett M, Nathan PJ, Innis RB. Pre- and postsynaptic dopamine imaging and its relation with frontostriatal cognitive function in Parkinson disease: PET studies with [11C]NNC 112 and [^{18}F] FDOPA. Psychiatry Res. 2008;163:171–82.
139. Pavese N, Evans AH, Tai YF, Hotton G, Brooks DJ, Lees AJ, Piccini P. Clinical correlates of levodopa-induced dopamine release in Parkinson disease: a PET study. Neurology. 2006;67:1612–7.
140. José López-Sendón MAM, Yébenes JG d. Drug induced parkinsonism. Expert Opin Drug Saf. 2013;12:487–96.
141. Yébenes MAMaJGd. Drug-induced parkinsonism. Expert Opin Drug Saf. 2006;5:759–71.
142. Burn DJ, Brooks DJ. Nigral dysfunction in drug-induced parkinsonism: an ^{18}F-dopa PET study. Neurology. 1993;43:552–6.
143. Ghaemi M, Hilker R, Rudolf J, Sobesky J, Heiss WD. Differentiating multiple system atrophy from Parkinson's disease: contribution of striatal and midbrain MRI volumetry and multi-tracer PET imaging. J Neurol Neurosurg Psychiatry. 2002;73:517–23.
144. Biessels GJ, Staekenborg S, Brunner E, Brayne C, Scheltens P. Risk of dementia in diabetes mellitus: a systematic review. Lancet Neurol. 2006;5:64–74.
145. van Harten B, de Leeuw FE, Weinstein HC, Scheltens P, Biessels GJ. Brain imaging in patients with diabetes: a systematic review. Diabetes Care. 2006;29:2539–48.
146. Last D, Alsop DC, Abduljalil AM, Marquis RP, de Bazelaire C, Hu K, Cavallerano J, Novak V. Global and regional effects of type 2 diabetes on brain tissue volumes and cerebral vasoreactivity. Diabetes Care. 2007;30:1193–9.
147. Baker LD, Cross DJ, Minoshima S, Belongia D, Watson GS, Craft S. Insulin resistance and Alzheimer-like reductions in regional cerebral glucose metabolism for cognitively normal adults with prediabetes or early type 2 diabetes. Arch Neurol. 2011;68:51–7.
148. Luchsinger JA, Small S, Biessels GJ. Should we target insulin resistance to prevent dementia due to Alzheimer disease? Arch Neurol. 2011;68:17–8.
149. Cardoso de Almeida JR, Phillips ML. Distinguishing between unipolar depression and bipolar depression: current and future clinical and neuroimaging perspectives. Biol Psychiatry. 2013;73:111–8.
150. Phillips ML, Swartz HA. A critical appraisal of neuroimaging studies of bipolar disorder: toward a new conceptualization of underlying neural circuitry and a road map for future research. Am J Psychiatry. 2014;171:829–43.
151. Oxenkrug GF. Tryptophan–Kynurenine metabolism as a common mediator of genetic and environmental impacts in major depressive disorder: the serotonin hypothesis revisited 40 years later. Isr J Psychiatry Relat Sci. 2010;47:56–63.
152. Drevets WC, Videen TO, Price JL, Preskorn SH, Carmichael ST, Raichle ME. A functional anatomical study of unipolar depression. J Neurosci. 1992;12:3628–41.
153. Drevets WC, Price JL, Bardgett ME, Reich T, Todd RD, Raichle ME. Glucose metabolism in the amygdala in depression: relationship to diagnostic subtype and plasma cortisol levels. Pharmacol Biochem Behav. 2002;71:431–47.
154. Ressler KJ, Mayberg HS. Targeting abnormal neural circuits in mood and anxiety disorders: from the laboratory to the clinic. Nat Neurosci. 2007;10:1116–24.
155. Wu J, Buchsbaum MS, Gillin JC, Tang C, Cadwell S, Wiegand M, Najafi A, Klein E, Hazen K, Bunney WE Jr, Fallon JH, Keator D. Prediction of antidepressant effects of sleep deprivation by metabolic rates in the ventral anterior cingulate and medial prefrontal cortex. Am J Psychiatry. 1999;156:1149–58.
156. Fu CH, Steiner H, Costafreda SG. Predictive neural biomarkers of clinical response in depression: a meta-analysis of functional and structural neuroimaging studies of pharmacological and psychological therapies. Neurobiol Dis. 2013;52:75–83.
157. McGrath CL, Kelley ME, Holtzheimer PE, Dunlop BW, Craighead WE, Franco AR, Craddock RC, Mayberg HS. Toward a neuroimaging treatment selection biomarker for major depressive disorder. JAMA Psychiat. 2013;70:821–9.

10 Fatty Liver Disease

Scott C. Beeman and Joel R. Garbow

10.1 Introduction

Fatty liver disease is a devastating pathology whose global incidence is increasing rapidly. Interest in nonalcoholic fatty liver disease (NAFLD), the most common form of fatty liver disease and the one that is primarily associated with metabolic syndrome (characterized by any three of obesity, elevated serum triglycerides, low high-density lipoprotein, elevated blood pressure, and/or elevated fasting plasma glucose), has grown substantially in recent decades as the incidence of metabolic syndrome has increased. Indeed, it is currently estimated that metabolic syndrome affects ~35% of the US adult population and that ~12–25% of the US population is affected by NAFLD [1]. Left unchecked, NAFLD can progress to cirrhosis and/or cancer, the treatment of which often requires a liver transplant. The incidence of NAFLD can be expected to rise as incidences of obesity, type 2 diabetes, and heart disease grow.

NAFLD encompasses a spectrum of increasingly severe liver abnormalities, beginning with typically benign simple steatosis, defined by excessive intrahepatic triglyceride (IHTG). From steatosis, NAFLD can progress to nonalcoholic steatohepatitis (NASH), which is characterized by further increases in IHTG and liver inflammation at its early stages, and fibrosis at late stage. The prevailing hypothesis describing the mechanism leading to liver fibrosis is called the "multi-hit" hypothesis. First described by Day et al. in 1998 [2], the multi-hit hypothesis postulates that dysregulation of free fatty acid (FFA) metabolism due to metabolic syndrome leads to IHTG accumulation (steatosis). In response to increased IHTG, expressions of inflammatory and lipid metabolism mediators shift, oxidative damage increases, and apoptosis is dysregulated, leading to increased stellate cell activity and hepatocyte death. In this poorly regulated mechanism, the stellate cells will produce extracellular matrix (ECM) faster than the rate at which hepatocytes can be regenerated, and the massive deposition of ECM into the cavities left by the dead hepatocytes will lead to fibrosis. Left unchecked, the disease will progress to cirrhosis, characterized primarily by massive fibrosis of the liver, leading to restriction of portal vein blood flow and, potentially, liver failure. In addition to these primary complications, steatosis, fibrosis, and cirrhosis can also lead to hepatic encephalopathy,

S.C. Beeman
Mallinckrodt Institute of Radiology,
Washington University, St. Louis, MO, USA
e-mail: scbeeman@wustl.edu

J.R. Garbow (✉)
Mallinckrodt Institute of Radiology,
Washington University, St. Louis, MO, USA

The Alvin J. Siteman Cancer Center, Washington
University, St. Louis, MO, USA
e-mail: garbow@wustl.edu

J.S. Lewis, K.R. Keshari (eds.), *Imaging and Metabolism*, DOI 10.1007/978-3-319-61401-4_10

renal failure, and hepatocellular carcinoma. Fatty liver disease is a major indicator for liver transplant and is the primary cause of hepatocellular carcinoma [3].

The current gold standard methods for detection and diagnosis of fatty liver disease are serum-based liver function tests and biopsy. Elevated serum levels of the enzymes aspartate transaminase (AST) and alanine transaminase (ALT) are the most common biomarkers of liver dysfunction. Although these tests are noninvasive and cost-effective, measures of ALT and AST are not specific to fatty liver disease. Dramatic elevation of ALT and AST is also seen in hepatitis B and C, autoimmune hepatitis, drug-induced toxicity, and hepatic ischemia. Thus, evaluation of these biomarkers demands comparison against a patient's symptoms, anthropometrics, medical history, and histologic findings. Beyond the standard measurements of AST and ALT are more sophisticated tests such as SteatoTest [4] and FibroTest [5], which combine serologic measures of ALT, total bilirubin, triglyceride, and glucose (among other serum biomarkers) with age, gender, and body mass index to differentiate NAFLD and NASH from other liver diseases and to predict a patient's susceptibility to advanced NASH or cirrhosis. Despite advances in multi-parametric, serum-based measures, histologic examination of liver biopsy samples remains the best way to assess the extent/severity of steatosis and fibrosis. Still, while the value of invasive biopsy is clear, steatosis and fibrosis are diffuse in nature and, thus, biopsy is subject to sampling errors. In addition, biopsy is not without pain and potential serious complications. Thus, imaging techniques assume a critical role in the noninvasive detection and characterization of NAFLD in both humans and preclinical animal models.

Herein, we describe the application of a number of imaging modalities for detecting and characterizing NAFLD, its precursors, and its downstream complications. Special emphasis will be placed on ultrasound (US), computed tomography (CT), and magnetic resonance (MR) techniques, which are routinely available in the clinic, though positron emission tomography (PET) and optical imaging methods will also be discussed.

10.2 Ultrasound

Ultrasound (US) imaging is the cheapest and, often, the most accessible imaging modality for detecting, characterizing, and diagnosing fatty liver. Additionally, US does not employ ionizing radiation and is considered safe for repeated usage. US devices are portable and can be moved between exam rooms, making the imaging procedure convenient and comfortable for medical staff and patients. Typical B-mode US imaging and US transient elastography are the primary US-based methods for detecting and staging fatty liver disease.

10.2.1 Typical B-Mode Ultrasound Imaging

Because it is cheap and ubiquitous, B-mode US imaging is often the preferred radiologic method for initial screening for fatty liver. In practice, the dominant radiologic feature of steatosis is increased echogenicity and, thus, "bright" signal in fatty liver, relative to normal liver [6]. However, the robustness of US for detecting and staging fatty liver disease remains subject to debate. The sensitivity of US to liver steatosis has been cited at values ranging from 64% to 100% [7–12]. The sensitivity of US to liver steatosis is highly dependent upon the severity of fat infiltration, the size and shape of the patient, and the sonographer. Indeed, Stauss et al. [13] measured the intra- and inter-operator agreement rates for detecting the presence of excess fat in the liver to be only 76% and 72%, respectively. The intra- and inter-operator agreement rates for assessing the extent of fatty liver were worse, 68% and 55%, respectively. While the large variance in the reported sensitivity of US to steatosis is disappointing, it is important to note that a study by Palmentieri et al. [11] showed that US is highly sensitive and predictive of severe liver steatosis (>30%). In this study, the authors report sensitivity, specificity, positive predictive value, and negative predictive values of 91%, 93%, 89%, and 94%, respectively, for liver steatosis of >30%. Because the fat-related US signal enhancement is small at levels lower than 30% steatosis, B-mode

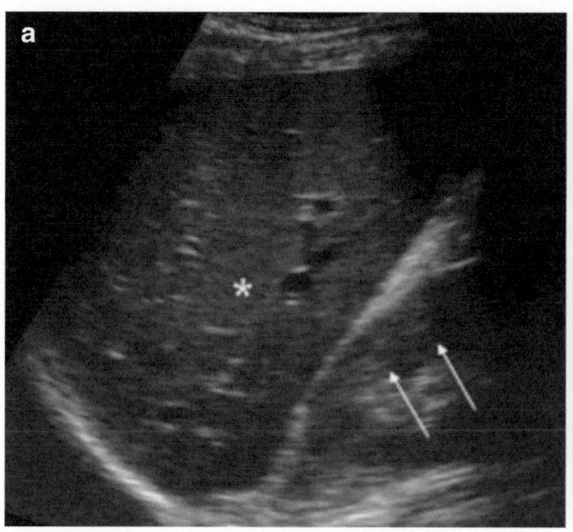

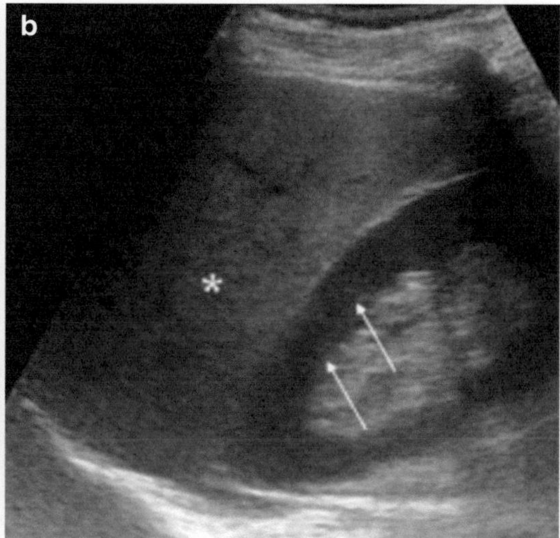

Fig. 10.1 Ultrasound images of a non-steatotic (**a**) and a steatotic liver (**b**). In these images, the liver parenchyma is identified by a *star* and the renal cortex is identified by *two arrows*. Echogenicity in healthy (non-steatotic) liver is similar to that of healthy renal cortex, while that in steatotic liver is increased relative to renal cortex. Figure from Schwenzer et al. J Hepatology, 2009 51:3433–45 [15]

ultrasonography struggles to accurately detect and characterize low-to-moderate levels of fat accumulation in the liver. Thus, typical B-mode ultrasound might be best suited for detecting >30% liver steatosis [14].

It has been suggested that the relative signal difference between the liver and kidney might serve as a more reliable metric for detecting liver steatosis (Fig. 10.1), particularly at levels of steatosis lower than 30%. The superiority of this so-called hepatorenal contrast in detecting low-to-moderate levels of liver steatosis depends on the similarity in the echo textures of healthy liver and kidney. For liver steatosis, in which the liver signal is slightly brightened, the healthy renal cortex provides a constant reference against which the brightened steatotic liver signal can be compared. Osawa et al. pioneered this technique and showed that fatty liver could be diagnosed with a sensitivity of 91% and a specificity of 84%, though the extent of fat infiltration into the liver was not measured in this study [16]. Webb et al. showed that by calculating the hepatorenal contrast, steatosis less than 25% could be detected reliably [17]. Expanding on the hepatorenal index, Hamaguchi et al. [18] have developed a simple scoring system, based on hepatorenal contrast, liver brightness, echo penetration into deep regions of the liver, and vascular blurring, to evaluate patients for visceral fat accumulation, metabolic syndrome, and the severity of fatty liver disease. In this method, ultrasonography is scored on a scale of 1–3, with a score of 1 reflecting *either* hepatorenal contrast *or* brightening of the liver, a score of 2 reflecting *both* hepatorenal contrast *and* brightening of the liver, and a score of 3 reflecting a significant brightening of the liver relative to a score of 2. The authors conclude that this scoring system, which accounts for a number of US feature within a single metric, might inform on metabolic syndrome, visceral obesity, and liver steatosis in patients who appear otherwise healthy. Such scoring of US provides a reliable and semi-quantitative method for detection and characterization of steatosis and its complications.

10.2.2 Measuring Liver Stiffness with Ultrasound

The development of transient elastography (TE, FibroScan) has been a major advance in noninvasively detecting and measuring the extent of liver fibrosis. TE is a mono-dimensional technique that measures the propagation of an applied, low-frequency (typically 50 Hz) shear wave through the liver tissue [19]. TE yields a single measure of tissue elasticity over a cylindrical volume of roughly 3 cm^3. Liver stiffness, characterized by the elastic modulus of the liver, E, is approximately proportional to the square of the measured velocity at which the applied, low-frequency shear wave propagates through the tissue, v:

$$E = 3\rho v^2 \tag{10.1}$$

where ρ is the density of the tissue, assumed to be constant and approximately that of water, ~1 g/ml. It should be noted that Eq. (10.1) is a first approximation to the elastic modulus of the tissue that is based on the assumption that the liver is nonviscous, isotropic, and a soft elastic medium. E is typically expressed in units of kilopascals, kPa, and ranges between 2.5 and 75 kPa. A healthy, unscarred liver will typically have a TE-measured elastic modulus of less than 7 kPa, whereas the elastic modulus of cirrhotic liver ranges from 14 kPa to 69 kPa. TE measurements of liver elasticity are highly reproducible, with a coefficient of variance of ~3%. Furthermore, TE-based liver elasticity measures are well correlated with METAVIR fibrosis grade [19]. To date, TE is the most widely used and, thus, best validated method for measuring liver elasticity/fibrosis. Nonetheless, deriving meaningful results is challenging, particularly for patients with metabolic syndrome. In a study of >13,000 TE examinations, Castera et al. [20] concluded that nearly one in five liver stiffness measurements were uninterpretable. The authors attributed this high failure rate to large waist circumference, a major problem for the application of TE to fatty liver disease, and operator inexperience. Recent advances in probe design have led to the XL probe [21], a probe designed specifically for liver elasticity measurements in obese subjects.

10.3 Computed Tomography

Computed tomography (CT), which has better spatial resolution and depth of penetration than ultrasound and is cheaper and more accessible than magnetic resonance techniques, is an important tool in the noninvasive detection and characterization of fatty liver disease. The use of CT for diagnosing hepatic steatosis dates back to 1979 [22]. Liver steatosis can be diagnosed from absolute measures of CT attenuation. Since lipid attenuates X-rays less than water, fat-infiltrated liver demonstrates less CT attenuation than normal liver. The apparent negative, linear relationship between liver triglyceride content and CT attenuation was first observed by Ducommun et al. [22], in a study of rabbits with fat-infiltrated liver. Piekarski et al. [23] established an attenuation range of 50–57 Hounsfield units (HU) for normal liver. More recently, it has been suggested that attenuation values of <40 HU are indicative of liver steatosis [24–26] (Fig. 10.2).

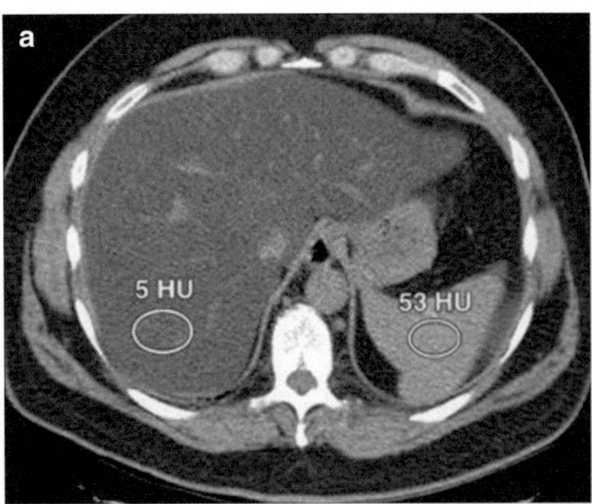

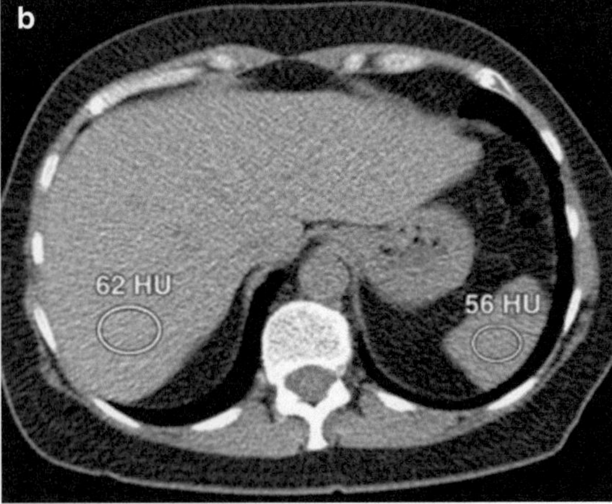

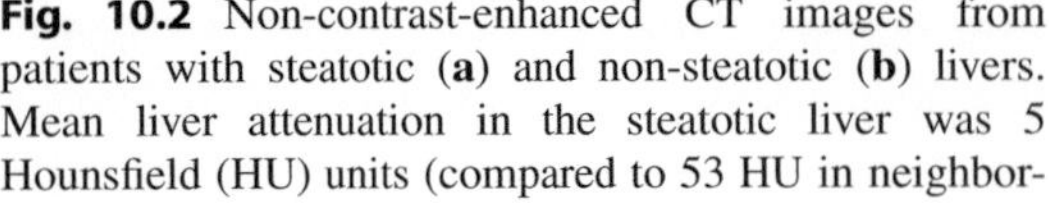

Fig. 10.2 Non-contrast-enhanced CT images from patients with steatotic (**a**) and non-steatotic (**b**) livers. Mean liver attenuation in the steatotic liver was 5 Hounsfield (HU) units (compared to 53 HU in neighboring spleen). Mean liver attenuation in the non-steatotic (normal) liver was 62 HU (compared to 56 HU in neighboring spleen). Figure from Boyce et al. AJR 2010; 194,623–8 [26].

Because there is an inherent variation in *absolute* CT attenuation in patients due to variations in body size and shape, it has been suggested that *relative* measures of liver attenuation might provide a more robust measure of steatosis. The spleen, being proximal to liver, has been proposed as an internal control for CT-based detection of liver steatosis. Normal liver typically appears brighter on CT than the neighboring spleen (healthy liver attenuation is ~10 HU *higher* than spleen), whereas moderately steatotic liver appears darker than spleen (steatotic liver attenuation is ~10 HU *lower* than spleen). Iwasaka et al. [27] have suggested that a liver-to-spleen attenuation ratio of 0.9 or greater is indicative of moderate steatosis. In work published in 2006, Park et al. [24] characterized thoroughly the diagnostic performance of unenhanced CT in detecting macrovesicular steatosis in potential liver donors. In this study, a cohort of 154 subjects underwent liver CT examinations and ultrasound-guided biopsy (for gold standard histologic grading of steatosis). From the CT data, the liver-to-spleen attenuation ratio, the difference between liver and spleen attenuation, and (blood-free) hepatic parenchymal attenuation were calculated and evaluated as metrics for liver steatosis. Using cutoff values optimized for sensitivity and specificity, the authors found the limits of agreement to be −14–14% for both the liver/spleen attenuation ratio and attenuation difference and −13–13% for the hepatic parenchymal attenuation metric, concluding that CT-based measures are insufficient for quantitative assessment of liver steatosis. When more relaxed cutoff values were used, the data demonstrated 100% specificity for steatosis greater than 30%, supporting the conclusion that CT performs well when charged with qualitative assessment of moderate to severe steatosis.

Contrast-enhanced CT has been explored as an alternative to the non-enhanced CT techniques described above. Studies by Johnston et al. [28] and Jacobs et al. [29] were conducted to establish robust methodologies for the diagnosis of fatty liver disease. In both studies, the authors sought to establish a quantitative liver-minus-spleen metric based on liver/spleen CT images enhanced with iodine-based contrast agents. Both of these studies reported a low sensitivity (~54–70%) of contrast-enhanced CT to steatosis, attributing the poor performance of contrast-enhanced CT to the significant influence of poorly controlled variables, including contrast agent injection rate and timing, during the measurement. Both concluded that non-enhanced CT is preferred to contrast-enhanced CT for detection of liver steatosis of greater than 30%. More recently, Varenika et al. [30] explored the utility of contrast-enhanced CT for detecting liver fibrosis in rats. Using both standard iodine-based contrast materials and a novel macromolecular CT contrast agent, hepatic fractional extracellular space and macromolecular contrast material uptake were calculated as measures of liver fibrosis. The authors found a positive correlation between measures of hepatic fractional extracellular space and histology-based Ishak fibrosis scores ($R^2 = 0.75$, $P < 0.001$) and histology-based fibrosis area ($R^2 = 0.80$, $P < 0.001$) and a negative correlation between macromolecular contrast material uptake and Ishak fibrosis scores ($R^2 = 0.83$, $P < 0.001$) and fibrosis area ($R^2 = 0.64$, $P < 0.001$), concluding that contrast-enhanced CT may be useful in detecting and grading liver fibrosis.

10.4 Magnetic Resonance

^{1}H magnetic resonance (MR)-based techniques, which employ nonionizing radiation, are ideally suited for the measurement of liver steatosis and its complications. Magnetic resonance imaging (MRI) has unmatched soft tissue contrast and MRI, and magnetic resonance spectroscopy (MRS) techniques can detect/measure tissue lipid content by exploiting the chemical shift effect, which generates a detectable difference in resonance frequency between water protons and lipid protons. In addition to standard MRI and MRS techniques, magnetic resonance elastography (MRE) has demonstrated considerable promise for the noninvasive measurement of liver elasticity and, thus, liver fibrosis. MRI, MRS, and MRE are indispensable tools in the study of liver steatosis.

10.4.1 ^{1}H MRS and Fat Fraction

MRS is a standard analytical technique that can quantitatively assess the chemical composition of tissues in vivo [31, 32]. Taking advantage of differences in resonance frequencies (chemical shifts) of protons in different chemical environments, MRS can readily quantify ^{1}H signal fractions from protons on fatty acids (0.9, 1.3, 2.1, 4.2, and 5.3 ppm) and those on water (4.7 ppm), in vivo (Fig. 10.3). Applying these principles, ^{1}H MRS has long been used as a tool for noninvasive quantification of hepatic lipid content [33–67]. In its simplest form, MRS-based fat fraction estimation involves collection of localized spectroscopy data in liver using either a *st*imulated *e*cho *a*cquisition *m*ode (STEAM) [68] or *p*oint-*res*olved *s*pectroscopy (PRESS) [69] pulse sequence. Data are collected at a minimum of two echo times (TE) in order to calculate and correct for T_2 relaxation of water and lipid and with an experiment repetition time (TR) much greater than that of the longitudinal relaxation time constant (T_1) of the "slowest relaxing" component of the signal (typically TR > 3.5 s). T_2 and proton density values for water and lipid are typically calculated via the standard mono-exponential transverse relaxation model:

$$S_{W,L}(t) = S(0)_{W,L}\, e^{\frac{-t}{T_{2,W,L}}}, \tag{10.2}$$

in which $S_{W,L}(t)$ is the measured spectral peak amplitude at sampled echo time t for water, *W*, and lipid, *L*, *S*(0) is the calculated peak amplitude

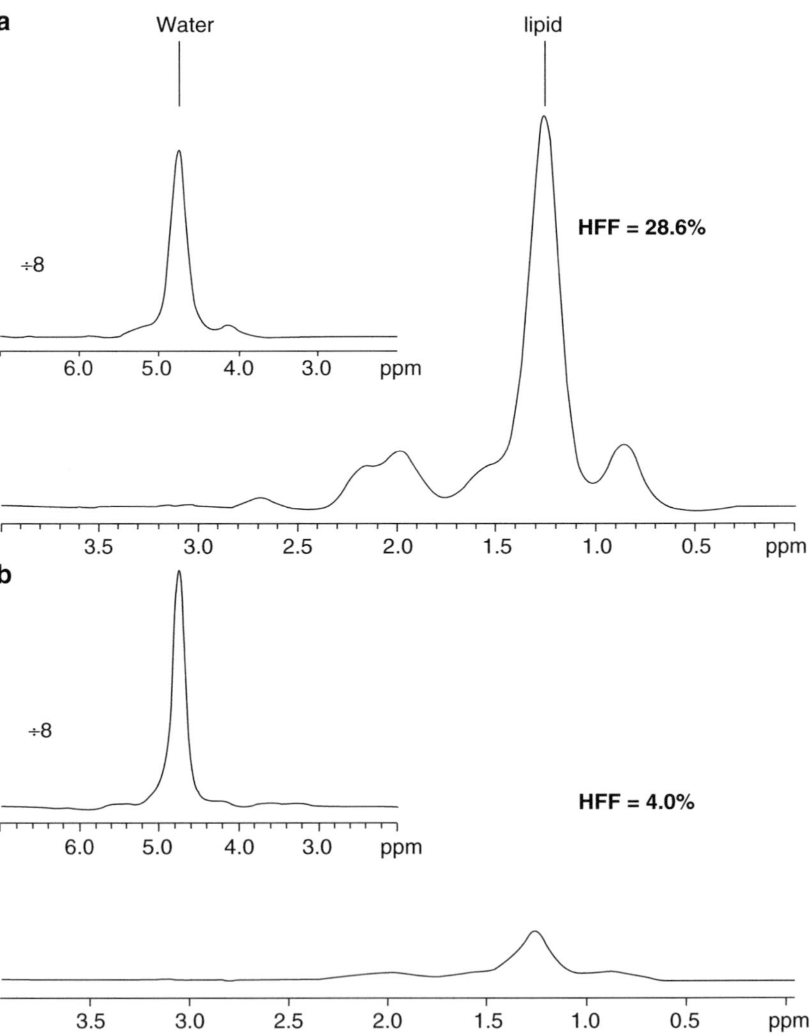

Fig. 10.3 Magnetic resonance spectra from a liver with high fat content (**a**) and a liver with low fat content (**b**). Spectra are split in order to scale down the water resonance by a factor of 8. Lipid-related peaks at 0.9, 1.3, 2.1, 4.2, and 5.3 ppm are especially apparent in the spectrum from the liver with high fat content. From these spectra, the hepatic fat fraction (HFF) for the liver with high fat content was calculated to be 28.6%, while in the lean liver, it was calculated to be 4%. Figure from Kim et al. Magn Reson Med, 2008; 59:521–7 [33]

in the absence of relaxation, and $T_{2,W,L}$ is the calculated transverse relaxation time constant for water or lipid. The signal fat fraction, SFF, can be calculated directly from the extrapolated $S(0)$ values:

$$SFF = \frac{S(0)_f}{S(0)_f + S(0)_w}, \tag{10.3}$$

in which $S(0)_f$ is the calculated peak amplitude of the methylene (1.3 ppm) peak (used as a single representative lipid peak). The challenges associated with MRS-based fat quantification and efforts to mitigate/eliminate these challenges were recently reviewed [70]. Among these challenges are (i) signal biases related to inhomogeneous longitudinal magnetization polarization due to short experiment repetition times (TR) relative to the longest T_1 component in the tissue, (ii) spatially inhomogeneous transverse relaxation intrinsic to the tissue, (iii) the spectral complexity of lipid (i.e., the spectral signature of lipid involves more than just the 1.3 ppm peak), and (iv) j-coupling among ^1H spins on the lipid chains. To mitigate T_1 biases, it is advised that one wait a minimum of 3 T_1 of the longest relaxing component of the spectrum, the time at which at least 95% of equilibrium magnetization polarization has been recovered. (Ideally, one would wait 5 T_1 values, though scans of this length are often not practical in a clinical setting). To account for transverse relaxation, data are often collected with several echo times (typically five) to precisely calculate T_2 and S(0) via Eq. (10.2). Spectral complexity is accounted for by applying Eqs. (10.2) and (10.3) to all identifiable lipid-related spectral peaks. While the ability to identify individual spectral peaks depends on the quality of the acquired spectroscopy data, the most commonly observed signals from the liver are those at 4.7 ppm (H_2O) and those at 0.9, 1.3, and 2.1 ppm, all of which arise from lipid. Other peaks of interest are those at 4.2 and 5.3 ppm, though these are often difficult to discern from the large and overlapping water signal and often must be calculated based on the measured spectral peak amplitudes at 0.9, 1.3, and 2.1 ppm and prior knowledge (assumptions) about the structure of triglycerides. Finally, J-coupling among ^1H spins can be mitigated during acquisition by an appropriate choice of echo times. If each of these potential confounds is properly accounted for, the signal fat fraction can then be regarded as the proton density fat fraction (PDFF), which is strictly defined as the ratio of the proton density of mobile lipid (the sum of all resolvable lipid-related peak amplitudes, $\Sigma\rho L$) to the sum of the proton densities from all mobile lipid and mobile water, ρ_w:

$$PDFF = \frac{\Sigma\rho L}{\Sigma\rho L + \rho w} \tag{10.4}$$

PDFF is considered the most accurate metric for noninvasive quantification of tissue fat. Importantly, accurate PDFF quantification is, in principle, insensitive to magnetic field strength, allowing for broad implementation of the technique and comparison of data across imaging centers.

10.4.2 Fat Imaging and the Dixon Method

In 1984, Dixon applied spectroscopy principles to MR imaging to generate maps of fat fraction by assuming a simplified system in which (i) ^1H signal only comes from water and lipid, (ii) water and lipid signals are separated by ~3.4 ppm (i.e., water is at a chemical shift of 4.7 ppm and lipid is represented only by the methylene resonance at 1.3 ppm), and (iii) T_2^* relaxation is negligible. This technique is referred to as the two-point Dixon technique [71]. Based on Dixon's assumptions, one collects gradient-recalled echo (GRE) or spin-echo (SE) images at two different echo times, one in which the water and lipid signal are in phase (zero-degree image, S_{IP}) with respect to one another and the acquired signal amplitude is the sum of the fractional water (S_W) and lipid (S_L) signal amplitudes, Eq. (10.5a), and one in which the water and lipid signal are out of phase (180-degree image, S_{OP}) and the acquired signal amplitude is the difference between fractional water and lipid signal amplitudes, Eq. (10.5b):

$$S_{IP} = S_W + S_L \tag{10.5a}$$

$$S_{OP} = S_W - S_L \tag{10.5b}$$

The echo times at which water and lipid are completely in and out of phase with respect to one another can be calculated directly from the magnetic field strength of the instrument and the chemical shift difference between water and methylene protons. Rearranging Eqs. (10.5a) and (10.5b), the water and lipid fractional signal amplitudes can be expressed in terms of measured in- and out-of-phase signals:

$$S_W = \frac{S_{IP} + S_{OP}}{2} \tag{10.6a}$$

$$S_L = \frac{S_{IP} - S_{OP}}{2} \tag{10.6b}$$

S_w and S_L are calculated on a voxel-wise basis and, when plotted, provide images of only water and fat, respectively (Fig. 10.4). Further, from Eqs. (10.6a) and (10.6b), one can calculate and map signal fat fraction, SFF:

$$SFF = \frac{S_L}{S_W + S_L}, \tag{10.7a}$$

or, equivalently, from the original acquired in- and out-of-phase data:

$$SFF = \frac{S_{IP} - S_{OP}}{2S_{IP}} \tag{10.7b}$$

The two-point Dixon method remains the foundation for many of the fat mapping and quantification experiments performed today, though significant modifications to the technique have been made since its original implementation. Importantly, the assumption of negligible signal decay between in-phase and out-of-phase echoes due to T_2^* is often not valid. In 1991, Glover added a third echo to the Dixon method to correct for T_2^* [73] and a susceptibility image to the output of the Dixon method [74]. It is also now recognized that measures of fat fraction can be biased by spatial heterogeneity in longitudinal relaxation (T_1 bias) within the tissue. Low flip angle (~10 degree) GRE experiments are now commonly used to mitigate T_1 bias while still permitting rapid data collection (e.g., experiment repetition every ~125 msec). Recently, more sophisticated data acquisition and signal modeling techniques have been investigated, including studies in which as many as six echoes are collected and, from these data, multiple spectral peaks and T_2^* relaxation are modeled [33–38, 48, 50, 54, 56, 58, 61, 62, 66, 67]. Because typical GRE MRI does not provide the same robust spectral information as MRS, multi-resonance signal modeling of MRI-based fat quantification data requires substantial prior knowledge (assumptions) about lipid composition. A particularly elegant example of fat quantification

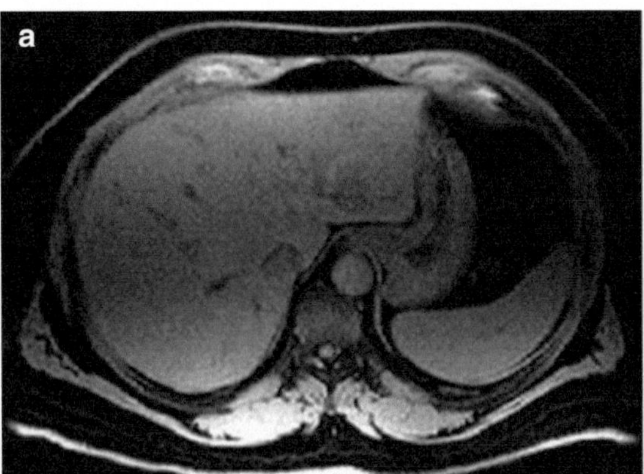

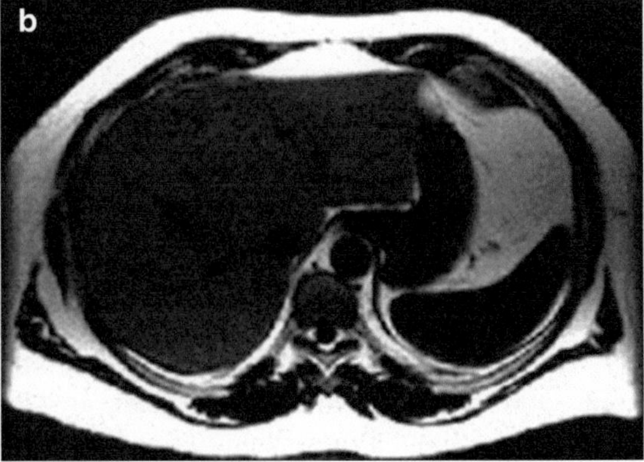

Fig. 10.4 Phase-corrected water- (**a**) and fat-only (**b**) images calculated from dual-echo, two-point Dixon data. Data were collected on a patient with a metastatic carcinoid tumor and likely steatosis. Indeed, signal in the liver on the fat image was elevated to ~6x that of a healthy, non-steatotic liver. Figure from Ma, Magn Reson Med. 2004;52:415–9 [72]

by MR imaging can be found in the work of Yokoo et al. [36], in which the authors assume that their six-echo, gradient-recalled echo MRI signal is comprised of six resonant frequencies: one water resonance (4.7 ppm, an apparent large DC contribution to the signal because the MRI instrument is tuned to transmit/receive at the water frequency) and five lipid resonances at frequencies 0.9, 1.3, 2.1, 4.2, and 5.3 ppm, having normalized weights of 0.09, 0.70, 0.12, 0.04, and 0.05, respectively. The resolvable, lipid-based resonant frequencies, and their relative weights, were determined from previous MRS studies [75]. The authors show a near-perfect correlation between MRS-quantified PDFF, considered the gold standard in the study, and MRI-based quantification of fat.

10.4.3 Magnetic Resonance Elastography

MRI and MRS are not sensitive to liver fibrosis and, thus, cannot fully characterize the more advanced stages of fatty liver disease. Like ultrasound transient elastography, magnetic resonance elastography (MRE) is a quantitative method for measuring the shear modulus (stiffness) of tissue. MRE has substantial advantages over ultrasound-based elastography techniques; it is inherently capable of mapping tissue stiffness in two and three dimensions and retains similar spatial resolution to MRI. Further, the hardware and software required to perform MRE experiments are becoming more routinely available on clinical MRI scanners, increasing the applicability of the technique.

MRE permits the mechanical properties (e.g., shear modulus) of tissue to be measured and requires a mechanical transducer to induce audio frequency shear waves in the tissue. Typically, these shear waves are driven by one of three different mechanical transducers: (i) an electromechanical transducer driven by the magnetic field of the MRI magnet [76], (ii) a piezoelectric transducer [77], (iii) or an acoustic speaker system [78, 79]. Among these commonly used MRE transducers, the acoustic speaker system is of particular interest in liver applications. Because the drivers of acoustic speaker systems employ permanent magnets, these transducers must be located remote from the MRI instrument. A pneumatic tube system is used to conduct pressure waves from the remote speaker system to the abdomen of the patient. These air pressure waves terminate at a drum that is in contact with the patient's abdomen and applies the shear waves to the liver.

MRE experiments to measure liver stiffness require the application of bipolar, motion-encoding gradients in synchrony with the mechanical shear waves. Using motion-encoding gradients, MRI sequences can be made sensitive to small, submicron displacements of ^{1}H spins in tissue. This effect has long been applied to measure the apparent diffusion of water through tissue and the flow of blood plasma in vessels. In 1995, Muthupillai et al. applied these same principles to measure tissue displacement resulting from the application of shear waves [76]. For both diffusion MRI and MRE, displacement is measured by the "accumulation of phase" of displaced ^{1}H spins during the application of the bipolar, motion-encoding gradients. The phase accumulation during the MRE experiment is linearly proportional to the proton displacement:

$$\varnothing(\vec{r},\theta) = \frac{\gamma NT\left(\vec{G}\cdot\vec{\xi}_0\right)}{2}\cos\left(\vec{k}\cdot\vec{r}+\theta\right) \tag{10.8}$$

where $\varnothing$ is the MR-measured phase contribution from motion and motion-encoding gradients, θ is the phase offset between motion and the motion-encoding gradient, $\vec{r}$ is the position vector, γ is the magnetogyric ratio of ^{1}H protons (~42.6 MHz T^{-1}), N is the number of motion-encoding gradient pairs, T is the period of the motion-encoding gradient waveform, $\vec{G}$ is the motion-encoding gradient amplitude, ξ_0 is the peak motion amplitude, and $\vec{k}$ is the wave number. The propagation of mechanical waves through the tissue is sampled in "snapshots", collected at 4–8 phase offsets equally spaced across the period of the mechanical wave. It is important to note that shear wave-induced proton displacement is not the only mechanism by which phase is accumulated. Thus, it is critical to perform a second MRE experiment, with gradients of opposite polarity, to remove static de-phasing elements. From the resultant images, which have encoded in them the propagation of the applied

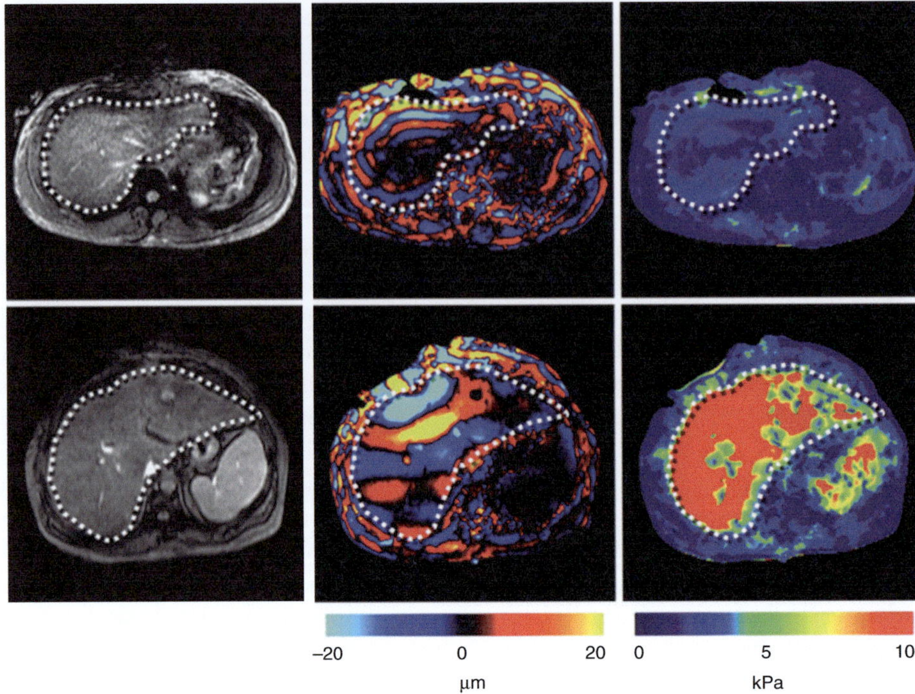

Fig. 10.5 Magnetic resonance elastography data from a patient with normal liver (**a–c**) and a patient with cirrhotic liver (**d–f**). Typical magnitude MR images show little difference between healthy and cirrhotic liver (**a**, **d**). Images of acoustic shear wave propagation reveal a substantially longer wavelength in the cirrhotic liver compared to the normal liver (**b**, **e**). Calculated elastograms reveal that the cirrhotic liver is much stiffer (18.83 kPa) than normal liver (1.7 kPa). Figure from Mariappan et al. Clin Anat. 2010; 23:497–511 [80]

mechanical wave, one can apply, for example, an inversion algorithm in concert with assumptions about isotropy, homogeneity, and incompressibility, to calculate and map the shear modulus of the tissue (Fig. 10.5). While mathematical inversion algorithms and other methods for calculating the mechanical properties of tissue are highly complex and outside of the scope of this chapter, further information can be found in [80–83].

MRE is now used clinically to detect and characterize liver fibrosis [84, 85]. In 2007, Yin et al. [78] thoroughly characterized the sensitivity and specificity of MRE to liver fibrosis. In this study, 35 healthy volunteers and 50 patients with chronic liver disease were examined with MRE- and MR-based fat fraction measures, and it was found that MRE-based liver stiffness measures were directly related to liver fibrosis stage (Fig. 10.6), as determined by biopsy. The sensitivity and specificity of MRE to all stages of liver fibrosis were found to be 98% and 99%, respectively. Further, the authors showed that MRE can

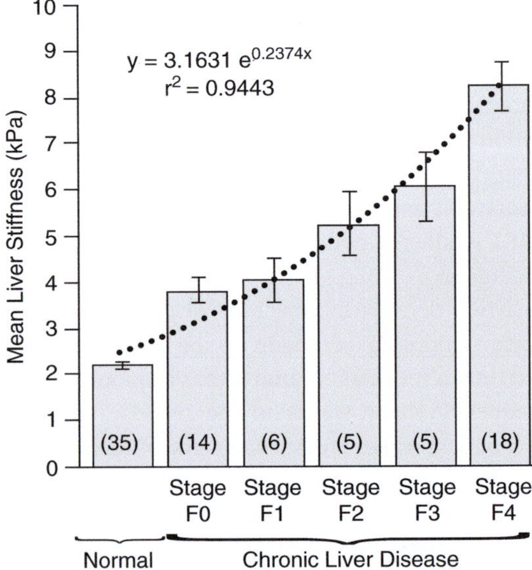

Fig. 10.6 MRE-measured mean liver stiffness versus fibrosis stage in a cohort of 35 normal volunteers and 48 patients with liver fibrosis. Liver stiffness correlates with the extent of liver fibrosis (r^2 = 0.94). Figure from Yin et al. Clin Gastroenterology and Hepatology. 2007; 5:1144–6 [78]

discern patients with moderate-to-severe fibrosis from those with mild fibrosis with a sensitivity and specificity of 86% and 85%, respectively. More recently, Singh et al. [86] evaluated the diagnostic performance of MRE in staging liver fibrosis via a systematic review of the literature and a meta-analysis of patient data. Based on the pooled data, the authors conclude that MRE is highly accurate in diagnosing significant and advanced fibrosis and cirrhosis. In short, MRE has significant potential for routine use in the clinic for the detection and characterization of liver fibrosis in patients with fatty liver disease.

10.4.4 Other MRI-Based Techniques

A number of more common clinical MR techniques, including diffusion-weighted imaging (DWI), magnetization transfer contrast (MTC) imaging, and contrast-enhanced T_1- and T_2^*-weighted imaging, have been applied to the detection/characterization of fatty liver disease and fibrosis. However, none have achieved the successes of the methods discussed above. Nonetheless, these techniques deserve brief mention here due to their ubiquity in the clinic. DWI has been investigated for characterization of steatosis and fibrosis [87–93]. While the results of these studies are mixed, typically, ADC values in steatotic and fibrotic livers are lower than those of healthy liver. For example, in a recent study, steatotic livers were shown to have a lower apparent diffusion coefficient (ADC; $1.20 \pm 0.22 \times 10^{-3}$ mm^2/s) than healthy livers ($1.32 \pm 0.23 \times 10^{-3}$ mm^2/s) [94]. MTC imaging, which serves as a surrogate measure of macromolecular concentration, should, in principle, be sensitive to the excessive deposition of collagen and other extracellular matrix constituents associated with liver fibrosis. The results of MTC as applied to liver fibrosis have, thus far, been disappointing [95–97]. Contrast-enhanced T_1- and T_2-weighted imaging techniques, which use gadolinium chelates and superparamagnetic iron oxide (SPIO) nanoparticles, respectively, to generate contrast at the sites of their accumulation, can identify regions of advanced fibrosis. While these protocols are typically more sensitive to fibrosis than CT, it is not clear that they can robustly detect early fibrosis [98].

10.5 Preclinical and Investigational Imaging

Rodent models of fatty liver disease have played a critical role in the study of fatty liver pathogenesis. Preclinical imaging techniques, including those described above, positron emission tomography (PET), and optical imaging methods, are uniquely informative for the study of fatty liver pathogenesis, as they allow for repeated and nondestructive longitudinal investigation of disease development. In addition, imaging results from preclinical studies can be correlated and validated via histology and immunohistochemistry. Imaging instrumentation designed specifically for small-animal studies can provide exquisite spatial resolution, and all of the clinical imaging techniques described above can be applied to the study of fatty liver pathogenesis in a preclinical setting. Importantly, experimental MR, PET, and optical techniques can inform on fatty liver biomarkers that are sometimes unavailable clinically, including direct measurement of the critical metabolic markers glucose, lactate, and pyruvate. In this section, we describe cutting-edge MR, PET, and optical techniques that are advancing the understanding of fatty liver disease in the preclinical setting. In the future, many of these techniques may find translation to the clinic.

10.5.1 Magnetic Resonance

MR-visible gadolinium- and iron oxide-based contrast agents have been designed or repurposed to enable measurements of fatty liver-related changes to specific liver structures and functions. For example, Tsuda et al. used the liver-specific gadolinium-ethoxybenzyl-diethylenetriamine pentaacetic acid (Gd-EOB-DTPA) contrast agent, which selectively accumulates in hepatocytes, to stage fatty liver disease in rats [99]. In this study, dynamic contrast-enhanced MRI principles, in which the influx, uptake, and clearance of a gadolinium-based MRI contrast agent are observed with rapidly acquired T_1-weighted MRI images (typically 1–5 s per acquisition), were used to observe the differential time-activity curves between cohorts of rats with simple steatosis and NASH. The observed Gd-EOB-DTPA dynamics were much slower in NASH livers compared to those with simple steatosis. Super paramagnetic iron oxide (SPIO) nanoparticles are also useful in detecting and measuring Kupffer cell function. While SPIOs have long been used for measuring Kupffer cell function in livers with focal lesions like hepatocellular carcinoma, a recent study showed that SPIOs are also effective in measuring Kupffer cell activity in steatotic livers. Indeed, through intravenous injection and MRI detection of SPIOs, decreased Kupffer cell activity in steatotic livers was demonstrated [100]. More recently, targeted iron oxide nanoparticles were employed to noninvasively detect ultrastructural (submicron-scale) changes in steatotic liver. In this study, intravenously administered cationized ferritin (CF), a chemically modified version of the endogenous iron storage ferritin protein, was used to measure plasma access to the hepatic perisinusoidal space, the space underlying the fenestrated endothelia of the liver that is the site of direct exchange between the blood and liver parenchyma [101]. Further, CF-enhanced MRI showed that NASH-related microstructural changes to the perisinusoidal space serve to restrict plasma access to the hepatic parenchyma.

Hyperpolarized carbon-13 (HP) MRS is cutting-edge technology that allows direct and rapid in vivo measurement of metabolism and metabolic fluxes. Molecules typically studied using HP methods include pyruvate, glucose, lactate, malate, and aspartate. While standard ^{13}C MRS has been used for decades to measure metabolic biomarkers in vivo in the steady state, the technique is challenged by the low natural abundance of ^{13}C (~1.1%), relatively low in vivo concentrations of carbon-bearing molecules (millimolar, compared to a concentration of ~55 M for the water molecules typically observed with ^{1}H MRI and MRS), and a relatively low magnetogyric ratio, conditions that combine to yield very low measured signal-to-noise ratio per unit time. The recent introduction of dissolution dynamic nuclear polarization (DNP) technology permits a massive (up to 100,000-fold), though transient, increase in ^{13}C signal to noise [102]. The DNP method employs microwaves to transfer polarization from electrons to carbon spins in a frozen glass matrix at very low temperatures (~1.2 K). The resulting hyperpolarized, carbon-containing species is dissolved rapidly using hot water, with retention of the spin polarization, and the solution can then be used for metabolic studies in vivo in animals and humans, and in cell culture and bioreactors. HP MR, as applied to biological systems, is a young, but rapidly developing field, with much work remaining for characterizing and optimizing its use in the liver. Still, recent hepatic studies of HP ^{13}C MRS hint at its promise for direct measurement of metabolite concentrations and in vivo observation of metabolic pathways. In 2008, Hu et al. used hyperpolarized ^{13}C-pyruvate and MRS to noninvasively and dynamically interrogate differential alanine production in normal and fasted livers [103]. Shortly afterward, Speilman et al. quantified ethanol metabolism in livers in vivo via HP ^{13}C-pyruvate MRS [104]. Merritt et al. expanded upon these studies in experiments designed to monitor the metabolism of pyruvate in the tricarboxylic acid cycle (TCA) in isolated, perfused livers using HP ^{13}C-pyruvate MRS [105]. The production of a number of metabolites, including [1-^{13}C]lactate, [1-^{13}C]alanine, [1-^{13}C]malate, [4-^{13}C]malate, [1-^{13}C]aspartate, [4-^{13}C]aspartate, and [^{13}C]bicarbonate, was observed. To date, this study provides the most comprehensive assessment of HP ^{13}C-pyruvate MRS-monitored metabolism in the liver and highlights the great potential of hyperpolarized ^{13}C-pyruvate MRS for interrogating liver metabolism. Finally, Lee et al. used HP ^{13}C-pyruvate MRS to measure liver glucose production in a high-fat diet-induced model of fatty liver and insulin resistance [106]. These experiments showed differential production of downstream metabolites [1-^{13}C]malate and [1-^{13}C]aspartate and, importantly, demonstrated a correlation between the MRS-measured exchange rate between [1-^{13}C]pyruvate and [1-^{13}C]aspartate and gluconeogenic pyruvate carboxylase (PC) activity in hepatocytes.

10.5.2 Positron Emission Tomography (PET)

The majority of PET studies of fatty liver have used the tracer [^{18}F]fluorodeoxyglucose (FDG). While some of these studies have been directed at identifying and characterizing NASH and NAFLD, many have instead been associated with oncology and have focused on the suitability of using the liver as a reference tissue for PET tumor studies [107, 108]. FDG PET is an emerging technique for imaging inflammation, and it has been observed that hepatic FDG uptake is elevated in liver tissue with steatosis compared with controls [109, 110], probably the result of irreversible tracer uptake into inflammatory cells. Nonetheless, recent results in the PET literature for NAFLD have been varied and somewhat contradictory. Some studies have reported a positive correlation between standard uptake volume (SUV) of FDG and the degree of steatosis [111], others a negative relationship [108], and some no relationship [107, 112]. A recent study reexamining these effects posited that the conflicting literature results were due to ignoring the contributions of normal liver FDG kinetics and blood glucose levels. Hepatic FDG uptake is closely associated with elevated triglyceride (TG) and gamma-glutamyl transpeptidase (GGT) levels, independent of the presence of FLD. Thus, inflammation may play a major role in increased hepatic glucose uptake [113]. High hepatic FDG uptake may be a useful prognostic factor for cardiovascular events in individuals with NAFLD [114]. A relatively few number of PET studies of liver that do not involve FDG have also been reported. Fatty acid (FA) metabolism was measured in the livers of pigs using [^{11}C]palmitate, in which it was observed that obese individuals have increased hepatic oxidation of FA and increased FA flux from visceral fat [115]. A recent study explored whether translocator protein (TSPO) (inflammation) can serve as an imaging marker for noninvasive diagnosis and staging of NAFLD. A correlation was found between the uptake of [^{18}F]N-benzyl-N-methyl-2-[7,8-dihydro-7-(2-(18)F-fluoroethyl)-8-oxo-2-phenyl-9H-purin-9-yl]acetamide (^{18}F-FEDAC), a TSPO ligand, and NAFLD activity score, as assessed by histology on excised tissue, in mice [116].

10.5.3 Optical Imaging

Optical imaging methods have been applied primarily to the study of ex vivo tissue samples; only a few in vivo optical imaging studies of fatty liver have been reported. The combination of integrated coherent anti-Stokes Raman scattering (CARS), second harmonic generation (SHG), and two-photon excitation fluorescence (TPEF) microscopy imaging was used to monitor the progression of liver steatosis and fibrosis in a bile duct ligation rat model [117], and liver steatosis and fibrosis were found to develop at different rates. Diffuse reflectance spectroscopy (DRS) has been employed to assess steatosis in vivo in liver tissue during surgery and ex vivo on liver resection specimens. For steatosis quantification, correlations were found between in vivo and ex vivo DRS analysis (Spearman's rank correlation coefficient, $r_s = 0.925$) and between DRS and histology ($r_s = 0.854$) in ex vivo tissue [118]. Good correlation was also demonstrated between DRS-estimated hepatic steatosis vs. steatosis as determined by a pathologist in a series of ex vivo liver tissue immediately following resection [119]. Dual-phase, nonlinear photoacoustic contrast has been used to characterize excised, fresh liver tissue [120], while precise evaluation of liver histology via optical analysis and computerized morphometry has demonstrated that steatosis influences liver stiffness [121]. Conventional light microscopy is used routinely for histologic examination of tissue, including liver. For example, analysis of liver biopsy samples permitted measurement of fat droplets in patients with NAFLD [122] and allowed semiquantitative histologic grading of steatosis via assessment of the % of fatty hepatocytes (i.e., those containing lipid vacuoles) [123].

10.6 Summary

Fatty liver disease is a costly pathology of increasing worldwide incidence. Liver biopsy remains the gold standard for assessment of fat infiltration and fatty liver-related fibrosis, but is not an ideal tool—infection, bleeding, and pain are all potential complications of biopsy. Furthermore, steatosis and fibrosis can manifest in a heterogeneous manner, and, thus, focal biopsy might miss or improperly characterize the presence or extent of liver disease. Imaging techniques, which can non-invasively measure and/or map liver fat and fibrosis, are being used increasingly in the investigation and diagnosis of liver disease. Herein, we have detailed the most common and well-investigated ultrasound, computed tomography, and magnetic resonance techniques for detecting and measuring liver steatosis and fibrosis.

Ultrasound is an inexpensive and ubiquitous modality that is often employed for initial assessment of liver when steatosis is suspected. By exploiting the increased echogenicity caused by lipid droplets, standard B-mode ultrasound is able to reliably detect steatosis of greater than 30%. Because ultrasound-based detection of steatosis is highly dependent on abdominal size and shape, and prone to operator error, it has been suggested that assessing *relative* liver signal, by referencing to signal from a neighboring kidney, might better detect steatosis. While B-mode ultrasound cannot directly detect liver fibrosis, it can be used to measure fibrosis-related morphologic changes to the liver and, thus, indirectly detect fibrosis. Ultrasound can also be used to measure the rate at which shear waves propagate through tissue—a metric that is related to the stiffness of the tissue. This so-called transient elastography technique can directly detect and measure liver fibrosis.

Computed tomography (CT) has long been used for detecting liver steatosis. CT has significantly better spatial resolution than ultrasound and typically costs much less than magnetic resonance studies. CT measures liver steatosis by exploiting the negative linear relationship between CT attenuation and tissue lipid content. Like ultrasound, CT-based measures of steatosis are dependent upon body morphology; thus, a liver-to-spleen ratio measurement has been proposed for more reliable detection of liver steatosis. Using the liver-to-spleen ratio approach, levels of steatosis greater than 30% are reliably detected. More recently, CT contrast agents have been employed to quantify liver extracellular space and macromolecular uptake in the liver—measures that are sensitive to severity of liver fibrosis. Novel implementations of contrast-enhanced CT hold promise for grading of fibrosis by CT, though repeated use of CT is limited due to exposure to ionizing radiation.

Despite their relatively high cost, magnetic resonance-based techniques have several unique advantages in the assessment of fatty liver disease. Magnetic resonance spectroscopy is inherently sensitive to the molecular composition of tissue and can quantify the so-called proton density fat fraction of the liver with extremely high accuracy and precision. Through careful collection of data and a priori assumptions about the molecular composition of liver fat, measures of proton density fat fraction can be extended to magnetic resonance imaging techniques, thereby producing maps of liver fat and water and proton density fat fraction. Like ultrasound, MRI can be made sensitive to the propagation of shear waves through tissue via application of motion-encoding magnetic field gradients, introduced synchronously with applied shear waves, a technique referred to as magnetic resonance elastography. MRE is capable of mapping liver stiffness and, thus, fibrosis. Despite its cost, MR-based assessment offers the most sensitive and reliable quantitative data for diagnosing and staging fatty liver disease. The value of a combined and repeated MRS- and MRI-based assessment of steatosis and fibrosis, enabled by MR's use of nonionizing radiation, is substantial.

References

1. NIDDK. Nonalcoholic Steatohepatitis. In: NIH, editor. www.digestive.niddk.nih.gov: U.S. Department of Health and Human Services; 2006.
2. Day CP, James OF. Steatohepatitis: a tale of two "hits"? Gastroenterology. 1998;114(4):842–5.
3. Dyson J, Jaques B, Chattopadyhay D, Lochan R, Graham J, Das D, et al. Hepatocellular cancer: the

impact of obesity, type 2 diabetes and a multidisciplinary team. J Hepatol. 2014;60(1):110–7.
4. Poynard T, Ratziu V, Naveau S, Thabut D, Charlotte F, Messous D, et al. The diagnostic value of biomarkers (SteatoTest) for the prediction of liver steatosis. Comp Hepatol. 2005;4:10.
5. Ratziu V, Massard J, Charlotte F, Messous D, Imbert-Bismut F, Bonyhay L, et al. Diagnostic value of biochemical markers (FibroTest-FibroSURE) for the prediction of liver fibrosis in patients with nonalcoholic fatty liver disease. BMC Gastroenterol. 2006;6:6.
6. Taylor KJ, McCready VR. A clinical evaluation of grey-scale ultrasonography. Br J Radiol. 1976;49(579):244–52.
7. Yilmaz Y, Dolar E, Ulukaya E, Akgoz S, Keskin M, Kiyici M, et al. Soluble forms of extracellular cytokeratin 18 may differentiate simple steatosis from nonalcoholic steatohepatitis. World J Gastroenterol. 2007;13(6):837–44.
8. Wieckowska A, Feldstein AE. Nonalcoholic fatty liver disease in the pediatric population: a review. Curr Opin Pediatr. 2005;17(5):636–41.
9. Tarantino G, Conca P, Coppola A, Vecchione R, Di Minno G. Serum concentrations of the tissue polypeptide specific antigen in patients suffering from non-alcoholic steatohepatitis. Eur J Clin Investig. 2007;37(1):48–53.
10. Saadeh S, Younossi ZM, Remer EM, Gramlich T, Ong JP, Hurley M, et al. The utility of radiological imaging in nonalcoholic fatty liver disease. Gastroenterology. 2002;123(3):745–50.
11. Palmentieri B, de Sio I, La Mura V, Masarone M, Vecchione R, Bruno S, et al. The role of bright liver echo pattern on ultrasound B-mode examination in the diagnosis of liver steatosis. Dig Liver Dis. 2006;38(7):485–9.
12. Mottin CC, Moretto M, Padoin AV, Swarowsky AM, Toneto MG, Glock L, et al. The role of ultrasound in the diagnosis of hepatic steatosis in morbidly obese patients. Obes Surg. 2004;14(5):635–7.
13. Strauss S, Gavish E, Gottlieb P, Katsnelson L. Interobserver and intraobserver variability in the sonographic assessment of fatty liver. AJR Am J Roentgenol. 2007;189(6):W320–3.
14. Lewis JR, Mohanty SR. Nonalcoholic fatty liver disease: a review and update. Dig Dis Sci. 2010;55(3):560–78.
15. Schwenzer NF, Springer F, Schraml C, Stefan N, Machann J, Schick F. Non-invasive assessment and quantification of liver steatosis by ultrasound, computed tomography and magnetic resonance. J Hepatol. 2009;51(3):433–45.
16. Osawa H, Mori Y. Sonographic diagnosis of fatty liver using a histogram technique that compares liver and renal cortical echo amplitudes. J Clin Ultrasound. 1996;24(1):25–9.
17. Webb M, Yeshua H, Zelber-Sagi S, Santo E, Brazowski E, Halpern Z, et al. Diagnostic value of a computerized hepatorenal index for sonographic quantification of liver steatosis. AJR Am J Roentgenol. 2009;192(4):909–14.
18. Hamaguchi M, Kojima T, Itoh Y, Harano Y, Fujii K, Nakajima T, et al. The severity of ultrasonographic findings in nonalcoholic fatty liver disease reflects the metabolic syndrome and visceral fat accumulation. Am J Gastroenterol. 2007;102(12):2708–15.
19. Sandrin L, Fourquet B, Hasquenoph JM, Yon S, Fournier C, Mal F, et al. Transient elastography: a new noninvasive method for assessment of hepatic fibrosis. Ultrasound Med Biol. 2003;29(12):1705–13.
20. Castera L, Foucher J, Bernard PH, Carvalho F, Allaix D, Merrouche W, et al. Pitfalls of liver stiffness measurement: a 5-year prospective study of 13,369 examinations. Hepatology. 2010;51(3):828–35.
21. de Ledinghen V, Vergniol J, Foucher J, El-Hajbi F, Merrouche W, Rigalleau V. Feasibility of liver transient elastography with FibroScan using a new probe for obese patients. Liver Int. 2010;30(7):1043–8.
22. Ducommun JC, Goldberg HI, Korobkin M, Moss AA, Kressel HY. The relation of liver fat to computed tomography numbers: a preliminary experimental study in rabbits. Radiology. 1979;130(2):511–3.
23. Piekarski J, Goldberg HI, Royal SA, Axel L, Moss AA. Difference between liver and spleen CT numbers in the normal adult: its usefulness in predicting the presence of diffuse liver disease. Radiology. 1980;137(3):727–9.
24. Park SH, Kim PN, Kim KW, Lee SW, Yoon SE, Park SW, et al. Macrovesicular hepatic steatosis in living liver donors: use of CT for quantitative and qualitative assessment. Radiology. 2006;239(1):105–12.
25. Hamer OW, Aguirre DA, Casola G, Sirlin CB. Imaging features of perivascular fatty infiltration of the liver: initial observations. Radiology. 2005;237(1):159–69.
26. Boyce CJ, Pickhardt PJ, Kim DH, Taylor AJ, Winter TC, Bruce RJ, et al. Hepatic steatosis (fatty liver disease) in asymptomatic adults identified by unenhanced low-dose CT. AJR Am J Roentgenol. 2010;194(3):623–8.
27. Iwasaki M, Takada Y, Hayashi M, Minamiguchi S, Haga H, Maetani Y, et al. Noninvasive evaluation of graft steatosis in living donor liver transplantation. Transplantation. 2004;78(10):1501–5.
28. Johnston RJ, Stamm ER, Lewin JM, Hendrick RE, Archer PG. Diagnosis of fatty infiltration of the liver on contrast enhanced CT: limitations of liver-minus-spleen attenuation difference measurements. Abdom Imaging. 1998;23(4):409–15.
29. Jacobs JE, Birnbaum BA, Shapiro MA, Langlotz CP, Slosman F, Rubesin SE, et al. Diagnostic criteria for fatty infiltration of the liver on contrast-enhanced helical CT. AJR Am J Roentgenol. 1998;171(3):659–64.
30. Varenika V, Fu Y, Maher JJ, Gao D, Kakar S, Cabarrus MC, et al. Hepatic fibrosis: evaluation with semiquantitative contrast-enhanced CT. Radiology. 2013;266(1):151–8.

31. Haacke EM. Magnetic resonance imaging: physical principles and sequence design. New York: John Wiley & Sons; 1999. p. 914.
32. Levitt MH. Spin dynamics : basics of nuclear magnetic resonance. Chichester. New York: John Wiley & Sons; 2001. p. 686.
33. Kim H, Taksali SE, Dufour S, Befroy D, Goodman TR, Petersen KF, et al. Comparative MR study of hepatic fat quantification using single-voxel proton spectroscopy, two-point dixon and three-point IDEAL. Magn Reson Med. 2008;59(3):521–7.
34. Meisamy S, Hines CD, Hamilton G, Sirlin CB, McKenzie CA, Yu H, et al. Quantification of hepatic steatosis with T1-independent, T2-corrected MR imaging with spectral modeling of fat: blinded comparison with MR spectroscopy. Radiology. 2011;258(3):767–75.
35. Yokoo T, Bydder M, Hamilton G, Middleton MS, Gamst AC, Wolfson T, et al. Nonalcoholic fatty liver disease: diagnostic and fat-grading accuracy of low-flip-angle multiecho gradient-recalled-echo MR imaging at 1.5 T. Radiology. 2009;251(1):67–76.
36. Yokoo T, Shiehmorteza M, Hamilton G, Wolfson T, Schroeder ME, Middleton MS, et al. Estimation of hepatic proton-density fat fraction by using MR imaging at 3.0 T. Radiology. 2011;258(3):749–59.
37. Pineda N, Sharma P, Xu Q, Hu X, Vos M, Martin DR. Measurement of hepatic lipid: high-speed T2-corrected multiecho acquisition at 1H MR spectroscopy—a rapid and accurate technique. Radiology. 2009;252(2):568–76.
38. Reeder SB, Cruite I, Hamilton G, Sirlin CB. Quantitative assessment of liver fat with magnetic resonance imaging and spectroscopy. J Magn Reson Imaging. 2011;34(4):729–49.
39. Cowin GJ, Jonsson JR, Bauer JD, Ash S, Ali A, Osland EJ, et al. Magnetic resonance imaging and spectroscopy for monitoring liver steatosis. J Magn Reson Imaging. 2008;28(4):937–45.
40. d'Assignies G, Ruel M, Khiat A, Lepanto L, Chagnon M, Kauffmann C, et al. Noninvasive quantitation of human liver steatosis using magnetic resonance and bioassay methods. Eur Radiol. 2009;19(8):2033–40.
41. Hamilton G, Middleton MS, Bydder M, Yokoo T, Schwimmer JB, Kono Y, et al. Effect of PRESS and STEAM sequences on magnetic resonance spectroscopic liver fat quantification. J Magn Reson Imaging. 2009;30(1):145–52.
42. Hamilton G, Yokoo T, Bydder M, Cruite I, Schroeder ME, Sirlin CB, et al. In vivo characterization of the liver fat (1)H MR spectrum. NMR Biomed. 2011;24(7):784–90.
43. Longo R, Pollesello P, Ricci C, Masutti F, Kvam BJ, Bercich L, et al. Proton MR spectroscopy in quantitative in vivo determination of fat content in human liver steatosis. J Magn Reson Imaging. 1995;5(3):281–5.
44. Longo R, Ricci C, Masutti F, Vidimari R, Croce LS, Bercich L, et al. Fatty infiltration of the liver. Quantification by 1H localized magnetic resonance spectroscopy and comparison with computed tomography. Investig Radiol. 1993;28(4):297–302.
45. McPherson S, Jonsson JR, Cowin GJ, O'Rourke P, Clouston AD, Volp A, et al. Magnetic resonance imaging and spectroscopy accurately estimate the severity of steatosis provided the stage of fibrosis is considered. J Hepatol. 2009;51(2):389–97.
46. Thomsen C, Becker U, Winkler K, Christoffersen P, Jensen M, Henriksen O. Quantification of liver fat using magnetic resonance spectroscopy. Magn Reson Imaging. 1994;12(3):487–95.
47. Borra RJ, Salo S, Dean K, Lautamaki R, Nuutila P, Komu M, et al. Nonalcoholic fatty liver disease: rapid evaluation of liver fat content with in-phase and out-of-phase MR imaging. Radiology. 2009;250(1):130–6.
48. Bydder M, Yokoo T, Hamilton G, Middleton MS, Chavez AD, Schwimmer JB, et al. Relaxation effects in the quantification of fat using gradient echo imaging. Magn Reson Imaging. 2008;26(3):347–59.
49. Fishbein MH, Gardner KG, Potter CJ, Schmalbrock P, Smith MA. Introduction of fast MR imaging in the assessment of hepatic steatosis. Magn Reson Imaging. 1997;15(3):287–93.
50. Guiu B, Petit JM, Loffroy R, Ben Salem D, Aho S, Masson D, et al. Quantification of liver fat content: comparison of triple-echo chemical shift gradient-echo imaging and in vivo proton MR spectroscopy. Radiology. 2009;250(1):95–102.
51. He T, Gatehouse PD, Kirk P, Mohiaddin RH, Pennell DJ, Firmin DN. Myocardial T*2 measurement in iron-overloaded thalassemia: an ex vivo study to investigate optimal methods of quantification. Magn Reson Med. 2008;60(2):350–6.
52. Hussain HK, Chenevert TL, Londy FJ, Gulani V, Swanson SD, McKenna BJ, et al. Hepatic fat fraction: MR imaging for quantitative measurement and display—early experience. Radiology. 2005;237(3):1048–55.
53. Kawamitsu H, Kaji Y, Ohara T, Sugimura K. Feasibility of quantitative intrahepatic lipid imaging applied to the magnetic resonance dual gradient echo sequence. Magn Reson Med Sci. 2003;2(1):47–50.
54. Kovanlikaya A, Guclu C, Desai C, Becerra R, Gilsanz V. Fat quantification using three-point dixon technique: in vitro validation. Acad Radiol. 2005;12(5):636–9.
55. Levenson H, Greensite F, Hoefs J, Friloux L, Applegate G, Silva E, et al. Fatty infiltration of the liver: quantification with phase-contrast MR imaging at 1.5 T vs biopsy. AJR Am J Roentgenol. 1991;156(2):307–12.
56. Liu CY, McKenzie CA, Yu H, Brittain JH, Reeder SB. Fat quantification with IDEAL gradient echo imaging: correction of bias from T(1) and noise. Magn Reson Med. 2007;58(2):354–64.
57. Mitchell DG, Kim I, Chang TS, Vinitski S, Consigny PM, Saponaro SA, et al. Fatty liver. Chemical shift

phase-difference and suppression magnetic resonance imaging techniques in animals, phantoms, and humans. Investig Radiol. 1991;26(12):1041–52.
58. O'Regan DP, Callaghan MF, Wylezinska-Arridge M, Fitzpatrick J, Naoumova RP, Hajnal JV, et al. Liver fat content and T2*: simultaneous measurement by using breath-hold multiecho MR imaging at 3.0 T—feasibility. Radiology. 2008;247(2):550–7.
59. Pacifico L, Celestre M, Anania C, Paolantonio P, Chiesa C, Laghi A. MRI and ultrasound for hepatic fat quantification: relationships to clinical and metabolic characteristics of pediatric nonalcoholic fatty liver disease. Acta Paediatr. 2007;96(4):542–7.
60. Qayyum A, Goh JS, Kakar S, Yeh BM, Merriman RB, Coakley FV. Accuracy of liver fat quantification at MR imaging: comparison of out-of-phase gradient-echo and fat-saturated fast spin-echo techniques—initial experience. Radiology. 2005;237(2):507–11.
61. Reeder SB, McKenzie CA, Pineda AR, Yu H, Shimakawa A, Brau AC, et al. Water-fat separation with IDEAL gradient-echo imaging. J Magn Reson Imaging. 2007;25(3):644–52.
62. Reeder SB, Robson PM, Yu H, Shimakawa A, Hines CD, McKenzie CA, et al. Quantification of hepatic steatosis with MRI: the effects of accurate fat spectral modeling. J Magn Reson Imaging. 2009;29(6):1332–9.
63. Rinella ME, McCarthy R, Thakrar K, Finn JP, Rao SM, Koffron AJ, et al. Dual-echo, chemical shift gradient-echo magnetic resonance imaging to quantify hepatic steatosis: implications for living liver donation. Liver Transpl. 2003;9(8):851–6.
64. Schuchmann S, Weigel C, Albrecht L, Kirsch M, Lemke A, Lorenz G, et al. Non-invasive quantification of hepatic fat fraction by fast 1.0, 1.5 and 3.0 T MR imaging. Eur J Radiol. 2007;62(3):416–22.
65. Yoshimitsu K, Kuroda Y, Nakamuta M, Taketomi A, Irie H, Tajima T, et al. Noninvasive estimation of hepatic steatosis using plain CT vs. chemical-shift MR imaging: significance for living donors. J Magn Reson Imaging. 2008;28(3):678–84.
66. Yu H, McKenzie CA, Shimakawa A, AT V, Brau AC, Beatty PJ, et al. Multiecho reconstruction for simultaneous water-fat decomposition and T2* estimation. J Magn Reson Imaging. 2007;26(4):1153–61.
67. Yu H, Shimakawa A, McKenzie CA, Brodsky E, Brittain JH, Reeder SB. Multiecho water-fat separation and simultaneous R2* estimation with multifrequency fat spectrum modeling. Magn Reson Med. 2008;60(5):1122–34.
68. Haase A, Frahm J, Matthaei D, Hanicke W, Bomsdorf H, Kunz D, et al. MR imaging using stimulated echoes (STEAM). Radiology. 1986;160(3):787–90.
69. Bottomley PA, inventor. General electric company, assignee. Selective volume method for performing localized NMR spectroscopy; 1984.
70. Reeder SB, HH H, Sirlin CB. Proton density fat-fraction: a standardized MR-based biomarker of tissue fat concentration. J Magn Reson Imaging. 2012;36(5):1011–4.
71. Dixon WT. Simple proton spectroscopic imaging. Radiology. 1984;153(1):189–94.
72. Ma JF. Breath-hold water and fat imaging using a dual-echo two-point dixon technique with an efficient and robust phase-correction algorithm. Magn Reson Med. 2004;52(2):415–9.
73. Glover GH, Schneider E. Three-point Dixon technique for true water/fat decomposition with B0 inhomogeneity correction. Magn Reson Med. 1991;18(2):371–83.
74. Glover GH. Multipoint Dixon technique for water and fat proton and susceptibility imaging. J Magn Reson Imaging. 1991;1(5):521–30.
75. Middleton M, Hamilton G, Bydder M, Sirlin C, editors. How much fat is under the water peak in liver fat MR spectroscopy? Honolulu, Hawaii: International Society for Magnetic Resonance in Medicine; 2009.
76. Muthupillai R, Lomas DJ, Rossman PJ, Greenleaf JF, Manduca A, Ehman RL. Magnetic resonance elastography by direct visualization of propagating acoustic strain waves. Science. 1995;269(5232):1854–7.
77. Othman SF, Xu H, Royston TJ, Magin RL. Microscopic magnetic resonance elastography (microMRE). Magn Reson Med. 2005;54(3):605–15.
78. Yin M, Talwalkar JA, Glaser KJ, Manduca A, Grimm RC, Rossman PJ, et al. Assessment of hepatic fibrosis with magnetic resonance elastography. Clin Gastroenterol Hepatol. 2007;5(10):1207–13. e2.
79. Asbach P, Klatt D, Hamhaber U, Braun J, Somasundaram R, Hamm B, et al. Assessment of liver viscoelasticity using multifrequency MR elastography. Magn Reson Med. 2008;60(2):373–9.
80. Mariappan YK, Glaser KJ, Ehman RL. Magnetic resonance elastography: a review. Clin Anat. 2010;23(5):497–511.
81. Manduca A, Oliphant TE, Dresner MA, Mahowald JL, Kruse SA, Amromin E, et al. Magnetic resonance elastography: non-invasive mapping of tissue elasticity. Med Image Anal. 2001;5(4):237–54.
82. Oliphant TE, Manduca A, Ehman RL, Greenleaf JF. Complex-valued stiffness reconstruction for magnetic resonance elastography by algebraic inversion of the differential equation. Magn Reson Med. 2001;45(2):299–310.
83. Manduca A, Lake DS, Kruse SA, Ehman RL. Spatiotemporal directional filtering for improved inversion of MR elastography images. Med Image Anal. 2003;7(4):465–73.
84. Rouviere O, Yin M, Dresner MA, Rossman PJ, Burgart LJ, Fidler JL, et al. MR elastography of the liver: preliminary results. Radiology. 2006;240(2):440–8.
85. Venkatesh SK, Yin M, Glockner JF, Takahashi N, Araoz PA, Talwalkar JA, et al. MR elastography of liver tumors: preliminary results. AJR Am J Roentgenol. 2008;190(6):1534–40.

86. Singh S, Venkatesh SK, Wang Z, Miller FH, Motosugi U, Low RN, et al. Diagnostic performance of magnetic resonance elastography in staging liver fibrosis: a systematic review and meta-analysis of individual participant data. Clin Gastroenterol Hepatol. 2015;13(3):440–51. e6.
87. Koinuma M, Ohashi I, Hanafusa K, Shibuya H. Apparent diffusion coefficient measurements with diffusion-weighted magnetic resonance imaging for evaluation of hepatic fibrosis. J Magn Reson Imaging. 2005;22(1):80–5.
88. Ichikawa T, Haradome H, Hachiya J, Nitatori T, Araki T. Diffusion-weighted MR imaging with a single-shot echoplanar sequence: detection and characterization of focal hepatic lesions. AJR Am J Roentgenol. 1998;170(2):397–402.
89. Ichikawa T, Haradome H, Hachiya J, Nitatori T, Araki T. Diffusion-weighted MR imaging with single-shot echo-planar imaging in the upper abdomen: preliminary clinical experience in 61 patients. Abdom Imaging. 1999;24(5):456–61.
90. Muller MF, Prasad P, Siewert B, Nissenbaum MA, Raptopoulos V, Edelman RR. Abdominal diffusion mapping with use of a whole-body echo-planar system. Radiology. 1994;190(2):475–8.
91. Namimoto T, Yamashita Y, Sumi S, Tang Y, Takahashi M. Focal liver masses: characterization with diffusion-weighted echo-planar MR imaging. Radiology. 1997;204(3):739–44.
92. Taouli B, Vilgrain V, Dumont E, Daire JL, Fan B, Menu Y. Evaluation of liver diffusion isotropy and characterization of focal hepatic lesions with two single-shot echo-planar MR imaging sequences: prospective study in 66 patients. Radiology. 2003;226(1):71–8.
93. Yamada I, Aung W, Himeno Y, Nakagawa T, Shibuya H. Diffusion coefficients in abdominal organs and hepatic lesions: evaluation with intravoxel incoherent motion echo-planar MR imaging. Radiology. 1999;210(3):617–23.
94. Poyraz AK, Onur MR, Kocakoc E, Ogur E. Diffusion-weighted MRI of fatty liver. J Magn Reson Imaging. 2012;35(5):1108–11.
95. Aisen AM, Doi K, Swanson SD. Detection of liver fibrosis with magnetic cross-relaxation. Magn Reson Med. 1994;31(5):551–6.
96. Alanen A, Komu M, Leino R, Toikkanen S. MR and magnetisation transfer imaging in cirrhotic and fatty livers. Acta Radiol. 1998;39(4):434–9.
97. Chen JH, Chai JW, Shen WC. Magnetization transfer contrast imaging of liver cirrhosis. Hepato-Gastroenterology. 1999;46(29):2872–7.
98. Lall CG, Aisen AM, Bansal N, Sandrasegaran K. Nonalcoholic fatty liver disease. AJR Am J Roentgenol. 2008;190(4):993–1002.
99. Tsuda N, Okada M, Murakami T. Potential of gadolinium-ethoxybenzyl-diethylenetriamine pentaacetic acid (Gd-EOB-DTPA) for differential diagnosis of nonalcoholic steatohepatitis and fatty liver in rats using magnetic resonance imaging. Investig Radiol. 2007;42(4):242–7.
100. Asanuma T, Ono M, Kubota K, Hirose A, Hayashi Y, Saibara T, et al. Super paramagnetic iron oxide MRI shows defective Kupffer cell uptake function in non-alcoholic fatty liver disease. Gut. 2010;59(2):258–66.
101. Beeman SC, Mandarino LJ, Georges JF, Bennett KM. Cationized ferritin as a magnetic resonance imaging probe to detect microstructural changes in a rat model of non-alcoholic steatohepatitis. Magn Reson Med. 2013;70(6):1728–38.
102. Ardenkjaer-Larsen JH, Fridlund B, Gram A, Hansson G, Hansson L, Lerche MH, et al. Increase in signal-to-noise ratio of >10,000 times in liquid-state NMR. Proc Natl Acad Sci U S A. 2003;100(18):10158–63.
103. Hu S, Chen AP, Zierhut ML, Bok R, Yen YF, Schroeder MA, et al. In vivo carbon-13 dynamic MRS and MRSI of normal and fasted rat liver with hyperpolarized 13C-pyruvate. Mol Imaging Biol. 2009;11(6):399–407.
104. Spielman DM, Mayer D, Yen YF, Tropp J, Hurd RE, Pfefferbaum A. In vivo measurement of ethanol metabolism in the rat liver using magnetic resonance spectroscopy of hyperpolarized [1-13C]pyruvate. Magn Reson Med. 2009;62(2):307–13.
105. Merritt ME, Harrison C, Sherry AD, Malloy CR, Burgess SC. Flux through hepatic pyruvate carboxylase and phosphoenolpyruvate carboxykinase detected by hyperpolarized 13C magnetic resonance. Proc Natl Acad Sci U S A. 2011;108(47):19084–9.
106. Lee P, Leong W, Tan T, Lim M, Han W, Radda GK. In vivo hyperpolarized carbon-13 magnetic resonance spectroscopy reveals increased pyruvate carboxylase flux in an insulin-resistant mouse model. Hepatology. 2013;57(2):515–24.
107. Abele JT, Fung CI. Effect of hepatic steatosis on liver FDG uptake measured in mean standard uptake values. Radiology. 2010;254(3):917–24.
108. Abikhzer G, Alabed YZ, Azoulay L, Assayag J, Rush C. Altered hepatic metabolic activity in patients with hepatic steatosis on FDG PET/CT. AJR Am J Roentgenol. 2011;196(1):176–80.
109. Ceulemans G, Ilsen B, Verdries D, de Mey J, Everaert H. Focal eosinophilic hepatitis simulating a solitary metastatic lesion on FDG-PET/CT in a patient with history of head and neck cancer. JBR-BTR. 2011;94(2):94.
110. Nakahara T, Takagi Y, Takemasa K, Mitsui Y, Tsuyuki A, Shigematsu N, et al. Dose-related fluorodeoxyglucose uptake in acute radiation-induced hepatitis. Eur J Gastroenterol Hepatol. 2008;20(10):1040–4.
111. Bural GG, Torigian DA, Burke A, Houseni M, Alkhawaldeh K, Cucchiara A, et al. Quantitative assessment of the hepatic metabolic volume product in patients with diffuse hepatic steatosis and normal controls through use of FDG-PET and MR imaging: a novel concept. Mol Imaging Biol. 2010;12(3):233–9.

112. Dostbil Z, Varoglu E, Serdengecti M, Kaya B, Onder H, Sari O. Evaluation of hepatic metabolic activity in non-alcoholic fatty livers on 18FDG PET/CT. Rev Esp Med Nucl Imagen Mol. 2013;32(3):156–61.
113. Hong SP, Noh TS, Moon SH, Cho YS, Lee EJ, Choi JY, et al. Hepatic glucose uptake is increased in association with elevated serum gamma-glutamyl transpeptidase and triglyceride. Dig Dis Sci. 2014;59(3):607–13.
114. Moon SH, Hong SP, Cho YS, Noh TS, Choi JY, Kim BT, et al. Hepatic FDG uptake is associated with future cardiovascular events in asymptomatic individuals with non-alcoholic fatty liver disease. J Nucl Cardiol. 2015. doi:10.1007/s12350-015-0297-y.
115. Iozzo P, Bucci M, Roivainen A, Nagren K, Jarvisalo MJ, Kiss J, et al. Fatty acid metabolism in the liver, measured by positron emission tomography, is increased in obese individuals. Gastroenterology. 2010;139(3):846–56, 56.e1–6.
116. Xie L, Yui J, Hatori A, Yamasaki T, Kumata K, Wakizaka H, et al. Translocator protein (18 kDa), a potential molecular imaging biomarker for non-invasively distinguishing non-alcoholic fatty liver disease. J Hepatol. 2012;57(5):1076–82.
117. Lin J, Lu F, Zheng W, Xu S, Tai D, Yu H, et al. Assessment of liver steatosis and fibrosis in rats using integrated coherent anti-Stokes Raman scattering and multiphoton imaging technique. J Biomed Opt. 2011;16(11):116024.
118. Evers DJ, Westerkamp AC, Spliethoff JW, Pully VV, Hompes D, Hendriks BH, et al. Diffuse reflectance spectroscopy: toward real-time quantification of steatosis in liver. Transpl Int. 2015;28(4):465–74.
119. Evers DJ, Nachabe R, Hompes D, van Coevorden F, Lucassen GW, Hendriks BH, et al. Optical sensing for tumor detection in the liver. Eur J Surg Oncol. 2013;39(1):68–75.
120. Tian C, Xie Z, Fabiilli ML, Wang X. Imaging and sensing based on dual-pulse nonlinear photoacoustic contrast: a preliminary study on fatty liver. Opt Lett. 2015;40(10):2253–6.
121. Boursier J, de Ledinghen V, Sturm N, Amrani L, Bacq Y, Sandrini J, et al. Precise evaluation of liver histology by computerized morphometry shows that steatosis influences liver stiffness measured by transient elastography in chronic hepatitis C. J Gastroenterol. 2014;49(3):527–37.
122. Hatta T, Fujinaga Y, Kadoya M, Ueda H, Murayama H, Kurozumi M, et al. Accurate and simple method for quantification of hepatic fat content using magnetic resonance imaging: a prospective study in biopsy-proven nonalcoholic fatty liver disease. J Gastroenterol. 2010;45(12):1263–71.
123. Leiber LM, Boursier J, Michalak S, Roullier V, Fizanne L, Chaigneau J, et al. MRI versus histological methods for time course monitoring of steatosis amount in a murine model of NAFLD. Diagn Interv Imaging. 2015;96(9):915–22.

Imaging Myocardial Metabolism

11

Robert J. Gropler and Craig R. Malloy

Abbreviations

ATP	Adenosine triphosphate
DNP	Dynamic nuclear polarization
HP	Hyperpolarization
LV	Left ventricle
MRI	Magnetic resonance imaging
MRS	Magnetic resonance spectroscopy
PDH	Pyruvate dehydrogenase
PET	Positron emission computed tomography
PPP	Pentose phosphate pathway
RV	Right ventricle
SPECT	Single photon emission computed tomography
TCA	Tricarboxylic acid
TG	Triglycerides

R.J. Gropler (✉)
Division of Radiological Sciences, Mallinckrodt Institute of Radiology, Washington University School of Medicine, St. Louis, MO, USA
e-mail: groplerr@mir.wustl.edu

C.R. Malloy
Departments of Radiology and Internal Medicine, Advanced Imaging Research Center, University of Texas Southwestern Medical Center, Dallas, TX, USA

VA North Texas Health Care System, Dallas, TX, USA
e-mail: craig.malloy@utsouthwestern.edu

11.1 Introduction

Metabolism of exogenous and endogenous substrates, under baseline conditions and in response to metabolic and physiological stimuli, is central to cardiac myocyte health. The ever-burgeoning body of evidence demonstrating the primacy of perturbations in intermediary metabolism in the pathogenesis of common cardiovascular diseases such as ischemic heart disease, heart failure, and diabetic cardiomyopathy further supports this contention. It is becoming increasingly apparent that chronic adaptations in cellular metabolism initiate a host of pleiotropic actions detrimental to cellular health such as impaired energetics, increases in inflammation, oxidative stress, and apoptosis. Indeed the importance of altered intermediary metabolism underlying human cardiovascular disease is exemplified by the robust drug discovery and development efforts to identify new metabolic modulators.

Radionuclide imaging by positron emission tomography (PET) and single photon emission computed tomography (SPECT) are the most powerful used methods to perform in vivo assessments of myocardial metabolism. PET is currently the gold standard for imaging myocardial metabolism in humans. Its high sensitivity, resulting in the administration of nano- to picomolar concentrations of various radiotracers, and inherent quantitative capability permit the measurement of fluxes in

J.S. Lewis, K.R. Keshari (eds.), *Imaging and Metabolism*, DOI 10.1007/978-3-319-61401-4_11

absolute rates through key metabolic processes without perturbing the biochemical system. SPECT can also measure myocardial metabolism under baseline conditions but is nonquantitative and lacks the availability of an extensive portfolio of metabolic radiotracers. Both methods suffer from the inability to simultaneously measure multiple metabolic processes which is certainly desirable given the complexity of cellular metabolism in health and disease.

Nuclear magnetic resonance (NMR) spectroscopy and imaging methods are valuable tools, but their use in humans is practically impossible due to the combination of the low concentration of the relevant metabolites plus low NMR sensitivity of these nuclei with a detection threshold of millimolar concentrations. Hyperpolarization produces a temporary redistribution of nuclear spin populations and partially overcomes this sensitivity limitation while preserving the chemical specificity inherent in NMR. This technology was well known within the physics community for decades, but it was not until Ardenkjaer-Larsen, Golman, and colleagues demonstrated that the hyperpolarized state could be achieved temporarily under physiologically relevant conditions that potential in vivo assessments could be realized [1, 2]. Since this technology is applicable at conventional MR fields, it is possible to utilize standard MR scanners, coils, and other technologies, which are safe for humans [3]. There is considerable interest in developing hyperpolarized MR-based contrast agents for cardiac studies in humans. From a metabolic perspective, specific substrates labeled with ^{13}C offer the potential to simultaneously assess diverse metabolic pathways. However, MR imaging of hyperpolarized ^{13}C (^{13}C-HP) does present significant challenges for routine imaging such as the significant time constraints due to a short T_1. Furthermore, due to the administration of millimolar concentrations of material, metabolic conditions are perturbed which complicates the interpretation of the measurements.

This first portion of this chapter will summarize the fundamentals of myocardial metabolism and important regulatory mechanisms, highlighting aspects that are relevant to design and interpretation of PET or ^{13}C-HP studies. Although intermediary metabolism, energy capture, and biosynthetic pathways in the heart are complex, the key features can be understood as interacting modules and pathways. The second portion will detail the relative strengths and weaknesses of radionuclide imaging focusing on PET and ^{13}C-HP to assess myocardial metabolism. Compared to hyperpolarization methods, clinical radionuclide methods are far more mature. There is no experience with hyperpolarization methods in heart disease in humans. PET and ^{13}C-HP may be able to provide complementary information on myocardial metabolism. Accordingly, the final portion of the chapter will briefly discuss the metabolic perturbations associated with some common cardiovascular diseases and present potential scenarios whereby synergies may be realized by combining these two technologies.

11.2 Energy Production and Related Metabolic Pathways

Every metabolic pathway is complex, and control mechanisms operate at the level of enzyme expression, the interactions with cofactors, and the concentrations of substrates and products in the local environment. A useful generalization is to separate heart metabolism into distinct modules such as the citric acid cycle, glycolysis, the pentose phosphate pathway, and β-oxidation linked by a few key molecules at metabolic crossroads. These critical molecules are acetyl-CoA (the final common product of multiple pathways), pyruvate (linking the product of glycolysis with exogenous pyruvate and lactate), and glucose-6-phosphate (linking glycolysis, glycogenolysis, and the pentose phosphate pathway). This section presents a brief overview of helpful concepts for understanding the design and interpretation of studies with tracers in the heart. It will also serve to point out important aspects of cardiac metabolism that are currently difficult to probe. The focus is on key metabolites at metabolic crossroads since these molecules or their analogues are targeted in metabolic imaging.

The vast majority of the energy driving cardiac function comes from the oxidation of acetyl-CoA in the citric acid cycle. The heart normally generates acetyl-CoA from a complex mixture of exogenous substrates including fatty acids of various chain lengths, glucose, lactate, pyruvate and the ketones, acetoacetate, and β-hydroxybutyrate (Fig. 11.1). The relative concentrations may vary dramatically under both physiological and pathological conditions. Studies of isolated hearts in which only a single substrate or perhaps two substrates are supplied do not reflect the pattern of energy production observed in vivo. In general, the heart readily switches among substrates to generate acetyl-CoA [4, 5]. If glucose is the only substrate available to the heart, it is readily oxidized to acetyl-CoA, but the contribution of glucose to acetyl-CoA is negligible when a physiological mixture of substrates is available [6, 7]. Under normal conditions of perfusion and oxygen tension, the majority of energy production in the heart is derived from oxidation of long-chain fatty acids. A significant contribution is also derived from ketones and lactate [6, 7]. During a fast, the contribution of ketones to energy production increases substantially, and the contribution of lactate may increase markedly during exercise [8]. Under abnormal conditions, for example, left

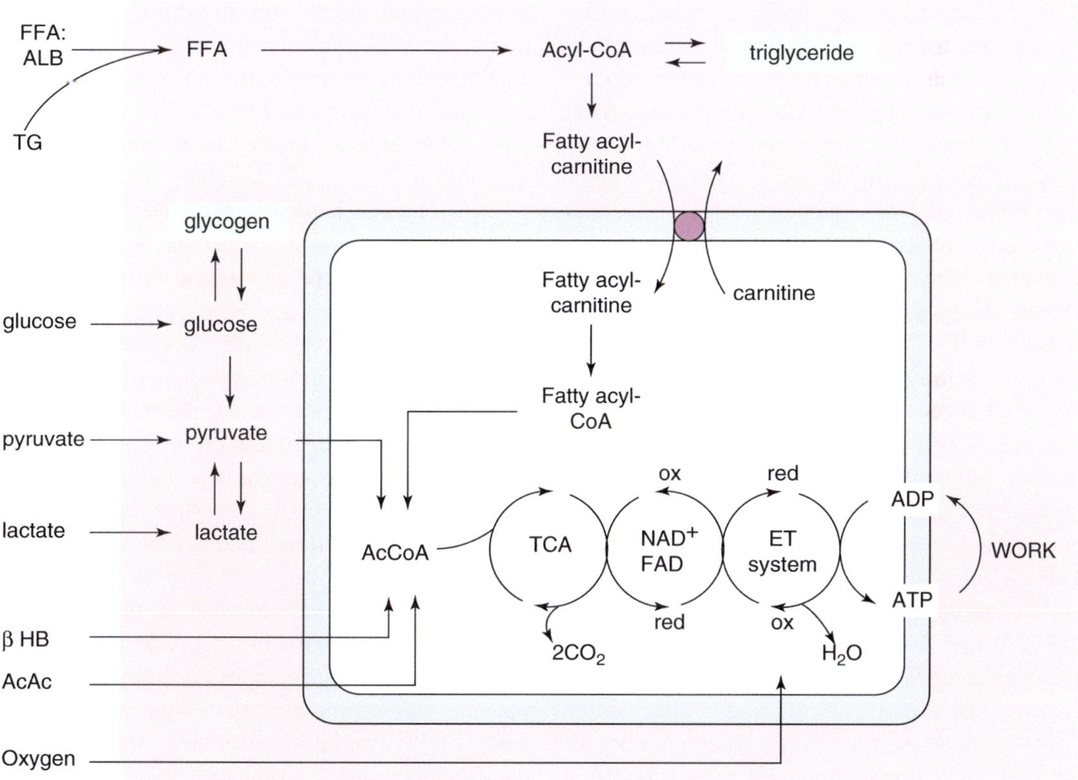

Fig. 11.1 Processes for energy capture in the heart. The heart in vivo is provided with a complex mixture of substrates including long-chain fatty acids, glucose, ketones, lactate, and pyruvate in varying combinations. The normal heart rapidly shifts among these available substrates as well as the stored energy sources, triglycerides, and glycogen, depending on the concentrations of substrates, the presence of insulin and other hormones, and the workload. *AcAc* acetoacetate, *βHB* β-hydroxybutyrate, *ET* electron transport, *FFA* free fatty acids

ventricular (LV) pressure-overload hypertrophy, oxidation of glucose increases substantially. Consequently, one of the challenges of understanding cardiac energy metabolism is that it is governed by at least three factors – plasma substrate concentration, normal physiological responses to energy demands, and disease.

11.2.1 Acetyl-CoA from β-Oxidation of Ketones and Fatty Acids

The concentration of fatty acids in plasma strongly influences the rate of uptake by the heart. The normal range of free fatty acids is roughly 0.2–0.8 mM but can reach 1.0 mM due to stress or conditions such as diabetes or starvation. Actually, long-chain fatty acids are water insoluble and therefore are always bound to albumin or incorporated into triglyceride (TG), either as chylomicrons or very low-density lipoproteins. After transport across the sarcolemma, a long-chain fatty acid is transiently bound to a fatty acid binding protein and subsequently activated by fatty acyl-CoA synthase. The product of this reaction, long-chain fatty acyl-CoA, may either be esterified to TG by glycerophosphate acyltransferase or converted to long-chain fatty acylcarnitine by carnitine palmitoyltransferase (Fig. 11.1). The fate of a fatty acid – esterification and storage vs. oxidation – is a critical branch point in metabolism of long-chain fatty acids. About 80% of radiolabeled oleate or palmitate is rapidly metabolized via ß-oxidation and the citric acid cycle. This suggests that about 20% of fatty acids entering a cardiomyocyte must enter the intracardiac TGTCA pool. However recent observations suggest preferential oxidation of fatty acids may occur via continuous mixing and cycling within the TG pool, suggesting the preferential route for fatty acid oxidation is still an open question [9]. It is important to be aware that cardiomyocytes may store TGs because these fatty acids can be mobilized during adrenergic stimulation and may provide a source of fatty acids for oxidation [10].

As noted above, the majority of long-chain fatty acids are oxidized for energy production. The cytoplasmic long-chain fatty acyl-CoA cannot penetrate the inner mitochondrial membrane and for this reason is converted to a fatty acyl carnitine, described above, by carnitine palmitoyl transferase I (CPT-1). Carnitine acyltranslocase transports this long-chain acylcarnitine across the inner mitochondrial membrane. Finally, the long-chain acyl-CoA is regenerated in the mitochondrial matrix by CPT-2. Within the mitochondria, fatty acids undergo repeated cycles of ß-oxidation to generate acetyl-CoA for oxidation in the citric acid cycle.

[1-^{11}C]acetate has been studied [11] as a tracer for the assessment of citric acid cycle flux in the myocardium. The time-activity curve of ^{11}C may be interpreted in terms of the tricarboxylic acid cycle (TCA) flux and oxygen consumption. Unlike long-chain fatty acids, acetate may be oxidized without the need for the carnitine palmitoyl transferase (CPT) system to cross the inner mitochondrial membrane. In addition to oxidation in the TCA cycle, acetate also participates in an important energy-buffering system in the myocardium catalyzed by carnitine acetyltransferse. This enzyme, located in the mitochondria, interconverts acetyl-CoA with acetylcarnitine [12, 13, 21]. Consequently, the excess concentration of acetyl groups, whether derived from infused acetate, carbohydrates, or fatty acids, can be buffered.

β-Hydroxybutyrate and acetoacetate are ketones that arise from metabolism of fatty acids in the liver. Like fatty acids, the heart oxidizes ketones at a rate dependent on the concentration in plasma. Consequently, the contribution of ketones to acetyl-CoA can shift dramatically depending on nutritional and neurohumoral conditions. The concentration of ketones is normally low in a fed, rested mammal, in the range of 0.03–0.06 millimolar [14, 15]. Considering the low concentration of ketones normally present in plasma, approximately 10x lower than fatty acids, it is perhaps surprising that ketones contribute to energy production at all [6]. During starvation, heart failure, or poorly managed type 1 diabetes, the concentrations can rise dramatically into the millimolar range and markedly suppress oxidation of both fatty acids and carbohydrates. Hence, under these conditions ketones may provide essentially all acetyl-CoA in the myocardium. For this reason it is important to be aware of the nutritional conditions when interpreting metabolic imaging studies.

11.2.2 Pyruvate and Lactate

Pyruvate is a substrate for pyruvate dehydrogenase (PDH), a regulatory site in cellular metabolism that links the TCA cycle and subsequent oxidative phosphorylation with key steps in glucose, lipid, and amino acid metabolism. Pyruvate levels in the blood are typically low (normally ~0.1 mM). Under normal physiological conditions, intracellular pyruvate is readily produced by conversion from lactate. However, after bolus administration, the heart rapidly oxidizes pyruvate. Like the concentration of ketones, the concentration of lactate (normally 1.0–1.2 mM) may vary substantially depending on the physiological response to exercise or disease. The heart is normally a net consumer of lactate, although during ischemia it may actually produce lactate. The enzyme interconverting lactate and pyruvate, lactate dehydrogenase, is highly active in the myocardium, so the heart readily metabolizes lactate (after conversion to pyruvate) when the plasma concentration rises. Pyruvate has four fates in the heart: decarboxylation to form acetyl-CoA for subsequent oxidation in the citric acid cycle, transamination to alanine, reduction to lactate, and carboxylation to form oxaloacetate.

Decarboxylation by PDH is irreversible, and this reaction plays a key role in regulating fatty acid and carbohydrate oxidation. PDH is located in the mitochondrial matrix and flux is regulated by both covalent modification and feedback inhibition [16]. Interestingly, certain fatty acids may paradoxically stimulate PDH [17, 18]. The cycle of covalent modification, phosphorylation-dephosphorylation, is controlled by PDH kinase and PDH phosphatase, respectively. High concentrations of pyruvate favor flux through PDH which is consistent with inhibition of the kinase (less phosphorylation of PDH). Flux through PDH is also stimulated by a low [acetyl-CoA]/[free CoA] and a low NADH/NAD^+ ratio. In the heart, the dominant isoform of PDH kinase is PDH kinase 4; its expression is induced by diabetes, starvation, and peroxisome proliferator activator receptor ligands. Under all these conditions, PDH phosphorylation is expected to increase, thereby inhibiting oxidation of pyruvate or upstream carbohydrates. Under starvation conditions, this effect is teleologically appropriate since it would have the effect of preserving carbohydrates for brain metabolism. Dephosphorylation of PDH (activation of PDH) by the phosphatase is increased by calcium, which in turn is sensitive to adrenergic stimulation or other interventions that drive increased [Ca^{++}] in the mitochondria and are associated with increased myocardial contractility.

Carboxylation of pyruvate to form oxaloacetate is quantitatively a minor pathway in pyruvate metabolism compared to potential flux through PDH [19–21]. Nevertheless, this pathway is likely important in understanding cardiac metabolism. The sum of TCA cycle intermediates varies substantially depending on available substrates and work state. Since the concentration of citrate may play a role in regulation of glycolysis, the total mass of TCA cycle intermediates may influence glucose metabolism. The myocardium has the capacity to remodel and hypertrophy; thus, metabolic pathways necessary for biosynthetic and degradation reactions involving amino acids are likely important. However, no imaging method is available to directly assess this reaction in vivo.

In addition to these two reactions in the mitochondria, decarboxylation to acetyl-CoA and carboxylation to oxaloacetate, pyruvate may also undergo exchange reactions in the cytosol. Transamination to alanine is catalyzed by alanine aminotransferase in the overall reaction: pyruvate + glutamate → alanine + α-ketoglutarate. Pyruvate may also be reduced to lactate by lactate dehydrogenase, a reaction requiring NADH as a cofactor. Consequently the rate of conversion of pyruvate to lactate (but not alanine) should be sensitive to redox conditions.

11.2.3 Glucose and Glycogen

Glucose and glycogen are mentioned last because at physiological concentrations of fatty acids, ketones, and lactate, both substrates contribute little to the overall energy production in the healthy, well-oxygenated myocardium. Nevertheless, glucose metabolism plays an important role in myocardial energetics, for a number of reasons. First, glycolysis and glycogenolysis provide energy buffers during periods of stress and protect the myocardium during periods of brief ischemia. Second, the pentose phosphate pathway (PPP) is an important source of NADPH which is required for protection of the myocardium from oxidative stress. Third, adenosine triphosphate (ATP) derived from glycolysis may preferentially drive membrane bound ion pumps.

Transport of glucose across the sarcolemma is sensitive to the concentration of extracellular glucose and the activity of glucose transporters in the cell membrane. The main transporter, GLUT-4, is translocated from intracellular vesicles to the membrane in response to ischemia, insulin, increased work load, or activation of AMP-activated protein kinase. The net effect is to increase the availability of intracellular glucose during periods of hyperglycemia or myocardial stress. Once glucose enters the cytosol, it is rapidly phosphorylated, effectively trapping the carbon skeleton in the cytosol because the highly charged phosphate group prevents diffusion or transport out of the cardiomyocyte. Another source of glucose-6-phosphate is degradation of glycogen. Glycogenolysis is stimulated in the heart by increases in cAMP (due to adrenergic stimulation or glucagon), increases in [Ca^{++}], increased [inorganic phosphate], or reduced ATP.

The overall regulation of glycolysis has been intensively investigated and reviewed in detail [22]. Two sites of regulation may be mentioned briefly. First, phosphofructokinase-1 (PFK-1) uses ATP to convert fructose-1-phosphate to fructose 1,6-bisphosphate. This reaction is activated by adenosine diphosphate, adenosine monophosphate, and inorganic phosphate (ADP, AMP, and Pi). Consequently, during periods of myocardial stress (defined by an increased concentration of ATP breakdown products), the reaction is accelerated. Citrate is a negative regulator of PFK-1, and Philip Randle initially proposed that accumulation of citrate due to fatty acid oxidation may inhibit glycolysis, thus linking mitochondrial metabolism to glycolysis at an early step. A second important component in regulation of glycolysis is glyceraldehyde-3-phosphate dehydrogenase (GAPDH). Glyceraldehyde 3-phosphate is converted to 1,3-diphosphoglycerate and in the process generates the NADH produced in glycolysis. A high concentration of NADH in the cytosol will inhibit glycolysis at this step, as is the case during ischemia. Glycolysis is inhibited by accumulation of NADH unless NAD^+ can be regenerated by conversion of pyruvate to lactate and export of lactate.

Other than the generation of pyruvate and energy, glucose metabolism may be important for other processes. Glucose-6-phosphate is the substrate for the PPP (also termed the hexose monophosphate shunt or the phosphogluconate pathway). The PPP has two functions: the generation of NADPH, which is used in virtually all biosynthetic pathways and also reduces oxidized glutathione, and the generation of pentoses which are necessary for nucleotide synthesis. Since these are essential cellular processes, it seems likely that the PPP is important in the heart [23–25]. However, no imaging method is available to specifically probe the PPP.

11.2.4 Anaplerosis

Anaplerosis refers to any reaction that provides a net addition of a carbon skeleton to the TCA cycle [21, 26] . This is in contrast to the oxidation of acetyl-CoA in which two carbons are added to the TCA cycle with release of two molecules of CO_2 per cycle. Anaplerosis is required to maintain the concentration of TCA cycle intermediates which may be lost at a slow rate during biosynthetic reactions or leakage of intermediates from the cardiomyocyte. Pyruvate carboxylation is probably the most important pathway for anaplerosis with carboxylation of propionate, an odd-carbon fatty acid, being a lesser contributor [21, 27, 28]. Flux through pyruvate carboxylase is low, roughly 5–10% of TCA flux [29]. Although most metabolic imaging research has focused on oxidative pathways, it is likely that methods to specifically detect propionate or pyruvate carboxylation will be relevant in understanding cardiac remodeling disorders.

11.2.5 Compartmentation of Pyruvate Metabolism

There is strong evidence from tracer studies with exogenous pyruvate, lactate, and glucose that intracellular pyruvate cannot be treated as one fully mixed pool, even under steady-state conditions [30]. Years ago, Hassinen and colleagues reported that there are two intracellular pools of pyruvate, a pool derived from glycolysis and a peripheral pool that communicates with extracellular pyruvate, intracellular alanine, and intramitochondrial pyruvate [27]. These results were confirmed by others using the radiotracer technique [31, 32] that demonstrated some intracellular pyruvate is inaccessible to extracellular lactate. The production ratio of [^{14}C]bicarbonate relative to [1-^{14}C]lactate activity after administration of [1-^{14}C]]pyruvate was sensitive to the presence of glucose and was interpreted as evidence for multiple kinetically distinct pools of pyruvate in the heart [19]. Furthermore, acetyl-CoA derived from pyruvate originating from glucose is channeled preferentially to acetylcarnitine compared to acetyl-CoA [33].

^{13}C NMR isotopomer studies also found evidence for intracellular compartmentalization of glycolytic and glycogenolytic enzymes in isolated rat hearts perfused with [1-^{13}C]glucose [34]. Studies with [1-^{13}C]glucose [30] found that alanine and acetyl-CoA enrichments were similar under steady-state conditions, but the enrichment in intracellular lactate was less than alanine [35]. These observations strongly suggest that rapid exchange of extracellular labeled pyruvate and lactate with all intracellular pools is not consistent with experimental results. Hyperpolarization has the potential to monitor evolution of labeled lactate and bicarbonate from enriched pyruvate with high temporal resolution, offering the opportunity to probe subcellular compartments and examine the kinetic flexibility of the heart in response to stress and physiological stimuli.

11.3 Radionuclide Methods to Image Metabolism

Imaging of myocardial metabolism using radionuclides is widely applied in cardiovascular investigation as well as the clinical management of the cardiac patient. Detection of viable myocardium based on the metabolic signature of enhanced glucose metabolism in hypoperfused myocardium is the most prominent example used in cardiovascular investigation [36]. Some currently available radionuclide approaches to quantify key aspects of myocardial metabolism are summarized in Table 11.1 and will be described with examples of their application in cardiovascular investigation.

Table 11.1 Radiopharmaceuticals and ^{13}C-labeled compounds for cardiac metabolism

Metabolic process	Radiopharmaceutical[a]	^{13}C-labeled compound
Oxygen consumption	$^{15}O_2$, [1-^{11}C]acetate	[1-^{13}C]acetate, [2-^{13}C]pyruvate, [1-^{13}C]pyruvate
Long-chain fatty acid metabolism		
Uptake, oxidation, and storage	[1-^{11}C]palmitate, ^{18}F-F7, ^{123}I-IPPA[2]	
Uptake and oxidation	^{18}F-FTHA, ^{18}F-FTP, ^{18}F-FTO, ^{18}F-FCPHA	
Uptake and storage	^{123}I-BMIPP[b]	
Short-chain fatty acid metabolism		
Acetylcarnitine metabolism	–	[1-^{13}C]acetate
Butyrate oxidation	–	[1-^{13}C]butyrate
Carbohydrate metabolism		
Uptake	^{18}FDG	
Uptake, glycolysis, oxidation	[1-^{11}C]glucose	
Lactate metabolism	[3-^{11}C]Lactate	
pH determination		
CO_2 – bicarbonate ratio		[1-^{13}C]pyruvate

[a]Abbreviations defined in text
[b]SPECT radiopharmaceutical

11.3.1 Single Photon Emission Computed Tomography

The advantages of SPECT for cardiac metabolic imaging include a wide distribution of the technology, the potential for multiphoton energy imaging permitting simultaneous assessment of multiple processes, and the long physical half-life of SPECT radiotracers which facilitates delivery of a radiotracer from a central radiopharmacy to multiple geographical locations. To determine the human relevance of the metabolic phenotypes of rodent models of various forms of cardiovascular disease, numerous small animal imaging SPECT and SPECT/CT systems have been developed. The major current disadvantage of SPECT is the inability to quantify cellular metabolic processes primarily because of the relatively poor temporal resolution of the technology. However, new designs in SPECT technology may permit dynamic data acquisitions allowing quantitative or semiquantitative measurements of substrate metabolism.

Currently, there are few available SPECT approaches for measuring myocardial metabolism. One of the earliest and most promising SPECT radiotracers of fatty acid metabolism was 15-(*p*-iodophenyl)-pentadecanoic acid (^{123}I-IPPA) [37–39]. This radiotracer demonstrated myocardial kinetics similar to ^{11}C-palmitate. However, the poor temporal resolution of SPECT systems could not take advantage of the rapid turnover of IPPA. However, the recent introduction of higher temporal resolution SPECT cameras may result in the reemergence of this radiotracer. Currently, the most widely used SPECT radiotracer is the alkyl branched-chain FA analogue, ^{123}I-beta-methyl-P-iodophenylpentadecanoic acid (^{123}I-BMIPP) (Fig. 11.1 and Table 11.1) [39–42]. Alkyl branching inhibits β-oxidation, shuttling the radiolabel to the TG pool, thereby increasing radiotracer retention and improving image quality. No specific SPECT radiotracers are currently available to measure myocardial glucose metabolism. However, when combined with the appropriate detection scheme and collimator design, myocardial glucose metabolism can be assessed with SPECT and ^{18}F-fluorodexoyglucose (^{18}FDG) [43].

11.3.2 Positron Emission Tomography

The major advantage of PET is a detection scheme that permits quantification of radioactivity within the field of view by utilizing radiotracers labeled with positron-emitting radionuclides. Several of these radionuclides are biologically ubiquitous elements such as oxygen (^{15}O), carbon (^{11}C), and nitrogen (^{13}N). Fluorine (^{18}F) can be substituted for hydroxyl groups which allow for its incorporation into a wide variety of substrates or substrate analogues that participate in diverse biochemical pathways. Moreover, because these radiotracers are administered at tracer doses, they do not alter the metabolic processes of interest (Tables 11.1 and 11.2). The general principle to quantify a myocardial metabolic process based on the tracer method is to measure both the delivery of material from blood, or input, and the tissue response. The latter represents the metabolic process of interest (Fig. 11.2). With PET, the radiolabeled metabolite-corrected input function is derived and used in conjunction with a mathematical model, or

Table 11.2 Summary of the effects of heart disease on myocardial substrate metabolism. Little is known about the effects of various disorders on ketone metabolism

	Fatty acids	Glucose	Pyruvate or lactate	Ketones
LV hypertrophy	↓	↑	↑	–
Ischemia	↓↓	↑	↓	↓
Insulin resistance and diabetes	↑	↓	–	–

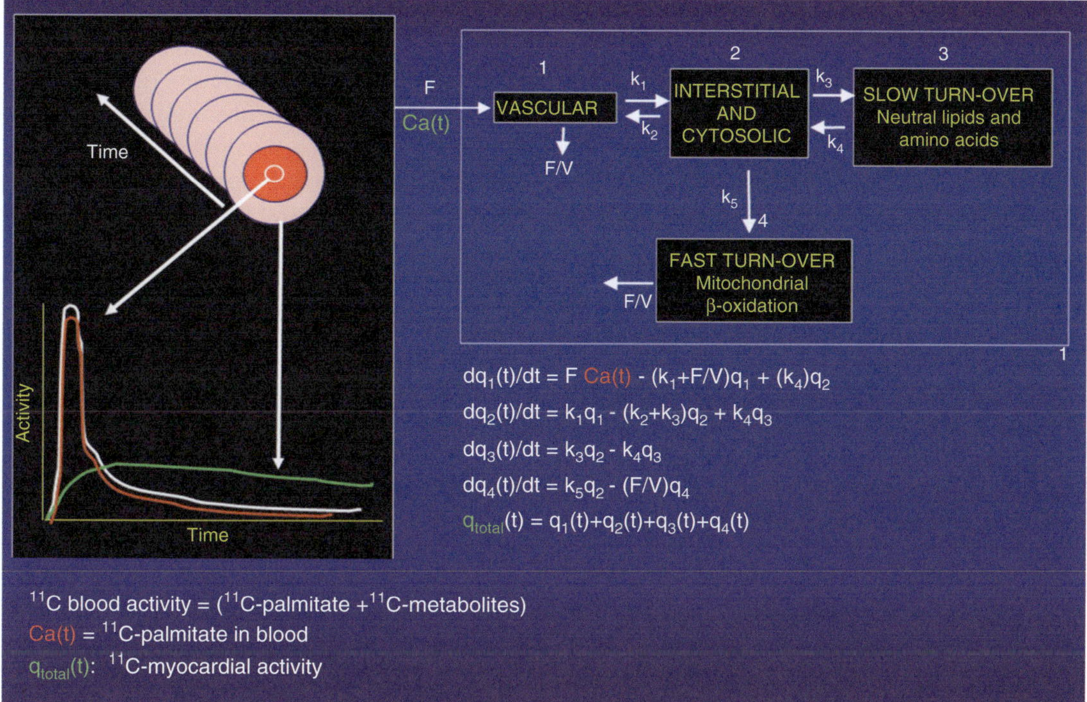

Fig. 11.2 Processes to quantify metabolic flux by PET. Shown here are the steps used to quantify flux through various pathways with PET using measurements of myocardial fatty acid with [1-^{11}C]palmitate as an example [59]. The left side of this figure again shows the conversion of idealized serial PET images from which both arterial and regional myocardial time-activity curves can be generated. The arterial time-activity curve is corrected for ^{11}C-labeled blood metabolites (in this case $^{11}CO_2$) to generate the arterial input function which reflects the delivery of [1-^{11}C]palmitate to the heart. The myocardial time-activity curve reflects the sum total of activity from all radiolabeled species in the myocardium. Movement of [1-^{11}C]palmitate into the myocardium is corrected for myocardial blood flow (F). The kinetic model for [1-^{11}C]palmitate has been divided into four key compartments of fatty acid metabolism with movement between the compartments determined by various rate constants (ks). The kinetic model fits the myocardial time-activity curve with the arterial input function to estimate the various rate constants. The rate constants are then included in the various differential equations to solve for different components of fatty acid metabolism

some variation, to quantify the metabolic processes by optimizing the model against PET-measured tissue response data (Fig. 11.2). Because of the poor spatial resolution of PET, both the input and tissue need to be corrected for geometric considerations such as partial volume and spillover effects. The measured tissue response in PET imaging reflects the sum total of radioactivity from all radiolabeled species in the tissue of interest. As such, the contribution of individual species and metabolic rates must be determined from the model parameters. PET cannot reliably characterize metabolism of substrates emanating from intracellular storage sites such as TG and glycogen pools. Other disadvantages of PET are its complexity in radiotracer design, image quantification schemes, and expense.

11.3.3 Myocardial Oxygen Consumption

Because oxygen is the final electron acceptor in all pathways of myocardial oxidative metabolism, PET with ^{15}O-oxygen has also been used to measure myocardial oxygen consumption (MVO_2). The approach provides a measure of myocardial oxygen extraction which when combined with measurements of myocardial blood flow and arterial oxygen content directly measures MVO_2. Due to its short physical half-life, ^{15}O-oxygen is readily applicable in studies requiring repetitive assessments, such as those with an acute pharmacologic intervention. Its major disadvantages are the requirement for an on-site cyclotron, the need for a multiple tracer study to account for myocardial blood flow and blood volume, and the fairly complex compartmental modeling to obtain the measurements [44–46].

Acetate is a two-carbon fatty acid whose primary metabolic fate is rapid conversion to acetyl-CoA and metabolism through the TCA cycle. Because the TCA cycle and oxidative phosphorylation are tightly coupled, myocardial turnover of ^{11}C-acetate reflects overall oxidative metabolism or MVO_2. Either exponential curve fitting or compartmental modeling can be used to calculate MVO_2. Modeling is typically preferable when cardiac output is low because marked dispersion of the input function and spillover of activity from the lungs to the myocardium is present, which decreases the accuracy of the curve-fitting method [11, 47–50]. However, it is more complex than exponential curve fitting and requires correction of blood radioactivity for $^{11}CO_2$.

11.3.4 Carbohydrate Metabolism

^{18}F-Fluorodeoxyglucose, an analogue of glucose, is transported into the cytosol where it undergoes hexokinase-mediated phosphorylation. In general, ^{18}FDG-6-phosphate is trapped in the cytosol, and the myocardial uptake of ^{18}FDG is thought to reflect overall anaerobic and aerobic myocardial glycolytic flux [51–54]. Myocardial glucose uptake can be assessed in either relative or absolute terms (i.e., in nanomoles $\cdot$ g^{-1} $\cdot$ min^{-1}). For quantification, a mathematical correction called the "lumped constant" that accounts for the differences in glucose transport and hexokinase-mediated phosphorylation between FDG and glucose must be used to calculate rates of glucose uptake. This value may vary depending upon the prevailing plasma substrate and hormonal conditions, decreasing the accuracy of the measurement of myocardial glucose uptake [53, 55–57]. The limited kinetics of FDG in tissue precludes determination of the metabolic fate (i.e., glycogen formation versus glycolysis) of the extracted tracer and glucose.

Quantification of myocardial glucose metabolism has been performed with PET using glucose radiolabeled in the one-carbon position with ^{11}C, [1-^{11}C]glucose. Advantages of this approach include the lack of need for a lumped constant correction because [1-^{11}C]glucose is chemically identical to unlabeled glucose and thus has the same metabolic fate as glucose, more accurate measurements of myocardial glucose uptake compared with FDG, and the ability to estimate the metabolic fate of extracted glucose. Disadvantages of this method include a fairly complex synthesis of the tracer, the short physical half-life of ^{11}C (requiring an on-site cyclotron), compartmental modeling that is more demanding with ^{11}C-glucose than it is with FDG, and the need to correct the arterial input function for the production of $^{11}CO_2$ and ^{11}C-lactate.

Lactate metabolism in the heart can be measured with L-[3-^{11}C]lactate. A multi-compartmental model is used to estimate the extraction of lactate which correlates well with lactate oxidation measured by arterial and coronary sinus sampling over a wide range of conditions (Fig. 11.3) [58].

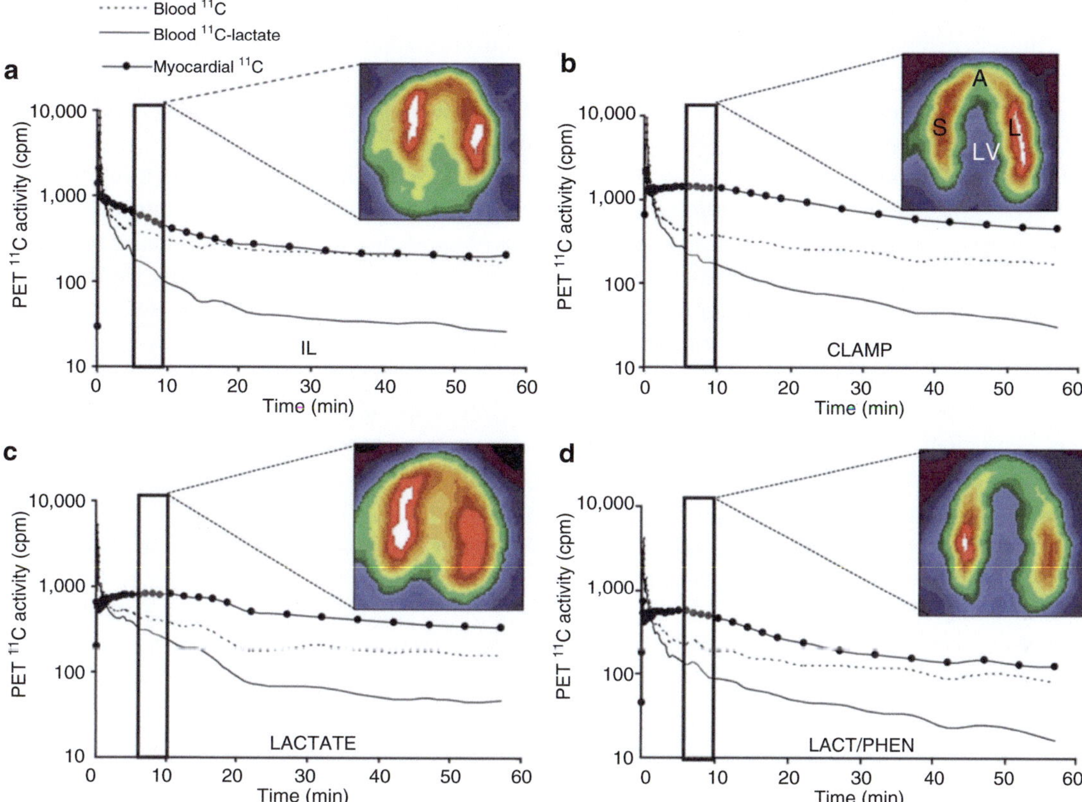

Fig. 11.3 PET measurement lactate metabolism. Representative PET time-activity curves of L-3-^{11}C-lactate obtained from intralipid (IL), insulin clamp (CLAMP), lactate infusion (LACTATE), or lactate and phenylephrine (LAC/PHEN) studies and corresponding myocardial images obtained 5–10 min after tracer injection and depicting primarily early tracer uptake. Images are displayed on horizontal long axis. Blood ^{11}C = ^{11}C time-activity curves obtained from region of interest (ROI) placed on the left atrium; blood ^{11}C-lactate = blood ^{11}C time-activity curves after removing $^{11}CO_2$, ^{11}C-neutral, and ^{11}C-basic metabolites; myocardial ^{11}C = ^{11}C time-activity curves obtained from ROI placed on the lateral wall. *A* apical wall, *S* septal wall, *L* lateral wall, *LV* left ventricle. Reproduced with permission Herrero P, et al. J Nucl Med. Dec 2007;48:2046-2055

11.3.5 Fatty Acid Metabolism

Palmitate is a saturated 16-carbon physiological long-chain fatty acid. A major advantage of [1-^{11}C]palmitate is that its myocardial kinetics including flux through β-oxidation and the TCA cycle are representative of oxidation of long-chain fatty acids. Currently, mathematical modeling techniques of the myocardial kinetics are used to measure various aspects of myocardial fatty acid metabolism uptake, oxidation, and storage [59–61]. The use of [1-^{11}C]palmitate does suffer from several disadvantages including sub-optimal image quality, complex analysis, and the need for an on-site cyclotron and radiopharmaceutical production capability.

To increase the dissemination potential for measuring fatty acid metabolism, numerous

^{18}F- radiotracers have been developed. Most of the PET tracers in this category have been designed to reflect myocardial β-oxidation. The largest number of radiotracers has been developed as ^{18}F-radiolabeled thia fatty acids (Table 11.1). 14-(R,S)-^{18}F-fluoro-6-thiaheptadecanoic acid (^{18}FTHA) was one of the first radiotracers developed using this approach. Although in preclinical models myocardial uptake and retention tracked accordingly with changes in substrate delivery, blood flow, and workload, the uptake and retention of ^{18}FTHA were insensitive to the inhibition of β-oxidation by hypoxia [62–64]. To circumvent this problem, 16-^{18}F-fluoro-4-thia-palmitate (^{18}FTP) was developed and demonstrated a metabolic trapping function that is proportional to fatty acid oxidation under normal oxygenation and hypoxic conditions [64, 65]. Because fractional oxidation may be greater for oleate than for palmitate, a 4-thia-substituted oleate analogue 18-^{18}F-fluoro-4-thia-oleate (^{18}FTO) was recently developed [66]. In rat heart, FTO demonstrated a greater specificity for mitochondrial fatty acid oxidation and superior imaging characteristics than ^{18}FTP. Further studies are needed to confirm its utility in measuring myocardial FA metabolism in humans. The F-18-labeled fatty acid radiotracer, *trans*-9(*RS*)-^{18}F-fluoro-3,4(*RS*,*RS*) methyleneheptadecanoic acid (^{18}FCPHA), a beta-methyl fatty acid analogue, has also been developed [67]. This radiotracer is also trapped after undergoing several steps of β-oxidation with uptake in rat heart approaching 1.5% injected dose per gram of tissue at 5 min postinjection. However, the impact of alterations in plasma substrates, work load, and blood flow on myocardial kinetics is unknown even though the radiotracer has undergone preliminary evaluation in humans [68]. There are some limitations with this class of radiotracers. Similar to ^{18}FDG, quantification of myocardial fatty acid metabolism requires the use of a lumped constant to correct for kinetic differences between the radiotracer and unlabeled palmitate. Furthermore, the extent to which myocardial fatty acid uptake can be separated from oxidation based on the myocardial kinetics of these radiotracers is unknown.

Other measurements of myocardial fatty acid metabolism are also accessible. Typically, PET measurements of myocardial FA metabolism only reflect the contribution of extracted FA bound to albumin or free fatty acids. However, myocardial fatty acid metabolism is dependent on the plasma delivery of fatty acid not just as free fatty acids but also in the form bound to TG, either as chylomicrons or very low-density lipoproteins. Fatty acids bound to TGs are made available to the myocardium via their release by lipoprotein lipase located on capillary endothelium. A noninvasive protocol for the assessment of TG-bound fatty acids has proven elusive. One proposed method to circumvent this problem is to administer the radiotracer orally to permit its incorporation into chylomicrons which can then be delivered to the heart. Using ^{18}FTHA, the approach has shown some promise in both rats and humans [69, 70]. Consistent with the mode of administration, most of the ^{18}F activities were recovered in the chylomicron fraction and with myocardial uptake occurring by 1 h and peaking 3 h post-administration. However, there remain technical challenges in quantifying the response from multiple sources of radiolabeled metabolites in the blood (radiolabeled TGs, chylomicrons, and nonesterified fatty acids), all of which contribute to the signal in PET imaging [71].

The contribution of intracellular or endogenous TG-derived fatty acids to overall energy metabolism appears to be altered in various animal models of cardiac disease such as heart failure and diabetes. However, relatively little is known about regulation of myocardial TG metabolism in humans [72, 73]. The lack of information is primarily due to the lack of adequate methods for its measurement [74, 75]. To help circumvent this problem, two strategies have been investigated. The first involves pre-labeling the myocardial TG pool with [1-^{11}C]palmitate, and once equilibrium is reached, measure the washout of activity under various substrate and hormonal conditions [76]. The approach was evaluated in dog heart where the rate of ^{11}C washout from the myocardium was correlated with arterial and coronary sinus measurements of the ^{11}C-metabolic species under varying metabolic conditions such as fasting and hyperinsulinemic-euglycemic clamp with and without intralipid. However, the method suffers from the limitations of providing only an index of myocardial TG turnover and requiring the administration of a relatively high dose level of ^{11}C-plamitate which may preclude human use. A second approach to measure the turnover of the myocardial endogenous TG pool integrates the quantification of myocardial lipids by ^{1}H-MRS with PET-derived measurement (using [1-^{11}C] palmitate) of the oxidation rates for extracted fatty acids that either enter β-oxidation directly or after traversing the TG pool [77]. Using the method in obese humans demonstrated that the contribution to myocardial β-oxidation from fatty acids derived from intracellular TGs was at least equal to that of fatty acids extracted from plasma. The method is intriguing but does require validation with independent measurements of TG turnover. This is particularly important given the recent observations of the preferential oxidation of FAs derived from endogenous TGs compared with extracted fatty acids [9].

11.4 Hyperpolarized ^{13}C

The need for imaging specific metabolic pathways is clear from the complex interactions between disease and intermediary metabolism. Hyperpolarized ^{13}C technology takes advantage of the chemical specificity of ^{13}C NMR to probe multiple specific pathways plus the improved sensitivity afforded by various hyperpolarization methods. Dissolution dynamic nuclear polarization (DNP) is the most commonly used method to hyperpolarize ^{13}C, and its principles are summarized elsewhere [78–83]. The potential value of HP methods is illustrated in Fig. 11.4 where the kinetics of metabolism of HP[1-^{13}C]pyruvate to HP$^{13}CO_2$, HP[^{13}C]bicarbonate, [1-^{13}C]lactate and [1-^{13}C]alanine were monitored in a single exam of an isolated heart, enabling detection of flux through multiple pathways important in cardiac physiology.

Integration of hyperpolarized nuclei into a human imaging work flow will require the solution of three engineering problems. One problem is that instruments to generate hyperpolarized materials

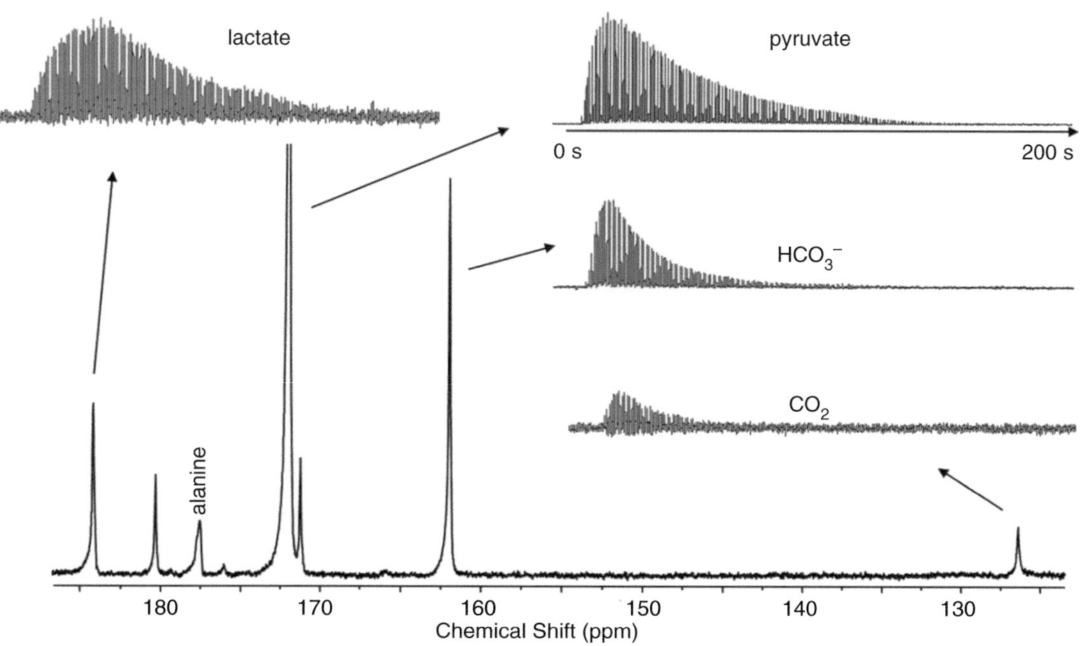

Fig. 11.4 ^{13}C NMR spectroscopy of an isolated rat heart. An isolated Langendorff-perfused rat heart was injected with hyperpolarized [1-^{13}C]pyruvate. Spectra were acquired every 2 s over an observation period of 200 seconds. Each inset is the ^{13}C NMR signal from a specific metabolite: lactate, pyruvate, bicarbonate, or CO_2. These spectra illustrate the rapid metabolism of [1-^{13}C]pyruvate to [^{13}C]CO_2 and other products. The total duration of data acquisition was 200 seconds. Data were redrawn from Merritt et al. Proc Natl Acad Sci USA. 2007; 104: 19,773-7

are prototypes with respect to clinical needs. A clinical instrument to rapidly and conveniently supply sterile, highly polarized (>80%) materials in sufficient mass for human exams is not available. A second challenge is that regardless of the details of the DNP process, once generated, the metabolite must be rapidly injected to minimize T_1 losses of polarization. Since the polarization state only exists in a magnetic field, it is essential to transfer the material from the site of generation to the subject through a slowly varying magnetic field. Passage through a region with zero field or a region with strong magnetic field gradients may eliminate polarization. Finally, optimal methods for data acquisition are necessary because once the hyperpolarized materials are no longer frozen at low temperatures, nuclear polarization will irreversibly decay to its thermal equilibrium value. One of the best molecules for HP exams is [1-^{13}C]pyruvate with a carbonyl T_1 of ~40 s, so there is generally a critical limit of 1–2 min for completion of the entire injection and image acquisition. Furthermore, the details of the imaging sequence are critical because each radiofrequency pulse depletes the available ^{13}C magnetization. The duration of available signal is therefore a combination of the nucleus (generally ^{15}N has a longer T_1 than ^{13}C), the chemical nature of the ^{13}C (generally carbonyls and carboxyls have a longer T_1 than protonated carbons), and the pulse sequence.

In addition to technical challenges, interpretation of ^{13}C-HP signals is not straightforward. Aside from technical issues, the ^{13}C NMR signal from any metabolite is proportional to [metabolite] (concentration of metabolite) · (fractional enrichment in ^{13}C) · (polarization). Consequently, for example, an increase in HP[1-^{13}C]lactate signal could be due to an increase in the pool size of lactate, an increase in the ^{13}C enrichment of the lactate pool, or an increase in the ^{13}C polarization as a consequence of better perfusion or more rapid transport of HP[1-^{13}C]pyruvate. In addition, it will be important to consider the multiple interacting biochemical events that could influence signals from HP products.

11.4.1 Probes and Pathways

The ideal ^{13}C-labeled probe for DNP must have four properties: safety after intravenous injection, long T_1, simple handling and efficient polarization, and rapid metabolism or the capacity to rapidly provide useful information. Characteristically these molecules are low molecular weight and water soluble. Thus an important challenge is to consider the metabolic pathway of interest and to match the possible probes to the pathway, as summarized in Tables 11.1 and 11.2. Glycolysis, for example, is important in understanding cardiac metabolism during ischemia, and it would be valuable to be able to compare studies of HP glucose to ^{18}FDG exams by PET. Glucose fulfills the other criteria: it is safe and water soluble and polarizes efficiently. However the T_1 of ^{13}C in glucose is short, on the order of a few seconds, so human imaging HP with glucose will be challenging, although not impossible. On the other hand, [1-^{13}C]pyruvate, [1-^{13}C]lactate, or [1-^{13}C]acetate all indirectly probe different aspects of glucose metabolism and offer simplicity, relatively long T_1 value, and the potential to probe important pathways. Unlike PET, multiple hyperpolarized ^{13}C probes may be injected in a single experiment. Multi-probe polarization or co-polarization refers to the simultaneous polarization of more than one probe as a single solution injection [84, 85]. This approach takes advantage of the chemical shift information encoded in the ^{13}C spectrum.

11.4.2 Pyruvate

Pyruvate is the reference molecule for DNP of the heart because of its central role in cardiac metabolism, convenience, ready polarization, and relatively long T_1 in carbons 1 and 2. [1-^{13}C]pyruvate is avidly metabolized in the heart to [1-^{13}C]lactate, [1-^{13}C]alanine, and [^{13}C]bicarbonate (Figs. 11.4 and 11.5); each product can be separately imaged in vivo because of the inherent chemical shift dispersion of ^{13}C [86–89]. Although interpreting each signal is a challenge because of the interacting effects of pool sizes and level of polarization, the capacity to image lactate, alanine, and bicarbonate provides direct information about key metabolic events in the heart. For example, the appearance of HP[1-^{13}C]lactate reflects activity of lactate dehydrogenase and the redox state of the cytosol. The appearance of HP[1-^{13}C]alanine reflects activity of another cytosolic enzyme,

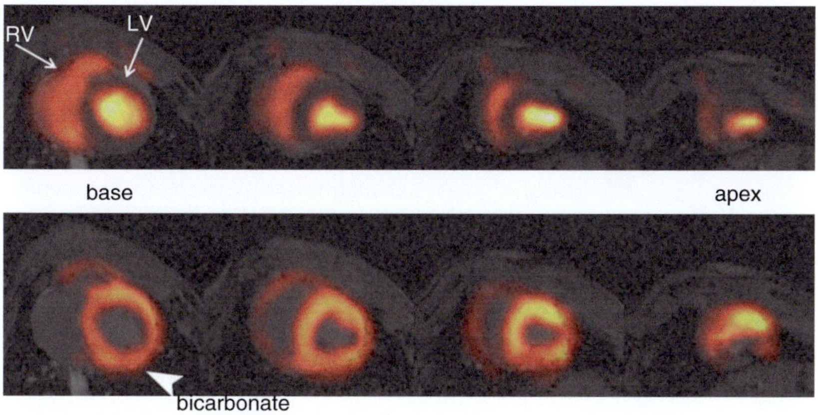

Fig. 11.5 Short axis hyperpolarized [1-^{13}C]pyruvate and [^{13}C]bicarbonate images of the pig heart. ^{13}C images were overlain on the corresponding anatomical images, arranged from the mid-left ventricle to the apex, left to right. In the upper panel, HP[1-^{13}C]pyruvate is seen filling the cavities of the right and left ventricles. In the lower panel, HP[^{13}C]bicarbonate was imaged throughout the left ventricular myocardium plus small regions of the right ventricular free wall. Redrawn from Dominguez-Viqueira et al. Magn Reson Med. 2016; 75: 859-65

alanine aminotransferase. Since activity of this enzyme is high and independent of redox potential, perhaps the HP[1-^{13}C]alanine signal reflects perfusion and transport of pyruvate. The decarboxylation of [1-^{13}C]pyruvate via PDH generates $^{13}CO_2$. Dissolved HP $^{13}CO_2$ may be directly detected in isolated rat [90] and mouse [18] hearts. In vivo, HP $^{13}CO_2$ exchanges rapidly with [^{13}C]bicarbonate via carbonic anhydrase and enables detection of flux through PDH. Since an HP exam can detect both dissolved HP $^{13}CO_2$ and [^{13}C]bicarbonate in the heart, pH can be calculated from the Henderson-Hasselbalch relationship [91]. The capacity to detect four specific enzyme-catalyzed reactions – pyruvate dehydrogenase, alanine aminotransferase, lactate dehydrogenase, and carbonic anhydrase – in a single exam illustrates the potential of HP technology.

One high-impact cardiac application of HP will likely be the detection of PDH flux; the biomarker in HP exams is the appearance of HP[^{13}C] bicarbonate from HP[1-^{13}C]pyruvate [90]. Noninvasive detection of flux through PDH would be of value in understanding heart disease because pharmacologic and metabolic interventions that target flux through PDH have been examined with the goal of protecting ischemic myocardium or improving function in the failing heart. Since ischemic heart disease is by definition a regional abnormality of perfusion due to coronary artery disease, the capacity for multislice imaging is critical for clinical translation and was demonstrated recently in a large animal model [88, 92] and illustrated in Fig. 11.5. Reduced [^{13}C]bicarbonate signal in hearts after coronary occlusion and reflow was previously attributed to an effect of transient ischemia on flux into the TCA cycle [86, 87].

[1-^{13}C]pyruvate also serves as an indirect probe of the TCA cycle because the HP products related to mitochondrial metabolism, $^{13}CO_2$ and [^{13}C]bicarbonate, are generated during flux through PDH. The product entering the TCA cycle, acetyl-CoA, is not ^{13}C labeled. Flux of pyruvate into the TCA cycle flux may be detected directly by placing the ^{13}C in position 2 of pyruvate (Fig. 11.6), which via PDH is converted to the product [1-^{13}C]acetyl-CoA. After condensation with oxaloacetate in the reaction catalyzed by citrate synthase, [5-^{13}C]citrate is produced. With further metabolism in the TCA cycle, α-ketoglutarate is produced and exchanges rapidly with glutamate; both metabolites are labeled in position 5 and glutamate can be detected [93, 94]. Since the biochemical pathways involved in [1-^{13}C]pyruvate and [2-^{13}C]pyruvate are identical, any difference in the rate of appearance of [^{13}C]bicarbonate from [1-^{13}C]pyruvate compared to the rate of appearance of [5-^{13}C]glutamate from [2-^{13}C] pyruvate presumably would be due to T_1 effects or metabolite pool sizes in the TCA cycle.

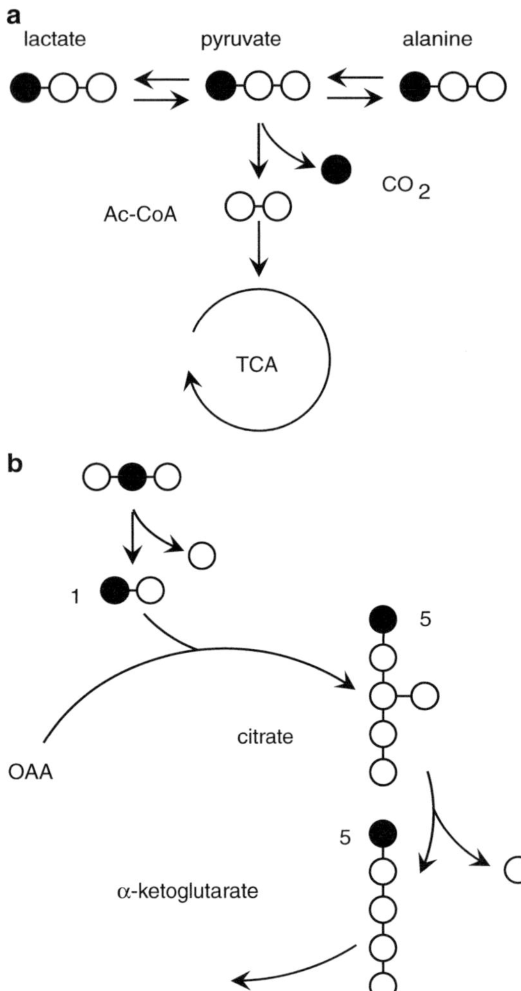

Fig. 11.6 Effect of ^{13}C labeling on detection of metabolism of pyruvate in the TCA cycle. Panel A illustrates conversion of [1-^{13}C]pyruvate to acetyl-CoA via pyruvate dehydrogenase with release of $^{13}CO_2$. PDH flux is detected directly from the appearance of $^{13}CO_2$ which is proportional to oxidation of pyruvate in the TCA cycle. Metabolism of [2-^{13}C]pyruvate in the heart, illustrated in Panel B, does not immediately yield $^{13}CO_2$, but ^{13}C will be transferred to position 5 of citrate and glutamate. Appearance of [5-^{13}C]glutamate directly demonstrates flux through citrate synthase

11.4.3 Lactate

As noted above, the ability to monitor flux through PDH may provide important information related to mitochondrial function. HP [1-^{13}C]pyruvate is safe in human subjects, but the endogenous plasma concentration is low. Therefore a bolus markedly alters plasma redox ratios, and arrhythmias have been reported at very high concentrations during intracoronary infusions. An alternative may be [1-^{13}C]lactate since lactate is also readily oxidized in the heart and the plasma concentration is roughly 10× pyruvate. Consequently, a bolus of an equivalent mass of lactate in principle has much less effect on redox potential. It is feasible to hyperpolarize [1-^{13}C]lactate using procedures similar to [1-^{13}C]pyruvate [95].

11.4.4 Acetate and Butyrate: Substrates That Bypass PDH

Pyruvate, in any of the labeling patterns described, is the reference molecule for DNP because of its central role in cell metabolism, ready polarization, and relatively long T_1 in carbons 1 and 2. However, fatty acids are the preferred substrate for energy production in the heart, and it would be ideal to probe TCA cycle metabolism directly. Acetate, the shortest chain fatty acid, is present only in low concentration in plasma but it is avidly oxidized by the heart. After conversion to acetyl-CoA by carnitine acetyltransferase, it also exchanges into acetylcarnitine. Thus, [1-^{13}C]acetate could in principle probe both the TCA cycle via metabolism to [5-^{13}C]glutamate and the kinetics of enrichment in acetylcarnitine [96, 97]. In healthy rats, HP[1-^{13}C]acetate was converted to both HP[1-^{13}C]acetylcarnitine and HP[5-^{13}C]citrate [97]. The kinetics of appearance of HP[1-^{13}C]acetylcarnitine have been studied in a pig model [98], but [5-^{13}C]glutamate could not be detected.

Fatty acid oxidation may be studied indirectly by examining the inhibition of pyruvate oxidation due to the presence of fatty acids. Hyperpolarized acetate bypasses PDH and may be considered a marker of fatty acid oxidation since it competes effectively against pyruvate and it interconverts with acetylcarnitine. However, because it bypasses β-oxidation, acetate fails to probe a key aspect of cardiac metabolism. [1-^{13}C]butyrate is a water-soluble four-carbon fatty acid that polarizes well. Normally it is present in very low concentrations in plasma and is thought to be derived from colonic bacteria. Since [1-^{13}C]butyrate is metabolized through β-oxidation to [1-^{13}C]acetoacetyl-CoA and [1-^{13}C]acetyl-CoA (plus unlabeled acetyl-CoA), in principle [5-^{13}C]glutamate, [1-^{13}C]acetylcarnitine, and the redox pair, [1-^{13}C]acetoacetate and [1-^{13}C] beta-hydroxybutyrate, should all be detected. Indeed, this is the case in isolated perfused heart despite the hyperpolarized ^{13}C having passed through a minimum of nine enzyme-catalyzed reactions: [1-^{13}C]butyrate → [1-^{13}C]butyryl-CoA → [1-^{13}C]β-hydroxybutyryl-CoA → [1-^{13}C] acetoacetyl-CoA → [1-^{13}C]acetyl-CoA → [5-^{13}C] citrate → [5-^{13}C]isocitrate → [5-^{13}C]aconitate → [5-^{13}C]α-ketoglutarate → [5-^{13}C]glutamate [99].

11.4.5 Substrate Competition in Hyperpolarization Exams

The heart is exquisitely adapted to adjust fluxes in metabolic pathways almost instantaneously in response to changes in hemodynamic load as well as fluctuating concentrations of extracellular substrates. In general, an increase in extracellular concentration of a readily oxidized substrate is matched rapidly by an increase in oxidation of that substrate [105, 106]. This inherent flexibility of substrate selection is important in the design and interpretation of HP exams.

The normal concentration of pyruvate in plasma is ~0.1 mM, and pyruvate at this concentration contributes little to acetyl-CoA because of competing substrates [10]. Consequently, the capacity of the heart to rapidly switch to pyruvate, as after a bolus of HP[1-^{13}C]pyruvate, enables HP imaging of the heart. The rate of $^{13}CO_2$ production is proportional to the rate of acetyl-CoA production × the fractional contribution of [1-^{13}C]pyruvate to acetyl-CoA. Other factors being equal, the appearance of $^{13}CO_2$ or [^{13}C]bicarbonate in the heart is proportional to the fractional contribution of pyruvate to acetyl-CoA. Conversely, a high concentration of other circulating substrates, ketones, or fatty acids, for example, can inhibit oxidation of [1-^{13}C]pyruvate even in the high concentrations of pyruvate present after a bolus. In isolated hearts under conditions mimicking the fed state, 3 mM pyruvate was sufficient to produce ~80% of the acetyl-CoA [10]. At fatty acid and ketone concentrations present in fasting, pyruvate at 6 mM was oxidized at a significantly higher rate than at baseline, but oxidation of fats and ketones still provided the majority of acetyl-CoA. Consequently and not unexpectedly, the plasma concentration of HP [1-^{13}C]pyruvate (or other metabolizable substrate) will influence results. Further, the concentration of competing substrates will also influence pyruvate metabolism. Because the TCA cycle can oxidize acetyl-CoA from any source, there is no strict linkage between flux in the TCA cycle and flux in any one of the feeding pathways. Hence, the rate of appearance of HP $^{13}CO_2$ from HP[1-^{13}C]pyruvate may index flux through pyruvate dehydrogenase but not necessarily the TCA cycle.

11.5 Complementary Information

The purpose of this section is to consider how the unique and complementary attributes of PET and HP could be used to better understand myocardial metabolism. The first component will describe the potential for methodologic advancements, whereas the second component will provide a few examples where our understanding of metabolism could be enhanced.

PET provides the evolution over time of tissue radioactivity with very high sensitivity, measurable in three dimensions. Since the accessible information is total tissue radioactivity, detection of flux (in nanomoles · g^{-1} · min^{-1}) in a particular pathway relies on a tracer kinetic model that relates externally observed signal to an underlying metabolic network. Once the model is described mathematically and the relation between individual rate constants for each reaction and externally observed signal is established by validation experiments, typically performed in perfused tissues and large animal models, results from human patients can be derived. This approach, although well accepted, has several limitations. *First*, the arterial input function influences the kinetics of a tracer in heart muscle. The arterial input function is in turn sensitive to multiple factors including the cardiac output, the rate of tracer injection, and the mix of radiolabeled entities in the blood. *Second*, kinetic models rely on knowledge of tissue metabolite pool sizes which, in the heart, are sensitive to normal physiological changes and disease. This limitation would presumably be most important for complex multi-compartment processes such as the oxidation of [1-^{11}C]acetate in the TCA cycle rather than the one-step phosphorylation of ^{18}FDG. In studies of MVO_2 over a wide range, an index of TCA cycle flux, there is a good correlation between the rate constant describing acetate oxidation and oxygen consumption, implying that the sum of metabolite concentrations involved in the TCA cycle remains more or less constant under normal physiological conditions. Nonetheless, the relevance of these measurements in healthy myocardium to patients with disease is uncertain. *Third*, it is difficult to build up experience in healthy volunteers or subjects with mild disease because of concerns related to exposure to ionizing radiation. Thus, much of the literature is based on patients with known significant heart disease.

In principle, MR imaging of hyperpolarized ^{13}C tracers overcomes some of these constraints. For example, after the injection of HP[1-^{13}C] pyruvate, the appearance of [1-^{13}C]lactate, [1-^{13}C] alanine, and [^{13}C]bicarbonate in the myocardium can only be interpreted as transit through lactate dehydrogenase, alanine aminotransferase, and pyruvate dehydrogenase, respectively, without the need for any mathematical models. Of course, conversion of HP-^{13}C signals to flux information will require kinetic models as well. Furthermore, the HP ^{13}C signal is depleted by the imaging sequence itself in a complex manner depending on the interpulse delay, flip angles, and whether individual metabolites are irradiated. Intracellular T_1 values in various tissue compartments are uncertain and perhaps even unknowable in intact tissues. If absolute flux information is desired, then all the factors that influence kinetic measurements by PET – the arterial input function and knowledge of tissue metabolite pool sizes – will be equally important for analysis of HP data.

11.5.1 Methodologic Advances

Based on the aforementioned discussion, it appears exploiting the complementary nature of PET and HP MR can provide potential advances. Perhaps PET can be used to help advance the quantitative capabilities of HP MR. For example, a properly calibrated arterial input function and tissue response on PET could be used as a gold standard to test the accuracy of new MR approaches that account for loss of polarization due to both the acquisition and the T_1 of the hyperpolarized molecule in order to derive similarly accurate measurements by HP MR, setting the stage for quantitative capability with this technology. Conversely, could knowledge of downstream metabolic partitioning of an extracted substrate measured with HP MR cross-validate a proposed mathematical model designed to interrogate certain metabolic pathways with PET? In addition, since PET measures myocardial metabolism without perturbing the system, it could be used to provide insight into the return of metabolic pathways of interest to baseline conditions following the administration of a ^{13}C HP molecule. Such information is fundamental to the successful advancement and application of serial HP MR studies. Finally, with the advent of PET/MR, it may be possible to link metabolic dose response by HP to the underlying baseline metabolic conditions measured by PET.

11.5.2 Applications and Potential Synergies

11.5.2.1 Myocardial Ischemia

The classic metabolic signature for myocardial ischemia is a decline in fatty acid uptake and oxidation and an increase in overall glucose metabolism via augmented anaerobic glycolysis and continued, albeit, diminished oxidative metabolism [107]. This metabolic switch permits continued energy production and cell survival in the setting of reduced tissue oxygen. However, unless NAD^+ can be regenerated by conversion of pyruvate to lactate and export of lactate, glycolysis will be inhibited by accumulation of NADH, and myocardial necrosis will ensue. When the ischemic insult is resolved, oxygen availability increases and oxidative metabolism resumes. Abnormalities in myocardial substrate metabolism present initially may persist well after the resolution of ischemia, a pattern termed "ischemic memory."

PET and SPECT

Demonstration of either accelerated myocardial glucose metabolism or reduced fatty acid metabolism using ^{18}FDG and ^{123}I-BMIPP, respectively, has been used to document ischemic memory. For example, over 20 years ago, it was shown that PET myocardial FDG uptake was increased in patients with unstable angina during pain-free episodes [108]. An example is shown in Fig. 11.7. Moreover, in patients with stable angina, increased FDG uptake was demonstrated following exercise-induced ischemia, in the absence of either perfusion deficits or ECG abnormalities [109]. Similar observations have been made with SPECT using ^{123}I-BMIPP. Results of numerous studies have

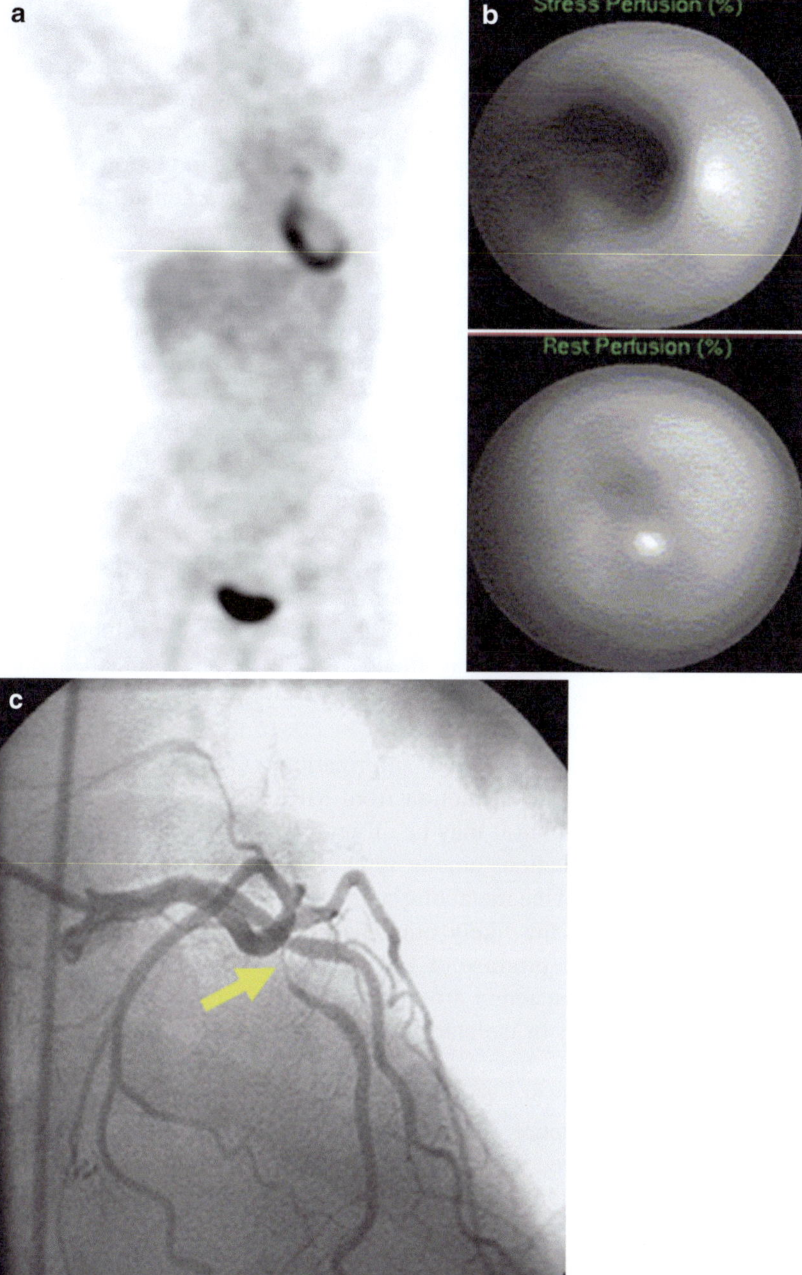

Fig. 11.7 Myocardial ischemia detected by FDG-PET. A patient with non-Hodgkin's lymphoma undergoing whole-body FDG-PET imaging for detection of recurrence. (**a**) Images acquired under fasting conditions demonstrate localized uptake in septal, anterior, and inferior walls of the myocardium, suggestive of either ischemia in these walls or infarction of the lateral wall. (**b**) Rest/stress SPECT myocardial perfusion imaging demonstrates inducible ischemia in the same distribution as the FDG uptake. (**c**) Coronary angiography demonstrates a high-grade stenosis in the left anterior descending artery (*yellow arrow*)

demonstrated in patients with acute chest pain that reductions in myocardial BMIPP uptake may persist 24–36 h following the resolution of symptoms [110, 111]. Moreover, this "metabolic fingerprint" may be superior to perfusion imaging for either identifying coronary artery disease as the cause of the chest pain or assigning prognosis [112]. It also appears that rest ^{123}I-BMIPP imaging may provide unique prognostic information in patients with end-stage renal dialysis receiving hemodialysis, a patient cohort with a high cardiovascular risk [113]. Metabolic imaging with either ^{18}FDG or ^{123}I-BMIPP has also been used for direct ischemia detection during stress testing. Abnormalities in vasodilator reserve with perfusion tracers will underestimate ischemia if oxygen and supply remain balanced. Results of initial studies where ^{18}FDG was injected during exercise demonstrated greater detection rate for moderately severe coronary artery stenoses compared with perfusion imaging [48, 114]. Despite the promising results with these radiotracers, numerous questions still remain such as the optimal imaging protocols and the impact of alterations in the plasma substrate environment on diagnostic accuracy, whether added diagnostic and prognostic information is provided over perfusion imaging and whether this information alters clinical management.

^{13}C Hyperpolarization

Clinicians can acquire detailed information about LV function and wall motion from MRI and echocardiography, but it may be difficult to readily identify the relations among symptoms, coronary anatomy, and the metabolic state of the tissue and to predict the likely outcome after revascularization. The promise of HP methods to probe myocardial ischemia arose early in its development [91, 92]. In isolated hearts where the timing of ischemia, reperfusion, and delivery of HP[1-^{13}C]pyruvate can be controlled, there is already evidence that spectra of the products [1-^{13}C]lactate, $^{13}CO_2$, and [^{13}C]bicarbonate can provide highly specific information about myocardial ischemia. Necrotic myocardium cannot produce lactate, CO_2, or bicarbonate from HP [1-^{13}C]pyruvate. Brief ischemia not sufficient to cause irreversible injury was associated with rapid recovery of high-energy phosphates, mechanical function, and oxygen consumption [115]. Yet even under these conditions where conventional physiological studies indicate that the myocardium is "normal," the HP ^{13}C NMR spectrum was dramatically abnormal. Flux through PDH was undetectable, and the concentration of lactate was dramatically increased, likely due to the strongly reducing environment in both the mitochondria, causing inhibition of PDH, and in the cytosol, causing accumulation of lactate. This profile, absent bicarbonate and abnormally high lactate, demonstrates that the cardiomyocytes were functional in the sense that pyruvate is being delivered to the cells and that lactate dehydrogenase is highly active. Thus, a low ratio of HP bicarbonate to HP lactate appears to indicate recent brief ischemia when all other conventional measures are normal.

The effects of brief (15 min) or prolonged (45 min) occlusion of the circumflex coronary artery followed by reperfusion were examined in a pig model in vivo [92]. Ejection fraction was not measurably altered in this study, indicating that the volume of ischemic myocardium was relatively small, and the concentration of creatine kinase MB was elevated after 45 min but not after 15 min of ischemia. Delayed enhancement after Gd was not detected after brief ischemia. Nevertheless (Fig. 11.8) a small but distinct volume of reduced HP [^{13}C]bicarbonate was observed in the circumflex territory 2 h after reperfusion. The HP[1-^{13}C]alanine image was not influenced by brief ischemia. This study demonstrated that while a map of perfusion and cytosolic function, HP[1-^{13}C]alanine, was normal after brief ischemia with 2 h of reperfusion, the HP[^{13}C]bicarbonate image was abnormal. This finding illustrates the potential sensitivity of HP methods for ischemia and is an example of ischemic memory: metabolism was abnormal even when perfusion and function were apparently preserved.

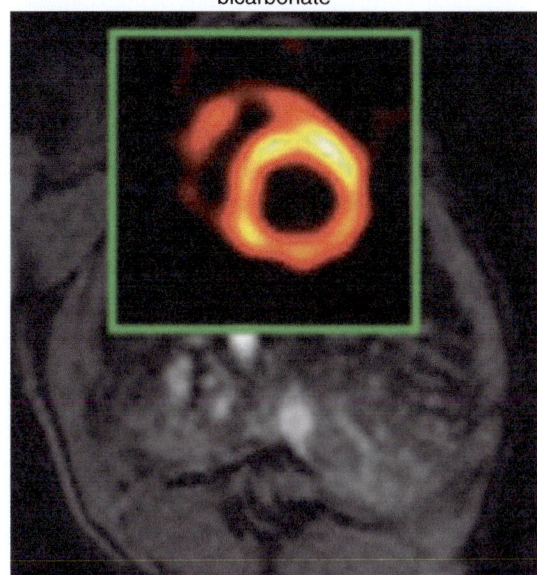

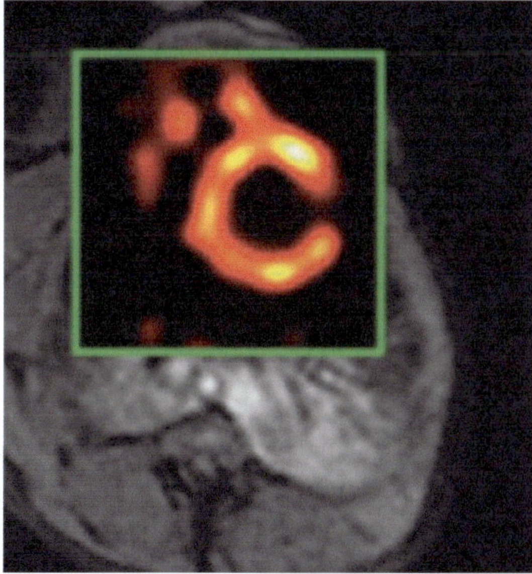

Fig. 11.8 Influence of brief ischemia in the circumflex territory on appearance of hyperpolarized [^{13}C] bicarbonate. The left circumflex artery of a pig was occluded for 15 min followed by 2 h. of reperfusion and intravenous injection of HP[1-^{13}C]pyruvate. The bicarbonate signal in the circumflex territory was significantly reduced. Images from Golman et al. Magn Reson Med. 2008; 59: 1005-13

Potential Synergies

The metabolic fate of a carbohydrate is very sensitive to normal physiological changes and pathological conditions; a good example is oxidation of glucose via glycolysis in the TCA cycle under normal aerobic conditions compared to export as lactate during ischemia. ^{18}FDG accumulates prior to the split between aerobic and anaerobic carbohydrate metabolisms and therefore cannot distinguish these pathways. Preserved uptake of ^{18}FDG and trapping as a phosphorylated product indicate ischemic myocardium, but it is not known if this biomarker is detecting preserved mitochondrial metabolism (glucose → pyruvate → CO_2) or preserved cytosolic functions (glucose → lactate). Having the capability to measure the proportional contributions of the cytosolic and mitochondrial partitioning of glucose metabolism (measured by ^{13}C-HP) normalized to overall glucose metabolism (measured with PET and ^{18}FDG) would permit delineation of the relative importance of these two pathways in maintaining cardiomyocyte health in humans with coronary artery disease, perhaps laying the foundation for novel clinical management paradigms.

11.5.2.2 Myocardial Hypertrophy and Cardiomyopathies

The metabolic phenotype of a reduction in the expression of β-oxidation enzymes, leading to a fall in myocardial fatty acid oxidation and an increase in glucose use, characterizes both LV and right ventricular (RV) hypertrophy [116–119]. This adaptive response is considered beneficial to cardiac function under acute conditions, but under exposure to sustained pressure overload, the metabolic switch becomes more permanent, impairing flexibility in myocardial substrate use and inducing mitochondrial dysfunction [120]. Indeed, interventions in animals that involve inhibition of mitochondrial fatty acid β-oxidation result in cardiac hypertrophy [116]. Further support for this linkage arises from observations in humans, where variants in genes regulating key aspects of myocardial fatty acid metabolism ranging from PPARα to various key β-oxidative enzymes are associated with LV hypertrophy [121, 122].

In addition to LV hypertrophy, alterations in myocardial substrate metabolism have been implicated in the pathogenesis of contractile dysfunction and heart failure. Animal models of heart failure have shown that in the progression from cardiac hypertrophy to ventricular dysfunction, the expression of genes encoding for enzymes regulating β-oxidation is coordinately decreased, resulting in a shift in myocardial substrate metabolism to primarily glucose use, similar to that seen in the fetal heart [123, 124]. The reactivation of the metabolic fetal gene program may have numerous detrimental consequences on myocardial contractile function ranging from energy deprivation to the inability to process fatty acids leading to accumulation of nonoxidized toxic fatty acid derivatives, resulting in lipotoxicity. It should be noted this metabolic adaptation becomes more complex when there is concomitant insulin resistance [125].

SPECT and PET

In preclinical models of LV hypertrophy, PET with FDG has demonstrated that myocardial glucose uptake tracks directly with increasing hypertrophy and provides evidence that metabolic changes are one of the first myocardial responses to increased stress, and these metabolic adaptations may drive the hypertrophic response with respect to its functional and structural consequences [126–130]. Similar results have been found in man. PET with [1-^{11}C]palmitate in humans has shown the reduction in myocardial fatty acid oxidation is an independent predictor of LV mass in hypertension [131]. Measurements of myocardial glucose metabolism with PET and ^{18}FDG and myocardial structure and function by echocardiography were performed in a cross-sectional study of normal controls and hypertensive patients without or with LV hypertrophy [132]. Consistent with the aforementioned observations obtained in preclinical studies, the rate of myocardial glucose uptake PET was higher in patients without LV hypertrophy compared with controls suggesting the metabolic remodeling preceded structural remodeling in these patients. But surprisingly, the rate of myocardial glucose uptake was lower in hypertensive patients with LV hypertrophy when compared with the hypertensive patients without LV hypertrophy. Furthermore, it appeared the decline in the rate of glucose uptake paralleled the decline in diastolic function. These latter findings are at odds with preclinical observations and may be attributable to the greater preponderance of females and diabetics in the LV hypertrophy cohort.

Similar observations of increased myocardial ^{18}FDG uptake have been obtained in patients with RV hypertrophy due to pulmonary hypertension [133–135]. The increase in ^{18}FDG uptake correlates with the level of pulmonary hypertension, plasma NT-pro-brain natriuretic peptide levels, as well as circulating levels of bone marrow-derived proangiogenic progenitors (CD34+ and CD133+ cells) which are markers of generalized hypoxia-inducible factor 1-alpha activation, a known driver of the hypertrophic response [133]. Moreover, an increase RV glucose uptake appears to be a marker of poorer prognosis [135, 136]. It also appears that measuring RV ^{18}FDG uptake can be used to follow therapeutic responses as treatment of pulmonary hypertension (e.g., epoprostenol or sildenafil) results in a decline in pulmonary hypertension that is paralleled by a decrease in RV myocardial glucose uptake [135, 137]. Finally, alterations in RV myocardial metabolism also occur in RV dysfunction, secondary to left heart failure [138].

In summary, these studies raise the possibility of using metabolic imaging for both prognosis assignment and treatment monitoring for patients with pressure-overload conditions of either the left or right ventricle. However, they also highlight the complexity of metabolic imaging and the need to control the many determinants of myocardial metabolism in order to accurately attribute a unique metabolic signature to a specific disease process.

SPECT with BMIPP has demonstrated reduced myocardial uptake and increased radiotracer clearance in patients with dilated cardiomyopathy compared with controls [139]. Moreover, the magnitude of these metabolic abnormalities correlated with other measurements of severe heart failure such as left ventricular size and plasma β-natriuretic peptide levels. It appears these abnormalities in BMIPP kinetics reflect the combined effects of reduced fatty acid uptake and oxidation as evidenced by PET with [1-^{11}C]palmitate studies in a similar patient population. In this same study, myocardial glucose metabolism was higher in the cardiomyopathic patients compared with controls confirming the metabolic shift [140]. Moreover, it appears sex impacts the metabolic phenotype in nonischemic cardiomyopathy with women exhibiting higher levels of myocardial fatty acid uptake (and blood flow) compared with males as measured by PET using [1-^{11}C]palmitate (Fig. 11.9) [141]. However, it should be noted that the presence of concomitant insulin resistance appears to be a major contributor to the variability in levels of myocardial glucose and fatty acid metabolism in these patients [142, 143].

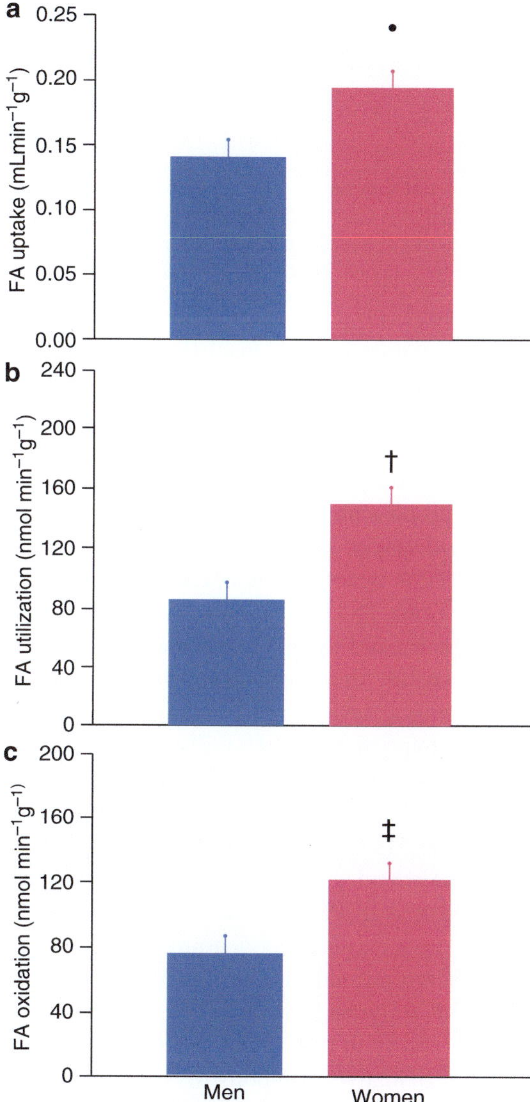

Fig. 11.9 PET measurements in nonischemic cardiomyopathy. Sex differences in myocardial fatty acid (FA) uptake and metabolism in heart failure. Myocardial FA uptake (**a**), utilization (**b**), and oxidation (**c**) averages in men (*blue bars*) and women (*pink bars*) with nonischemic heart failure. Reproduced with permission Kadkhodayan A, et al. J Nucl Cardiol. 2016;epub

Metabolic imaging can also be used to study the mechanisms responsible for the effectiveness of treatment in dilated cardiomyopathy. For example, the administration of the nonselective β-blocker, carvedilol, results in a 20% decline in myocardial fatty acid uptake [144]. Theoretically, decreasing myocardial fatty acid oxidation should increase the oxidation of glucose leading to a more favorable energetic state and improved LV function. Alterations in myocardial substrate use are now becoming attractive targets for novel treatments for heart failure with prime examples being the partial fatty acid oxidation antagonists and the insulin sensitizer glucagon-like peptide-1 [145, 146]. The administration of trimetazidine to patients with dilated cardiomyopathy resulted in a significant improvement in LV ejection fraction [147]. However, the improvement in LV function appeared to reflect the complex interplay between a mild decrease in myocardial FA oxidation, improved whole-body insulin resistance, and synergistic effects with β-blockade. More recently the effects of the GLP-1 agonist, albiglutide, on myocardial glucose and oxidative metabolism were assessed with PET and ^{18}FDG and [1-^{11}C]acetate, respectively, in patients with NYHA Class II–III heart failure. Although there was no detectable effect of albiglutide on cardiac function or myocardial glucose and oxygen use, there was a modest increase in peak oxygen consumption, which could have been mediated by noncardiac effects [148]. However, the study does highlight the potential of PET-derived metabolic biomarkers as endpoints for CV drug development.

^{13}C Hyperpolarization

Even at this relatively early stage in the development of technology for HP studies, preclinical models of heart failure have been examined. Hypertrophy, induced by thyroxine administration in rats, was associated with a reduction in PDH flux measured by metabolism of HP[1-^{13}C] pyruvate [149]. Pacing-induced dilated cardiomyopathy was examined over time in a pig model [94]. Early in the period of rapid pacing, HP[^{13}C] bicarbonate production from HP-[1-^{13}C]pyruvate was preserved (Fig. 11.10). The metabolism of

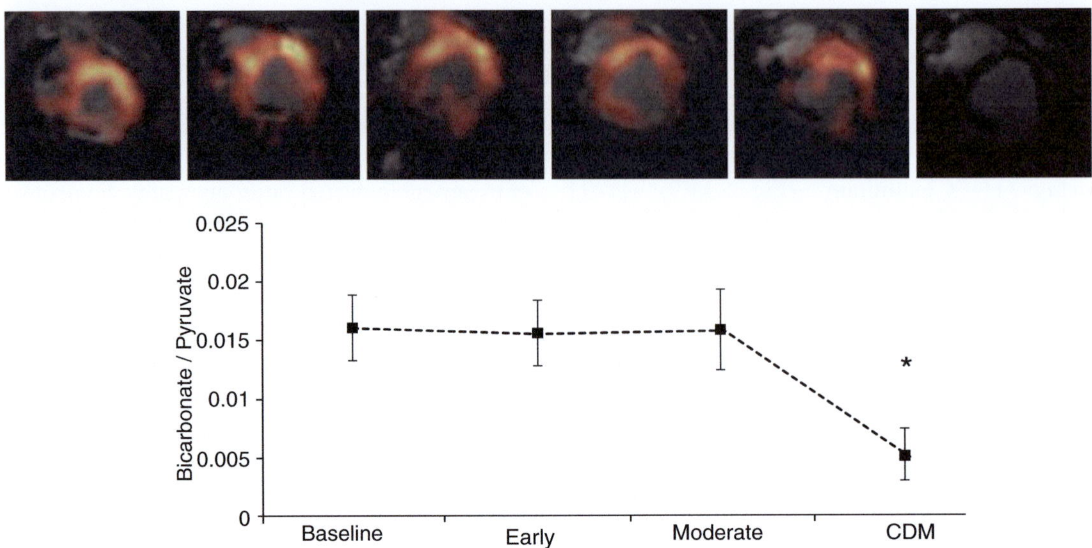

Fig. 11.10 Influence of pacing-induced dilated cardiomyopathy on appearance of hyperpolarized [^{13}C] bicarbonate. ^{13}C MR images were taken from the same pig at weekly intervals during the evolution of a dilated cardiomyopathy (DCM) induced by rapid pacing. *Upper panel*: The appearance of HP[1-^{13}C]bicarbonate was preserved in the left ventricular myocardium until late in the progression to heart failure. *Lower panel*: Bicarbonate signal normalized to pyruvate. "Early" and "moderate" refer to the duration of pacing, 1–2 weeks and 2–5 weeks, respectively. DCM refers to the appearance of overt heart failure. Data from Schroeder et al. Eur J Heart Fail. 2013; 15: 130-40

HP[2-^{13}C]pyruvate was used to examine production of [5-^{13}C]glutamate in the TCA cycle to directly probe citrate synthase. Surprisingly, the signal of HP[5-^{13}C]glutamate decreased early during hemodynamic stress, demonstrating a dissociation between bicarbonate production from [1-^{13}C]pyruvate and [5-^{13}C]glutamate production from [2-^{13}C]pyruvate. It is conceivable that mitochondrial water content or other structural changes may modify the T_1 of metabolites early in the citric acid cycle, or exchange of metabolite upstream from α-ketoglutarate may delay the transfer of HP [1-^{13}C]acetyl-CoA to glutamate. These data suggest that an integrated investigation using HP probes could provide new insights into the pathophysiology of heart failure.

Potential Synergies

PET with [1-^{11}C]acetate has been investigated extensively as a tool to measure myocardial oxygen consumption [52, 53, 64, 150–152]. A challenge is that regional measurements of acetate clearance are converted to oxygen consumption or, equivalently, TCA cycle flux by a predetermined relationship. However, it is not feasible to model all possible conditions that may influence that relationship. The use of HP [1-^{13}C]acetate to assess TCA cycle flux is attractive because the signal from HP[5-^{13}C]citrate can be resolved from the acetate signal in perfused heart models, and kinetic analyses have been reported. Interestingly, several reports described metabolism of hyperpolarized [1-^{13}C]acetate → [1-^{13}C] acetyl-CoA → [1-^{13}C]acetylcarnitine in a reaction catalyzed by carnitine acetyltransferase [102, 103, 153]. The buffering capacity of the carnitine-acetylcarnitine system has not been incorporated in PET kinetic models. As anticipated, both [1-^{13}C]acetylcarnitine and [1-^{13}C] butyrylcarnitine are detected in the presence of HP[1-^{13}C]butyrate [154].

The ability to distinguish metabolism of acetate via oxidative metabolism vs. entry into the acetylcarnitine pool may be important in myopathies. Carnitine is absolutely required for normal oxidation of fatty acids in the heart, and abnormalities of carnitine metabolism have been associated with heart failure [155] or abnormal mitochondrial function in the heart [156, 157]. Reports of heart failure are presumably due to interference with fatty acid oxidation. Dietary carnitine supplementation has been suggested in heart failure [158]. Since the conversion of hyperpolarized [1-^{13}C]acetate to [1-^{13}C]acetylcarnitine is readily detected, HP methods may prove useful in understanding carnitine metabolism and indirectly fatty acid metabolism. As described previously, metabolism of hyperpolarized [1-^{13}C] butyrate into the TCA cycle also provides information about TCA cycle kinetics [104].

11.5.2.3 Obesity, Insulin Resistance, and Diabetes

Obesity is a major risk factor for heart failure [159]. Moreover, it appears an "obesity cardiomyopathy" is a distinct clinical entity characterized by LV remodeling, reduced cardiac efficiency, and diastolic dysfunction, which may progress to systolic dysfunction [160]. The mechanisms responsible for the relation between obesity and heart failure in humans are not well understood but may, in part, involve altered myocardial substrate metabolism. Preclinical models demonstrate obesity increases myocardial fatty acid metabolism, lipid accumulation, and MVO_2 leading to increased oxidative stress, cardiac dysfunction, and apoptosis [161, 162]. Interventions that reduce fatty acid accumulation and/or oxidative stress in cardiac myocytes prevent the development of myocardial dysfunction in these models [161].

Overdependence on fatty acid metabolism and a decrease in glucose use typifies the metabolic phenotype in diabetes mellitus [163, 164]. The increase in plasma fatty acid delivery due to peripheral insulin resistance leads to increased myocardial fatty acid uptake. This activates key transcriptional pathways such as the PPARα/PGC-1 signaling network resulting in a further increase in myocardial fatty acid uptake and oxidation with reciprocal reduction in glucose oxidation [165–167]. However, additional mechanisms are also likely at play. Insulin-mediated stimulation of glucose transport is impaired by intramyocardial lipid accumulation likely through activation of various isoforms of protein kinase C [168–170]. Excess fatty acid oxidation may also be associated with a decrease in the metabolic flexibility of the heart which as noted above is a characteristic of the normal myocardium [171, 172]. Through poorly understood mechanisms, increased fatty acid oxidation is associated with excess myocardial oxygen consumption [173–178]. This effect is generally modest, perhaps an increase in oxygen consumption of a few percent up to 30% for the same myocardial work. This change is much less than the normal variation in oxygen consumption by the heart during minimal exercise. However under perfusion-limiting conditions such as ischemic heart disease or with impaired subendocardial capillary flow during hypertrophy, this effect is conceivably significant. Moreover, these chronic metabolic adaptations can initiate a cascade of events that acting either individually or synergistically are detrimental to cardiac myocyte health such as an increase in oxidative stress, inflammation, and increased cell death, all of which can lead to diastolic dysfunction [163, 166].

PET

Imaging of obese young women with PET and [1-^{11}C]acetate and [1-^{11}C]palmitate has demonstrated that an increase in body mass index is associated with a shift in myocardial substrate metabolism toward greater fatty acid use that increased with worsening insulin resistance [173]. Of note, little change in myocardial glucose metabolism was observed. Paralleling the preferential use of FAs was an increase in MVO_2 and a decrease in energy transduction. The myocardial metabolic response to obesity appears to be sex dependent. For example, using similar PET techniques, it has been demonstrated that in contrast to obese women, obese men have a greater impairment in myocardial glucose metabolism [179, 180]. In addition, obesity had less effect on myocardial fatty acid metabolism in men. In contrast, MVO_2 was higher in the obese women compared with obese men. PET studies have now documented the salutary effects of weight loss on myocardial metabolism, structure, and function [181, 182].

Small animal PET imaging has helped clarify the mechanisms responsible for the metabolic alterations that occur in diabetes mellitus. For example, PET studies with [1-^{11}C]palmitate and FDG in relevant genetic models demonstrate that PPARα and PPARβ/σ drive different metabolic regulatory programs in the diabetic heart [183, 184]. In a more clinically relevant model of type 2 diabetes mellitus, the Zucker diabetic fat rat, myocardial glucose uptake correlates directly and closely with GLUT 4 gene expression, demonstrating the quantitative capability of the technique [185]. PET measurements in the same model demonstrated a decline in myocardial glucose uptake and an increase in fatty acid uptake and oxidation. The metabolic adaptations were associated with a decline in insulin-mediated phosphorylation of Akt which is indicative of reduced insulin action and an increase in abundance at the sarcolemma of the fatty acid transporter CD36, respectively [186]. Of note, these PET techniques have now been optimized for mouse heart [187].

The results of several imaging studies in humans have generally reproduced the observations from preclinical studies and as a result greatly expanded our understanding of the chronic metabolic adaptations in the diabetic heart. PET and [1-^{11}C]palmitate and [1-^{11}C]glucose in patients with type 1 diabetes mellitus demonstrate higher levels of fatty acid uptake and oxidation compared with nondiabetics primarily due to increased plasma FA levels. In contrast, glucose uptake is reduced in these patients primarily due to decreased glucose transport mechanisms [65]. Moreover, the metabolic fate of extracted glucose is impaired in diabetes with reduced rates of glycolysis and glucose oxidation which become more pronounced with increases in cardiac work induced by dobutamine [188]. However, the myocardium in type 1 diabetic patients is responsive to changes in plasma insulin and fatty acid levels but at a cost. Higher insulin levels are needed to achieve the same level of glucose uptake and glucose oxidation compared with nondiabetics, consistent with myocardial insulin resistance. Similarly, in response to higher fatty acid plasma levels, myocardial fatty acid uptake is increased at the cost of a greater esterification rate [189].

Results of metabolic imaging studies in patients with type 2 diabetes mellitus that were composed of various combinations of PET, ^{1}H-MRS, ^{31}P-MRS, MRI, and echocardiography have yielded remarkably consistent results that in general parallel preclinical observations and support the mechanistic framework for diabetes-induced chronic metabolic adaptations. These observations include a systemic environment typified by reduced whole-body insulin sensitivity and increased plasma fatty acid and TG levels that is paralleled by a PET-derived myocardial metabolic profile that includes increased fatty acid uptake and oxidation and reduced glucose uptake, the magnitude of which is dependent upon whether the measurements are performed in the fasted state or during insulin clamp [190–193]. In general, results of ^{1}H-MRS studies demonstrate an increase in myocardial lipid content and decline in energetics that are associated with LV diastolic and in some cases systolic dysfunction [194–196]. It appears changes in the myocardial metabolic-functional relationship parallel the progressive worsening in the systemic profile as one transitions from a lean condition to obesity without diabetes to concomitant obesity [191, 193]. It also appears the sexual dimorphism in myocardial metabolism that exists in lean subjects and obese nondiabetics is present in patients with concomitant obesity and type 2 diabetes mellitus. In these patients, women appear to have more pronounced augmentation in myocardial fatty acid metabolism and a greater propensity to form TG compared with diabetic men [191]. In contrast, diabetic men appear to have a greater impairment in myocardial glucose uptake and oxidation compared with diabetic women (Figs. 11.11 and 11.12) [180]. These results are intriguing given the greater susceptibility of females with type 2 diabetes mellitus to develop heart failure and exhibit a poorer prognosis when compared with male diabetics [197–199].

The effects of antidiabetic therapies in humans on myocardial metabolism have been evaluated by PET. For example, differential effects of the PPARγ agonists pioglitazone,

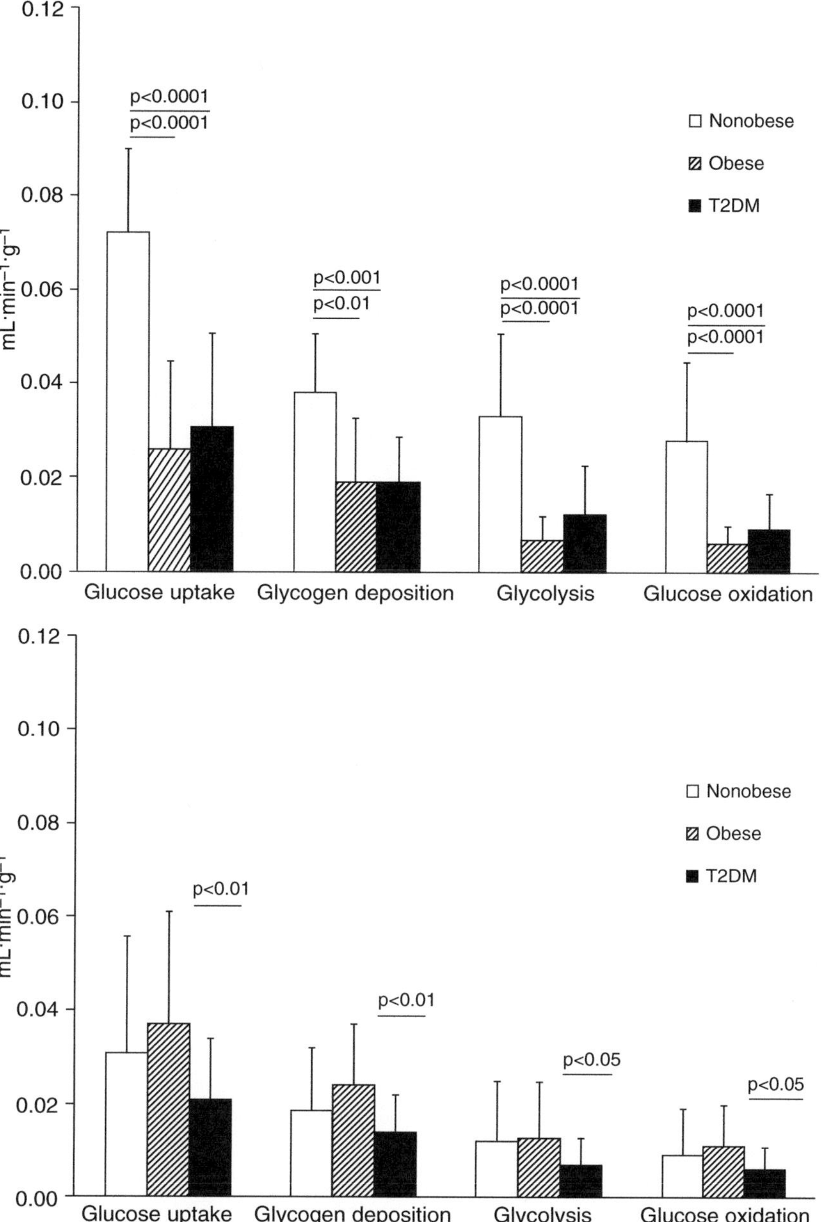

Fig. 11.11 Sexual dimorphism in myocardial metabolism in obesity and diabetes. Measurements of the fractional uptake of glucose, glycogen deposition, glycolysis, and oxidation measured by PET with [1-^{11}C]glucose in lean, obese, and diabetic men (*Top*) and women (*Bottom*). Data suggest that men exhibit a greater decline in glucose metabolism compared with women as one transitions from lean to obese to diabetes. Reproduced with permission Peterson LP et al., Am J Physiol Heart Circ Physiol 308: H1510–H15

rosiglitazone, and the biguanide and metformin on myocardial glucose and fatty acid metabolism have been assessed using PET with FDG or [1-^{11}C]glucose and [1-^{11}C]palmitate, respectively. Treatment with either rosiglitazone or pioglitazone results in an increase in insulin-stimulated myocardial glucose uptake. In contrast, insulin-stimulated myocardial glucose uptake is either unchanged or reduced with metformin therapy [200, 201]. In male diabetics,

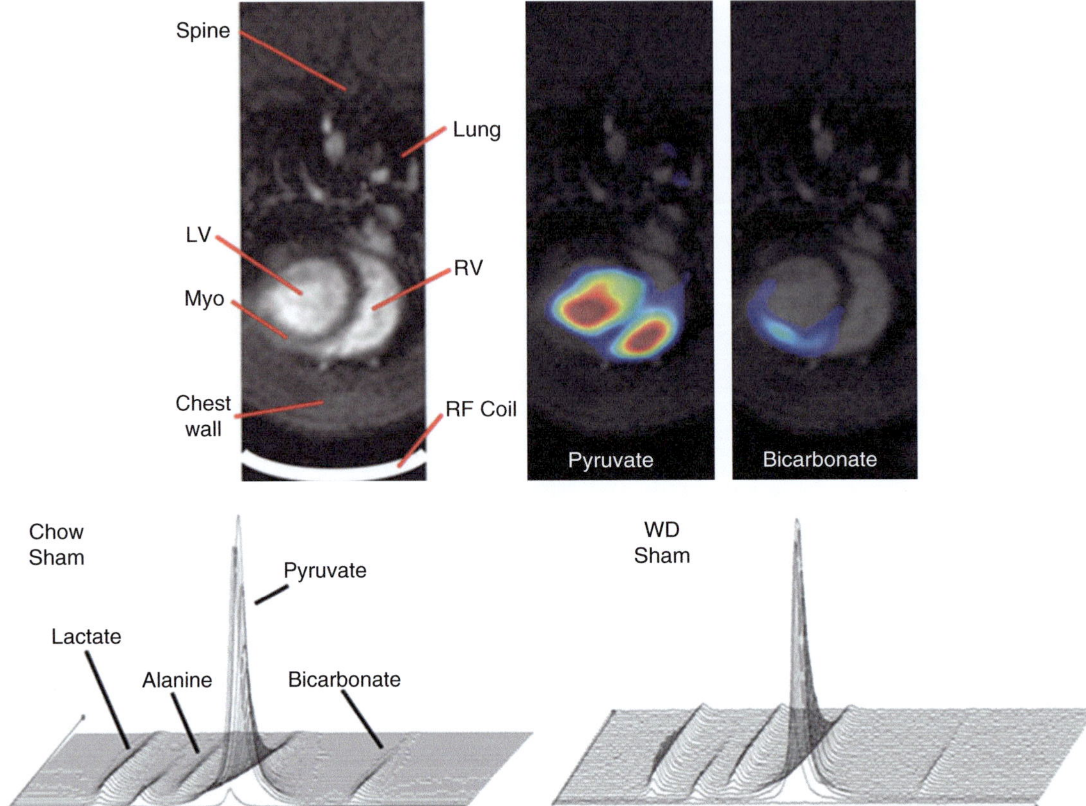

Fig. 11.12 Effects of a Western diet on appearance of hyperpolarized [^{13}C]bicarbonate in the rat heart. *Upper panel* shows, left to right, a conventional MRI, a ^{13}C MR image of pyruvate in the right and left ventricular cavities, and a ^{13}C MR image of HP[^{13}C]bicarbonate in the anterior wall of the myocardium. The inhomogeneous [^{13}C]bicarbonate signal is due to the high local sensitivity of the surface coil. *Bottom panel*: Stacked plots showing the evolution of HP[^{13}C]bicarbonate and other metabolites in the myocardium after infusion of HP[1-^{13}C]bicarbonate. Eating a high-fat, high-sucrose Western diet (WD) was associated with suppression of HP[^{13}C]bicarbonate appearance, presumably due to increased oxidation of fatty acids. Data from Seymour et al. Cardiovasc Res. 2015; 106: 249-60

pioglitazone therapy does not have a significant effect on myocardial fatty acid metabolism [200]. The lack of a decrease in fatty acid metabolism and variable response in myocardial glucose uptake with these therapies may be explained by different responses in men and women. In men, metformin alone decreases whole-body fatty acid clearance, which results in increased plasma fatty acid levels, myocardial fatty acid uptake and oxidation, and lower myocardial glucose uptake. In women, myocardial glucose uptake is increased. When metformin and rosiglitazone are combined, women exhibit increased whole-body fatty acid clearance, which decreases plasma fatty acid levels and myocardial fatty acid uptake. This effect is much less pronounced in men. Group and sex also interacted in determining myocardial glucose uptake. Thus, in diabetes, different therapeutic regimens impact myocardial metabolism in a sex-specific manner. Of note for all of the studies above, metabolic response could not be predicted by changes in the plasma glucose or $HgBA1_C$ levels. Although requiring further evaluation in larger studies, these observations suggest metabolic imaging may be used to follow the effects of therapies designed to alter myocardial substrate metabolism in patients with diseases such as diabetes mellitus where more readily available clinical parameters are not predictive of a therapeutic response. Moreover, they suggest more personalized approaches that incorporate patient gender may be useful in designing diabetic therapies.

HP MR

Compared to PET technology, there are limited examples of studies in vivo using HP-^{13}C to examine cardiac lipotoxicity in insulin resistance and diabetes mellitus. Nonetheless, early-stage investigations have begun to explore the metabolic consequences of diabetes and high fat diets. For example, it is known that malonyl-CoA is a critical regulator of fatty acid oxidation and the concentration of malonyl-CoA in diabetic myocardium is reduced. Since carnitine acetyltransferase is inhibited by malonyl-CoA, the rate of conversion of acetate to acetylcarnitine could be increased, potentially providing an important imaging biomarker of abnormal fatty acid oxidation. Metabolism of [1-^{13}C]acetate has been examined by hyperpolarization methods in perfused hearts and in vivo demonstrating the capacity to detect metabolism to [1-^{13}C]acetylcarnitine [101, 103, 153]. The effect of type 1 diabetes, modeled by administration of streptozotocin to rats, was examined using HP[1-^{13}C]acetate [202]. As outlined above, after activation by acetyl-CoA synthetase to acetyl-CoA, [1-^{13}C]acetate may be metabolized to [1-^{13}C]acetylcarnitine or [5-^{13}C]citrate. The focus of this study was on detection of [1-^{13}C]acetylcarnitine because the chemical shift difference between [5-^{13}C]citrate and [1-^{13}C]acetate is too small for resolution in vivo at clinical fields, although sufficient resolution is achievable in perfused hearts [102]. However, in spite of marked hyperglycemia after 3 weeks, induced by streptozotocin, there was no effect of type 1 diabetes on HP[1-^{13}C]acetylcarnitine/HP[1-^{13}C]acetate. Although further study is necessary to interpret this finding, these results may indicate that flux through the acetyl-CoA pool is small compared to the activity of an exchange reaction and that a reduction in activity of carnitine acetyltransferase is for this reason undetectable. These results were consistent with other exams detecting the products of [1-^{13}C]acetate metabolism: signal is modest compared to results from HP[1-^{13}C]pyruvate.

"Western" diets, modeled in rodents by high saturated lipid and sucrose content, are associated with insulin resistance and reduced left ventricular function [203–205]. In its early stages, exposure to an excess of dietary fat may result in lipotoxicity. High fat diets rapidly inhibit PDH flux [206], at least in part due to selective increase in the expression of pyruvate dehydrogenase kinase. This effect is very rapid and sustained, occurring within the first day on a diet, and implies that PDH flux will be sensitized to the inhibitory effects of fatty acids, presumably due to high [acetyl-CoA]/[CoA]. These observations predict that an imaging biomarker of PDH flux and conversion of HP[1-^{13}C]pyruvate to HP[^{13}C] bicarbonate will be inhibited. High-quality [^{13}C] bicarbonate images were achieved, and as anticipated, PDH flux was reduced [207]. This occurred in the absence of structural or functional deterioration, suggesting that HP methods may be a very sensitive indicator of early changes in metabolism due to diet.

Potential Synergies

As emphasized above, the heart must be capable of quickly managing major shifts in the demand for energy production as well as discontinuities in the hormonal and substrate environment. This adaptability has been termed "metabolic flexibility" which in the context of type 2 diabetes is equivalent to insulin resistance. There is little information about the evolution of metabolic inflexibility in the hearts of adolescents at risk for type 2 diabetes and cardiac lipotoxicity because studies with ionizing radiation are difficult to justify. There is a significant need for imaging technology enabling metabolic exams in children that can be used over time to assess baseline physiology as well as the response to interventions. Combined PET and ^{13}C-HP studies employing PET/MR may help this regard. Strategies are currently designed and evaluated to permit whole-body PET/MR imaging with very low injectable doses of ^{18}FDG and MR attenuation resulting in significantly reduced radiation exposure. As a consequence, the PET component of the PET/MR study could be used for both baseline metabolic measurements and identifying key organs or specific regions of interest where glucose metabolism is altered. In the latter, more in-depth metabolic interrogation could be performed with ^{13}C-HP.

11.6 The Future: Validation and the Potential of Combined PET and ^{13}C-HP

By dint of the aforementioned discussion, the combining of capabilities of PET and HPMR to simultaneously measure both imaging readouts with PET/MR has the potential to open entirely new avenues of scientific discovery. For example, it would now be possible to cross-calibrate and cross-validate both imaging technologies. From HPMR perspective, metabolic measurements using various ^{13}C tracers can be compared with their PET ^{11}C radiotracer counterparts to determine impact of non-tracer doses of substrate on myocardial metabolism. Conversely, measurements of various components of myocardial metabolism measured with PET and compartmental modeling (e.g., oxidation and storage) can be referenced to the true metabolic fate of the exogenous substrate measured with HPMR. Most exciting is the potential use of the quantitative capabilities of PET to facilitate the HPMR quantification of substrate flux through metabolic pathways of interest. Such information is attainable from a PET-derived input function, an MR tissue response, and knowledge of the MR tracer blood concentration. Such information is critical for the accurate interpretation of HPMR-derived measurements of disease effects and dose response. Finally, it is conceivable that investigations using hyperpolarized compounds may actually enable further development of new PET agents and further encourage the development of PET/MR. Clearly, significant technical developments in probe development and image acquisition, analysis, and display are going to be required to move these examples from theory to practice.

Even with these major advances, translation to clinical application of these combined imaging approaches will require overcoming several challenges. The typical paradigm for developing new imaging tests has been used to perform the exam in patients with suspected or known disease and then to compare the results to a "gold standard" metric which may be an accepted exam or results from pathology [208]. These studies typically report sensitivity, specificity, or receiver operating characteristic (ROC) analysis. More recently, investigators and policy makers have recognized that the number of potential imaging approaches and probes is steadily increasing and recognizing appropriate use may be difficult. Questions of clinical utility are premature at this point in the development of hyperpolarization because the technology is still evolving rapidly and numerous refinements are anticipated in the next few years. Nevertheless investigators should consider that the technology will likely be evaluated based on three classes of data to support clinical translation: analytical validity, clinical validity, and clinical utility [209, 210]. Analytic validity means the reproducibility and reliability of a measurement. Does an HP image really measure what it claims? Can the measurement be performed reliably? Clinical validity refers to the relation between the imaging results and a clinical outcome or diagnosis of interest. Does an HP image detect clinically meaningful information, as judged by a reference standard? Very importantly, has HP imaging been tested against a technology with which clinicians are comfortable? Clinical utility is the most difficult challenge and tests whether the use of HP imaging results in a favorable redistribution of benefits compared to risks and costs. Does the use of HP imaging lead to improved outcomes, compared to nonuse? Eventually, these questions will need to be addressed, presumably through large multicenter prospective trials.

References

1. Ardenkjaer-Larsen JH, et al. Increase in signal-to-noise ratio of > 10,000 times in liquid-state NMR. Proc Natl Acad Sci U S A. 2003;100(18):10158–63.
2. Golman K, et al. Molecular imaging with endogenous substances. Proc Natl Acad Sci U S A. 2003;100(18):10435–9.
3. Nelson SJ, et al. Metabolic imaging of patients with prostate cancer using hyperpolarized [1-(1)(3)C] pyruvate. Sci Transl Med. 2013; 5(198): 198ra108.

4. Taegtmeyer H. Six blind men explore an elephant: aspects of fuel metabolism and the control of tricarboxylic acid cycle activity in heart muscle. Basic Res Cardiol. 1984;79(3):322–36.
5. Moreno KX, et al. Competition of pyruvate with physiological substrates for oxidation by the heart: implications for studies with hyperpolarized [1-13C]pyruvate. Am J Physiol Heart Circ Physiol. 2010;298(5):H1556–64.
6. Jeffrey FM, et al. Substrate selection in the isolated working rat heart: effects of reperfusion, afterload, and concentration. Basic Res Cardiol. 1995;90(5):388–96.
7. Jeffrey FM, et al. Direct evidence that perhexiline modifies myocardial substrate utilization from fatty acids to lactate. J Cardiovasc Pharmacol. 1995;25(3):469–72.
8. Drake AJ, Haines JR, Noble MI. Preferential uptake of lactate by the normal myocardium in dogs. Cardiovasc Res. 1980;14(2):65–72.
9. Banke NH, et al. Preferential oxidation of triacylglyceride-derived fatty acids in heart is augmented by the nuclear receptor PPARalpha. Circ Res. 2010;107(2):233–41.
10. Saddik M, Lopaschuk GD. Myocardial triglyceride turnover and contribution to energy substrate utilization in isolated working rat hearts. J Biol Chem. 1991;266(13):8162–70.
11. Armbrecht JJ, Buxton DB, Schelbert HR. Validation of [1-11C]acetate as a tracer for noninvasive assessment of oxidative metabolism with positron emission tomography in normal, ischemic, postischemic, and hyperemic canine myocardium. Circulation. 1990;81(5):1594–605.
12. Abbas AS, Wu G, Schulz H. Carnitine acetyltransferase is not a cytosolic enzyme in rat heart and therefore cannot function in the energy-linked regulation of cardiac fatty acid oxidation. J Mol Cell Cardiol. 1998;30(7):1305–9.
13. Bakker A, et al. Ultrastructural localisation of carnitine acetyltransferase activity in mitochondria of rat myocardium. Biochim Biophys Acta. 1994;1185(1):97–102.
14. Remesy C, Demigne C. Changes in availability of glucogenic and ketogenic substrates and liver metabolism in fed or starved rats. Ann Nutr Metab. 1983;27(1):57–70.
15. Owen OE, et al. Liver and kidney metabolism during prolonged starvation. J Clin Invest. 1969;48(3):574–83.
16. Hansford RG, Cohen L. Relative importance of pyruvate dehydrogenase interconversion and feedback inhibition in the effect of fatty acids on pyruvate oxidation by rat heart mitochondria. Arch Biochem Biophys. 1978;191(1):65–81.
17. Latipaa PM, et al. Regulation of pyruvate dehydrogenase during infusion of fatty acids of varying chain lengths in the perfused rat heart. J Mol Cell Cardiol. 1985;17(12):1161–71.
18. Purmal C, et al. Propionate stimulates pyruvate oxidation in the presence of acetate. Am J Physiol Heart Circ Physiol. 2014;307(8):H1134–41.
19. Bunger R. Compartmented pyruvate in perfused working heart. Am J Phys. 1985;249(3 Pt 2):H439–49.
20. Malloy CR, Sherry AD, Jeffrey FM. Evaluation of carbon flux and substrate selection through alternate pathways involving the citric acid cycle of the heart by 13C NMR spectroscopy. J Biol Chem. 1988;263(15):6964–71.
21. Peuhkurinen KJ, et al. Role of pyruvate carboxylation in the energy-linked regulation of pool sizes of tricarboxylic acid-cycle intermediates in the myocardium. Biochem J. 1982;208(3):577–81.
22. Depre C, Vanoverschelde JL, Taegtmeyer H. Glucose for the heart. Circulation. 1999;99(4):578–88.
23. Zimmer HG. Regulation of and intervention into the oxidative pentose phosphate pathway and adenine nucleotide metabolism in the heart. Mol Cell Biochem. 1996;160-161:101–9.
24. Zimmer HG. The oxidative pentose phosphate pathway in the heart: regulation, physiological significance, and clinical implications. Basic Res Cardiol. 1992;87(4):303–16.
25. Vimercati C, et al. Beneficial effects of acute inhibition of the oxidative pentose phosphate pathway in the failing heart. Am J Physiol Heart Circ Physiol. 2014;306(5):H709–17.
26. Nuutinen EM, et al. Elimination and replenishment of tricarboxylic acid-cycle intermediates in myocardium. Biochem J. 1981;194(3):867–75.
27. Peuhkurinen KJ, Hiltunen JK, Hassinen IE. Metabolic compartmentation of pyruvate in the isolated perfused rat heart. Biochem J. 1983;210(1):193–8.
28. Peuhkurinen KJ, Hassinen IE. Pyruvate carboxylation as an anaplerotic mechanism in the isolated perfused rat heart. Biochem J. 1982;202(1):67–76.
29. Sherry AD, et al. Propionate metabolism in the rat heart by 13C n.M.R. Spectroscopy. Biochem J. 1988;254(2):593–8.
30. Chatham JC, Forder JR. Metabolic compartmentation of lactate in the glucose-perfused rat heart. Am J Phys. 1996;270(1 Pt 2):H224–9.
31. Mowbray J, Ottaway JH. The flux of pyruvate in perfused rat heart. Eur J Biochem. 1973;36(2):362–8.
32. Mowbray J, Ottaway JH. The effect of insulin and growth hormone on the flux of tracer from labelled lactate in perfused rat heart. Eur J Biochem. 1973;36(2):369–79.
33. Li Q, et al. Multiple mass isotopomer tracing of acetyl-CoA metabolism in Langendorff-perfused rat hearts: channeling of acetyl-CoA from pyruvate dehydrogenase to carnitine acetyltransferase. J Biol Chem. 2015;290(13):8121–32.
34. Anousis N, et al. Compartmentation of glycolysis and glycogenolysis in the perfused rat heart. NMR Biomed. 2004;17(2):51–9.
35. Khemtong C, et al. Hyperpolarized 13C NMR detects rapid drug-induced changes in cardiac metabolism. Magn Reson Med. 2015;74(2):312–9.
36. Schinkel AF, et al. Hibernating myocardium: diagnosis and patient outcomes. Curr Probl Cardiol. 2007;32(7):375–410.

37. DeGrado TR, et al. Quantitative analysis of myocardial kinetics of 15-p-[iodine-125] iodophenylpentadecanoic acid. J Nucl Med. 1989;30(7):1211–8.
38. Dormehl IC, et al. Planar myocardial imaging in the baboon model with iodine-123-15-(iodophenyl) pentadecanoic acid (IPPA) and iodine-123-15-(P-iodophenyl)-3-R,S-methylpentadecanoic acid (BMIPP), using time-activity curves for evaluation of metabolism. Nucl Med Biol. 1995;22(7):837–47.
39. Eckelman WC, Babich JW. Synthesis and validation of fatty acid analogs radiolabeled by nonisotopic substitution. J Nucl Cardiol. 2007;14(3 Suppl):S100–9.
40. Ambrose KR, et al. Evaluation of the metabolism in rat hearts of two new radioiodinated 3-methyl-branched fatty acid myocardial imaging agents. Eur J Nucl Med. 1987;12(10):486–91.
41. Goodman MM, Kirsch G, Knapp FF Jr. Synthesis and evaluation of radioiodinated terminal p-iodophenyl-substituted alpha- and beta-methyl-branched fatty acids. J Med Chem. 1984;27(3):390–7.
42. Reske SN, et al. Metabolism of 15 (p 123I iodophenyl-)pentadecanoic acid in heart muscle and noncardiac tissues. Eur J Nucl Med. 1985;10(5-6):228–34.
43. He ZX, et al. Direct imaging of exercise-induced myocardial ischemia with fluorine-18-labeled deoxyglucose and Tc-99m-sestamibi in coronary artery disease. Circulation. 2003;108(10):1208–13.
44. Iida H, et al. Noninvasive quantification of regional myocardial metabolic rate for oxygen by use of 15O2 inhalation and positron emission tomography. Theory, error analysis, and application in humans. Circulation. 1996;94(4):792–807.
45. Laine H, et al. Myocardial oxygen consumption is unchanged but efficiency is reduced in patients with essential hypertension and left ventricular hypertrophy. Circulation. 1999;100(24):2425–30.
46. Yamamoto Y, et al. Noninvasive quantification of regional myocardial metabolic rate of oxygen by 15O2 inhalation and positron emission tomography, experimental validation. Circulation. 1996;94(4):808–16.
47. Brown M, et al. Delineation of myocardial oxygen utilization with carbon-11-labeled acetate. Circulation. 1987;76(3):687–96.
48. Brown MA, Myears DW, Bergmann SR. Noninvasive assessment of canine myocardial oxidative metabolism with carbon-11 acetate and positron emission tomography. J Am Coll Cardiol. 1988;12(4):1054–63.
49. Buck A, et al. Effect of carbon-11-acetate recirculation on estimates of myocardial oxygen consumption by PET. J Nucl Med. 1991;32(10):1950–7.
50. Sun KT, et al. Simultaneous measurement of myocardial oxygen consumption and blood flow using [1-carbon-11]acetate. J Nucl Med. 1998;39(2):272–80.
51. Choi Y, et al. Parametric images of myocardial metabolic rate of glucose generated from dynamic cardiac PET and 2-[18F]fluoro-2-deoxy-d-glucose studies. J Nucl Med. 1991;32(4):733–8.
52. Gambert S, et al. Adverse effects of free fatty acid associated with increased oxidative stress in post-ischemic isolated rat hearts. Mol Cell Biochem. 2006;283(1-2):147–52.
53. Iozzo P, et al. Regional myocardial blood flow and glucose utilization during fasting and physiological hyperinsulinemia in humans. Am J Physiol Endocrinol Metab. 2002;282(5):E1163–71.
54. Krivokapich J, et al. Fluorodeoxyglucose rate constants, lumped constant, and glucose metabolic rate in rabbit heart. Am J Phys. 1987;252(4 Pt 2):H777–87.
55. Botker HE, et al. Glucose uptake and lumped constant variability in normal human hearts determined with [18F]fluorodeoxyglucose. J Nucl Cardiol. 1997;4(2 Pt 1):125–32.
56. Hariharan R, et al. Fundamental limitations of [18F]2-deoxy-2-fluoro-D-glucose for assessing myocardial glucose uptake. Circulation. 1995;91(9):2435–44.
57. Hashimoto K, et al. Lumped constant for deoxyglucose is decreased when myocardial glucose uptake is enhanced. Am J Phys. 1999;276(1 Pt 2):H129–33.
58. Herrero P, et al. L-3-11C-lactate as a PET tracer of myocardial lactate metabolism: a feasibility study. J Nucl Med. 2007;48(12):2046–55.
59. Bergmann SR, et al. Quantitation of myocardial fatty acid metabolism using PET. J Nucl Med. 1996;37(10):1723–30.
60. Herrero P, et al. Increased myocardial fatty acid metabolism in patients with type 1 diabetes mellitus. J Am Coll Cardiol. 2006;47(3):598–604.
61. Kisrieva-Ware Z, et al. Assessment of myocardial triglyceride oxidation with PET and 11C-palmitate. J Nucl Cardiol.
62. DeGrado TR. Synthesis of 14(R,S)-[18F]fluoro-6-thia-heptadecanoic acid (FTHA). J Label Comp Radiopharm. 1991;29:989–95.
63. DeGrado TR, Coenen HH, Stocklin G. 14(R,S)-[18F]fluoro-6-thia-heptadecanoic acid (FTHA): evaluation in mouse of a new probe of myocardial utilization of long chain fatty acids. J Nucl Med. 1991;32(10):1888–96.
64. DeGrado TR, et al. Synthesis and preliminary evaluation of (18)F-labeled 4-thia palmitate as a PET tracer of myocardial fatty acid oxidation. Nucl Med Biol. 2000;27(3):221–31.
65. DeGrado TR, et al. Validation of 18F-fluoro-4-thia-palmitate as a PET probe for myocardial fatty acid oxidation: effects of hypoxia and composition of exogenous fatty acids. J Nucl Med. 2006;47(1):173–81.
66. DeGrado TR, et al. Synthesis and preliminary evaluation of 18-(18)F-fluoro-4-thia-oleate as a PET probe of fatty acid oxidation. J Nucl Med. 2010;51(8):1310–7.
67. Shoup TM, et al. Evaluation of trans-9-18F-fluoro-3,4-Methyleneheptadecanoic acid as a PET tracer for myocardial fatty acid imaging. J Nucl Med. 2005;46(2):297–304.

68. Demeure F, et al. A new F-18 labeled PET tracer for fatty acid imaging. J Nucl Cardiol. 2015;22(2):391–4.
69. Labbe SM, et al. Increased myocardial uptake of dietary fatty acids linked to cardiac dysfunction in glucose-intolerant humans. Diabetes. 2012;61(11):2701–10.
70. Labbe SM, et al. Organ-specific dietary fatty acid uptake in humans using positron emission tomography coupled to computed tomography. Am J Physiol Endocrinol Metab. 2011;300(3):E445–53.
71. Shoghi KI, Gropler RJ. PET measurements of organ metabolism: the devil is in the details. Diabetes. 2015;64(7):2332–4.
72. O'Donnell JM, et al. The absence of endogenous lipid oxidation in early stage heart failure exposes limits in lipid storage and turnover. J Mol Cell Cardiol. 2008;44(2):315–22.
73. Saddik M, Lopaschuk GD. Triacylglycerol turnover in isolated working hearts of acutely diabetic rats. Can J Physiol Pharmacol. 1994;72(10):1110–9.
74. Wisneski JA, et al. Myocardial metabolism of free fatty acids. Studies with 14C-labeled substrates in humans. J Clin Invest. 1987;79(2):359–66.
75. Wicklmayr M, et al. Inhibition of muscular triglyceride lipolysis by ketone bodies: a mechanism for energy-preservation in starvation. Horm Metab Res. 1986;18(7):476–8.
76. Kisrieva-Ware Z, et al. Assessment of myocardial triglyceride oxidation with PET and 11C-palmitate. J Nucl Cardiol. 2009;16(3):411–21.
77. Bucci M, et al. Trimetazidine reduces endogenous free fatty acid oxidation and improves myocardial efficiency in obese humans. Cardiovasc Ther. 2012;30(6):333–41.
78. Brindle KM. Imaging metabolism with hyperpolarized (13)C-labeled cell substrates. J Am Chem Soc. 2015;137(20):6418–27.
79. Comment A, Merritt ME. Hyperpolarized magnetic resonance as a sensitive detector of metabolic function. Biochemistry. 2014;53(47):7333–57.
80. Kurhanewicz J, et al. Analysis of cancer metabolism by imaging hyperpolarized nuclei: prospects for translation to clinical research. Neoplasia. 2011;13(2):81–97.
81. Bhattacharya P, Ross BD, Bunger R. Cardiovascular applications of hyperpolarized contrast media and metabolic tracers. Exp Biol Med (Maywood). 2009;234(12):1395–416.
82. Tyler DJ. Cardiovascular applications of hyperpolarized MRI. Curr Cardiovasc Imaging Rep. 2011;4(2):108–15.
83. Rider OJ, Tyler DJ. Clinical implications of cardiac hyperpolarized magnetic resonance imaging. J Cardiovasc Magn Reson. 2013;15:93.
84. Keshari KR, Wilson DM. Chemistry and biochemistry of 13C hyperpolarized magnetic resonance using dynamic nuclear polarization. Chem Soc Rev. 2014;43(5):1627–59.
85. Lau AZ, et al. Simultaneous assessment of cardiac metabolism and perfusion using copolarized [1-13 C]pyruvate and 13 C-urea. Magn Reson Med. 2016.
86. Golman K, Petersson JS. Metabolic imaging and other applications of hyperpolarized 13C1. Acad Radiol. 2006;13(8):932–42.
87. Golman K, et al. Cardiac metabolism measured noninvasively by hyperpolarized 13C MRI. Magn Reson Med. 2008;59(5):1005–13.
88. Lau AZ, et al. Rapid multislice imaging of hyperpolarized 13C pyruvate and bicarbonate in the heart. Magn Reson Med. 2010;64(5):1323–31.
89. Schroeder MA, et al. Hyperpolarized (13)C magnetic resonance reveals early- and late-onset changes to in vivo pyruvate metabolism in the failing heart. Eur J Heart Fail. 2013;15(2):130–40.
90. Merritt ME, et al. Hyperpolarized 13C allows a direct measure of flux through a single enzyme-catalyzed step by NMR. Proc Natl Acad Sci U S A. 2007;104(50):19773–7.
91. Lau, A.Z., J.J. Miller, and D.J. Tyler, Mapping of intracellular pH in the in vivo rodent heart using hyperpolarized [1-13C]pyruvate. Magn Reson Med, 2016.
92. Dominguez-Viqueira W, et al. Intensity correction for multichannel hyperpolarized 13C imaging of the heart. Magn Reson Med. 2016;75(2):859–65.
93. Schroeder MA, et al. Real-time assessment of Krebs cycle metabolism using hyperpolarized 13C magnetic resonance spectroscopy. FASEB J. 2009;23(8):2529–38.
94. Chen AP, et al. Simultaneous investigation of cardiac pyruvate dehydrogenase flux, Krebs cycle metabolism and pH, using hyperpolarized [1,2-(13)C2] pyruvate in vivo. NMR Biomed. 2012;25(2):305–11.
95. Chen AP, et al. Using [1-(13) C]lactic acid for hyperpolarized (13) C MR cardiac studies. Magn Reson Med. 2015;73(6):2087–93.
96. Jensen PR, et al. Tissue-specific short chain fatty acid metabolism and slow metabolic recovery after ischemia from hyperpolarized NMR in vivo. J Biol Chem. 2009;284(52):36077–82.
97. Bastiaansen JA, et al. Direct noninvasive estimation of myocardial tricarboxylic acid cycle flux in vivo using hyperpolarized (1)(3)C magnetic resonance. J Mol Cell Cardiol. 2015;87:129–37.
98. Flori A, et al. Real-time cardiac metabolism assessed with hyperpolarized [1-(13) C]acetate in a large-animal model. Contrast Media Mol Imaging. 2015;10(3):194–202.
99. Ball DR, et al. Hyperpolarized butyrate: a metabolic probe of short chain fatty acid metabolism in the heart. Magn Reson Med. 2014;71(5):1663–9.
100. Vary TC, Reibel DK, Neely JR. Control of energy metabolism of heart muscle. Annu Rev Physiol. 1981;43:419–30.
101. Neely JR, Morgan HE. Relationship between carbohydrate and lipid metabolism and the energy balance of heart muscle. Annu Rev Physiol. 1974;36:413–59.
102. Lopaschuk G. Regulation of carbohydrate metabolism in ischemia and reperfusion. Am Heart J. 2000;139(2 Pt 3):S115–9.
103. Araujo LI, et al. Abnormalities in myocardial metabolism in patients with unstable angina as assessed

by positron emission tomography. Cardiovasc Drugs Ther. 1988;2(1):41–6.
104. Camici P, et al. Increased uptake of 18F-fluorodeoxyglucose in postischemic myocardium of patients with exercise-induced angina. Circulation. 1986;74(1):81–8.
105. Tamaki N, et al. The role of fatty acids in cardiac imaging. J Nucl Med. 2000;41(9):1525–34.
106. Kawai Y, et al. Diagnostic value of 123I-betamethyl-p-iodophenyl-pentadecanoic acid (BMIPP) single photon emission computed tomography (SPECT) in patients with chest pain. Comparison with rest-stress 99mTc-tetrofosmin SPECT and coronary angiography. Circ J. 2004;68(6):547–52.
107. Kontos MC, et al. Iodofiltic acid I 123 (BMIPP) fatty acid imaging improves initial diagnosis in emergency department patients with suspected acute coronary syndromes: a multicenter trial. J Am Coll Cardiol. 2010;56(4):290–9.
108. Moroi M, et al. Association between abnormal myocardial fatty acid metabolism and cardiac-derived death among patients undergoing hemodialysis: results from a cohort study in Japan. Am J Kidney Dis. 2013;61(3):466–75.
109. Dou KF, et al. Myocardial 18F-FDG uptake after exercise-induced myocardial ischemia in patients with coronary artery disease. J Nucl Med. 2008;49(12):1986–91.
110. Merritt ME, et al. Inhibition of carbohydrate oxidation during the first minute of reperfusion after brief ischemia: NMR detection of hyperpolarized 13CO2 and H13CO3. Magn Reson Med. 2008;60(5):1029–36.
111. Rupp H, Jacob R. Metabolically-modulated growth and phenotype of the rat heart. Eur Heart J. 1992;13(Suppl D):56–61.
112. Barger PM, Kelly DP. Fatty acid utilization in the hypertrophied and failing heart: molecular regulatory mechanisms. Am J Med Sci. 1999;318(1):36–42.
113. Tuder RM, Davis LA, Graham BB. Targeting energetic metabolism: a new frontier in the pathogenesis and treatment of pulmonary hypertension. Am J Respir Crit Care Med. 2012;185(3):260–6.
114. Kolwicz SC Jr. And R. Tian, glucose metabolism and cardiac hypertrophy. Cardiovasc Res. 2011;90(2):194–201.
115. Taegtmeyer H, et al. Linking gene expression to function: metabolic flexibility in the normal and diseased heart. Ann N Y Acad Sci. 2004;1015:202–13.
116. Jamshidi Y, et al. Peroxisome proliferator-activated receptor alpha gene regulates left ventricular growth in response to exercise and hypertension. Circulation. 2002;105(8):950–5.
117. Blair E, et al. Mutations in the gamma(2) subunit of AMP-activated protein kinase cause familial hypertrophic cardiomyopathy: evidence for the central role of energy compromise in disease pathogenesis. Hum Mol Genet. 2001;10(11):1215–20.
118. Razeghi P, et al. Downregulation of myocardial myocyte enhancer factor 2C and myocyte enhancer factor 2C-regulated gene expression in diabetic patients with nonischemic heart failure. Circulation. 2002;106(4):407–11.
119. Buttrick PM, et al. Alterations in gene expression in the rat heart after chronic pathological and physiological loads. J Mol Cell Cardiol. 1994;26(1):61–7.
120. Ouwens DM, et al. Cardiac contractile dysfunction in insulin-resistant rats fed a high-fat diet is associated with elevated CD36-mediated fatty acid uptake and esterification. Diabetologia. 2007;50(9):1938–48.
121. Handa N, et al. Quantitative FDG-uptake by positron emission tomography in progressive hypertrophy of rat hearts in vivo. Ann Nucl Med. 2007;21(10):569–76.
122. Banke NH, et al. Sexual dimorphism in cardiac triacylglyceride dynamics in mice on long term caloric restriction. J Mol Cell Cardiol. 2012;52(3):733–40.
123. Hollingsworth KG, et al. Left ventricular torsion, energetics, and diastolic function in normal human aging. Am J Physiol Heart Circ Physiol. 2012;302(4):H885–92.
124. van der Meer RW, et al. The ageing male heart: myocardial triglyceride content as independent predictor of diastolic function. Eur Heart J. 2008;29(12):1516–22.
125. Zhong M, et al. Quantitative PET imaging detects early metabolic remodeling in a mouse model of pressure-overload left ventricular hypertrophy in vivo. J Nucl Med. 2013;54(4):609–15.
126. de las Fuentes L, et al. Myocardial fatty acid metabolism: independent predictor of left ventricular mass in hypertensive heart disease. Hypertension. 2003; 41(1): 83–7.
127. Hamirani YS, et al. Noninvasive detection of early metabolic left ventricular remodeling in systemic hypertension. Cardiology. 2016;133(3):157–62.
128. Lundgrin EL, et al. Fasting 2-deoxy-2-[18F]fluoro-D-glucose positron emission tomography to detect metabolic changes in pulmonary arterial hypertension hearts over 1 year. Ann Am Thorac Soc. 2013;10(1):1–9.
129. Bokhari S, et al. PET imaging may provide a novel biomarker and understanding of right ventricular dysfunction in patients with idiopathic pulmonary arterial hypertension. Circ Cardiovasc Imaging. 2011;4(6):641–7.
130. Fang W, et al. Comparison of 18F-FDG uptake by right ventricular myocardium in idiopathic pulmonary arterial hypertension and pulmonary arterial hypertension associated with congenital heart disease. Pulm Circ. 2012;2(3):365–72.
131. Tatebe S, et al. Enhanced [18F]fluorodeoxyglucose accumulation in the right ventricular free wall predicts long-term prognosis of patients with pulmonary hypertension: a preliminary obser-

vational study. Eur Heart J Cardiovasc Imaging. 2014;15(6):666–72.
132. Oikawa M, et al. Increased [18F]fluorodeoxyglucose accumulation in right ventricular free wall in patients with pulmonary hypertension and the effect of epoprostenol. J Am Coll Cardiol. 2005;45(11):1849–55.
133. Mielniczuk LM, et al. Relation between right ventricular function and increased right ventricular [18F]fluorodeoxyglucose accumulation in patients with heart failure. Circ Cardiovasc Imaging. 2011;4(1):59–66.
134. Nakae I, et al. Iodine-123 BMIPP scintigraphy in the evaluation of patients with heart failure. Acta Radiol. 2006;47(8):810–6.
135. Davila-Roman VG, et al. Altered myocardial fatty acid and glucose metabolism in idiopathic dilated cardiomyopathy. J Am Coll Cardiol. 2002;40(2):271–7.
136. Kadkhodayan, A., et al., Sex affects myocardial blood flow and fatty acid substrate metabolism in humans with nonischemic heart failure. J Nucl Cardiol, 2016.
137. Tuunanen H, et al. Decreased myocardial free fatty acid uptake in patients with idiopathic dilated cardiomyopathy: evidence of relationship with insulin resistance and left ventricular dysfunction. J Card Fail. 2006;12(8):644–52.
138. Sharma S, et al. Intramyocardial lipid accumulation in the failing human heart resembles the lipotoxic rat heart. FASEB J. 2004;18(14):1692–700.
139. Thackery J, dR, Beanlands R, DaSilva J. Early diabetes therapy does not prevent sympathetic dysinnervation in the streptozocin diabetic rat. J Nucl Cardiol. 2014.
140. Vinik AI, Maser RE, Ziegler D. Neuropathy: the crystal ball for cardiovascular disease? Diabetes Care. 2010;33(7):1688–90.
141. Boulton AJ, et al. Diabetic neuropathies: a statement by the American Diabetes Association. Diabetes Care. 2005;28(4):956–62.
142. Tuunanen H, et al. Trimetazidine, a metabolic modulator, has cardiac and extracardiac benefits in idiopathic dilated cardiomyopathy. Circulation. 2008;118(12):1250–8.
143. Lepore, J.J., et al., Effects of the novel long-acting GLP-1 agonist, Albiglutide, on cardiac function, cardiac metabolism, and exercise capacity in patients with chronic heart failure and reduced ejection fraction. JACC Heart Fail, 2016.
144. Atherton HJ, et al. Role of pyruvate dehydrogenase inhibition in the development of hypertrophy in the hyperthyroid rat heart: a combined magnetic resonance imaging and hyperpolarized magnetic resonance spectroscopy study. Circulation. 2011;123(22):2552–61.
145. Brown MA, Myears DW, Bergmann SR. Validity of estimates of myocardial oxidative metabolism with carbon-11 acetate and positron emission tomography despite altered patterns of substrate utilization. J Nucl Med. 1989;30(2):187–93.
146. Walsh MN, et al. Noninvasive estimation of regional myocardial oxygen consumption by positron emission tomography with carbon-11 acetate in patients with myocardial infarction. J Nucl Med. 1989;30(11):1798–808.
147. Buxton DB, et al. Radiolabeled acetate as a tracer of myocardial tricarboxylic acid cycle flux. Circ Res. 1988;63(3):628–34.
148. Koellisch U, et al. Metabolic imaging of hyperpolarized [1-(13) C]acetate and [1-(13) C]acetylcarnitine - investigation of the influence of dobutamine induced stress. Magn Reson Med. 2015;74(4):1011–8.
149. Bastiaansen JA, Merritt ME, Comment A. Measuring changes in substrate utilization in the myocardium in response to fasting using hyperpolarized [1-(13)C] butyrate and [1-(13)C]pyruvate. Sci Rep. 2016;6:25573.
150. Erguven M, et al. A case of early diagnosed carnitine deficiency presenting with respiratory symptoms. Ann Nutr Metab. 2007;51(4):331–4.
151. Rinaldo P, Matern D, Bennett MJ. Fatty acid oxidation disorders. Annu Rev Physiol. 2002;64:477–502.
152. Palmieri F. Diseases caused by defects of mitochondrial carriers: a review. Biochim Biophys Acta. 2008;1777(7-8):564–78.
153. Cave MC, et al. Obesity, inflammation, and the potential application of pharmaconutrition. Nutr Clin Pract. 2008;23(1):16–34.
154. Kenchaiah S, et al. Obesity and the risk of heart failure. N Engl J Med. 2002;347(5):305–13.
155. Wong CY, et al. Alterations of left ventricular myocardial characteristics associated with obesity. Circulation. 2004;110(19):3081–7.
156. Zhou YT, et al. Lipotoxic heart disease in obese rats: implications for human obesity. Proc Natl Acad Sci U S A. 2000;97(4):1784–9.
157. Commerford SR, et al. Fat oxidation, lipolysis, and free fatty acid cycling in obesity-prone and obesity-resistant rats. Am J Physiol Endocrinol Metab. 2000;279(4):E875–85.
158. Boudina S, Abel ED. Diabetic cardiomyopathy revisited. Circulation. 2007;115(25): 3213–23.
159. Severson DL. Diabetic cardiomyopathy: recent evidence from mouse models of type 1 and type 2 diabetes. Can J Physiol Pharmacol. 2004;82(10): 813–23.
160. Stanley WC, Lopaschuk GD, McCormack JG. Regulation of energy substrate metabolism in the diabetic heart. Cardiovasc Res. 1997;34(1):25–33.
161. Taegtmeyer H, McNulty P, Young ME. Adaptation and maladaptation of the heart in diabetes: part I: general concepts. Circulation. 2002;105(14):1727–33.
162. Young ME, McNulty P, Taegtmeyer H. Adaptation and maladaptation of the heart in diabetes: part II: potential mechanisms. Circulation. 2002;105(15):1861–70.
163. Itani SI, et al. Involvement of protein kinase C in human skeletal muscle insulin resistance and obesity. Diabetes. 2000;49(8):1353–8.

164. Ruderman NB, et al. Malonyl-CoA, fuel sensing, and insulin resistance. Am J Phys. 1999;276(1 Pt 1):E1–E18.
165. Schmitz-Peiffer C, Craig DL, Biden TJ. Ceramide generation is sufficient to account for the inhibition of the insulin-stimulated PKB pathway in C2C12 skeletal muscle cells pretreated with palmitate. J Biol Chem. 1999;274(34):24202–10.
166. Oakes ND, et al. Cardiac metabolism in mice: tracer method developments and in vivo application revealing profound metabolic inflexibility in diabetes. Am J Physiol Endocrinol Metab. 2006;290(5):E870–81.
167. Young ME, et al. Impaired long-chain fatty acid oxidation and contractile dysfunction in the obese Zucker rat heart. Diabetes. 2002;51(8):2587–95.
168. Peterson LR, et al. Effect of obesity and insulin resistance on myocardial substrate metabolism and efficiency in young women. Circulation. 2004;109(18):2191–6.
169. Buchanan J, et al. Reduced cardiac efficiency and altered substrate metabolism precedes the onset of hyperglycemia and contractile dysfunction in two mouse models of insulin resistance and obesity. Endocrinology. 2005;146(12):5341–9.
170. Mazumder PK, et al. Impaired cardiac efficiency and increased fatty acid oxidation in insulin-resistant ob/ob mouse hearts. Diabetes. 2004;53(9):2366–74.
171. Boudina S, Abel ED. Mitochondrial uncoupling: a key contributor to reduced cardiac efficiency in diabetes. Physiology (Bethesda). 2006;21:250–8.
172. Boudina S, et al. Reduced mitochondrial oxidative capacity and increased mitochondrial uncoupling impair myocardial energetics in obesity. Circulation. 2005;112(17):2686–95.
173. How OJ, et al. Increased myocardial oxygen consumption reduces cardiac efficiency in diabetic mice. Diabetes. 2006;55(2):466–73.
174. Peterson LR, et al. Impact of gender on the myocardial metabolic response to obesity. J Am Coll Cardiol Imaging. 2008;1:424–33.
175. Peterson LR, et al. Type 2 diabetes, obesity, and sex difference affect the fate of glucose in the human heart. Am J Physiol Heart Circ Physiol. 2015;308(12):H1510–6.
176. Viljanen AP, et al. Effect of caloric restriction on myocardial fatty acid uptake, left ventricular mass, and cardiac work in obese adults. Am J Cardiol. 2009;103(12):1721–6.
177. Lin CH, et al. Myocardial oxygen consumption change predicts left ventricular relaxation improvement in obese humans after weight loss. Obesity (Silver Spring). 2011;19(9):1804–12.
178. Finck BN, et al. The cardiac phenotype induced by PPARalpha overexpression mimics that caused by diabetes mellitus. J Clin Invest. 2002;109(1):121–30.
179. Burkart EM, et al. Nuclear receptors PPARbeta/delta and PPARalpha direct distinct metabolic regulatory programs in the mouse heart. J Clin Invest. 2007;117(12):3930–9.
180. Shoghi KI, et al. Time course of alterations in myocardial glucose utilization in the Zucker diabetic fatty rat with correlation to gene expression of glucose transporters: a small-animal PET investigation. J Nucl Med. 2008;49(8):1320–7.
181. van den Brom CE, et al. Altered myocardial substrate metabolism is associated with myocardial dysfunction in early diabetic cardiomyopathy in rats: studies using positron emission tomography. Cardiovasc Diabetol. 2009;8:39.
182. Thorn SL, et al. Repeatable noninvasive measurement of mouse myocardial glucose uptake with 18F-FDG: evaluation of tracer kinetics in a type 1 diabetes model. J Nucl Med. 2013;54(9):1637–44.
183. Herrero P, et al. PET detection of the impact of dobutamine on myocardial glucose metabolism in women with type 1 diabetes mellitus. J Nucl Cardiol. 2008;15(6):791–9.
184. Peterson LR, et al. Fatty acids and insulin modulate myocardial substrate metabolism in humans with type 1 diabetes. Diabetes. 2008;57(1):32–40.
185. Rijzewijk LJ, et al. Altered myocardial substrate metabolism and decreased diastolic function in nonischemic human diabetic cardiomyopathy: studies with cardiac positron emission tomography and magnetic resonance imaging. J Am Coll Cardiol. 2009;54(16):1524–32.
186. Peterson LR, et al. Sex and type 2 diabetes: obesity-independent effects on left ventricular substrate metabolism and relaxation in humans. Obesity (Silver Spring). 2012;20(4):802–10.
187. Monti LD, et al. Myocardial insulin resistance associated with chronic hypertriglyceridemia and increased FFA levels in type 2 diabetic patients. Am J Physiol Heart Circ Physiol. 2004;287(3):H1225–31.
188. McGill JB, et al. Potentiation of abnormalities in myocardial metabolism with the development of diabetes in women with obesity and insulin resistance. J Nucl Cardiol. 2011;18(3):421–9. quiz 432-3
189. Rijzewijk LJ, et al. Myocardial steatosis is an independent predictor of diastolic dysfunction in type 2 diabetes mellitus. J Am Coll Cardiol. 2008;52(22):1793–9.
190. Rijzewijk LJ, et al. Effects of hepatic triglyceride content on myocardial metabolism in type 2 diabetes. J Am Coll Cardiol. 2010;56(3):225–33.
191. Ng AC, et al. Myocardial steatosis and biventricular strain and strain rate imaging in patients with type 2 diabetes mellitus. Circulation. 2010;122(24):2538–44.
192. MacDonald MR, et al. Discordant short- and long-term outcomes associated with diabetes in patients with heart failure: importance of age and sex: a population study of 5.1 million people in Scotland. Circ Heart Fail. 2008;1(4):234–41.
193. Ho KK, et al. The epidemiology of heart failure: the Framingham study. J Am Coll Cardiol. 1993;22(4 Suppl A):6A–13A.
194. Gu K, Cowie CC, Harris MI. Diabetes and decline in heart disease mortality in US adults. JAMA. 1999;281(14):1291–7.

195. van der Meer RW, et al. Pioglitazone improves cardiac function and alters myocardial substrate metabolism without affecting cardiac triglyceride accumulation and high-energy phosphate metabolism in patients with well-controlled type 2 diabetes mellitus. Circulation. 2009;119(15):2069–77.
196. Hallsten K, et al. Enhancement of insulin-stimulated myocardial glucose uptake in patients with type 2 diabetes treated with rosiglitazone. Diabet Med. 2004;21(12):1280–7.
197. Koellisch U, et al. Investigation of metabolic changes in STZ-induced diabetic rats with hyperpolarized [1-13C]acetate. Physiol Rep. 2015;3(8):e12474.
198. Wilson CR, et al. Western diet, but not high fat diet, causes derangements of fatty acid metabolism and contractile dysfunction in the heart of Wistar rats. Biochem J. 2007;406(3):457–67.
199. Qin F, et al. The polyphenols resveratrol and S17834 prevent the structural and functional sequelae of diet-induced metabolic heart disease in mice. Circulation. 2012;125(14):1757–64. S1-6
200. Vasanji Z, et al. Alterations in cardiac contractile performance and sarcoplasmic reticulum function in sucrose-fed rats is associated with insulin resistance. Am J Physiol Cell Physiol. 2006;291(4):C772–80.
201. Crewe C, Kinter M, Szweda LI. Rapid inhibition of pyruvate dehydrogenase: an initiating event in high dietary fat-induced loss of metabolic flexibility in the heart. PLoS One. 2013;8(10):e77280.
202. Seymour AM, et al. In vivo assessment of cardiac metabolism and function in the abdominal aortic banding model of compensated cardiac hypertrophy. Cardiovasc Res. 2015;106(2):249–60.
203. Mankoff DA, et al. Molecular imaging research in the outcomes era: measuring outcomes for individualized cancer therapy. Acad Radiol. 2007;14(4):398–405.
204. McShane LM, Hayes DF. Publication of tumor marker research results: the necessity for complete and transparent reporting. J Clin Oncol. 2012;30(34):4223–32.
205. Henry NL, Hayes DF. Cancer biomarkers. Mol Oncol. 2012;6(2):140–6.

12 Other Metabolic Syndromes

Matthew T. Whitehead and Andrea L. Gropman

12.1 Introduction

Most inborn errors of metabolism (IEMs) have neurological symptoms, and many cause injury to the developing central nervous system (CNS). Diagnosis can be challenging, as a number of these neurometabolic disease processes manifest similar signs and symptoms. Disorders may present with acute encephalopathy and metabolic crisis; these are the most critical to recognize and prevent as the risk for repeated, intermittent, or ongoing injury is significant. On the other hand, some IEMS can cause progressive injury resulting in chronic encephalopathy and may be amenable to lifelong therapies.

While the etiologies of neurologic injury in the IEMs have not been fully established in many disorders, they may share common mechanisms of injury such as disrupted astrocyte function, excitotoxic cell damage, neuroinflammation, and energy failure. For many of the IEMs, there is a specific anatomical pattern of vulnerability, despite the entire brain being subject to the global metabolic insult. Selectivity for particular brain regions or even cell types based on morphology or neurotransmitter systems (astrocytes or neurons: glutamatergic and gamma-aminobutyric acid [GABA]-ergic) in IEMS is poorly understood.

Neuroimaging offers the ability to study the brain in a noninvasive manner and holds potential to improve diagnostic specificity. In addition to conventional MRI, several imaging platforms exist to evaluate differing aspects of disease including fMRI to study neural networks underlying cognitive processes, diffusion imaging, and diffusion tensor imaging (DTI) to study white matter or myelin microstructure, and spectroscopy (most commonly 1H, but also 31P and 13C) to study cerebral metabolism in vivo, providing tools to evaluate the extent and potential mechanisms of neurological damage. In any disease, there may be a number of imaging biomarkers that can serve as a measure of disease burden and may guide therapy. However, these advanced imaging techniques have yet to be employed universally in routine clinical practice.

From an imaging perspective, neurometabolic disorders affect the brain in various overlapping locations, degrees, and patterns. Many factors ultimately contribute to the final imaging appearance, including but not limited to genotype, phenotype, disease severity, duration, and comorbidities. Brain imaging may be variable,

M.T. Whitehead
Children's National Health System,
Washington, DC, USA
e-mail: mwhitehe@childrensnational.org

A.L. Gropman (✉)
The George Washington University School of Medicine, Washington, DC, USA
e-mail: agropman@childrensnational.org

J.S. Lewis, K.R. Keshari (eds.), *Imaging and Metabolism*, DOI 10.1007/978-3-319-61401-4_12

ranging from normal to severe diffuse brain disease. Shared features suggesting a metabolic brain disorder include symmetric brain involvement (abnormal density on CT, signal on MRI, and/or echogenicity on ultrasound) disrespecting arterial territories, and/or progressive atrophy. Lesions in multiple stages of temporal evolution reflecting multiphasic brain involvement are strong imaging signs of an IEM. While many neurometabolic diseases have a nonspecific appearance, especially in early and late phases, some have patterns that are more suggestive and even diagnostic in some circumstances [1–6].

A common approach is to classify the disorders by the presenting neurologic features that predominantly reflect either gray or white matter involvement, recognizing that many IEMs show elements of damage in both. Though the ultimate goal is accurate genotype-phenotype identification, this is not often achievable because the final imaging phenotype may be caused by several different genetic defects and different phenotypes can be caused by a common gene defect [3, 7].

Patients with cortical gray matter involvement may present with seizures, encephalopathy, or dementia, whereas deep gray matter injury may result in extrapyramidal movement disorders (dystonia, chorea, or athetosis). White matter disorders present with pyramidal signs (spasticity or hyperreflexia) and visual findings. Involvement of the cerebellum or its connecting tracts may lead to imbalance (ataxia or dysmetria), and involvement of tracts from basal ganglia or lesions to the nuclei (caudate, putamen, globus pallidus) may unmask movement disorders (dystonia, chorea, athetosis, hyperkinesias, or bradykinesias).

Patterns of brain injury in various IEMs may also be explained based on metabolic models of toxicity. For example, some IEMs lead to brain injury due to a substrate intoxication model of injury. This pattern is most characteristic of the aminoacidopathies, organic acidurias, urea cycle disorders (UCDs), carbohydrate intolerances, disorders of metal, and porphyrias. There is usually an acute, explosive clinical onset that can present at any stage of life from the neonatal period to adulthood (but is more common in the newborn period) or can be intermittent in a partial form, from infancy to late adulthood. Most of these disorders are treatable by dietary restriction and bulk dialysis by emergency removal of the neurotoxin or by scavenging drugs or vitamins serving as cofactors for enzymes [8].

The second major category of brain injury in IEMs is attributable to substrate-depletion model of injury, such as observed in creatine deficiencies. These disorders affect the cytoplasmic and mitochondrial energetic processes. In addition to creatine deficiencies, this group also includes disorders of glycolysis, glycogenesis, gluconeogenesis, hyperinsulinisms, and creatine and pentose phosphate pathways [9].

In some disorders, brain injury results from both toxicity and depletion. Additionally, anatomical patterns of brain injury may be discerned based on location. Although the entire brain is exposed to the insult, there are typically areas of increased vulnerability. The insult may be focal or diffuse having a predilection for neurons and an impact the gray matter versus the white matter. Additionally, gray matter injury may be cortical only, involve cortical and deep structures, or alternatively involve only the deep gray structures such as the thalamus and basal ganglia. Small molecule disorders and lysosomal disorders have a predilection for white matter involvement, but the location within the white matter often differs based on the individual disorder and may be restricted to deep centrum semiovale white matter, periventricular white matter, and/or the subcortical U-fibers.

This review will focus on some of the more commonly encountered neurometabolic disorders within these categories that have specific imaging features, organized by age of onset. Disorders that may present across the life span will be included in a separate category.

12.2 Neonatal-Onset Metabolic Disease

12.2.1 Acute Toxicity: Aminoacidopathies, Organic Acidemias, and Urea Cycle Disorders

12.2.1.1 Aminoacidopathies

Maple Syrup Urine Disease (MSUD)

MSUD is an autosomal recessive disorder caused by deficiency in a subunit of the branched-chain alpha-keto acid dehydrogenase complex [3, 10]. This enzyme complex is required for the oxidative decarboxylation of branched-chain keto acids. MSUD may present acutely in the newborn period and is a progressive disorder. Patients have the odor of maple syrup in the urine and cerumen even during health. Elevation of several plasma amino acids define this condition, specifically the branched-chain amino acids isoleucine, leucine, and valine. Studies suggest that leucine is the neurotoxic amino acid responsible for neural injury in this condition. MSUD is a rare condition in Caucasians, with an incidence of 1:185,000–1:290,000; however, it is much more common in Mennonites where it is 1:176 due to a common founder effect.

During the acute stages of MSUD, there is plasma accumulation of branched-chain amino acids. Why should the branched-chain keto acid accumulation exert brain toxicity? This question has been studied in cell culture models as a surrogate for MSUD. Results strongly indicate that oxidative stress might be involved in the cell morphological alterations and death, as well as in the cytoskeletal reorganization elicited by the branched-chain keto acids [11]. Additionally, alpha-ketoisocaproic acid derived from leucine is known to be neurotoxic, leading to acute brain edema which if untreated may lead to coma and death (by herniation) [12].

MSUD: Imaging

MR imaging demonstrates symmetric swelling, edema, decreased anisotropy, and markedly reduced diffusion reflecting intramyelinic edema predominantly in myelinating/myelinated areas including the perirolandic parenchyma, projectional fibers, optic radiations, thalami, globi pallidi, brainstem, dentate nuclei, and cerebellar white matter [3, 13–23] (Fig. 12.1). Vasogenic edema manifesting T2 prolongation and facilitated diffusion is present in nonmyelinated brain white matter. Water is pulled from the vascular and extracellular space into the intracellular spaces of the brain by intracellular metabolites with osmotic activity. This is similar to the mechanism of neural injury and edema in several of the urea cycle disorders including ornithine transcarbamylase deficiency (OTCD). To balance this osmotic effect, myoinositol (mI), an osmolyte, is depleted from the brain in both conditions. The imaging findings can predate symptoms [15, 17]. Over time with adequate treatment, diffusion reduction is reversible, but atrophy may develop if symptoms are severe and/or prolonged [13, 15, 20, 23].

MR spectroscopy is useful for diagnosis and monitoring of disease activity [3, 15, 24, 25]. It demonstrates a dominant metabolic peak or peaks at 0.9–1.1 ppm corresponding to elevated branched-chain amino acids (BCAA) and branched-chain alpha-keto acids (BCKA) as well as a lactate peak at 1.3 ppm in metabolic crises [15] (Fig. 12.1). The BCAA-/BCKA-associated 0.9 ppm metabolic peak differs from the normal macromolecular peak that co-resonates here by magnitude; the BCAA/BCKA peak is larger and, unlike normal macromolecules, remains visible on long TE spectra (288 ppm) [3] (Fig. 12.1). Furthermore, these amino and keto acid peak(s) can invert on intermediate echo time MRS due to J-coupling, similar to lactate (Fig. 12.1). The height of the BCAA/BCKA peak diminishes in patients under metabolic control on follow-up MRS though may or may not entirely resolve [3, 15, 24, 25].

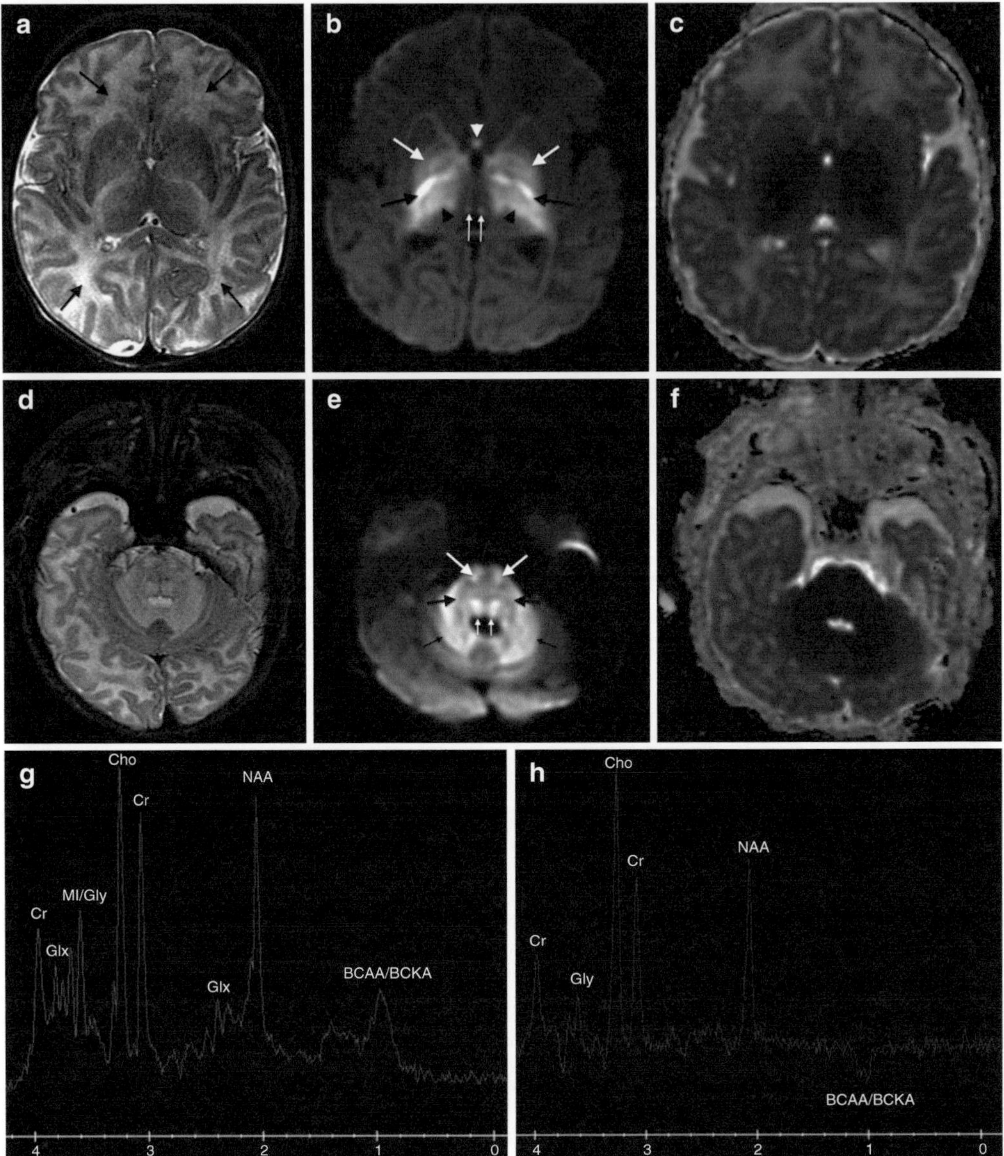

Fig. 12.1 12-day-old male with maple syrup urine disease. Axial T2WI (TR/TE ms, 3500/120) (**a**), axial diffusion-weighted image (DWI) (TR/TE ms, 8000/85) (**b**), and axial apparent diffusion coefficient map (ADC) (TR/TE ms, 8000/85) (**c**) through the basal ganglia demonstrate diffuse excessive hyperintense white matter signal consistent with vasogenic edema in nonmyelinated areas (**a**, *arrows*) and markedly reduced diffusion in myelinated/myelinating brain regions manifested by bright signal on DWI (**b**) and dark signal on ADC (**c**) in the internal capsules (*black arrows*), globi pallidi (*large white arrows*), thalami (*black arrowhead*), fornices (*white arrowhead*), and habenula (*small white arrows*), compatible with intramyelinic edema. Axial T2WI (**d**), DWI (**e**), and ADC (**f**) at the mid-pontine level show similar signal changes throughout the brainstem consistent with mixed vasogenic and intramyelinic edema involving the corticospinal tracts (*large white arrows*), pontine tegmental projectional fibers (*small white arrows*), transverse pontine/middle cerebellar peduncle fibers (*large black arrows*), and cerebellar white matter (*small black arrows*, **d–f**). The brain is diffusely swollen with diffusely small sulci and ventricles (**a–f**). Short echo time (TR/TE ms, 1500/35) (**g**) and intermediate echo time (TR/TE ms, 1500/144) (**h**) single-voxel MR spectroscopy over the left basal ganglia reveal branched-chain amino acids (BCAA) and branched-chain keto acids (BCKA) centered at 1 ppm shown as a positively reflected peak on short echo MRS (**g**) and inverted at 144 ms echo time (**h**). The choline (Cho) to creatine (Cr) ratio is mildly decreased. N-acetylacetate (NAA) and glutamine/glutamate (Glx) are within normal range. Glycine (gly), which co-resonates with myoinositol (MI) at 3.6 ppm, is mildly elevated

Nonketotic Hyperglycinemia (NKH)

Nonketotic hyperglycinemia is an autosomal recessive disease causing a glycine cleavage defect [4]. Glycine overabundance causes hyperexcitation in the brain and neural inhibition in the spinal cord. There are several different forms of glycine encephalopathy, which are characterized by the age of onset and severity of symptoms [26]. All forms present with exclusively neurological symptoms, including intellectual impairment, hypotonia, apneic seizures, and/or symptoms associated with cortical malformations.

The classical or neonatal presentation of glycine encephalopathy is the best described and is typified by an infant born after an unremarkable pregnancy but presents soon after with lethargy, hypotonia, apneic seizures, and myoclonic jerks, which can progress to the need for mechanical ventilation and often death. Apneic patients can regain spontaneous respiration in their second to third week of life but are left with intractable seizures and profound mental retardation. The phenomenon of fetal rhythmic "hiccuping" episodes during pregnancy, most likely reflecting seizure episodes in utero, has been described. Glycine encephalopathy can also present as a milder form with episodic seizures, ataxia, movement disorders, and gaze palsy during febrile illness. In the later-onset form, patients typically have normal intellectual function but present with spastic diplegia and optic atrophy.

NKH: Imaging

Neonatal presentations of NKH and MSUD share several imaging features. Both demonstrate symmetric T2 prolongation and restricted diffusion involving myelinating or myelinated cerebral, cerebellar, and brainstem parenchyma representing intramyelinic edema [27–31] (Fig. 12.2). However, signal alteration tends to be less extensive and severe in NKH and without overt swelling [27]. Excessive deep cerebral white matter hyperintensity on T2WI and absent T1 shortening in the posterior limb of the internal capsule in term neonates with NKH could reflect myelination delay [4, 28, 29] and/or gliosis [32] (Fig. 12.2). Unlike MSUD, structural brain defects may be present in patients with NKH including dysgenesis or hypogenesis of the corpus callosum [3, 4, 27, 28, 30, 33], malformations of cerebral cortical development [33], and cerebellar hypoplasia [33] (Fig. 12.2). MRS is confirmative, demonstrating glycine elevation at 3.6 ppm using intermediate or long echo times [27–29, 34] (Fig. 12.2).

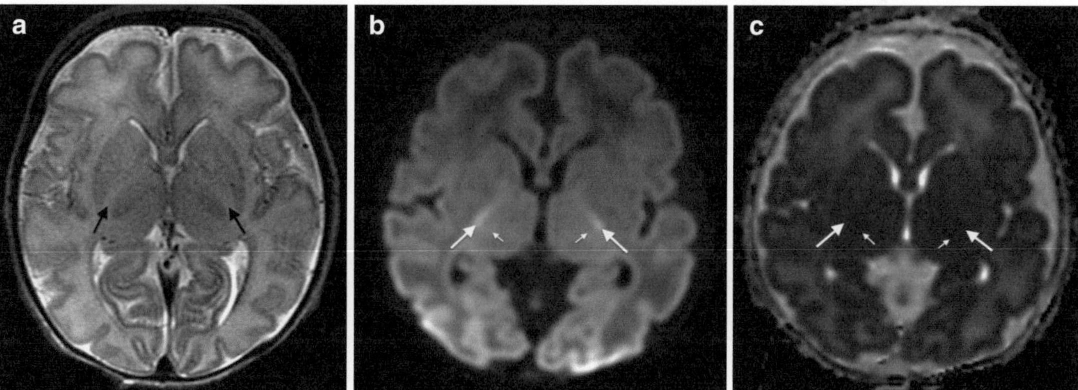

Fig. 12.2 4-day-old female with nonketotic hyperglycinemia. Axial T2WI (TR/TE ms, 3500/120) (**a**), axial diffusion-weighted image (DWI) (TR/TE ms, 8000/85) (**b**), and axial apparent diffusion coefficient map (ADC) (TR/TE ms, 8000/85) (**c**) through the basal ganglia demonstrate delayed myelination with lack of hypointense signal in the posterior limb of the internal capsule (PLIC) (*arrows*, **a**) and reduced diffusion in the PLIC (*large arrows*, **b** and **c**) and lateral thalami (*small arrows*, **b** and **c**). Axial T2WI (**d**), DWI (**e**), and ADC (**f**) at the midpontine level show reduced diffusion in several myelinated brainstem tracts in the dorsal tegmentum (*large white arrows*), central tegmental tracts (*small white arrows*), and dentate nuclei (*black arrows*). Sagittal spoiled gradient echo (SPGR) T1WI (TR/TE/IT ms, 7/2/700) (**g**) demonstrates a thin, mildly shortened corpus callosum consistent with hypogenesis (*arrow*). The vermis is also hypoplastic. Intermediate echo time (TR/TE ms, 1500/144) (**h**) single-voxel MR spectroscopy over the left basal ganglia reveals an abnormal peak at 3.6 ppm compatible with glycine. The choline (Cho) to creatine (Cr) ratio and N-acetylacetate (NAA) to Cr ratios are normal

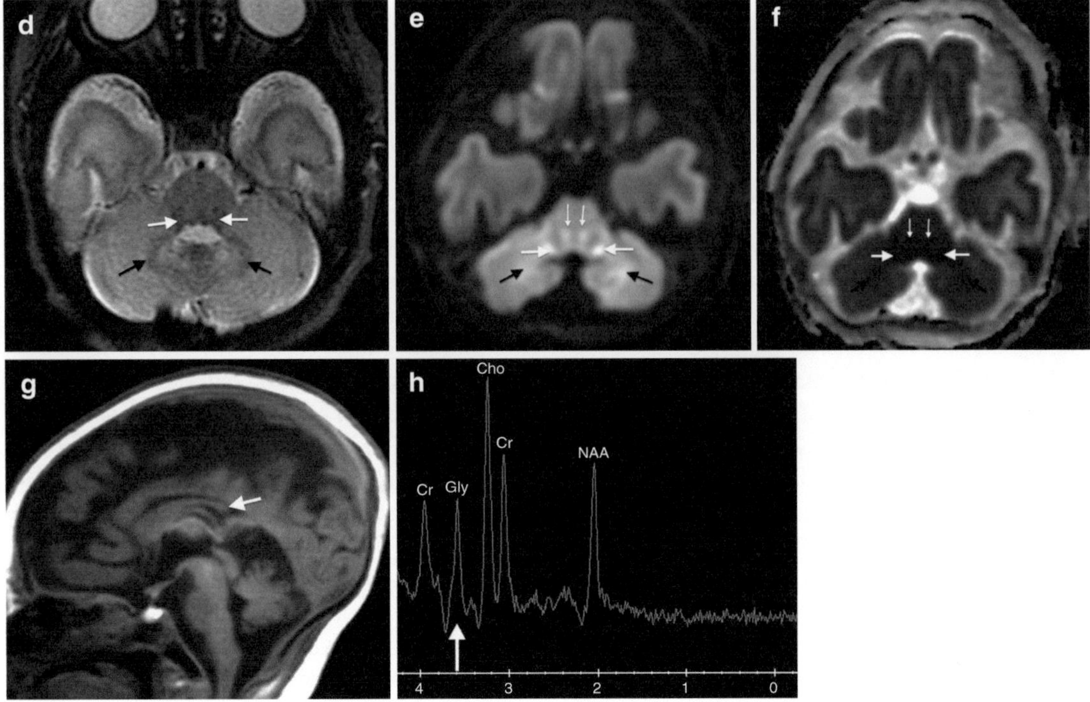

Fig. 12.2 (continued)

12.2.1.2 Organic Acidemias

Methylmalonic Acidemia (MMA)

MMA is a heterogeneous group of disorders characterized by accumulation and toxicity of methylmalonic acid and its by-products in biological fluids. The primary defect is due to intracellular cobalamin metabolism (coenzyme deficiency). MMA exhibits autosomal recessive inheritance. The approximate frequency for MMA is 1 per 48,000 infants. The main enzyme deficiency is due to deficiency of the adenosylcobalamin-dependent enzyme methylmalonyl-CoA mutase (apoenzyme deficiency) [3, 35–39]. A subset of children with defects of intracellular cobalamin metabolism also may have simultaneous homocystinuria. Based on complementation studies, there are eight different complementation groups (mut0, mut-, cblA, cblB, cblC, cblD, cblF, and cblH) causing MMA [40]. The most severe is mut0 showing undetectable mutase activity fibroblasts [40].

MMA typically presents in the newborn period after the first few days of life. The typical history is the newborn that was healthy for the first days to weeks of life (mut0 or MMA mut-) progresses to poor feeding, vomiting, progressive lethargy, floppiness, and hypotonia. In later onset, older children with one of the other forms of MMA or mild mut- may present after illness or stress with lethargy, seizures, and hypoglycemia. Metabolic changes include methylmalonic acid, methylcitrate, propionic acid, and 3-OH propionic acid in the urine, and plasma amino acids typically show elevation of glycine but may be normal. Acylcarnitine profile (dry blood spot or plasma) shows an elevation of propionylcarnitine (C3) and may show decreased free carnitine and total carnitine levels.

MMA: Imaging

Acute brain lesions manifest with hyperintensity on T2-weighted sequences and restricted diffusion during times of metabolic decompensation

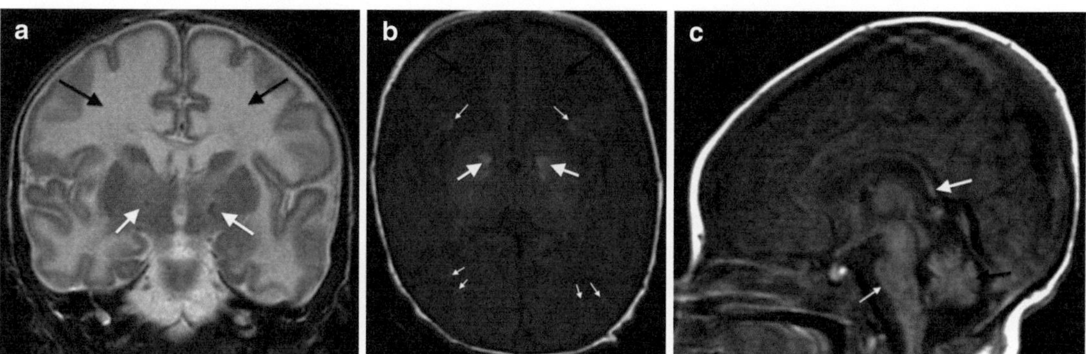

Fig. 12.3 25-day-old male with methylmalonic academia. Coronal T2WI (TR/TE ms, 3000/104) (**a**), axial T1WI (TR/TE ms, 500/14) (**b**), and sagittal T1WI (TR/TE ms, 467/14) (**c**). The cerebral white matter is diffusely hyperintense for age (*black arrows*, **a**). The globi pallidi are abnormally bright on T1WI and T2WI (*white arrows*, **a** and **b**), consistent with prior metabolic injury/infarctions. The cerebral cortex is also hyperintense in some areas on T1WI, representing laminar necrosis from prior metabolic injury (*small arrows*, **b**). The corpus callosum is thin, reflecting cerebral white matter volume loss or hypoplasia (*large white arrow*, **c**). The brainstem (*small white arrow*, **c**) and vermis (*black arrow*, **c**) are also mildly small, consistent with hypoplasia and/or volume loss

(Fig. 12.3). Basal ganglia lesions called "metabolic infarctions" may develop over time, especially or exclusively involving the globi pallidi, often in an asymmetric fashion and rarely isolated unilaterally [3, 36–39, 41–44] (Fig. 12.3). In a recent survey of 40 patients, 19 were noted to have GP infarcts [36]. Globus pallidus infarct prevalence by methylmalonic acidemia class revealed the following pattern: cblA (71%), cblB (43%), mut(o) (45%), and mut- (25%). Tiny lacunar infarcts in the pars reticulata of the substantia nigra, previously unrecognized in methylmalonic acidemia, were found in 17 patients, 13 of whom also had a globus pallidus infarctions [36]. Movement disorders, such as chorea and tremor, were common ($n = 31$, 83%), even among patients without evidence of basal ganglia injury [36]. In severe cases of methylmalonic acidemia, the globi pallidi can be damaged to the point of necrosis, appearing cystic on MRI images (hyperintense on T2WI and hypointense on T2 FLAIR sequences) [3]. In chronic stages, basal ganglia calcifications can develop in the lentiform nucleus [3, 35].

The differential diagnosis for hyperintense globi pallidi lesions on T2WI includes other organic acidemias (often with striatal lesions), mitochondrial diseases, profound hypoxic-ischemic injury, hypoglycemia, osmotic demyelination (generally other areas of the basal ganglia and thalami are also affected), post-viral injury, vitamin B12 (cobalamin) deficiency, Vigabatrin, and toxins such as carbon monoxide, methanol, and cyanide [37, 38, 42, 45, 46].

In addition to globi pallidi abnormalities, dentate nuclear injury may be present in patients with methylmalonic academia [3]. Delayed brain maturation (delayed myelination and immature gyral pattern), white matter signal changes, and progressive brain volume loss are also characteristic [3, 35, 44, 47] (Fig. 12.3). Occasionally, one also sees demyelination of corticospinal tracts in a pattern that resembles B12 deficiency of combined systems degeneration. Gao and colleagues found that for patients with negative MRI findings, compared with healthy infants, a statistically significant reduction in DTI FA value of the frontal, temporal, and occipital white matter was observed, thus contending that DTI is a useful tool for clinical monitoring [48].

MR spectroscopy may demonstrate elevated lactate and/or decreased NAA in active disease states that may normalize with resolution of symptoms [3, 49, 50].

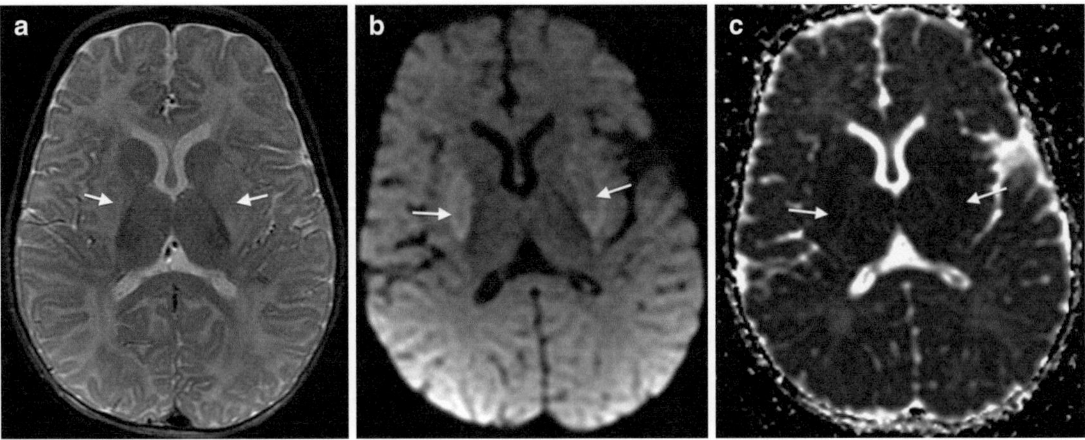

Fig. 12.4 5-month-old male with propionic academia. Axial T2WI (TR/TE ms, 3200/90) (**a**), DWI (TR/TE ms, 10,000/97) (**b**), and ADC (TR/TE ms, 10,000/97) (**c**) through the basal ganglia. Putamen are abnormally hyperintense on T2WI (*arrows*, **a**) and demonstrate restricted diffusion (*arrows*, **b** and **c**), consistent with ongoing metabolic injury

Propionic Academia (PA)

Propionic academia is an autosomal recessive inborn metabolic error caused by a propionyl-CoA carboxylase gene defect [3, 44]. Propionic acid toxicity damages brain structures, similar to MMA. Although both disorders commonly affect the basal ganglia, the striatum is preferentially involved in PMA, whereas the globi pallidi are more commonly involved in isolation in MMA [3, 44, 51] (Fig. 12.4). Delayed myelination, periventricular white matter signal changes, and progressive brain volume loss are also characteristic [3, 44]. Basal ganglia MRS may show altered glutamine/glutamate levels (increased or decreased) and decreased myoinositol and NAA levels [3, 51].

Glutaric Aciduria Type I

Autosomal recessively inherited defects involving the mitochondrial enzyme glutaryl-CoA dehydrogenase (GCDH) are responsible for glutaric aciduria type I [3, 52, 53]. Toxic metabolites are believed to overstimulate NMDA receptors, causing cellular injury. GCDH deficiency leads to accumulation of glutaric acid (GA) and 3-hydroxyglutaric acid (3-OHGA), two metabolites that are believed to be neurotoxic. Patients typically present clinically during a catabolic state such as an intercurrent illness with an acute encephalopathic crisis that results in striatal necrosis and in a permanent dystonic-dyskinetic movement disorder. The results of various in vitro and in vivo assays suggest three main mechanisms involved in the metabolite-mediated neuronal damage: excitotoxicity, impairment of energy metabolism, and oxidative stress. The metabolites are thought to be produced endogenously in the CNS and accumulate because of limiting transport mechanisms across the blood-brain barrier.

Glutaric Aciduria Type I: Imaging

Neuroimaging plays an important role in diagnosis because both structural brain defects and signal changes are common. Basal ganglia and/or cerebral white matter and corpus callosum may be involved with T2 prolongation and diffusion abnormalities [3, 52–54] (Fig. 12.5). Reduced diffusion appears in the acute phase and may improve with symptom control but can persist in asymptomatic patients [54–56]. Characteristic structural changes occur in almost all patients and include under-opercularization of the sylvian fissures, enlarged temporopolar extra-axial spaces, and macrencephaly, often preceding brain signal alterations [3, 53] (Fig. 12.5). In fact, if these temporo-insular changes are encountered in a patient with macrocephaly, the diagnosis is highly suggestive. If the basal ganglia are also involved, findings are nearly pathognomonic for glutaric aciduria type I [53]. Structural brain abnormalities may even be

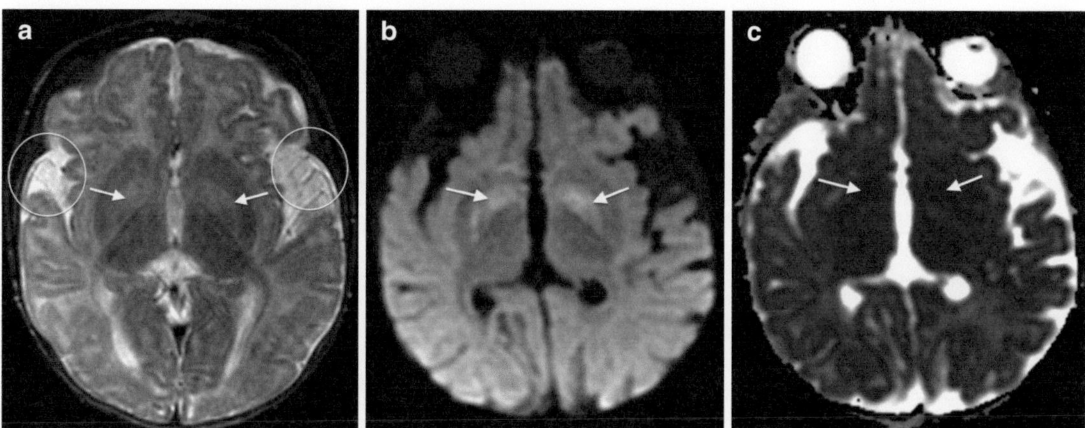

Fig. 12.5 5-month-old male with glutaric aciduria type I. Axial T2WI (TR/TE ms, 3100/90) (**a**), DWI (TR/TE ms, 10,000/84) (**b**), and ADC (TR/TE ms, 10,000/84) (**c**) through the basal ganglia. Globi pallidi are abnormally hyperintense on T2WI (*arrows*, **a**) and demonstrate restricted diffusion (*arrows*, **b** and **c**), consistent with ongoing metabolic injury. The temporal lobes are under-developed, the lateral sulci are broadened, and the insula are uncovered consistent with under-opercularization (*circles*, **a**), hallmarks of glutaric aciduria

detected on fetal MRI [3, 57]. Other findings include delayed myelination and signal abnormalities involving the cerebellar gray nuclei, central tegmental tracts, and midbrain [3, 58]. Progressive atrophy is typical, and subdural hemorrhages are not uncommon and may even be the presenting symptom on occasion [3, 44, 59].

MR spectroscopy may demonstrate lactate elevation and decreased NAA [3, 55, 60]. Choline and myoinositol levels may also be elevated [3]. Recent advances have allowed for direct identification of toxic metabolites glutaric acid and 3-hydroxyglutaric acid making follow-up monitoring with MRS more feasible [61].

12.2.1.3 Urea Cycle Disorders

Urea cycle disorders represent a group of rare inborn errors of metabolism that lead to accumulation of ammonia, a toxic product of protein metabolism. Individuals with urea cycle disorders cannot metabolize the ammonia that accumulates due to enzyme deficiency. The symptoms of these disorders may present at birth, childhood, or adulthood (milder deficiencies). Acute hyperammonemic (HA) coma in patients with proximal urea cycle disorders (UCD) such as ornithine transcarbamylase deficiency (OTCD) often results in cognitive impairment. Many of these patients also manifest chronic, albeit intermittent, elevations of plasma ammonia and glutamine (Gln) even while on dietary therapy and alternate pathway drugs.

While HA can lead to severe consequences in the CNS, the pathophysiology is unclear. Current theories have focused on (1) Gln accumulation leading to impaired cerebral osmoregulation and (2) glutamate/NMDA receptor activation and excitotoxic injury and energy deficit [62]. Neuropathological changes in UCD are similar to those in hepatic encephalopathy and hypoxic ischemic encephalopathy affecting not only gray matter but also the white matter (WM), reflecting astrocyte damage [62]. The extent of WM injury depends upon the disease severity. Neuropathological findings in patients with UCD demonstrate that late-onset disorders are associated with white matter injury and neonatal disorders show hypomyelination of WM, myelination delay, cystic changes of WM, gliosis of the deep gray matter nuclei, and gray matter heterotopia [63–66].

Urea Cycle Defects: Imaging

The pattern of brain injury in the proximal urea cycle disorders such as OTCD can be fairly specific [67]. Both cerebral gray matter (cortical and basal ganglia) and white matter are involved in neonatal-onset UCDs [64, 67–71]. In the acute phase, MRI demonstrates hyperintense signal on T2WI and proton density images with corresponding restricted diffusion in areas of brain involvement (Fig. 12.6). Later, regional

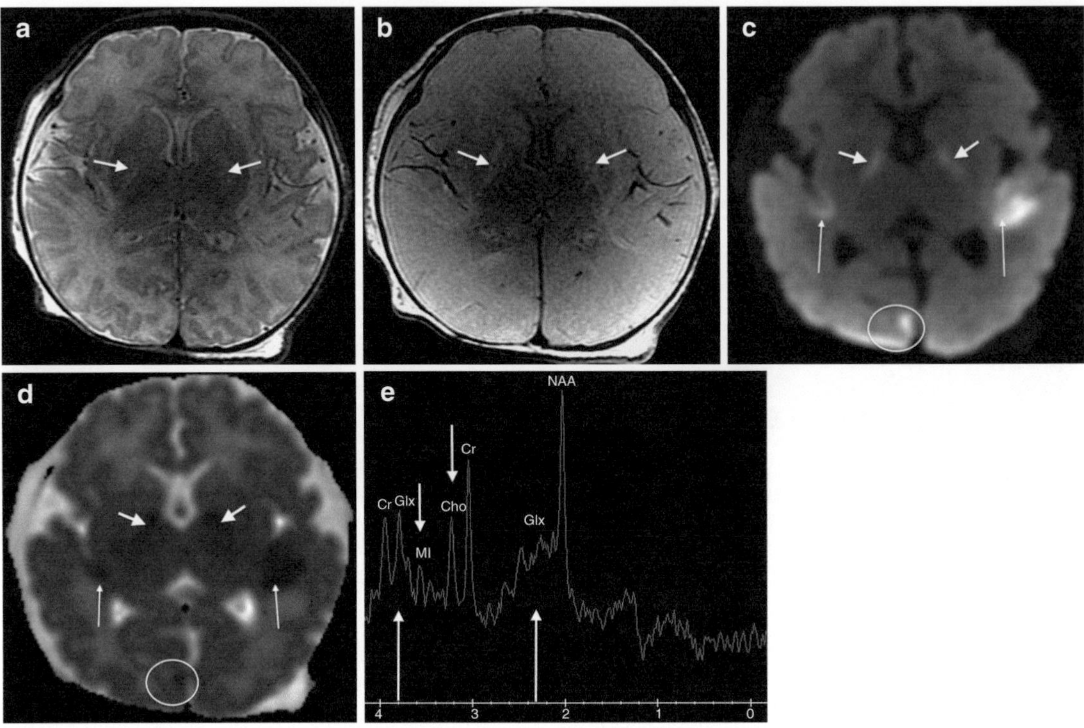

Fig. 12.6 9-day-old male with a urea cycle disorder (ornithine transcarbamylase deficiency). Axial T2WI (TR/TE ms, 3500/90) (**a**), proton density (TR/TE ms, 3500/30) (**b**), DWI (TR/TE ms, 8000/81) (**c**), and ADC (TR/TE ms, 8000/81) (**d**) through the basal ganglia. Collectively, the globi pallidi and PLIC are abnormally hyperintense on proton density and T2WI (*arrows*, **a** and **b**) and demonstrate restricted diffusion (*thick arrows*, **c** and **d**) consistent with ongoing metabolic injury. Cortical/subcortical restricted diffusion compatible with injury is also present in the insular/peri-insular regions (*thin arrows*, **c** and **d**) and right occipital cortex (*circle*, **c** and **d**). The thalami are normal in signal. Single-voxel MRS over the left basal ganglia (TR/TE ms, 1500/35) (**e**) reveals findings typical of urea cycle disorders: elevated glutamine/glutamate (Glx), decreased choline (Cho), and decreased myoinositol (MI). NAA and creatine (Cr) are within normal range

encephalomalacia/laminar necrosis, gliosis, and atrophy may develop depending on the duration and severity of the metabolic derangement. Two distinct general patterns have been described: "diffuse" and "central" [68]. In the diffuse form, a posterior predominant cerebral cortical disease occurs, whereas in the central form, involvement is more localized. Insular/peri-insular parenchyma is often firstly and more profoundly affected (Fig. 12.6). Frontoparietal perirolandic, temporal, and ultimately occipital lobes are then involved in this sequence. Concurrent symmetric cingulate gyri and basal ganglia abnormalities are frequent, often sparing the thalami (Fig. 12.6).

MR spectroscopy offers complementary information for diagnosis and disease monitoring. In metabolically decompensated patients, MRS reveals elevated glutamine/glutamate (2.1–2.4 and 3.8 ppm), decreased myoinositol (3.55 ppm), and decreased choline (3.2 ppm) (Fig. 12.6). Although these metabolites may remain abnormal after recovery, the degrees of spectroscopic alterations typically improve with symptom resolution making MRS a useful tool for temporal disease and therapeutic response monitoring [67, 70]. While MRI and MRS injury pattern partially overlaps with that of hypoxic ischemic encephalopathy, thalamic sparing and insular predilection would be atypical in HIE. Still, HIE is substantially more common; therefore, brain imaging should be interpreted within the context of the patient's clinical presentation.

12.3 Chronic Encephalopathies of Infancy

12.3.1 Aminoacidopathies, Peroxisomal Disorders, Mitochondrial Disorders, Lysosomal Disorders, and Lipidoses

12.3.1.1 Aminoacidopathies

Phenylketonuria (PKU)

PKU was first identified in 1934 by Norwegian physician Asbjørn Følling. Phenylketonuria is an autosomal recessive genetic disorder characterized by deficiency in the phenylalanine hydroxylase enzyme. Phenylalanine hydroxylase is necessary for the metabolism of the amino acid phenylalanine (Phe) to tyrosine (Tyr), an essential precursor for the neurotransmitter, dopamine (DA) that is important in cognitive functions of the frontal cortex. Early-treated phenylketonuria (PKU) is associated with a range of neuropsychological impairments believed to be due to dopamine depletion and white matter pathology. Patients who are diagnosed are placed on a low-Phe/low-protein diet yet despite this may have chronic encephalopathy.

PKU: Imaging

Histopathology and neuroimaging studies in humans have demonstrated extensive white matter damage, in both untreated and early-treated PKU cases. On MRI, high signal intensity is present in the periventricular white matter, often extending into subcortical and frontal regions in more severe cases (Fig. 12.7). White matter pathology in untreated PKU

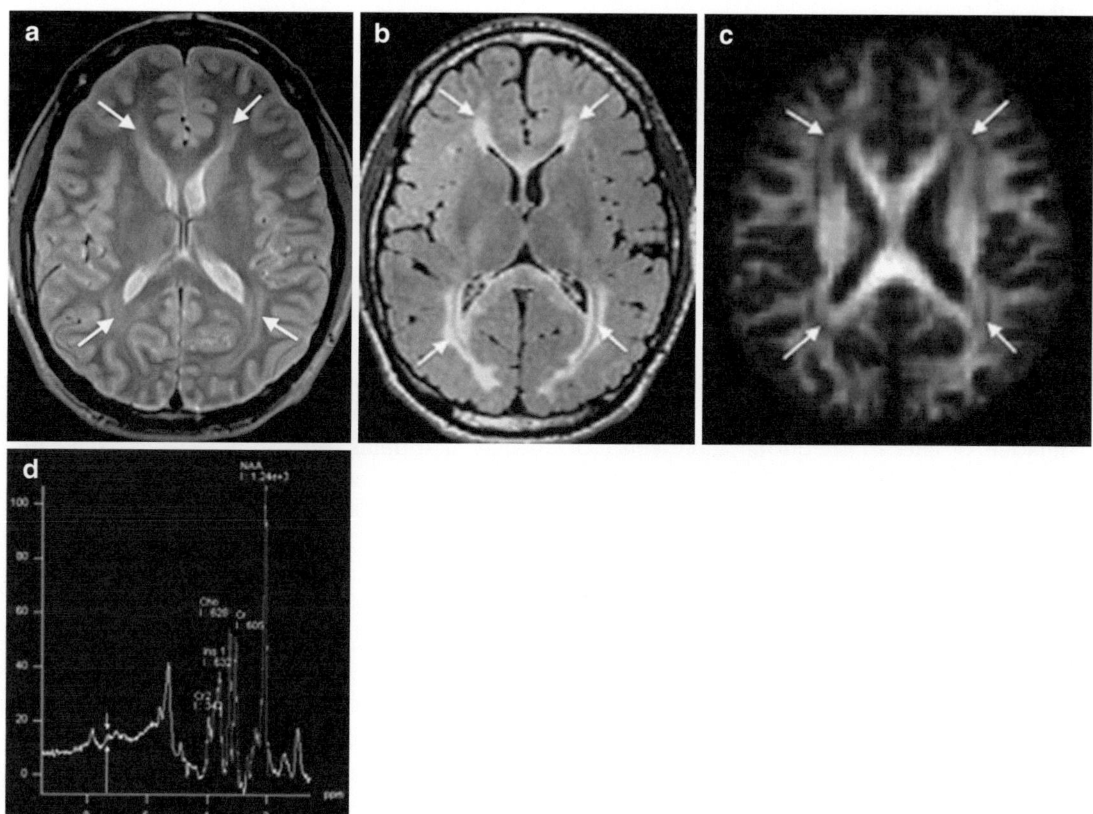

Fig. 12.7 27-year-old male with phenylketonuria (PKU). Axial T2WI (**a**), T2 FLAIR (**b**), and fractional anisotropy (FA) images through the level of the lateral ventricles. There is symmetric hyperintense signal involving the deep and periventricular cerebral white matter (*arrows*, **a** and **b**), with corresponding decreased anisotropy (*arrows*, **c**). Single-voxel MRS through the left parietal white matter (**d**) demonstrates a small phenylalanine peak at 7.37 ppm (*arrows*) in this patient at baseline under good dietary control

patients is likely to reflect hypomyelination, whereas in early-treated patients, white matter abnormalities observed on magnetic resonance imaging (MRI) are believed to be caused by intramyelinic edema. It has been estimated that over 90% of patients show white matter pathology on structural MRI scans and diffusion tensor imaging, and this is true even when T2 MRI appears normal [72–74] (Fig. 12.7). Research demonstrates that this pathology is associated with metabolic control and may be reversed with adherence to a strict low-phenylalanine (Phe) diet [75]. MR spectroscopy can demonstrate elevated phenylalanine (Phe) at 7.37 ppm. Brain Phe concentration has been shown to correlate with clinical, biochemical, and imaging disease [76].

12.3.1.2 Peroxisomal Disorders

Zellweger Syndrome

Zellweger syndrome is the most severe disease in the spectrum of peroxisomal defects and is due to absence of the organelle. Peroxisomes are organelles necessary for normal anabolic and catabolic cellular processes involving very long chain of fats. The major manifestations are in the liver and brain, but there is also a facial dysmorphism and skeletal manifestations that are rather common features. Zellweger presents a clinical and biochemical spectrum which is divided into three clinical phenotypes. Patients can present in the neonatal period with severe symptoms or later in life during adolescence or adulthood with only minor features. Neonates present with hepatic dysfunction and profound hypotonia resulting in prolonged jaundice and feeding difficulties. They also develop epileptic seizures that are usually present in these patients and are noted to have characteristic dysmorphic features. Patients with late onset have a more variable presentation with delayed developmental milestone achievement, retinitis pigmentosa, cataract, and glaucoma as well as deafness. In adolescents and adults, ocular abnormalities and a sensorineural hearing deficit are the most typical symptoms.

Zellweger Syndrome: Imaging

Typical neuroimaging findings include the triad of cerebral polymicrogyria (perirolandic and perisylvian predominant), germinolytic cysts, and diffuse cerebral white matter disease [3, 4, 27, 77, 78] (Fig. 12.8). Other characteristic imaging features include cerebellar white matter disease, cerebellar dysplasia, inferior olivary nucleus dysplasia, and corpus callosum dysgenesis. Fumaric aciduria and congenital muscular dystrophies with brain involvement (dystroglycanopathies) are differential diagnostic considerations on brain MRI [4]. However, these more commonly present with ventriculomegaly and brainstem abnormalities [27, 79].

MRS findings reflect the degree of hepatocellular dysfunction (elevated glutamine and glutamate, decreased myoinositol), decreased neurons and/or neuronal axonal integrity (decreased NAA/Cr), and increased cell membrane turnover (elevated Cho/Cr) [80, 81] (Fig. 12.8). Elevated lactate and lipids can also be detected; the latter may reflect accumulation of lipids or myelin destruction.

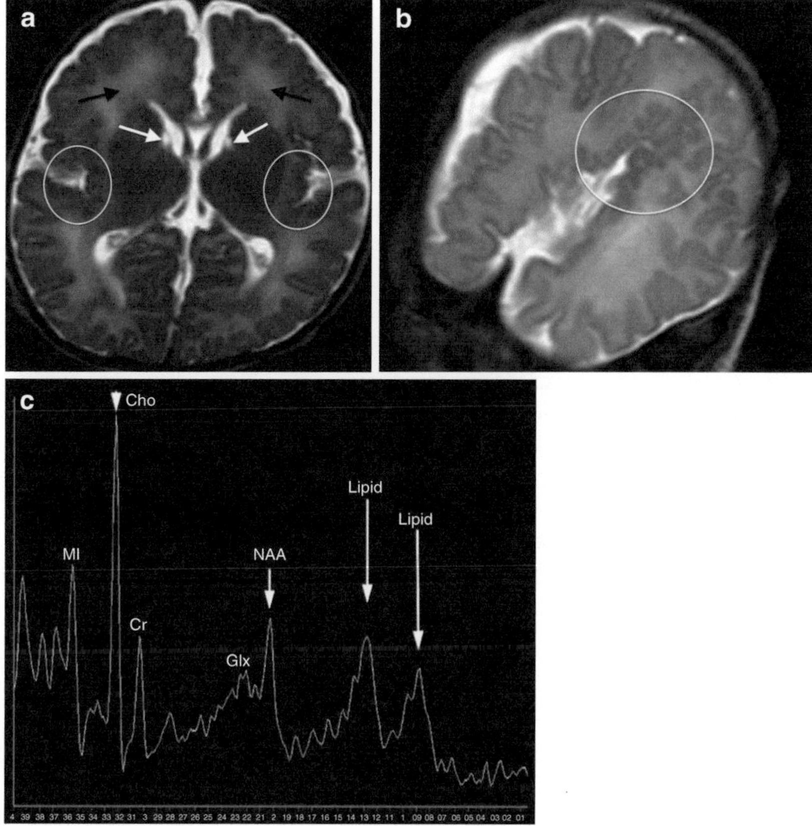

Fig. 12.8 4-day-old male with Zellweger syndrome. Axial (**a**) and sagittal (**b**) T2WI (TR/TE ms 3500/105) demonstrate perisylvian polymicrogyria (*circles*), caudothalamic groove germinolytic cysts (*white arrows*, **a**), and white matter disease with excessive signal for age (*black arrows*, **a**). Single-voxel MRS through the right frontal white matter (TR/TE ms, 1500/35) (**c**) reveals elevated lipids at 0.9 and 1.3 ppm (*long arrows*), increased choline (Cho; *arrowhead*), and decreased NAA (*short arrow*). Glutamine/glutamate (Glx) and myoinositol (MI) are within normal range

X-Linked ALD

X-linked adrenoleukodystrophy (X-ALD) is the most common peroxisomal disorder and is a neurodegenerative disorder involving predominantly white matter tracts. It has been demonstrated neuropathologically that demyelination typically begins in the parietal occipital regions and extends across the corpus callosum before it progresses anteriorly in the classic disease phenotype. Male patients present with symptoms in early childhood often misdiagnosed as ADHD. While ALD being an X-linked disease affects mostly males, some female carriers can have milder forms of the disease [82]. The condition results in the accumulation of VLCFAs in the nervous system, adrenal gland, and testes [82–85]. The three major categories of disease are the childhood cerebral form, appearing in mid-childhood with classic MRI imaging findings; an adrenomyeloneuropathy, occurring in men in their 20s or later; and a third category encompassing impaired adrenal gland function (called Addison's disease or Addison-like phenotype) where the adrenal gland does not produce enough steroid hormones [82–84].

X-Linked ALD: Imaging

The callosal splenium and forceps major are initially involved in most cases, with progression along a posteroanterior and centrifugal gradient [3, 82–84] (Fig. 12.9). Corticospinal tract, visual pathway, and auditory pathway involvement are also typical in the cerebrum and brainstem [3, 82, 86, 87]. Mild to severe cerebellar white matter involvement can also occur. A typical zonal pattern of signal alteration occurs in the involved deep posterior cerebral white matter with central gliosis/necrosis (zone A), an intermediate area of enhancing inflammation/demyelination (zone B), and peripheral demyelination alone (zone C) [3, 88] (Fig. 12.9). Contrast enhancement predicts clinical and MR disease progression [87]. A scoring system for location, extent, and severity of brain involvement has been developed and validated [89]. The Loes MRI score has proven to be a valuable marker for the degree of current and future neurologic impairment [83].

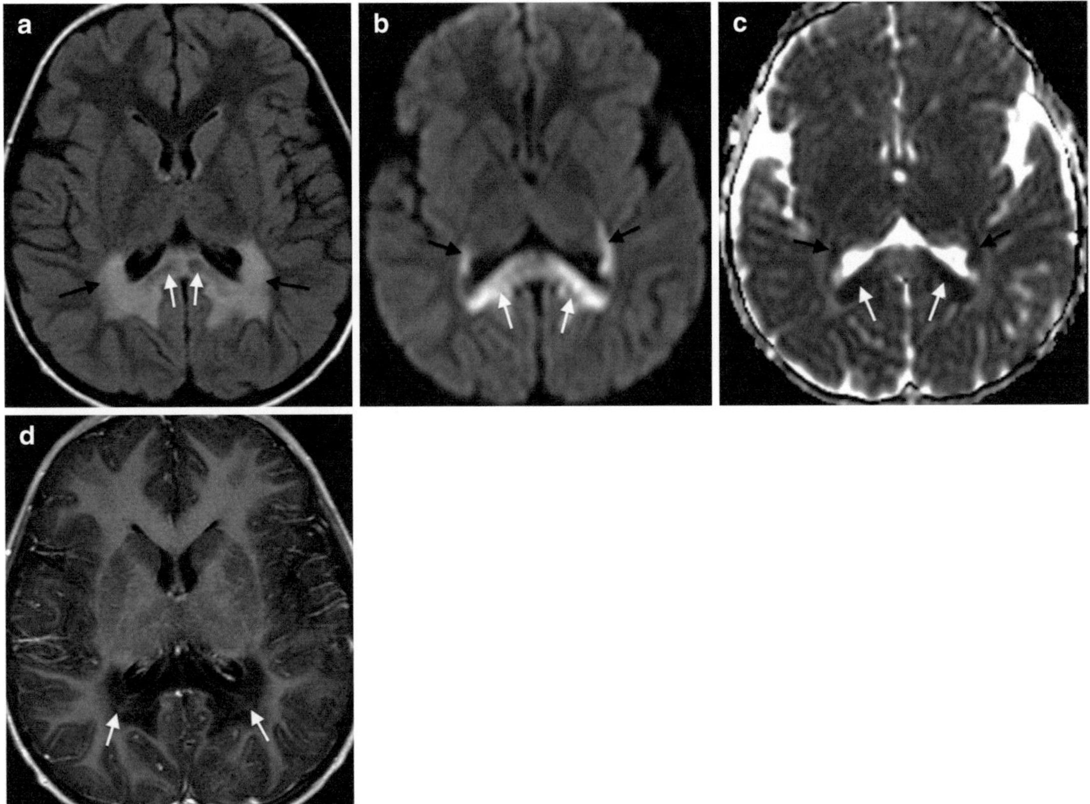

Fig. 12.9 7-year-old male with X-linked adrenoleukodystrophy. Axial T2 FLAIR (TR/TE/IT ms, 8000/120/2250) (**a**), DWI (TR/TE ms, 3566/74) (**b**), ADC (TR/TE ms, 3566/74) (**c**), and post-contrast T1WI (TR/TE ms, 1902/20) (**d**) through the level of the lateral ventricles. The callosal splenium signal is abnormal with mixed hyperintensity and hypointensity (*white arrows*, **a–c**), representing central necrosis/gliosis (zone A) and peripheral demyelination (zone B). Signal abnormality and restricted diffusion extend to involve the forceps major and retrolenticular internal capsules, representing zone C (*black arrows*, **a–c**). There is mild contrast enhancement along the leading edge of inflammation/demyelination reflecting local permeability of the blood-brain barrier in zone B (*arrows*, **d**)

Studies using DTI in X-ALD have shown that fractional anisotropy decreases and ADC increases over zones toward the center of the lesions [90–93]. Abnormalities in diffusion may be even observed in white matter appearing unaffected on routine anatomic MR sequences [93]. Regardless of the imaging modality, the ability to recognize characteristic MRI patterns is crucial in the diagnosis of leukodystrophy. Magnetic resonance spectroscopy (MRS) can be employed for prognostication; NAA/Cho less than 5 predicts deterioration over time [3].

12.3.1.3 Mitochondrial Disorders

The mitochondrial disorders can present across the life span and are due to mutations in either nuclear DNA (nDNA) or mitochondrial DNA (mtDNA). The result is a disruption of oxidative phosphorylation and mitochondrial dysfunction. Mitochondrial disease can be limited to central and peripheral nervous system or be multisystemic. The clinical manifestations will be related to the tissues and organs involved and the disease burden (mtDNA heteroplasmy) in those tissues. The consequences range from manifestations of a single organ or tissues, such as muscle fatigue, if confined only to muscle, seizures, intellectual disabilities, dementia, and stroke (if involving the central nervous system), leading to disability or even early death. The definitive diagnosis of a mitochondrial disorder can be difficult to establish and may depend on clinical history and examination, details of family history, imaging, biochemistry, tissue biopsy (typically muscle), and molecular genetics.

Neuroimaging is useful for the investigation and management of patients with mitochondrial disorders [94–98]. Depending upon which imaging platform is used, clinicians and researchers can evaluate the timing, extent, and potential of reversibility of neural injury. MRS and DTI can additionally serve as noninvasive and repeatable biomarker inquiry [95, 97, 99, 100].

There are several characteristic patterns of brain injury that MRI technologies can identify: focal deep gray nuclear involvement, stokes crossing vascular territories, and white matter changes [95, 96, 101].

12.4 Focal Lesions in Deep Gray Matter Structures

12.4.1 Leigh Disease

Focal, bilateral, symmetric brain lesions involving basal ganglia and periaqueductal gray matter are typical of Leigh syndrome (subacute necrotizing encephalomyelopathy), which can be caused by mutations in either mtDNA or nuclear DNA-encoded mitochondrial proteins [94, 98, 102–109] (Fig. 12.10). Symmetric basal ganglia involvement alone is not specific for Leigh disease; several other congenital and acquired metabolic diseases as well as toxic, demyelinating, ischemic, and infectious processes may result in a similar imaging pattern [46]. Diagnostic criteria for Leigh disease include typical symmetric cerebral and cerebellar deep gray nuclear and/or brainstem lesions in a patient with elevated lactate that exhibits characteristic clinical signs and symptoms [106–109]. Symptoms generally initiate in infancy with brainstem dysfunction leading to abnormal cranial nerve findings, respiration, global delay, and oral motor dysfunction interfering with feeding. Additionally, there are long tract signs leading to spasticity as well as multiple organ involvement. Indeed, concurrent white matter disease is often found on imaging. Lesions in multiple stages of temporal evolution reflecting multiphasic brain involvement can be found. Many brain lesions will evolve to necrosis. Progressive brain atrophy is typical.

Arterial spin labeling (ASL) MR sequence can depict perfusion alteration in brain lesions [110]. Hyperperfusion is seen with acute/active lesions and may relate to small-vessel proliferation and hyperlactic acidemia-induced vasodilation characteristic to Leigh disease [110] (Fig. 12.10).

MR spectroscopy demonstrates elevated lactate at 1.3 ppm, especially in patients imaged during metabolic decompensation [96, 97, 100–102] (Fig. 12.10). Destructive lesions have diminished NAA [97].

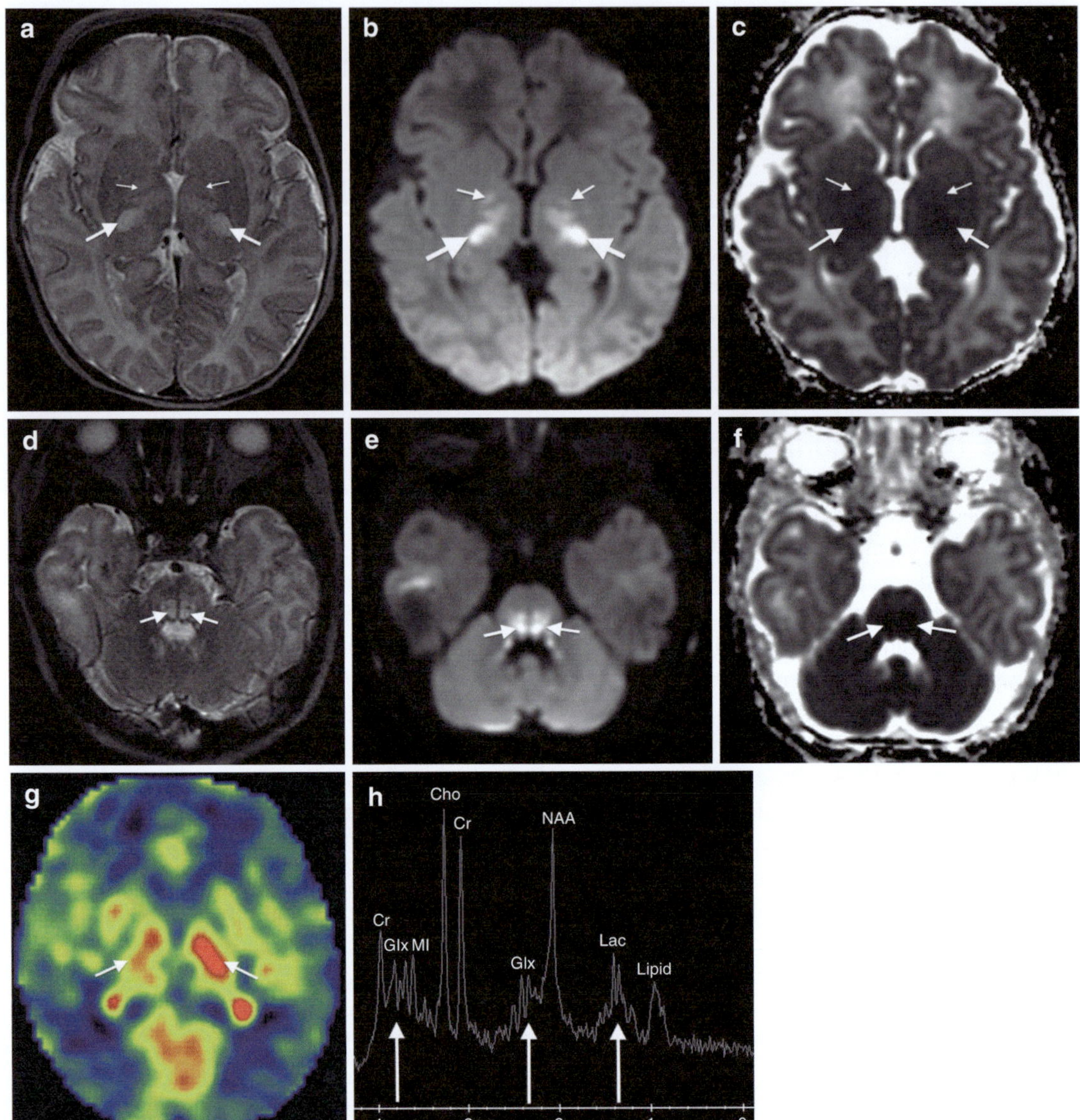

Fig. 12.10 48-day-old female with Leigh disease. Axial T2WI (TR/TE ms, 3500/120) (**a**), DWI (TR/TE ms, 8000/85) (**b**), and ADC (TR/TE ms, 8000/85) (**c**) images through the cerebral deep gray nuclei. T2 prolongation and reduced diffusion are present in the thalami (*large arrows*, **a–c**) and globi pallidi (*small arrows*, **a–c**). Axial T2WI (**d**), DWI (**e**), and ADC (**f**) images through the pons show T2 prolongation, swelling, and reduced diffusion involving multiple white matter tracts in the pontine tegmentum (*arrows*, **d–f**). Arterial spin labeling (ASL) perfusion images (TR/TE/post-label delay ms, 4371/11/1025) (**g**) through the deep gray nuclei show thalamic hyperperfusion (*arrows*). MR spectroscopy over the left basal ganglia (**h**) demonstrates elevated lactate (Lac) consistent with anaerobic metabolism. Glutamine/glutamate (Glx) is elevated, possibly from excitotoxic injury

12.5 Strokes Crossing Vascular Territories

MELAS (mitochondrial encephalomyopathy, lactic acidosis, and stroke-like episodes) is a progressive neurodegenerative disorder associated with migraine-like headaches, refractory partial or generalized seizures, short stature, muscle weakness, exercise intolerance, sensorineural deafness, diabetes, cardiac conduction defects, and slowly progressive dementia due to recurrent strokes [111].

Patients may present with a seizure that heralds a stroke, recurrent strokes, or difficult-to-control epilepsy as major symptoms. Approximately 80% of patients with MELAS have a common mutation (mitochondrial mt 3243 A>G within the $tRNA^{leu}$ transfer RNA (ribonucleic acid), leucine).

Patients with MELAS have a characteristic imaging pattern (Fig. 12.11). In the acute phase, neuroimaging patterns are reflective of symptomatology. The imaging correlates of seizures and stroke-like episodes are readily

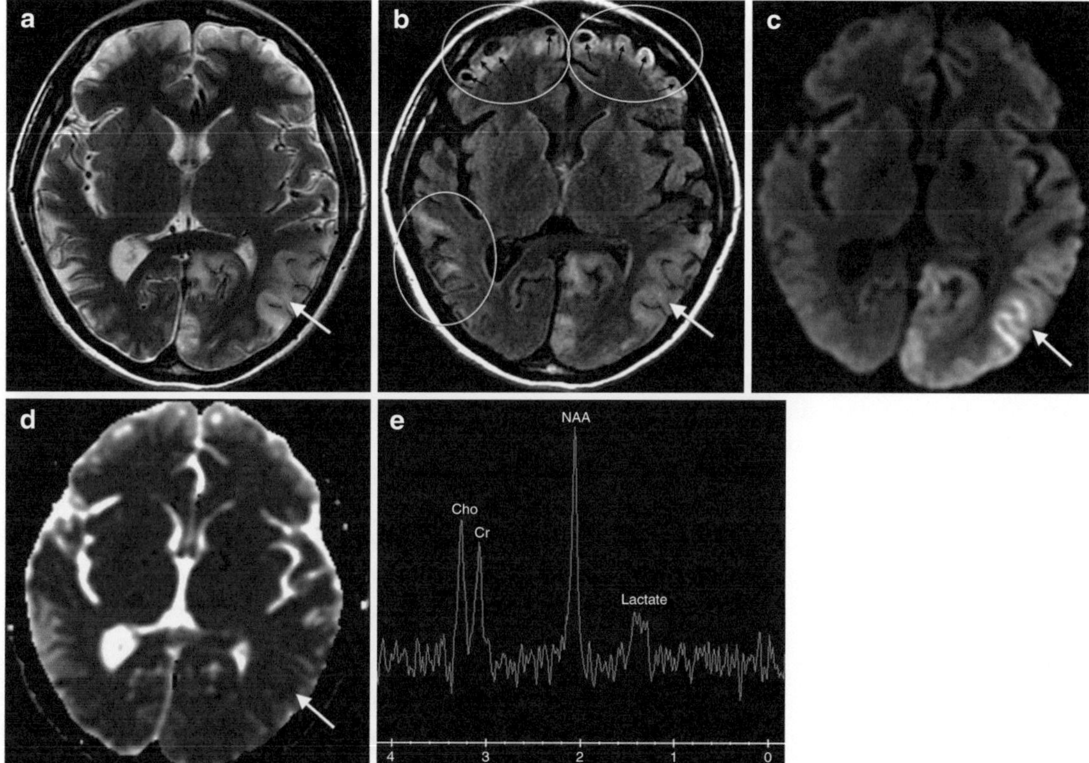

Fig. 12.11 18-year-old female with MELAS. Axial T2WI (TR/TE ms, 4041/103) (**a**), T2 FLAIR (TR/TE/IT ms, 10,000/126/2200) (**b**), DWI (TR/TE ms, 10,000/80) (**c**), and ADC (TR/TE ms, 10,000/80) (**d**) through the level of the lateral ventricles. There is cortical/subcortical hyperintensity and swelling affecting the left occipital lobe and posterior temporal lobe not confined to major arterial territories (*white arrows*, **a** and **b**), with cortical diffusion abnormality (combined reduced and intermediate diffusion; *arrows*, **c** and **d**). These findings are indicative of acute stroke-like and/or seizure-related edema. Old cortical/subcortical lesions are present in the right temporal lobe and frontal lobes (*circles*, **b**), demonstrating mixed hyperintense and hypointense signal consistent with areas of encephalomalacia and juxtacortical necrosis (*black arrows*, **b**). Single-voxel MRS (TR/TE ms, 1500/288) over the left basal ganglia demonstrates mild lactate at 1.33 ppm (**e**)

discernible and can overlap. Vasoconstriction from diminished nitric oxide in arterial wall smooth muscle cells has been shown to cause or contribute to stroke-like episodes [112]. Small arteries are more commonly involved; however, larger arteries of the circle of Willis can also be affected [112]. Stroke-like episodes manifest with cortical/subcortical edema and swelling, similar to an infarction but not confined to an arterial territory, most commonly in the parieto-occipital regions [3, 101, 113] (Fig. 12.11). Diffusion-weighted images demonstrate restricted or facilitated water movement depending on the magnitude of cytotoxic and vasogenic edema, often both [101, 114]. Whether or not acutely symptomatic patients with these types of brain signal changes will go on to permanent brain injury cannot be accurately predicted; follow-up is required to distinguish transient edema from more permanent brain injury. As with other mitochondrial disorders, the basal ganglia may be involved and manifest variable density and MR signal [3, 101, 113]. On the other hand, absence of basal ganglia involvement does not exclude the diagnosis as sparing is not uncommon. The cerebellum, brainstem, and/or spinal cord are less commonly involved [3]. Over time, accrued cerebral injury tends to occur along a posteroanterior gradient in patients with suboptimally controlled symptoms.

The argument to obtain DTI and MRS in MELAS is based on the fact that diffusion imaging is helpful to differentiate acute lesions with restricted diffusion from older/chronic lesions that often present with increased diffusion and to identify strokes before they are evident on T2-weighted images in order to initiate therapy. In addition, repeated MRI using DTI may show progressive spread of the cortical lesion to the surrounding cortex for a few weeks, even after the onset of symptoms [114]. In patients with mitochondrial disease, significant widespread reductions in fractional anisotropy (FA) values have been shown in white matter tracts and in some cases in normal-appearing white matter [99, 115].

Lactic acidosis is readily captured by MR spectroscopy [101, 113, 114, 116] (Fig. 12.11). Although other diseases in the differential diagnosis (i.e., infarction and non-MELAS-associated seizure-related edema) can manifest lactate in areas of signal abnormality on T2WI and diffusion-weighted images, lactate is also present in areas of normal signal in mitochondrial diseases such as MELAS [101, 114]. MRS may also show decreased NAA, glutamine/glutamate, and creatine and increased glucose [3, 116].

12.6 White Matter Changes

White matter changes are the hallmark of genetically defined leukodystrophies. White matter changes are frequently with many syndromes featuring developmental delay, several of which are metabolic syndromes. Cerebral white matter involvement is commonly seen in childhood-onset mitochondrial disorders [117]. Therefore, oxidative phosphorylation disorders should be considered when the MRI is suggestive of childhood leukoencephalopathy or leukodystrophy [117–119] (Fig. 12.12).

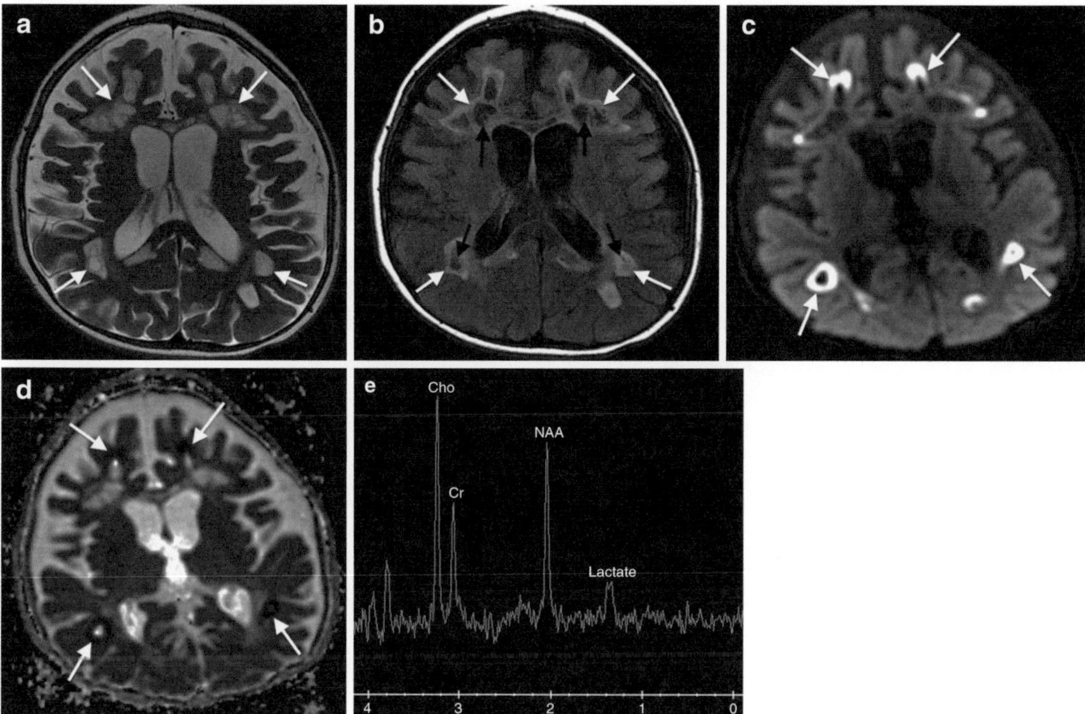

Fig. 12.12 22-month-old male with a mitochondrial disorder (cytochrome C oxidase deficiency). Axial T2WI (TR/TE ms, 3200/101) (**a**), T2 FLAIR (TR/TE/IT ms, 10,000/148/2250) (**b**), DWI (TR/TE ms, 10,000/82) (**c**), and ADC (TR/TE ms, 10,000/82) (**d**) through the lateral ventricular level. Extensive multifocal and coalescent subcortical, deep, paraventricular cerebral white matter and corpus callosum lesions are present. These demonstrate T2 prolongation (*arrows*, **a**) and hyperintense (*white arrows*, **b**) and hypointense signal (*black arrows*, **b**) on T2 FLAIR consistent with gliosis and necrosis. Mixed restricted diffusion (*arrows*, **c** and **d**) and facilitated diffusion are present, compatible with multiphasic injury. Single-voxel MRS (TR/TE ms, 1500/288) over the left basal ganglia demonstrates lactate at 1.33 ppm (**e**)

12.7 Pyruvate Dehydrogenase Deficiency

One of the mitochondrial disorders, pyruvate dehydrogenase deficiency, is due to the inability to convert pyruvate to acetyl-coenzyme A, which is integral for citric acid cycle energy production. Instead, excessive pyruvate is converted to lactate, which is considered neurotoxic. Normal neurogenesis, growth, migration, and organization require adequate energy production. Two distinct neuropathologic phenotypes have been recognized: prenatal onset with brain malformations (gender nonspecific) and postnatal-onset energy

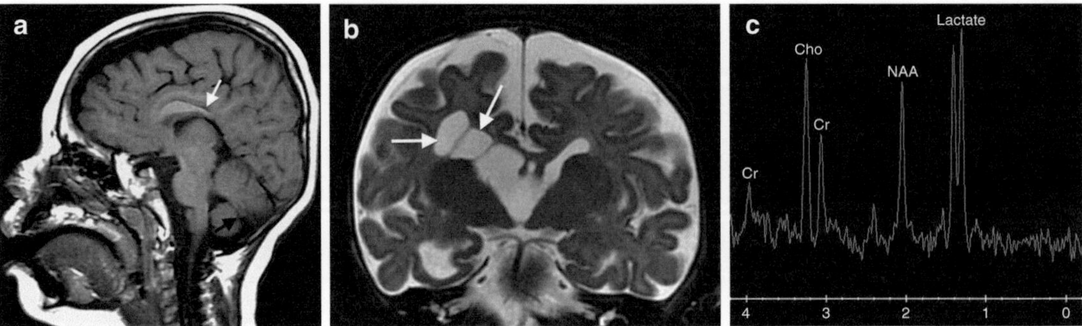

Fig. 12.13 5-month-old female with pyruvate dehydrogenase deficiency. Sagittal T1WI (TR/TE ms, 400/13) (**a**) shows a shortened, malformed corpus callosum consistent with hypogenesis/dysgenesis (*white arrow*), hypoplasia of the vermis (*black arrow*), and a small brain to face ratio compatible with micrencephaly. Coronal T2WI (TR/TE ms, 6300/103) (**b**) demonstrates asymmetric right cerebral white matter volume loss and necrotic, porencephalic cystic changes adjacent to the right lateral ventricle related to remote injury (*arrows*). Single-voxel MRS over the left basal ganglia (TR/TE ms, 1500/288) (**c**) shows a large double peak at 1.3 ppm consistent with markedly elevated lactate

failure with basal ganglia lesions (males only) [120]. The most common clinical features mimic a Leigh syndrome, which is defined by neurodegeneration caused by mitochondrial dysfunction and bilateral lesions in the central nervous system, usually in the deep gray matter structures.

On imaging, deep gray nuclear signal changes and white matter disease are typical [3, 121, 122]. Cerebral white matter signal may be diffusely hyperintense on T2WI, which may represent delayed myelination or injury depending on signal magnitude, occasionally without concurrent deep gray nuclei and brainstem involvement [3, 117, 122]. White matter may become severely injured with gliosis evolving to necrosis [3, 122, 123] (Fig. 12.13). Longstanding in utero alterations of energy metabolism can cause variable brain structure malformations depending on the timing and severity of disease. A dysgenetic corpus callosum is considered a hallmark for the condition in the correct clinical context [27] (Fig. 12.13). Neuronal migration abnormalities and brainstem dysplasia may also be present. Lactate is almost always elevated in the brain on MRS [3, 124–126] (Fig. 12.13). Elevated pyruvate may also be detectable at 2.36 ppm but may be difficult to distinguish from glutamine/glutamate [3]. Severely injured brain areas demonstrate decreased NAA, consistent with neuronal loss [3].

12.7.1 Lysosomal Disorders

12.7.1.1 Neuronal Ceroid Lipofuscinoses

The neuronal ceroid lipofuscinosis (NCL) disorders are a group of inherited, neurodegenerative, storage diseases with progressive intellectual decline, progressive loss of motor function, seizures, vision loss, and early death [127]. Many demonstrate vision loss. This group of disorders is subtyped by the age of onset. Infantile NCL (INCL), late-infantile NCL (LINCL), and Batten disease present in infancy or childhood, whereas Kufs' disease is an adult-onset disorder. Kufs' disease presents with behavioral abnormalities or progressive myoclonic epilepsy with subsequent dementia and cerebellar ataxia [128].

The infantile NCLs present between 6 and 24 months of life with developmental delay, myoclonic seizures, and abnormal EEG. The children progress to acquired microcephaly and blindness. The late-infantile form of this disorder is similar with later onset and symptoms at 2–4 years of age.

It may be heralded by epilepsy, regression of milestones and subsequent development of dementia, extrapyramidal and pyramidal signs, and visual impairment and blindness by age 4–6 years. Batten disease is the most common subtype (type 3). Clinically, these patients present with visual changes associated with retinitis pigmentosa. Subsequently, seizures and dementia manifest in late childhood.

12.7.1.2 Neuronal Ceroid Lipofuscinoses: Imaging

Early imaging may be normal in all forms of NCL. A progressive predominant gray matter volume loss then occurs, affecting both the cerebrum and cerebellum [3, 129–134] (Fig. 12.14). Cortical volume loss raises a differential diagnosis of transient volume loss (e.g., dehydration, malnutrition, steroid effect) and atrophy secondary to various types of neurodegeneration. Drastic cortical volume loss can even lead to subdural fluid collections in NCL [135]. Concurrent symmetric lateral thalamic hypointensity and periventricular/posterior limb internal capsule hyperintensity on T2WI can help support the diagnosis of NCL if present [129, 132–134] (Fig. 12.14). MRS typically demonstrates decreased NAA reflecting neuronal loss, decreased Cr, and variable lactate, myoinositol, and choline depending on the location of interrogation and stage of disease [3, 136, 137]. Spectroscopic alterations evolve over the disease course; NAA declines, whereas Cho and MI decrease in the cerebrum and increase in the brainstem and cerebellum [136].

12.7.1.3 Sphingolipidoses

Krabbe's Disease

Krabbe's disease (globoid cell leukodystrophy) is a lysosomal disorder caused by a galactocerebrosidase deficiency, psychosine toxicity, and subsequent giant cell accumulation in lysosomes [3, 4, 138]. The majority of patients come to clinical attention by age 6 months due to neurological deterioration, often with irritability or spasticity. Diagnosis is by enzymatic testing in cultured fibroblasts or molecular testing for the GALC gene mutations.

Krabbe's Disease: Imaging

Four distinct neuroimaging patterns have been described, correlating with disease onset: early infantile (0–6 months), late infantile (6–12 months), late onset (13 months to 10 years), and adult (>10 years) [139]. Early infantile disease most commonly manifests periventricular white matter, dentate hilus, and cerebellar white matter T2 prolongation (Fig. 12.15); less common variable signal changes may be found more diffusely in the deep posterior cerebral white matter, brainstem, thalamus, and optic pathway.

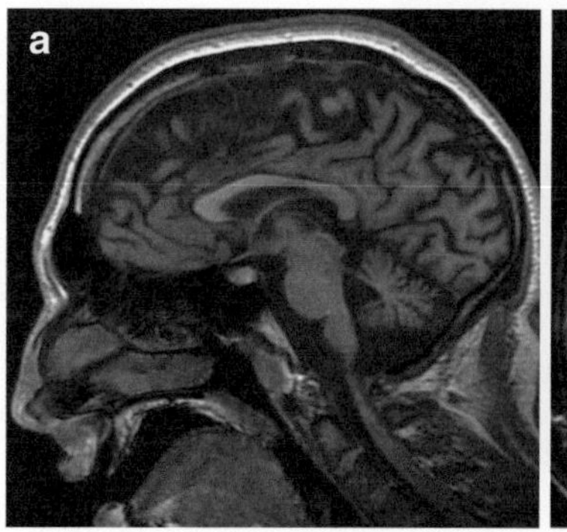

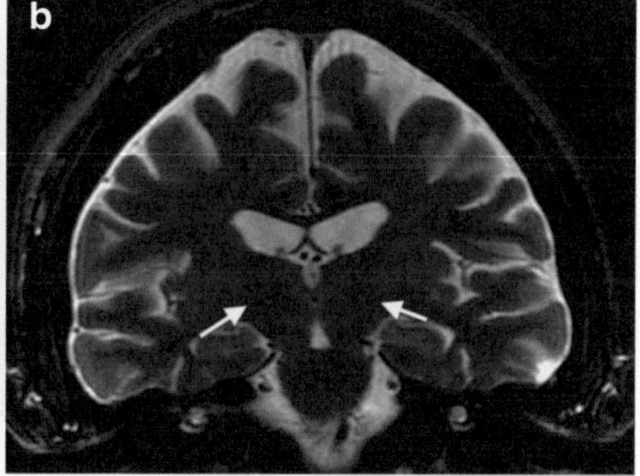

Fig. 12.14 17-year-old male with Batten disease (neuronal ceroid lipofuscinosis type 3). Sagittal T1WI (TR/TE/IT ms, 500/12/5) (**a**) and coronal fat-saturated T2WI (TR/TE ms, 4450/101) (**b**) demonstrate enlarged cerebral sulci and cerebellar fissures consistent with mild diffuse cortical atrophy. The corpus callosum maintains a relatively normal thickness. Abnormal hypointense signal is present in the thalami on T2WI (*arrows*, **b**)

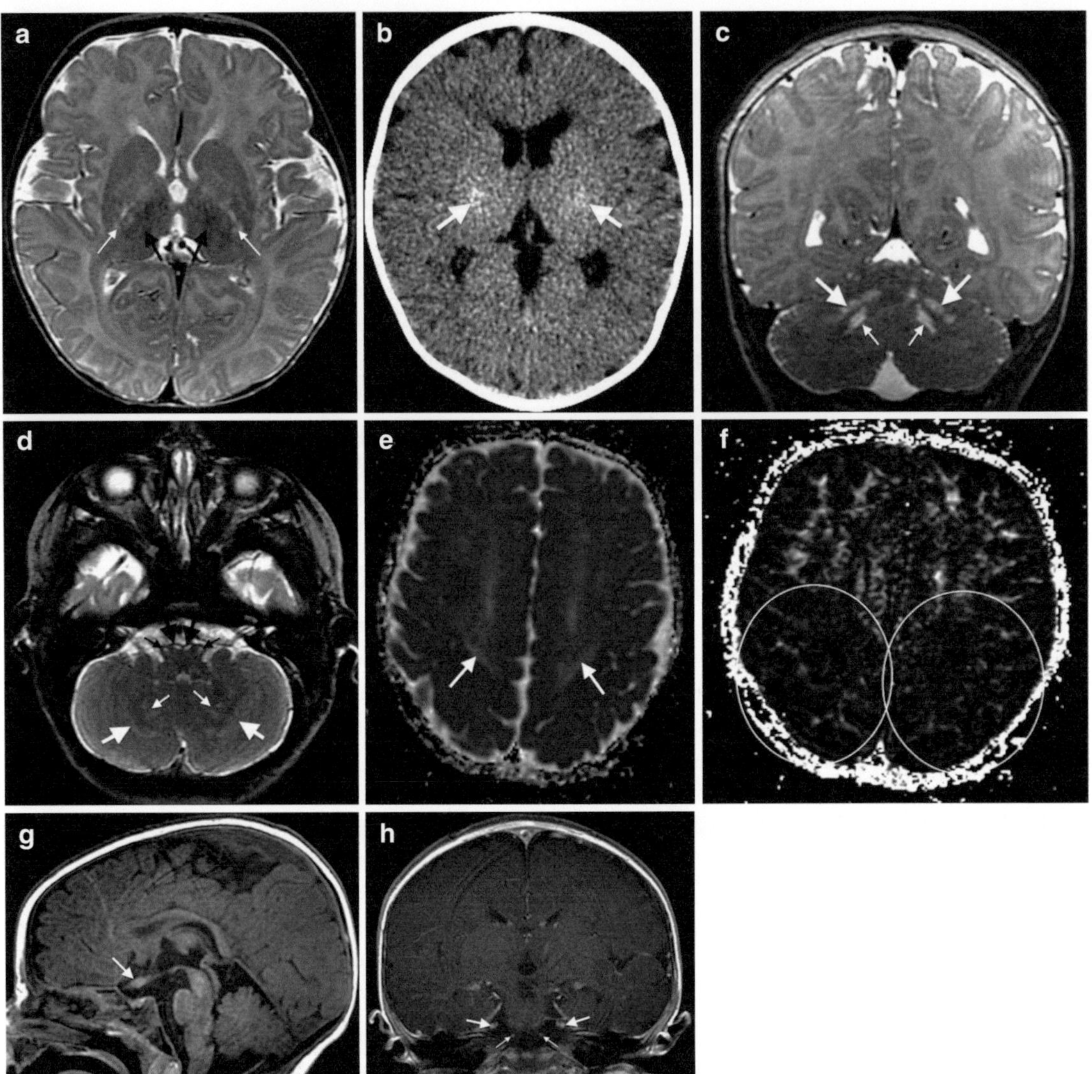

Fig. 12.15 4-month-old male with Krabbe's disease. Axial T2WI (TR/TE ms, 3375/103) (**a**) and axial CT (**b**) through the cerebral deep gray nuclei demonstrate abnormal mineralization of the thalami, hypointense on T2WI (*black arrows*, **a**) and hyperdense on CT (*arrows*, **b**). The PLIC is abnormally hyperintense (*white arrows*, **a**). Coronal T2WI (TR/TE ms, 3500/90) (**c**) and axial T2WI (TR/TE ms, 3375/103) (**d**) show hyperintense deep cerebral white matter (*large white arrows*, **c** and **d**) and dentate nuclear hila (*small white arrows*, **c** and **d**), marginating the dentate nuclei proper. The medullary pyramids (*large black arrows*, **d**) and inferior olivary nuclei (*small black arrows*, **d**) are also hyperintense. Axial ADC (TR/TE ms, 10,000/92) (**e**) and FA map (TR/TE ms, 10,000/92) (**f**) show deep posterior predominant cerebral white matter facilitated diffusion (*arrows*, **e**) and decreased anisotropy (*circles*, **f**). Sagittal T1WI (TR/TE/IT ms, 8/3/450) (**g**) and post-contrast coronal T1WI (TR/TE ms, 650/11) (**h**). Cranial nerve abnormalities include enlargement of the optic chiasm (*arrow*, **g**) and enhancement of the abducens (*small arrows*, **h**) and trigeminal nerves (*large arrows*, **h**)

Late-infantile and late-onset manifestations also include periventricular T2 prolongation, but more extensive deep posterior cerebral white matter disease along an anteroposterior and centrifugal gradient becomes more common over time (most prominent in late-onset forms) [139, 140]. Dentate hilus and cerebellar white matter signal changes are also more variable in older subtypes;

those found to have cerebellar abnormalities may have a worse prognosis [139]. Thalamic hypointensity on T2WI is most frequently observed in late-infantile cases [139]. Projectional fibers in the brainstem may be involved in all forms, especially in adult forms of the disease [141, 142] (Fig. 12.15). Microstructural changes may be demonstrable at an early age even in asymptomatic patients using DTI; diminished anisotropy may be present in the splenium and corticospinal tracts, correlating with treatment outcomes [143–146] (Fig. 12.15). Lowe's score and degree of midbrain atrophy have been found to correlate with the degree of functional deficits [147, 148].

An important distinguishing feature that may help define the diagnosis is basal ganglia and cerebral white matter calcification (Fig. 12.15). To that end, CT can be complimentary to identify or verify mineralization if Krabbe's disease is under consideration [3, 149, 150]. Basal ganglia calcifications can also occur in the gangliosidosis, another group of lysosomal disorders with leukodystrophy imaging patterns that may be entertained in the differential diagnosis; however, gangliosidoses often have concurrent cerebral deep gray nuclear T2 prolongation. In Krabbe's disease, giant cell accumulation in certain areas causes discernible mass effect, such as within the optic pathway (Fig. 12.15). After intravenous gadolinium administration, heterogeneous contrast enhancement of the peripheral cerebral white matter is typical. The spinal cord and cauda equina may also be affected; therefore, examination of the spinal column can be helpful in the workup.

MR spectroscopy may demonstrate nonspecific findings associated with cell membrane turnover (elevated choline) and astrogliosis (elevated choline and myoinositol) and decreased neuronal-axonal integrity (diminished NAA) [3, 81, 151, 152]. Lactate may also be found, especially in active disease presentations.

12.7.1.4 Metachromatic Leukodystrophy

Metachromatic leukodystrophy (MLD) is an inherited lysosomal disorder caused by mutations in the ARSA gene, causing arylsulfatase A deficiency [153, 154]. Low activity of arylsulfatase A subsequently results in the accumulation of sulfatides in both the central and peripheral nervous system leading to a demyelinating disorder [153, 154]. The disease is classified by age of onset into late-infantile, juvenile and adult-onset types, which manifest a variety of neurological symptoms and early death [153, 154]. Although there is no cure, new therapeutic approaches are emerging and include enzyme replacement, stem cell transplantation, and gene therapy [153, 154]. Gray matter volume is reduced in addition to the MRI changes that accompany demyelination [155].

12.7.1.5 Metachromatic Leukodystrophy: Imaging

Childhood-onset MLD causes a leukodystrophy. As a sphingolipidosis, it shares many neuroimaging similarities with one of the main items on the differential diagnosis, Krabbe's disease, namely, a non-enhancing cerebral white matter disease progresses along a centrifugal gradient (and often, a posteroanterior gradient, especially in the late-infantile subtype), optic pathway may be involved, and the brainstem and cerebellum may be affected in severe and/or long-standing disease [153, 156] (Fig. 12.16). Detailed assessment of the cerebral white matter demonstrates a peculiar pattern of involvement with perivenular sparing that creates a striated or "tigroid" appearance [3, 156–158] (Fig. 12.16). Although this pattern may also be present in patients with Krabbe's disease, gangliosidosis, and Alexander disease, it tends to be less common in these disorders. White matter diffusion restriction and facilitation may be present [159]. Cranial nerves, spinal nerves, and/or cauda equina nerve roots may enhance with gadolinium (Fig. 12.16). Unlike Krabbe's disease, basal ganglia calcifications are not a hallmark of MLD.

MR spectroscopy demonstrates decreased NAA, elevated choline and myoinositol, and lactate in acute disease [160]. Decreased choline has also been described and interpreted to represent dysmyelination [161].

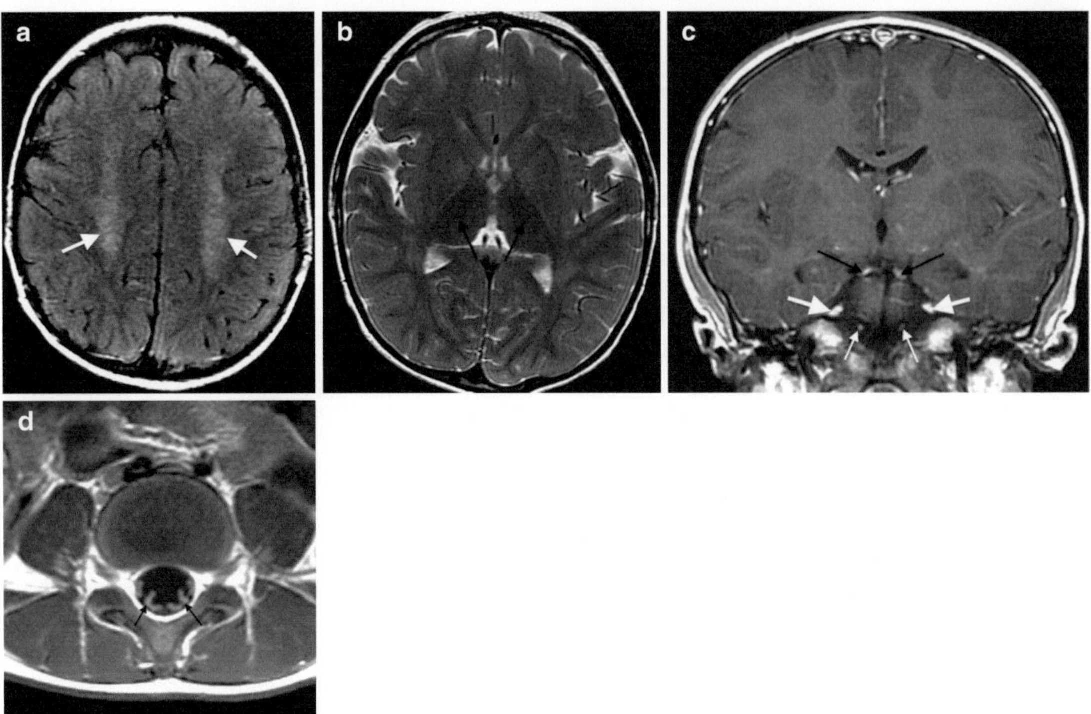

Fig. 12.16 2-year-old male with metachromatic leukodystrophy. Axial T2 FLAIR images (TR/TE/IT ms, 10,002/137/2200) (**a**) demonstrate hyperintense deep cerebral white matter signal sparing the U-fibers with a subtle striated, "tigroid" appearance (*arrows*). Axial T2WI (TR/TE ms, 4300/99) (**b**) shows abnormal hypointense signal in the thalami (*arrows*). Coronal post-contrast T1WI (TR/TE ms, 467/9) (**c**) depicts enhancement of multiple cranial nerves including trigeminal (*large white arrows*), abducens (*small white arrows*), and oculomotor (*black arrows*) nerves. Axial post-contrast T1WI (TR/TE ms, 550/9) (**d**) through the lumbar spine shows abnormal enhancement of all cauda equina nerve roots (*arrows*)

12.7.1.6 Gangliosidoses

Genetic defects in galactosidase (GM1) and hexosaminidase A or hexosaminidase A and B (GM2) are responsible for the heterogeneous group of lysosomal disorders called gangliosidoses.

In the most characterized lysosomal storage disease, Tay-Sachs, the alpha subunit of β-hexosaminidase, is defective [162]. The lesser known disorder, Sandhoff's disease, is caused by defective beta subunit, and the least common form is caused by deficiency of the GM2 activator activity [163]. In all three scenarios, children present with retinal cherry red spots, progressive weakness, regression of motor skills, and neurodegeneration with seizures, blindness, spasticity, and death. In all three disorders, initial loss of developmental milestones occurs at 3 to 6 months with death often before the age of 4 years. The juvenile- and adult-onset variants of this disorder are due to variants of the hexosaminidase A gene and have later onsets with similar outcomes. The infantile form of the disease is found most often in the Ashkenazi Jewish population with a carrier frequency of 1:27.

Neuroimaging demonstrates symmetric swelling and signal abnormalities in the cerebral deep gray nuclei in the acute phase. Calcifications may occur concurrently in the same areas. In contrast to conventional T1/T2 and MRS findings in these disorders, diffusion-weighted images are normal, suggesting that the demyelination progresses without myelin edema. Cerebral white matter involvement is also typical as is often seen in lysosomal disorders.

12.7.1.7 Tay-Sachs: Imaging

Neuroimaging in Tay-Sachs suggests similar changes to NCL, with thalamic signal abnormalities early on progressing to brain atrophy and increased T2 signal in white matter. ^{1}H MRS demonstrates similar findings as in INCL, reflecting the common features of brain atrophy and gliosis. ^{1}H MRS demonstrates an increase in myoinositol and choline with decrease in the NAA, again reflecting demyelination, gliosis, and neuronal loss in the neuropathological process of Tay-Sachs disease [164, 165].

12.7.1.8 Gaucher Disease

Gaucher disease is a group of disorders with variable ages of onset and symptoms ranging from a lethal neonatal form to one that can be asymptomatic at its mildest. Gaucher disease is due to deficiency of glucocerebrosidase that leads to accumulation of glucosylceramide. Gaucher disease type 1 is the most common and is clinically defined by bone manifestation (i.e., osteopenia and osteonecrosis), hepatosplenomegaly, anemia, thrombocytopenia, and lung disease. Certain genotypes can cause a Parkinson's-like neurological presentation [166]. Types 2 and 3 are characterized by neurological findings. Common neurological manifestations include horizontal gaze palsy, epilepsy, and ataxia. In type 2, onset is early with rapidly progressive course and death. In type 3, onset is in infancy to preschool years with a slower course and individuals living into the third and fourth decades. Early diagnosis is crucial for initiation of treatment prior to irreversible complications from the disease.

12.7.1.9 Gaucher Disease: Imaging

Periventricular white matter hyperintensity may be present on T2WI and T2 FLAIR images [167]. There are very few publications reporting quantitative imaging in the Gaucher brain. Abdel Razek et al. and Davies et al. used DTI to record white matter abnormalities with ADC measures and tract-based spatial statistics (TBSS) [168, 169]. The study groups included patients with types II and III Gaucher disease as well as three boys with type I Gaucher disease. These studies suggested decreased ADC and FA in the middle cerebellar peduncles. Diffuse nonspecific DTI changes were seen in the type I patients. Elevated choline has been found in otherwise normal-appearing type I Gaucher patients on MR spectroscopy [170].

12.7.1.10 Niemann-Pick Type C

Niemann-Pick disease type C is caused by abnormal cholesterol esterification, due to defective enzymatic activity of NPC1. There are two genes, *NPC1* and *NPC2* genes, which have been identified causes of Niemann-Pick disease type C. Presentation of this disorder is variable with infants presenting fetal ascites, neonatal liver disease, and hypotonia and children presenting with supranuclear gaze palsy, ataxia, dysarthria, dystonia, and seizures [171]. In adolescence and adults, psychiatric symptoms are common with depression or schizophrenia.

12.7.1.11 NPC: Imaging

A progressive brain atrophy occurs in patients with NPC, more prominent in the frontal lobes bilaterally but also in the cerebellum, as well as hyperintense signal on T2WI predominantly in bilateral parietal-occipital periventricular white matter representing hypomyelination and dysmyelination [167] (Fig. 12.17). ^{1}H MRS has shown decrease in NAA in the frontal and parietal cortex, centrum semiovale, and caudate nucleus. Choline is also increased in the frontal cortex and centrum semiovale suggesting membrane breakdown with release of free choline. Multimodal imaging was achieved in a subject with NPC who had two scans at ages 19 and 22 years demonstrating progressive atrophy [172]. His MRS (at age 19 years) revealed no significant decrease in N-acetyl aspartate/choline ratio in the left frontal central white matter.

Walterfang et al. used a combination of voxel-based morphometry and tract-based spatial statistics of diffusion tensor images to examine structural changes in gray and white matter volumes [173]. Subjects with NPC demonstrated decreased gray matter volume bilaterally in the hippocampus, thalamus, superior cerebellum,

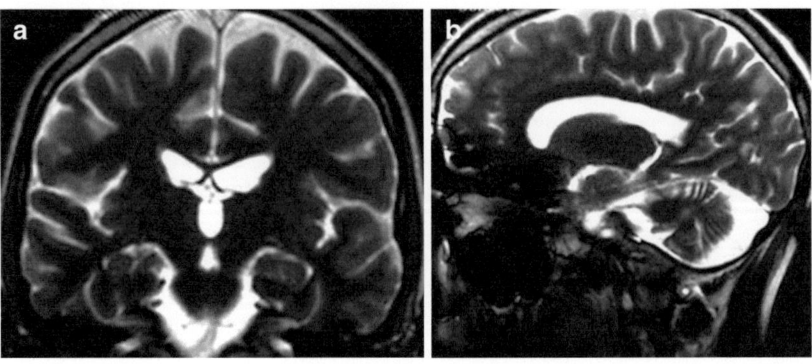

Fig. 12.17 Coronal (**a**) and sagittal (**b**) T2WI from a patient with Niemann-Pick disease type C show diffuse cerebral and cerebellar atrophy manifested by enlarged cerebral sulci, cerebellar fissures, and ventricles

and insula with reduced fractional anisotropy in several white matter tracts pointing to abnormalities in gray and white matter [173].

Recently, lower FA in the corpus callosum along with changes in volume and cross-sectional area has been shown to correlate with severity scores in the disease [174].

12.7.2 Lipid Storage Disorders

Lipid storage diseases are known as the lipidoses. These are a group of inherited metabolic disorders in which there is lipid accumulation in various cell types, including the central nervous system, due to the deficiency of a variety of enzymes required to break down complex lipid moieties. Accumulation over time with excessive storage can cause permanent cellular and tissue damage. The brain is particularly sensitive to lipid storage as the deposits will lead to pressure changes and interference with normal neurological function. In addition to primary lipid storage diseases, lysosomal storage diseases include the mucolipidoses (in which excessive amounts of lipids and carbohydrates are stored in the cells and tissues) and the mucopolysaccharidoses (in which abnormal glycosylated proteins cannot be broken down due to enzyme deficiency) [175].

The mucolipidoses (ML) and mucopolysaccharidoses (MPS) are both progressive storage disorders that share affect several organs including the brain, bone, and liver. As such, they present with multisystemic clinical features including facial dysmorphism, bone dysplasia, hepatosplenomegaly, and neurological abnormalities. They may present from childhood and vary in severity. In infancy they may present as developmental regression and a reduced life expectancy at the severe end of the clinical spectrum. Adults may have an almost normal clinical phenotype and normal life span due to an attenuated disease. Both MPS and ML are transmitted in an autosomal recessive manner, except for the MPS II (Hunter's syndrome), which is X-linked.

12.7.2.1 Mucolipidosis

In mucolipidoses, excessive amounts of lipids and carbohydrates are stored in the cells and tissues. The mucolipidoses were named due to the similar presentation to both the mucopolysaccharidoses and sphingolipidoses. There are four types of ML, which are type I also called sialidosis, type II (I-cell disease), and types III and IV.

Mucolipidosis type II (I-cell disease) is caused by a GNPTAB gene defect with resultant N-acetylglucosamine-1-phosphotransferase deficiency [176]. Facial dysmorphism and dysostosis multiplex are typical features, similar to other lysosomal disorders.

Mucolipidosis type IV is an autosomal recessive disorder caused by a defect in MCOLN1 [3, 177]. It typically presents with visual changes caused by corneal clouding, retinopathy, and optic atrophy, followed by nonprogressive psychomotor retardation [3, 177–179]. Gastrin level is frequently elevated in conjunction with achlorhydria [177, 179]. Unlike many lysosomal storage disorders, patients with mucolipidosis type IV lack skeletal manifestations and organomegaly [3, 178, 179].

12.7.2.2 Mucolipidosis: Imaging

Mucolipidosis Type II (I-Cell Disease)

Neuroimaging may be normal in some patients. Others show hypomyelination, atrophy, leukomalacia, and/or ventriculomegaly [176, 180] (Fig. 12.18). MR spectroscopy may show decreased choline [176].

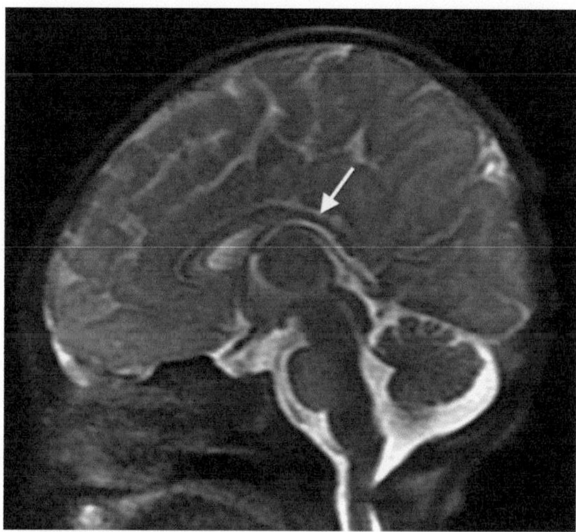

Fig. 12.18 9-day-old male with mucolipidosis type II (I-cell disease). Sagittal T2WI (TR/TE ms, 1087/60) demonstrates thinning of the corpus callosum (*arrow*), reflecting cerebral white matter volume loss

Mucolipidosis Type IV

Corpus callosum thinning is nearly universal, representing hypogenesis/hypoplasia, usually with superimposed commissural fiber volume loss [3, 177–179, 181] (Fig. 12.19). Corpus callosum dysgenesis has also been described [177, 178, 181]. Cerebral white matter volume is decreased [3]. Cerebral white matter lesions are variable in number and distribution and may represent gliosis, local hypomyelination, or demyelination [177, 178] (Fig. 12.19). White matter mean diffusivity and fractional anisotropy may also be decreased [182]. Like other lysosomal diseases, the basal ganglia (especially the globi pallidi) and thalami demonstrate excessive hypointense signal on T2WI, likely representing pathologic iron deposition [177, 178, 181] (Fig. 12.19). Cerebral and cerebellar atrophy tends to develop over time [177–179, 181]. MR spectroscopy may reveal decreased NAA correlating with the degree of motor deficits [183].

12.7.2.3 CPT II Deficiency

Carnitine palmitoyltransferase II (CPT II) deficiency is a disorder of fatty acid oxidation [184, 185]. CPT2 is a nuclear protein that is transported to the mitochondrial inner membrane, and with carnitine palmitoyltransferase I, oxidizes long-chain fatty acids in the mitochondria. Defects in

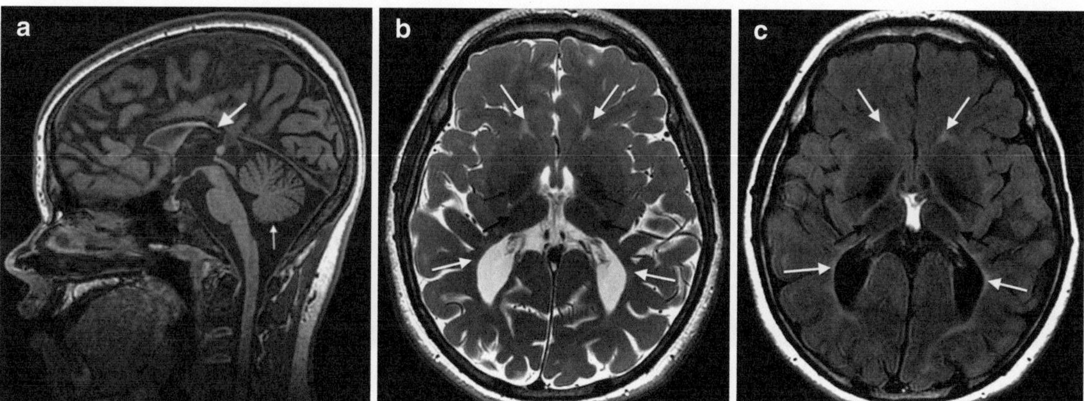

Fig. 12.19 19-year-old female with mucolipidosis type IV. Sagittal T1WI (TR/TE/IT ms, 8/3/450) (**a**) demonstrates a shortened, thinned corpus callosum consistent with hypogenesis and superimposed commissural fiber volume loss (*large arrow*) and hypoplasia of the vermis (*small arrow*). Axial T2WI (TR/TE ms, 3161/102) (**b**) and T2 FLAIR (TR/TE/IT ms, 10,000/147/2250) (**c**) show periventricular white matter hyperintensity (*white arrows*) and abnormal hypointensity in the globi pallidi (*small black arrows*) and thalami (*large black arrows*)

this gene are associated with mitochondrial long-chain fatty acid (LCFA) oxidation disorders and carnitine palmitoyltransferase II deficiency.

There are three clinical presentations including a lethal neonatal form, severe infantile hepatocardiomuscular form, and a myopathic form that is usually mild and can manifest from infancy to adulthood. The infantile forms tend to be multisystemic characterized by liver failure, hypoketotic hypoglycemia, cardiomyopathy, seizures, and early death. The myopathic form is associated with exercise-induced muscle pain and weakness often with myoglobinuria. The myopathic form of CPT II deficiency is the most common disorder of lipid metabolism affecting skeletal muscle and is the most frequent cause of hereditary myoglobinuria. Males are more likely to be affected than females.

12.7.2.4 CPT II Deficiency: Imaging

Few imaging reports have described periventricular cysts and calcifications, corpus callosum dysgenesis, malformations of cortical development, and cerebral infarctions [184, 186–190]. A postmortem MR performed to examine an infant that suffered sudden infant death syndrome (SIDS) demonstrated hepatosteatosis [191]. MR spectroscopy has demonstrated elevated lipid peaks at 0.9 and 1.3 ppm suggesting brain fat accumulation [190] (Fig. 12.20). Differential diagnosis of abnormal lipid peaks on MRS includes other disorders of fatty acid oxidation such as CPT I deficiency, peroxisomal disorders, and Sjogren-Larsson syndrome, among others [190].

12.7.3 Mucopolysaccharidoses

Mucopolysaccharidoses (MPS) are a heterogeneous group of disorders causing mucopolysaccharide (glycosaminoglycan) deposition in lysosomes throughout the body. In the brain, mucopolysaccharides accrue in various locations. As a result, perivascular and cerebrospinal fluid spaces may be dilated with or without hydrocephalus [3, 192–194] (Fig. 12.21). White matter may be diseased, with variable degrees of T2 prolongation in the periventricular and deep cerebral regions, reflecting demyelination, gliosis, and/or interstitial edema if hydrocephalus is present [3, 192–196] (Fig. 12.21). White matter changes and perivascular space abnormalities have been shown to improve after bone marrow transplantation [192]. Cerebral atrophy may develop over time [192–194]. Spinal imaging reveals dysostosis multiplex with vertebral

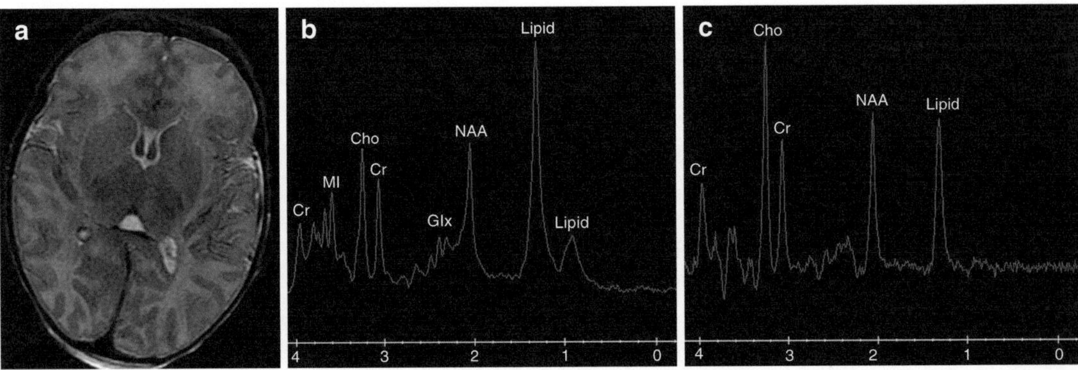

Fig. 12.20 3-day-old female with carnitine palmitoyltransferase 2 (CPT II) deficiency. Axial T2WI (TR/TE ms, 3500/120) (**a**) at basal ganglia level shows no brain parenchymal abnormality. However, basal ganglia single-voxel MRS (TR/TE ms, 1500/35) (**b**) and (TR/TE ms, 1500/144) (**c**) reveal a large peak at 1.3 ppm at 35 ms echo time (**b**) that remains positively deflected at 144 ms echo time (**c**). NAA, creatine (Cr), choline (Cho), glutamine/glutamate (Glx), and myoinositol (MI) are within normal range

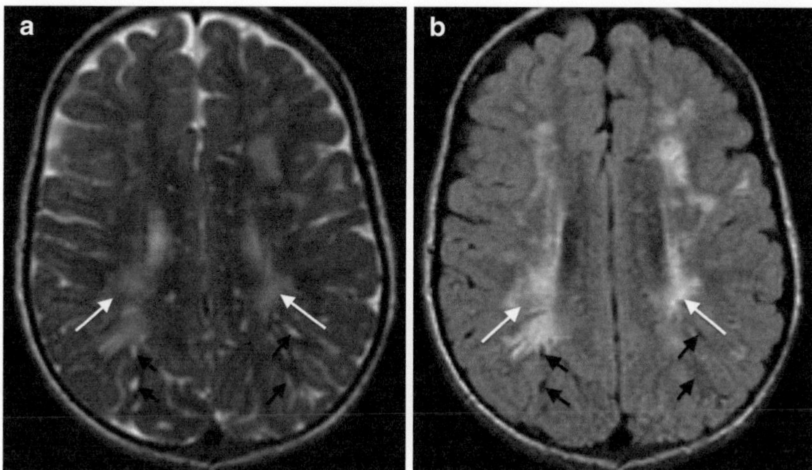

Fig. 12.21 6-year-old female with Hurler syndrome (mucopolysaccharidosis type I). Axial T2WI (TR/TE ms, 4700/83) (**a**) and T2 FLAIR (TR/TE/IT ms, 90,002/133/2200) (**b**) at the lateral ventricle superior margin shows white matter hyperintensity (*white arrows*) and multiple prominent perivascular spaces (*black arrows*) with signal suppression on T2 FLAIR

dysmorphism and may depict findings of spinal stenosis or craniocervical junction instability caused by a combination of bone dysplasia, extraosseous mucopolysaccharide deposition, and ligamentous laxity [3, 194]. MR spectroscopy can demonstrate accumulated mucopolysaccharides with an abnormal metabolic peak at 3.7 ppm, additional abnormal peaks beyond 3.3 ppm, and elevated choline [3, 195, 197]. Presumed mucopolysaccharide and choline peaks have been shown to decrease after marrow transplant [197].

12.8 Brain Injury due to Substrate Depletion

12.8.1 Creatine Deficiency

The cerebral creatine deficiency syndromes are inborn errors of creatine metabolism that include the two creatine biosynthesis disorders, guanidinoacetate methyltransferase (GAMT) deficiency and l-arginine/glycine amidinotransferase (AGAT or GATM) deficiency, as well as the creatine transporter (SLC6A8) deficiency [198–201]. All are associated with seizures and intellectual disability and autism spectrum disorders. Some may feature an extrapyramidal movement disorder. Onset is between ages 3 months and 3 years. The phenotype of SLC6A8 deficiency in affected males ranges from mild intellectual disability and speech delay to significant intellectual disability, seizures, and behavioral disorder. The disorder is recognized across the life span with the age at diagnosis ranging from 2 to 66 years. GAMT and AGAT deficiencies are autosomal recessive conditions, whereas the transport defect is an X-linked disorder.

The common feature of all creatine deficiency syndromes is the severe depletion of creatine or phosphocreatine in the brain. GAMT deficiency is characterized by accumulation of guanidinoacetic acid in the brain and body fluids. Guanidinoacetic acid seems to be responsible for intractable seizures and the movement disorder, both exclusively found in GAMT deficiency. Treatment with oral creatine supplementation is in part successful in GAMT and AGAT deficiencies, whereas in CrT1 defect, it is not able to replenish creatine in the brain.

12.8.2 Creatine Deficiency Disorders

The creatine (Cr)-phosphocreatine (PCr) system plays an important role in energy storage and transmission. Synthesis and transport of Cr are integral parts of cellular energy metabolism. Neuroimaging findings in creatine deficiency disorder are marked by the decrease or total lack of the creatine-phosphocreatine peak at 3.0 and 3.9 ppm in the patient's brain on in vivo proton MRS. Repletion with oral creatine can be followed by total Cr and phosphocreatine evaluated by 1H MRS and 31P MRS and shows a mild increase in brain creatine, although still below the normal range in small studies that have looked at this.

12.8.3 Cerebral Creatine Deficiency: Imaging

Structural imaging may be normal or demonstrate mild nonspecific changes such as volume loss and T2 prolongation in the globus pallidus [198] (Fig. 12.22). However, MRS is an important diagnostic tool, revealing low creatine and phosphocreatine at 3.0 and 3.9 ppm (Fig. 12.22).

12.8.4 Molybdenum Cofactor Deficiency

As the name implies, the molybdenum cofactor is deficient in molybdenum cofactor, an autosomal recessive disorder [3]. Severe neonatal encephalopathy and refractory epilepsy ensue in the first days of life, mimicking hypoxic ischemic encephalopathy with some precision.

12.8.5 Molybdenum Cofactor Deficiency: Imaging

Restricted diffusion preferentially affecting the cerebral cortex at the depths of sulci has been proclaimed as a distinctive disease pattern [202]. Destructive white matter and basal ganglia disease with rapidly progressive coagulative necrosis, atrophy, and delayed myelination in a neonate with a

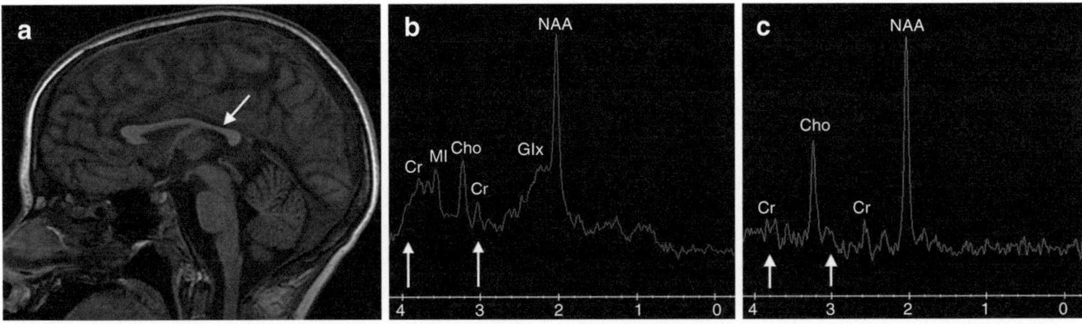

Fig. 12.22 11-year-old male with cerebral creatine deficiency due to a creatine transporter defect. Sagittal T1WI (TR/TE/IT ms, 11/5/500) (**a**) demonstrates thinning of the corpus callosum consistent with mild cerebral white matter volume loss or hypoplasia (*arrow*). Single-voxel MR spectroscopy (TR/TE ms, 1500/35) (**b**) and (TR/TE ms, 1500/144) (**c**) reveal markedly decreased creatine at 3.0 and 3.9 ppm (*arrows*). NAA, choline (Cho), glutamine/glutamate (Glx), and myoinositol (MI) are within normal range

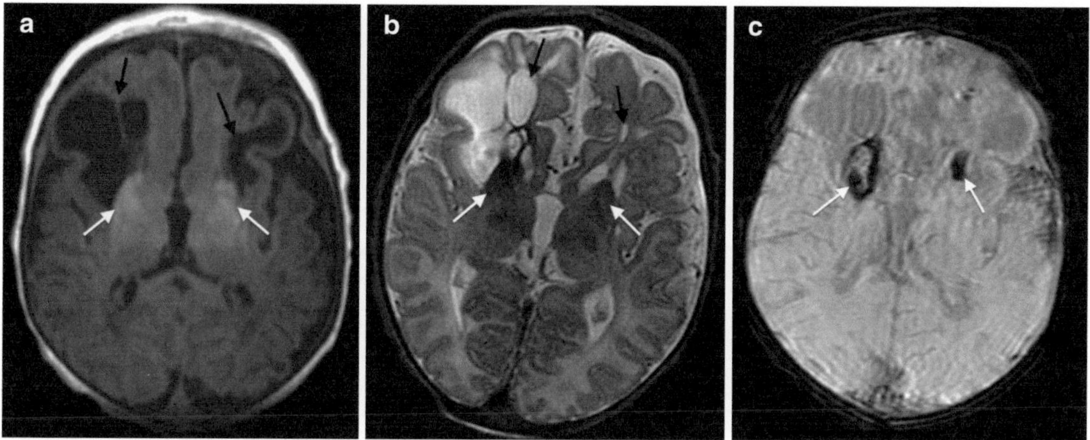

Fig. 12.23 3-day-old female with molybdenum cofactor deficiency. Axial T2WI (TR/TE ms, 3500/120) (**a**), T1WI (TR/TE/IT ms, 7/2/700) (**b**), and axial susceptibility-weighted angiography (SWAN) (TR/TE ms, 47/25) (**c**) through the basal ganglia demonstrate sequela of old basal ganglia injury and hemorrhage with T2 shortening (*white arrows*, **a**), T1 shortening (*white arrows*, **b**), and susceptibility hypointensity (*arrows*, **c**). Old necrotic white matter lesions are present in the frontal lobes bilaterally (*black arrows*, **a** and **b**)

presentation inconsistent with HIE are suggestive of molybdenum cofactor deficiency [3, 203, 204] (Fig. 12.23). Unlike HIE, the thalami are usually spared [3]. Furthermore, because hypoxic-ischemic injury most commonly occurs in the perinatal period, chronic-appearing lesions with necrosis, gliosis, and atrophy are uncommon (Fig. 12.23). Decreased uric acid in the blood and sulfite on urine dipstick will help confirm the diagnosis [3].

12.9 Other Disorders

12.9.1 Rett Syndrome (RS)

Rett syndrome is an X-linked neurodevelopmental disorder nearly exclusively affecting females. Most cases are caused by an MECP2 mutation. The classical presentation described by Andreas Rett is characterized by infantile developmental regression, seizures, and hand-wringing. With the advent of molecular testing, a spectrum of clinical findings is appreciated including milder phenotypes with some preserved language and head size. Histopathologically, progressive neuronal dendritic process atrophy occurs, mostly affecting projectional fibers [205]. Histopathologically, progressive neuronal dendritic process atrophy occurs, mostly affecting projectional fibers [205].

12.9.2 Rett Syndrome: Imaging

Neuroimaging demonstrates progressive parietal, cortical, thalamic, and caudate atrophy with relative occipital sparing [206–208] (Fig. 12.24). Disease severity correlates with the degree of anterior frontal lobe involvement [206].

MRS can be useful for diagnosis and disease monitoring. NAA, a marker of mature healthy neurons, may be decreased even prior to structural abnormalities on conventional MRI [208]. NAA progressively declines on follow-up studies [208, 209]. Cerebral choline and myoinositol are elevated in early disease but also diminish over time [208, 209].

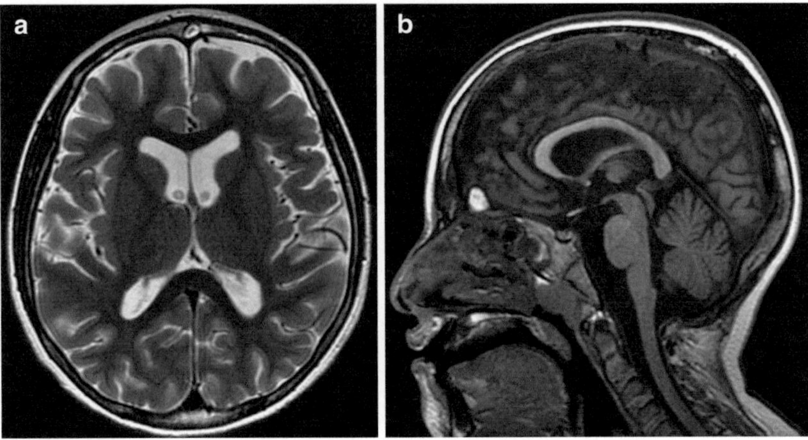

Fig. 12.24 8-year-old female with Rett syndrome. Sagittal T1WI (TR/TE/IT ms, 11/5/500) (**a**) and axial T2WI (TR/TE ms, 4548/102) (**b**) demonstrate mild diffuse cerebral cortical volume loss with prominent sulci and normal thickness of the corpus callosum

12.9.3 Smith-Lemli-Opitz Syndrome

Smith-Lemli-Opitz syndrome (SLOS) was identified initially as a dysmorphic syndrome and later found to be caused by deficiency of 7-dehydrocholesterol (7-DHC) reductase, the final step in the cholesterol synthetic pathway [210, 211]. Growth retardation with microcephaly, moderate to severe intellectual disability, and various severities of malformations are observed in this disorder. The spectrum of manifestation is wide with some patients having near-normal development and minor malformations. Second and third toe syndactyly and characteristic facial dysmorphism are clinical clues to the diagnosis [212]. With insufficient cholesterol, prechordal mesenchyme signaling is disturbed causing brain malformations along a centrifugal and ventrodorsal gradient mechanistically similar to classical holoprosencephaly (HPE) [213].

12.9.4 Smith-Lemli-Opitz Syndrome: Imaging

HPE features may be present with failed separation of parts of the ventral forebrain and/or diencephalon [213]. Multiple midline anomalies may include any combination of corpus callosum dysgenesis, anterior commissure hypoplasia, forniceal dysplasia, hypoplasia of a persistent cavum septum pellucidum/vergae, dysgenesis of the medulla oblongata, and vermian hypoplasia [27, 214] (Fig. 12.25). The degree of corpus callosum dysgenesis correlates with the clinical severity [215]. Other findings that have been described include polymicrogyria, hippocampal underrotation, extra-axial cysts, and volume loss [212–216]. On MRS, increased lipids and choline may be present in the cerebral white matter that may improve with treatment [217].

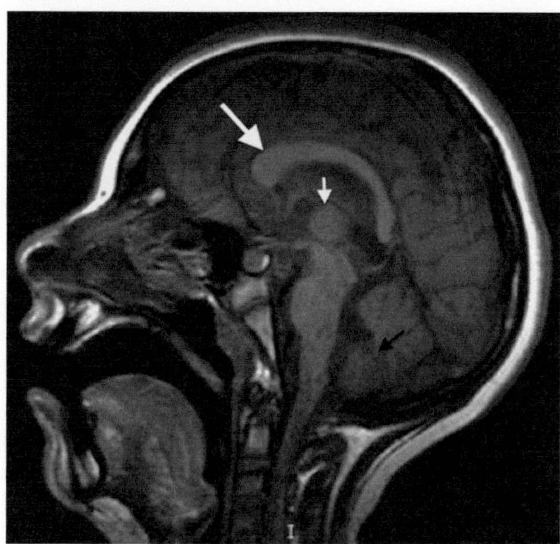

Fig. 12.25 Sagittal midline T1WI from a patient with Smith-Lemli-Opitz syndrome demonstrates a thickened, malformed corpus callosum lacking the normal rostrum (*large white arrow*), enlarged thalamic massa intermedia (*small white arrow*), and hypoplasia of the vermis (*black arrow*). The brainstem is also mildly hypoplastic. The brain to face ratio is small, consistent with micrencephaly

12.9.5 Alexander Disease

Alexander disease is a leukodystrophy associated with glial fibrillary acidic protein mutation(s) presenting in the neonatal, infantile, childhood (juvenile), or adult periods [218–222]. As with most inborn errors of metabolism, disease severity tends to correlate with symptom onset; younger patients have more severe disease [219, 223]. Type I (early onset) includes neonatal, infantile, and early childhood (up to age 4) presentations and dominantly manifests cerebral white matter disease [223]. Type II (late onset) includes patients older than age 4 years and presents mainly with infratentorial disease [223]. Abnormal Rosenthal fiber accumulation in the central nervous system is diagnostic.

12.9.6 Alexander: Imaging

Obviating the need for biopsy, diagnosis can be alternatively established on MRI when four of five of the following criteria are met: frontal predominant cerebral white matter disease (anteroposterior gradient of progression), differing signal of the periventricular white matter, basal ganglia involvement, brainstem involvement, and contrast enhancement [219] (Fig. 12.26). While fairly sensitive and specific, these imaging criteria are not met in all patients. Rare variant presentations can manifest predominant posterior fossa structure involvement, asymmetry, and milder cerebral leukoencephalopathy [224]. Rosenthal fiber aggregation at least partially causes these characteristic brain signal changes and abnormal enhancement. Spongiform changes cause regional swelling in active areas of disease, collectively contributing to macrencephaly/macrocephaly along with hydrocephalus that also may occur (Fig. 12.26). The latter is caused by subependymal periaqueductal Rosenthal fiber accumulation and secondary aqueductal stenosis [219, 225]. Facilitated diffusion is present in most of the involved white matter; periventricular and ependymal areas with dense Rosenthal fiber accumulation may demonstrate intermediate

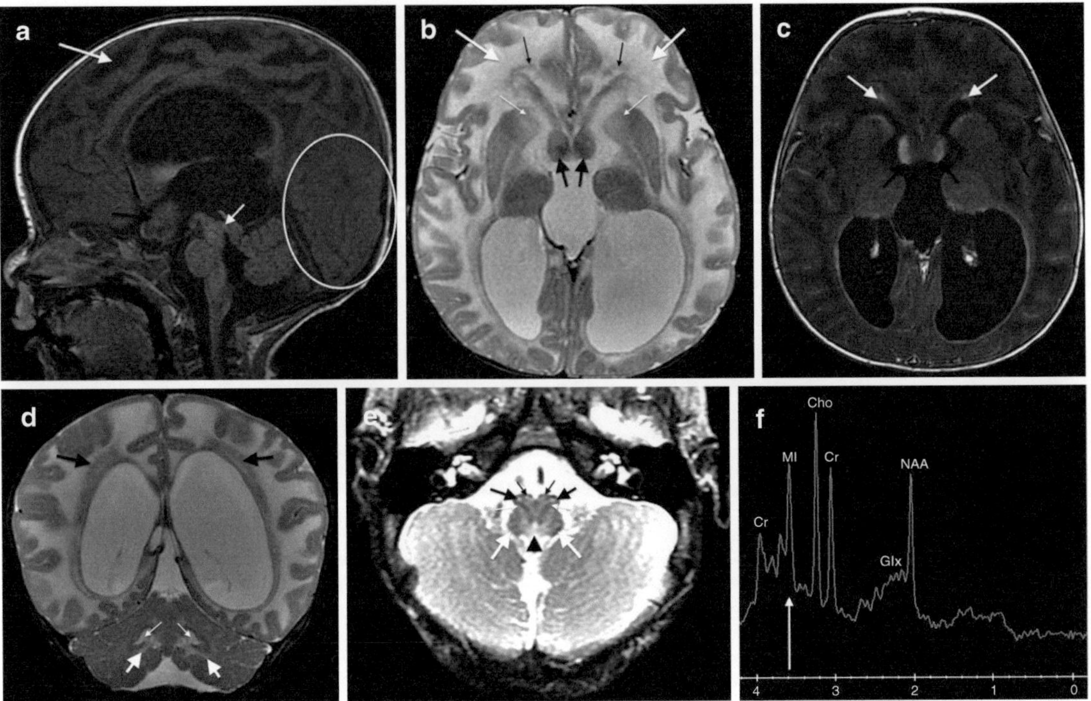

Fig. 12.26 5-month-old male with Alexander disease. Sagittal TWI (TR/TE/IT ms, 12/5/500) (**a**) demonstrates extensive frontal predominant hypointense cerebral subcortical white matter signal (*large white arrow*), relatively sparing the occipital lobes (*circle*), consistent with leukodystrophy. There is nodular thickening along and within the cerebral aqueduct causing aqueductal stenosis (*small white arrow*) and consequent hydrocephalus. There is mass-like enlargement of the optic chiasm (*black arrow*). Axial T2WI (TR/TE ms, 4500/100) (**b**) and post-contrast T1WI (TR/TE ms, 577/10) (**c**) show extensive white matter hyperintensity with an anteroposterior gradient (*large white arrows*, **b**), hyperintense signal in the striatum (*small white arrows*, **b**), an enhancing frontal paraventricular rim of signal intermediate to gray matter representing local Rosenthal fiber accumulation (*small black arrows*, **b** and *white arrows*, **c**), and thickening/enhancement of the fornices (*large black arrows*, **b** and *black arrows*, **c**). There is also thin ependymal signal alteration and enhancement along the remainder of the ventricles. Ventriculomegaly is consistent with hydrocephalus. Coronal T2WI (TR/TE ms, 4550/98) (**d**) demonstrates hyperintense signal in the cerebellar white matter (*large white arrows*) and hila of the dentate nucleus (*small white arrows*). There is striated signal alteration similar to gray matter signal in the parietal paraventricular white matter (*black arrows*). Axial T2WI (TR/TE ms, 577/10) (**e**) through the medulla oblongata shows multifocal hyperintense signal in the medullary pyramids (*small black arrows*) and central inferior olivary nuclear complexes (*large black arrows*) but sparing the olivary amiculum. The dorsal midline medulla is also involved (*arrowhead*), but the inferior peduncles are spared (*large white arrows*). Single-voxel MRS (TR/TE ms, 1500/35) (**f**) shows elevated myoinositol (MI, *arrow*)

diffusion characteristics. Mass-like/tumoral changes can occur in the cerebellum, brainstem, and optic pathway, simulating neoplasm [224, 226, 227] (Fig. 12.26). A "tigroid" cerebral white matter pattern has been demonstrated in some cases [228]. Myoinositol and lactate may be elevated, and NAA may be decreased in affected white matter [229–233] (Fig. 12.26).

Other macrocephalic leukodystrophies in the differential diagnosis include Canavan disease, glutaric aciduria type I, and megalencephalic leukodystrophy with subcortical cysts (MLSC). Canavan disease often has more widespread white matter disease without frontal predominance, sparing of the striatum, and, importantly, elevated NAA on MRS. Glutaric aciduria type I generally manifests incomplete opercularization and prominent temporopolar extra-axial spaces. Patients with MLSC generally have a milder clinical course and develop cystic changes in the anterior temporal and, sometimes also, the frontal lobes.

12.9.7 Biotinidase Deficiency

Biotinidase deficiency is the result of inability to recycle protein-bound biotin. Early recognition has profound implications for patient outcome because biotinidase deficiency is one of the few treatable neurometabolic disorders [234, 235]. If untreated, children with profound biotinidase deficiency exhibit early neurologic abnormalities including seizures, hypotonia, ataxia, developmental delay, vision problems, hearing loss, and skin and hair abnormalities. In milder cases, late onset is seen with limb weakness, spastic paresis, and decreased visual acuity. Early recognition and treatment are vital since once vision problems, hearing loss, and developmental delay occur, they are irreversible, even with supplementation. Symptoms of a biotinidase deficiency can appear just days after birth. If left untreated, the disorder can rapidly lead to coma and death [236]. Symptom severity is predictably correlated with the severity of the enzyme defect. Profound biotinidase deficiency refers to situations where enzyme activity is 10% or less. Individuals with partial biotinidase deficiency may have enzyme activity of 10–30% [237].

12.9.8 Biotinidase Deficiency: Imaging

Neuroimaging may demonstrate symmetric T2 prolongation and/or restricted diffusion in the mesial temporal lobes, medial thalami, central tegmental tracts, optic nerves, fornix, mammillary bodies, cerebellar white matter, brainstem, and/or spinal cord white matter [234, 238–242]. Reduced diffusion and increased anisotropy have been described in the perirolandic white matter and centrum semiovale [243]. Subcortical "cysts" probably representing white matter necrosis have also been shown [244]. Treatment reversible cerebral white matter hypodensity and hyperintensity on T2WI and progressive brain gray matter atrophy may also occur [245–248]. MR spectroscopy can reveal abnormal lactate that may persist during times of metabolic compensation [249].

References

1. Barkovich AJ. An approach to MRI of metabolic disorders in children. J Neuroradiol. 2007;34(2):75–88.
2. Barkovich AJ. A magnetic resonance approach to metabolic disorders in childhood. Rev Neurol. 2006;43(Suppl 1):S5–16.
3. Barkovich JA, Patay Z. Metabolic, toxic, and inflammatory brain disorders. In: Barkovich AJ, Raybaud C, editors. Pediatric neuroimaging. 5th ed. Philadelphia: Lippincott Williams & Wilkins; 2012.
4. Patay Z. Metabolic disorders. In: Tortori-Donati P, Rossi A, editors. Pediatric neuroradiology: brain, head, neck and spine. Berlin: Springer; 2009.
5. Vairo F, Vedolin L. The basis of inborn errors of metabolism for neuroradiologists. Top Magn Reson Imaging. 2011;22(5):209–14.
6. Edwards MK. Imaging of metabolic diseases of the brain. Curr Opin Radiol. 1991;3(1):25–30.
7. Longo MG, Vairo F, Souza CF, Giugliani R, Vedolin LM. Brain imaging and genetic risk in the pediatric population, part 1: inherited metabolic diseases. Neuroimaging Clin N Am. 2015;25(1):31–51.
8. Saudubray JM, Sedel F, Walter JH. Clinical approach to treatable inborn metabolic diseases: an introduction. J Inherit Metab Dis. 2006;29:261–74.
9. Banerjee S, Bhat MA. Neuron-glial interactions in blood-brain barrier formation. Annu Rev Neurosci. 2007;30:235–58.
10. Morton DH, Strauss KA, Robinson DL, Puffenberger EG, Kelley RI. Diagnosis and treatment of maple syrup disease: a study of 36 patients. Pediatrics. 2002;109:999–1008.
11. Funchal C, Gottfried C, De Almeida LM, Wajner M, Pessoa-Pureur R. Evidence that the branched-chain alpha-keto acids accumulating in maple syrup urine disease induce morphological alterations and death in cultured astrocytes from rat cerebral cortex. Glia. 2004;48:230–40.
12. Riviello JJ, Rezvani I, DiGeorge AM, Foley CM. Cerebral edema causing death in children with maple syrup urine disease. J Pediatr. 1991;119:42–5.
13. Brismar J, Aqeel A, Brismar G, Coates R, Gascon G, Ozand P. Maple syrup urine disease: findings on CT and MR scans of the brain in 10 infants. AJNR Am J Neuroradiol. 1990;11(6):1219–28.

14. Kar J, Nguyen FN, Moody SB. Pattern of restricted diffusion seen on magnetic resonance imaging in maple syrup urine disease. Pediatr Neurol. 2013;49(6):505–6.
15. Jain A, Jagdeesh K, Mane R, Singla S. Imaging in classic form of maple syrup urine disease: a rare metabolic central nervous system. J Clin Neonatol. 2013;2(2):98–100.
16. Indiran V, Gunaseelan RE. Neuroradiological findings in maple syrup urine disease. J Pediatr Neurosci. 2013;8(1):31–3.
17. Terek D, Koroglu O, Yalaz M, Gokben S, Calli C, Coker M, Kultursay N. Diagnostic tools of early brain disturbances in an asymptomatic neonate with maple syrup urine disease. Neuropediatrics. 2014;44(4):208–12.
18. Parmar H, Sitoh YY, Ho L. Maple syrup urine disease: diffusion-weighted and diffusion-tensor magnetic resonance imaging findings. J Comput Assist Tomogr. 2004;28(1):93–7.
19. Righini A, Ramenghi LA, Parini R, Triulzi F, Mosca F. Water apparent diffusion coefficient and T2 changes in the acute stage of maple syrup urine disease: evidence of intramyelinic and vasogenic-interstitial edema. J Neuroimaging. 2003;13(2):162–5.
20. Ha JS, Kim TK, Eun BL, Lee HS, Lee KY, Seol HY, Cha SH. Maple syrup urine disease encephalopathy: a follow-up study in the acute stage using diffusion-weighted MRI. Pediatr Radiol. 2004;34(2):163–6.
21. Schonberger S, Schweiger B, Schwahn B, et al. Dysmyelination in the brain of adolescents and young adults with maple syrup urine disease. Mol Genet Metab. 2004;82:69–75.
22. Klee D, Thimm E, Wittsack HJ, Schubert D, Primke R, Pentang G, Schaper J, Mödder U, Antoch A, Wendel U, Cohnen M. Structural white matter changes in adolescents and young adults with maple syrup urine disease. J Inherit Metab Dis. 2013;36(6):945–53.
23. Ferraz-Filho JR, Floriano VH, Quirici MB, Albuquerque RP, Souza AS. Contribution of the diffusion-weighted MRI in the diagnosis and follow-up of encephalopathy caused by maple syrup urine disease in a full-term newborn. Arq Neuropsiquiatr. 2009;67(3A):719–23.
24. Sato T, Muroya K, Hanakawa J, Asakura Y, Aida N, Tomiyasu M, Tajima G, Hasegawa T, Adachi M. Neonatal case of classic maple syrup urine disease: usefulness of (1) H-MRS in early diagnosis. Pediatr Int. 2014;56(1):112–5.
25. Felber SR, Sperl W, Chemelli A, Murr C, Wendel U. Maple syrup urine disease: metabolic decompensation monitored by proton magnetic resonance imaging and spectroscopy. Ann Neurol. 1993;33(4):396–401.
26. Hennermann JB. Clinical variability in glycine encephalopathy. Future Neurol. 2006;1:621–30.
27. Whitehead MT, Fricke ST, Gropman AL. Structural brain defects. Clin Perinatol. 2015;42(2):337–61.
28. Nicolasjilwan M, Ozer H, Wintermark M, Matsumoto J. Neonatal non-ketotic hyperglycinemia. J Neuroradiol. 2011;38(4):246–50.
29. Culjat M, Benjak V, Dasovic-Buljevic A, Ozretic D, Fumic K, Acquaviva C, Baric I. Magnetic resonance findings in a neonate with nonketotic hyperglycinemia: case report. J Comput Assist Tomogr. 2010;34(5):762–5.
30. Shah DK, Tingay DG, Fink AM, Hunt RW, Dargaville PA. Magnetic resonance imaging in neonatal nonketotic hyperglycinemia. Pediatr Neurol. 2005;33(1):50–2.
31. Khong PL, Lam BC, Chung BH, Wong KY, Ooi GC. Diffusion-weighted MR imaging in neonatal nonketotic hyperglycinemia. AJNR Am J Neuroradiol. 2003;24(6):1181–3.
32. Mourmans J, Majoie CB, Barth PG, Duran M, Akkerman EM, Poll-THE BT. Sequential MR imaging changes in nonketotic hyperglycinemia. AJNR Am J Neuroradiol. 2006;27(1):208–11.
33. Dobyns WB. Agenesis of the corpus callosum and gyral malformations are frequent manifestations of nonketotic hyperglycinemia. Neurology. 1989;39:817–20.
34. Gabis L, Parton P, Roche P, Lenn N, Tudorica A, Huang W. In vivo 1H magnetic resonance spectroscopic measurement of brain glycine levels in nonketotic hyperglycinemia. J Neuroimaging. 2001;11(2):209–11.
35. Radmanesh A, Zaman T, Ghanaati H, Molaei S, Robertson RL, Zamani AA. Methylmalonic acidemia: brain imaging findings in 52 children and a review of the literature. Pediatr Radiol. 2008;38(10):1054–61.
36. Baker EH, Sloan JL, Hauser NS, Gropman AL, Adams DR, Toro C, Manoli I, Venditti CP. MRI characteristics of globus pallidus infarcts in isolated methylmalonic acidemia. AJNR Am J Neuroradiol. 2015;36(1):194–201.
37. Işikay S, Temel L, Keskin M. Imaging findings associated with methylmalonic aciduria. Pediatr Neurol. 2014;50(4):435–6.
38. Andreula CF, De Blasi R, Carella A. CT and MR studies of methylmalonic acidemia. AJNR Am J Neuroradiol. 1991;12(3):410–2.
39. Ktena YP, Paul SM, Hauser NS, Sloan JL, Gropman A, Manoli I, Venditti CP. Delineating the spectrum of impairments, disabilities, and rehabilitation needs in methylmalonic acidemia (MMA). Am J Med Genet A. 2015;167A(9):2075–84.
40. Tanpaiboon P. Methylmalonic acidemia (MMA). Mol Genet Metab. 2005;85:2–6.
41. Sharrief AZ, Raffel J, Zee DS. Vitamin B(12) deficiency with bilateral globus pallidus abnormalities. Arch Neurol. 2012;69(6):769–72.
42. Yeşildağ A, Ayata A, Baykal B, Koroglu M, Yildiz H, Oral B, Oktem F, Oyar O. Magnetic resonance imaging and diffusion-weighted imaging in methylmalonic acidemia. Acta Radiol. 2005;46(1):101–3.

43. Michel SJ, Given CA, Robertson WC Jr. Imaging of the brain, including diffusion-weighted imaging in methylmalonic acidemia. Pediatr Radiol. 2004;34(7):580–2.
44. Brismar J, Ozand PT. CT and MR of the brain in disorders of the propionate and methylmalonate metabolism. AJNR Am J Neuroradiol. 1994;15(8):1459–73.
45. Pearl PL, Vezina LG, Saneto RP, McCarter R, Molloy-Wells E, Heffron A, Trzcinski S, McClintock WM, Conry JA, Elling NJ, Goodkin HP, de Menezes MS, Ferri R, Gilles E, Kadom N, Gaillard WD. Cerebral MRI abnormalities associated with vigabatrin therapy. Epilepsia. 2009;50(2):184–94.
46. Hegde AN, Mohan S, Lath N, Lim CC. Differential diagnosis for bilateral abnormalities of the basal ganglia and thalamus. Radiographics. 2011;31(1):5–30.
47. Harting I, Seitz A, Geb S, Zwickler T, Porto L, Lindner M, Kölker S, Hörster F. Looking beyond the basal ganglia: the spectrum of MRI changes in methylmalonic acidaemia. J Inherit Metab Dis. 2008;31(3):368–78.
48. Gao Y, Guan WY, Wang J, Zhang YZ, Li YH, Han LS. Fractional anisotropy for assessment of white matter tracts injury in methylmalonic acidemia. Chin Med J. 2009;122(8):945–9.
49. Takeuchi M, Harada M, Matsuzaki K, Hisaoka S, Nishitani H, Mori K. Magnetic resonance imaging and spectroscopy in a patient with treated methylmalonic acidemia. J Comput Assist Tomogr. 2003;27(4):547–51.
50. Trinh BC, Melhem ER, Barker PB. Multi-slice proton MR spectroscopy and diffusion-weighted imaging in methylmalonic acidemia: report of two cases and review of the literature. AJNR Am J Neuroradiol. 2001;22(5):831–3.
51. Davison JE, Davies NP, Wilson M, Sun Y, Chakrapani A, McKiernan PJ, Walter JH, Gissen P, Peet AC. MR spectroscopy-based brain metabolite profiling in propionic acidaemia: metabolic changes in the basal ganglia during acute decompensation and effect of liver transplantation. Orphanet J Rare Dis. 2011;6:19.
52. Desai NK, Runge VM, Crisp DE, Crisp MB, Naul LG. Magnetic resonance imaging of the brain in glutaric acidemia type I: a review of the literature and a report of four new cases with attention to the basal ganglia and imaging technique. Investig Radiol. 2003;38(8):489–96.
53. Brismar J, Ozand PT. CT and MR of the brain in glutaric acidemia type I: a review of 59 published cases and a report of 5 new patients. AJNR Am J Neuroradiol. 1995;16(4):675–83.
54. Citton V, Burlina A, Baracchini C, Gallucci M, Catalucci A, Dal Pos S, Burlina A, Manara R. Apparent diffusion coefficient restriction in the white matter: going beyond acute brain territorial ischemia. Insights Imaging. 2012;3(2):155–64.
55. Oguz KK, Ozturk A, Cila A. Diffusion-weighted MR imaging and MR spectroscopy in glutaric aciduria type 1. Neuroradiology. 2005;47(3):229–34.
56. Elster AW. Glutaric aciduria type I: value of diffusion-weighted magnetic resonance imaging for diagnosing acute striatal necrosis. J Comput Assist Tomogr. 2004;28(1):98–100.
57. Righini A, Fiori L, Parazzini C, Doneda C, Arrigoni F, Riva E, Triulzi F. Early prenatal magnetic resonance imaging of glutaric aciduria type 1: case report. J Comput Assist Tomogr. 2010;34(3):446–8.
58. Garbade SF, Greenberg CR, Demirkol M, Gökçay G, Ribes A, Campistol J, Burlina AB, Burgard P, Kölker S. Unravelling the complex MRI pattern in glutaric aciduria type I using statistical models-a cohort study in 180 patients. J Inherit Metab Dis. 2014;37(5):763–73.
59. Osaka H, Kimura S, Nezu A, Yamazaki S, Saitoh K, Yamaguchi S. Chronic subdural hematoma, as an initial manifestation of glutaric aciduria type-1. Brain and Development. 1993;15(2):125–7.
60. Cakmakci H, Pekcevik Y, Yis U, Unalp A, Kurul S. Diagnostic value of proton MR spectroscopy and diffusion-weighted MR imaging in childhood inherited neurometabolic brain diseases and review of the literature. Eur J Radiol. 2010;74(3):e161–71.
61. Harting I, Boy N, Heringer J, Seitz A, Bendszus M, Pouwels PJ, Kölker S. (1)H-MRS in glutaric aciduria type 1: impact of biochemical phenotype and age on the cerebral accumulation of neurotoxic metabolites. J Inherit Metab Dis. 2015;38(5):829–38.
62. Brusilow SW, Maestri NE. Urea cycle disorders: diagnosis, pathophysiology, and therapy. Adv Pediatr Infect Dis. 1996;43:127–70.
63. Yamanouchi H, Yokoo H, Yuhara Y, Maruyama K, Sasaki A, Hirato J, Nakazato Y. An autopsy case of ornithine transcarbamylase deficiency. Brain and Development. 2002;24(2):91–4.
64. Harding BN, et al. Ornithine carbamoyl transferase deficiency: a neuropathological study. Eur J Pediatr. 1984;141(4):215–20.
65. Kornfeld M, Woodfin BM, Papile L, Davis LE, Bernard LR. Neuropathology of ornithine carbamyl transferase deficiency. Acta Neuropathol. 1985;65(3–4):261–4.
66. Dolman CL, Clasen RA, Dorovini-Zis K. Severe cerebral damage in ornithine transcarbamylase deficiency. Clin Neuropathol. 1988;7(1):101–5.
67. Pacheco-Colón I, Fricke S, VanMeter J, Gropman AL. Advances in urea cycle neuroimaging: Proceedings from the 4th International Symposium on urea cycle disorders, Barcelona, Spain, September 2013. Mol Genet Metab. 2014;113(1–2):118–26.
68. Gunz AC, Choong K, Potter M, Miller E. Magnetic resonance imaging findings and neurodevelopmental outcomes in neonates with urea-cycle defects. Int Med Case Rep J. 2013;6:41–8.
69. Bireley WR, Van Hove JL, Gallagher RC, Fenton LZ. Urea cycle disorders: brain MRI and neurological outcome. Pediatr Radiol. 2012;42(4):455–62.

70. Gropman A. Brain imaging in urea cycle disorders. Mol Genet Metab. 2010;100(Suppl 1):S20–30.
71. Takanashi J, Barkovich AJ, Cheng SF, Weisiger K, Zlatunich CO, Mudge C, Rosenthal P, Tuchman M, Packman S. Brain MR imaging in neonatal hyperammonemic encephalopathy resulting from proximal urea cycle disorders. AJNR Am J Neuroradiol. 2003;24(6):1184–7.
72. White DA, Connor LT, Nardos B, Shimony JS, Archer R, Snyder AZ, Moinuddin A, Grange DK, Steiner RD, McKinstry RC. Age-related decline in the microstructural integrity of white matter in children with early- and continuously-treated PKU: a DTI study of the corpus callosum. Mol Genet Metab. 2010;99(Suppl 1):S41–6.
73. Anderson PJ, Leuzzi V. White matter pathology in phenylketonuria. Mol Genet Metab. 2010;99(Suppl 1):S3–9.
74. Ding XQ, Fiehler J, Kohlschutter B, Wittkugel O, Grzyska U, Zeumer H, Ullrich K. MRI abnormalities in normal-appearing brain tissue of treated adult PKU patients. J Magn Reson Imaging. 2008;27:998–1004.
75. Nardecchia F, Manti F, Chiarotti F, Carducci C, Carducci C, Leuzzi V. Neurocognitive and neuroimaging outcome of early treated young adult PKU patients: a longitudinal study. Mol Genet Metab. 2015;115(2–3):84–90.
76. Leuzzi V, Bianchi MC, Tosetti M, Carducci CL, Carducci CA, Antonozzi I. Clinical significance of brain phenylalanine concentration assessed by in vivo proton magnetic resonance spectroscopy in phenylketonuria. J Inherit Metab Dis. 2000;23(6):563–70.
77. Barkovich AJ, Peck WW. MR of Zellweger syndrome. AJNR Am J Neuroradiol. 1997;18(6):1163–70.
78. van der Knaap MS, Valk J. The MR spectrum of peroxisomal disorders. Neuroradiology. 1991;33(1):30–7.
79. Kerrigan JF, Aleck KA, Tarby TJ. Fumaric aciduria: clinical and imaging features. Ann Neurol. 2000;47(5):583–8.
80. Bruhn H, Kruse B, Korenke CG, Hanefeld F, Hanicke W, Merboldt KD, Frahm J. Proton NMR spectroscopy of cerebral metabolic alterations in infantile peroxisomal disorders. J Comput Assist Tomogr. 1992;16(3):335–44.
81. Cecil KM, Lindquist DM. Leukodystrophies. In: Bluml S, Panigrahy A, editors. MR spectroscopy of pediatric brain disorders. New York: Springer; 2013. p. 105–22.
82. Kim JH, Kim HJ. Childhood X-linked adrenoleukodystrophy: clinical-pathologic overview and MR imaging manifestations at initial evaluation and follow-up. Radiographics. 2005;25(3):619–31.
83. Moser HW. Adrenoleukodystrophy: phenotype, genetics, pathogenesis and therapy. Brain. 1997;120:1485–508.
84. Moser HW, Loes DJ, Melhem ER, Raymond GV, Bezman L, Cox CS, Lu SE. X-linked adrenoleukodystrophy: overview and prognosis as a function of age and brain magnetic resonance imaging abnormality. A study involving 372 patients. Neuropediatrics. 2000;31(5):227–39.
85. Berger J, Forss-Petter S, Eichler FS. Pathophysiology of X-linked adrenoleukodystrophy. Biochimie. 2014;98:135–42.
86. Barkovich AJ, Ferriero DM, Bass N, Boyer R. Involvement of the pontomedullary corticospinal tracts: a useful finding in the diagnosis of X-linked adrenoleukodystrophy. AJNR Am J Neuroradiol. 1997;18(1):95–100.
87. Melhem ER, Loes DJ, Georgiades CS, Raymond GV, Moser HW. X-linked adrenoleukodystrophy: the role of contrast-enhanced MR imaging in predicting disease progression. AJNR Am J Neuroradiol. 2000;21(5):839–44.
88. Melhem ER, Barker PB, Raymond GV, Moser HW. X-linked adrenoleukodystrophy in children: review of genetic, clinical, and MR imaging characteristics. AJR Am J Roentgenol. 1999;173(6):1575–81.
89. Loes DJ, Hite S, Moser H, Stillman AE, Shapiro E, Lockman L, Latchaw RE, Krivit W. Adrenoleukodystrophy: a scoring method for brain MR observations. AJNR Am J Neuroradiol. 1994;15(9):1761–6.
90. Eichler FS, Barker PB, Cox C, Edwin D, Ulug AM, Moser HM, Raymond GV. Proton MR spectroscopic imaging predicts lesion progression on MRI in X-linked adrenoleukodystrophy. Neurology. 2002;58:901–7.
91. ter Rahe BS, Majoie CB, Akkerman EM, den Heeten GT, Poll-The BT, Barth PG. Peroxisomal biogenesis disorder: comparison of conventional MR imaging with diffusion-weighted and diffusion-tensor imaging findings. AJNR Am J Neuroradiol. 2004;25(6):1022–7.
92. van der Voorn JP, Pouwels PJ, Powers JM, Kamphorst W, Martin JJ, Troost D, Spreeuwenberg MD, Barkhof F, van der Knaap MS. Correlating quantitative MR imaging with histopathology in X-linked adrenoleukodystrophy. AJNR Am J Neuroradiol. 2011;32(3):481–9.
93. Schneider JF, Il'yasov KA, Boltshauser E, Hennig J, Martin E. Diffusion tensor imaging in cases of adrenoleukodystrophy: preliminary experience as a marker for early demyelination? AJNR Am J Neuroradiol. 2003;24(5):819–24.
94. Friedman SD, Shaw DW, Ishak G, Gropman AL, Saneto RP. The use of neuroimaging in the diagnosis of mitochondrial disease. Dev Disabil Res Rev. 2010;16:129–35.
95. Saneto RP, Friedman SD, Shaw DW. Neuroimaging of mitochondrial disease. Mitochondrion. 2008;8(5–6):396–413.
96. Bianchi MC, Sgandurra G, Tosetti M, Battini R, Cioni G. Brain magnetic resonance in the diagnostic evaluation of mitochondrial encephalopathies. Biosci Rep. 2007;27(1–3):69–85.

97. Bianchi MC, Tosetti M, Battini R, Manca ML, Mancuso M, Cioni G, Canapicchi R, Siciliano G. Proton MR spectroscopy of mitochondrial diseases: analysis of brain metabolic abnormalities and their possible diagnostic relevance. Am J Neuroradiol. 2003;24:1958–66.
98. Haas R, Dietrich R. Neuroimaging of mitochondrial disorders. Mitochondrion. 2004;4:471–90.
99. Ishak GE, Poliakov AV, Poliachik SL, Saneto RP, Novotny EJ Jr, McDaniel S, Ojemann JG, Shaw DW, Friedman SD. Tract-based spatial statistical analysis of diffusion tensor imaging in pediatric patients with mitochondrial disease: widespread reduction in fractional anisotropy of white matter tracts. AJNR Am J Neuroradiol. 2012;33(9):1726–30.
100. Lin DD, Crawford TO, Barker PB. Proton MR spectroscopy in the diagnostic evaluation of suspected mitochondrial disease. AJNR Am J Neuroradiol. 2003;24:33–41.
101. Barkovich AJ, Good WV, Koch TK, Berg BO. Mitochondrial disorders: analysis of their clinical and imaging characteristics. AJNR Am J Neuroradiol. 1993;14(5):1119–37.
102. Dinopoulos A, Cecil KM, Schapiro MB, Papadimitriou A, Hadjigeorgiou GM, Wong B, deGrauw T, Egelhoff JC. Brain MRI and proton MRS findings in infants and children with respiratory chain defects. Neuropediatrics. 2005;36:290–301.
103. Gerards M, Sallevelt SC, Smeets HJ. Leigh syndrome: resolving the clinical and genetic heterogeneity paves the way for treatment options. Mol Genet Metab. 2016;117:300–12.
104. Baertling F, Rodenburg RJ, Schaper J, Smeitink JA, Koopman WJ, Mayatepek E, Morava E, Distelmaier F. A guide to diagnosis and treatment of Leigh syndrome. J Neurol Neurosurg Psychiatry. 2014;85(3):257–65.
105. Medina L, Chi TL, DeVivo DC, Hilal SK. MR findings in patients with subacute necrotizing encephalomyelopathy (Leigh syndrome): correlation with biochemical defect. AJR Am J Roentgenol. 1990;154(6):1269–74.
106. Ruhoy IS, Saneto RP. The genetics of Leigh syndrome and its implications for clinical practice and risk management. Appl Clin Genet. 2014;7:221–34.
107. Rahman S, Blok RD, Dahl HH, Danks DM, Kirby DM, Chow CW, Christodoulou J, Thorburn DR. Leigh syndrome: clinical features and biochemical and DNA abnormalities. Ann Neurol. 1996;39(3):343–51.
108. Parikh S, Goldstein A, Koenig MK, Scaglia F, Enns GM, Saneto R, Anselm I, Cohan BH, Falk MJ, Greene C, Gropman AL, Haas R, Hirano M, Morgan P, Sims K, Tarnopolsky MR, Van Hove L, Wolfe L, DiMauro S. Diagnosis and management of mitochondrial disease: a consensus statement from the Mitochondrial Medicine Society. Genet Med. 2015;17(9):689–701.
109. Arii J, Tanabe Y. Leigh syndrome: serial MR imaging and clinical follow-up. AJNR Am J Neuroradiol. 2000;21:1502–9.
110. Whitehead MT, Lee B, Gropman A. Lesional perfusion abnormalities in Leigh disease demonstrated by arterial spin labeling correlate with disease activity. Pediatr Radiol. 2016;46(9):1309–16.
111. Hirano M, Ricci E, Koenigsberger MR, Defendini R, Pavlakis SG, DeVivo DC, DiMauro S, Rowland LP. Melas: an original case and clinical criteria for diagnosis. Neuromuscul Disord. 1992;2(2):125–35.
112. Yoshida T, Ouchi A, Miura D, Shimoji K, Kinjo K, Sueyoshi T, Jonosono M, Rajput V. MELAS and reversible vasoconstriction of the major cerebral arteries. Intern Med. 2013;52(12):1389–92.
113. Pauli W, Zarzycki A, Krzyształowski A, Walecka A. CT and MRI imaging of the brain in MELAS syndrome. Pol J Radiol. 2013;78(3):61–5.
114. Abe K, Yoshimura H, Tanaka H, Fujita N, Hikita T, Sakoda S. Comparison of conventional and diffusion-weighted MRI and proton MR spectroscopy in patients with mitochondrial encephalomyopathy, lactic acidosis, and stroke-like events. Neuroradiology. 2004;46(2):113–7.
115. Brockmann K, Finsterbusch J, Schara U, Wilichowski E, Frahm J, Hanefeld F. Stroke-like pattern in DTI and MRS of childhood mitochondrial leukoencephalopathy. Neuroradiology. 2004;46:267–71.
116. Wilichowski E, Pouwels PJ, Frahm J, Hanefeld F. Quantitative proton magnetic resonance spectroscopy of cerebral metabolic disturbances in patients with MELAS. Neuropediatrics. 1999;30(5):256–63.
117. Moroni I, Bugiani M, Bizzi A, Castelli G, Lamantea E, Uziel G. Cerebral white matter involvement in children with mitochondrial encephalopathies. Neuropediatrics. 2002;33(2):79–85.
118. Weinstock A, Giglio P, Cohen ME, Bakshi R, Januario J, Balos L. Diffuse magnetic resonance imaging white-matter changes in a 15-year-old boy with mitochondrial encephalomyopathy. J Child Neurol. 2002;17(1):47–9.
119. Burgeois M, Goutieres F, Chretien D, Rustin P, Munnich A, Aicardi J. Deficiency in complex II of the respiratory chain, presenting as a leukodystrophy in two sisters with Leigh syndrome. Brain and Development. 1992;14:404–8.
120. Barnerias C, Saudubray JM, Touati G, De Lonlay P, Dulac O, Ponsot G, Marsac C, Brivet M, Desguerre I. Pyruvate dehydrogenase complex deficiency: four neurological phenotypes with differing pathogenesis. Dev Med Child Neurol. 2010;52(2):e1–9.
121. Ah Mew N, Loewenstein JB, Kadom N, Lichter-Konecki U, Gropman AL, Martin JM, Vanderver A. MRI features of 4 female patients with pyruvate dehydrogenase E1 alpha deficiency. Pediatr Neurol. 2011;45(1):57–9.
122. Cross JH, Connelly A, Gadian DG, Kendall BE, Brown GK, Brown RM, Leonard JV. Clinical diver-

sity of pyruvate dehydrogenase deficiency. Pediatr Neurol. 1994;10(4):276–83.
123. Sharma R, Sharrard MJ, Connolly DJ, Mordekar SR. Unilateral periventricular leukomalacia in association with pyruvate dehydrogenase deficiency. Dev Med Child Neurol. 2012;54(5):469–71.
124. Nissenkorn A, Michelson M, Ben-Zeev B, Lerman-Sagie T. Inborn errors of metabolism: a cause of abnormal brain development. Neurology. 2001;56(10):1265–72.
125. Prasad C, Rupar T, Prasad AN. Pyruvate dehydrogenase deficiency and epilepsy. Brain and Development. 2011;33(10):856–65.
126. Shevell MI, Matthews PM, Scriver CR, Brown RM, Otero LJ, Legris M, Brown GK, Arnold DL. Cerebral dysgenesis and lactic acidemia: an MRI/MRS phenotype associated with pyruvate dehydrogenase deficiency. Pediatr Neurol. 1994;11(3):224–9.
127. Kohlschütter A, Schulz A. Towards understanding the neuronal ceroid lipofuscinoses. Brain and Development. 2009;31(7):499–502.
128. Arsov T, Smith KR, Damiano J, Franceschetti S, Canafoglia L, Bromhead CJ, Andermann E, Vears DF, Cossette P, Rajagopalan S, McDougall A, Sofia V, Farrell M, Aguglia U, Zini A, Meletti S, Morbin M, Mullen S, Andermann F, Mole SE, Bahlo M, Berkovic SF. Kufs disease, the major adult form of neuronal ceroid lipofuscinosis, caused by mutations in CLN6. Am J Hum Genet. 2011;88(5):566–73.
129. Jadav RH, Sinha S, Yasha TC, Aravinda H, Rao S, Bindu PS, Satishchandra P. Magnetic resonance imaging in neuronal ceroid lipofuscinosis and its subtypes. Neuroradiol J. 2012;25(6):755–61.
130. Topçu M, Tan H, Yalnizoğlu D, Usubütün A, Saatçi I, Aynaci M, Anlar B, Topaloğlu H, Turanli G, Köse G, Aysun S. Evaluation of 36 patients from Turkey with neuronal ceroid lipofuscinosis: clinical, neurophysiological, neuroradiological and histopathologic studies. Turk J Pediatr. 2004;46(1):1–10.
131. D'Incerti L. MRI in neuronal ceroid lipofuscinosis. Neurol Sci. 2000;21(3 Suppl):S71–3.
132. Autti T, Joensuu R, Aberg L. Decreased T2 signal in the thalami may be a sign of lysosomal storage disease. Neuroradiology. 2007;49(7):571–8.
133. Autti T, Raininko R, Santavuori P, Vanhanen SL, Poutanen VP, Haltia M. MRI of neuronal ceroid lipofuscinosis. II. Postmortem MRI and histopathological study of the brain in 16 cases of neuronal ceroid lipofuscinosis of juvenile or late infantile type. Neuroradiology. 1997;39(5):371–7.
134. Autti T, Raininko R, Vanhanen SL, Santavuori P. MRI of neuronal ceroid lipofuscinosis. I. Cranial MRI of 30 patients with juvenile neuronal ceroid lipofuscinosis. Neuroradiology. 1996;38(5):476–82.
135. Levin SW, Baker EH, Gropman A, Quezado Z, Miao N, Zhang Z, Jollands A, Di Capua M, Caruso R, Mukherjee AB. Subdural fluid collections in patients with infantile neuronal ceroid lipofuscinosis. Arch Neurol. 2009;66(12):1567–71.
136. Baker EH, Levin SW, Zhang Z, Mukherjee AB. Evaluation of disease progression in INCL by MR spectroscopy. Ann Clin Transl Neurol. 2015;2(8):797–809.
137. Brockmann K, Pouwels PJ, Christen HJ, Frahm J, Hanefeld F. Localized proton magnetic resonance spectroscopy of cerebral metabolic disturbances in children with neuronal ceroid lipofuscinosis. Neuropediatrics. 1996;27(5):242–8.
138. Wenger DA. Krabbe disease: globoid cell leukodystrophy. 2003. In: Rosenberg RN, Prusiner SB, DiMauro S, Barchi RL, Nestler EJ, Eds. The molecular and genetic basis of neurologic and psychiatric disease. Philadelphia: Butterworth-Heinemann, 255-261.
139. Abdelhalim AN, Alberico RA, Barczykowski AL, Duffner PK. Patterns of magnetic resonance imaging abnormalities in symptomatic patients with Krabbe disease correspond to phenotype. Pediatr Neurol. 2014;50(2):127–34.
140. Romano A, De Simone R, Fasoli F, Ferrante M, Cipriani V, Fantozzi LM, Bozzoa A. Selective white matter involvement in a patient with late onset Krabbe disease: MR, MR spectroscopy, and diffusion tensor study. J Neuroimaging. 2009;19(2):191–3.
141. Wang C, Melberg A, Melberg A, Weis J, Månsson JE, Raininko R. The earliest MR imaging and proton MR spectroscopy abnormalities in adult-onset Krabbe disease. Acta Neurol Scand. 2007;116(4):268–72.
142. Henderson RD, MacMillan JC, Bradfield JM. Adult onset Krabbe disease may mimic motor neurone disease. J Clin Neurosci. 2003;10(5):638–9.
143. Gupta A, Poe MD, Styner MA, Panigrahy A, Escolar ML. Regional differences in fiber tractography predict neurodevelopmental outcomes in neonates with infantile Krabbe disease. Neuroimage Clin. 2014;7:792–8.
144. Poretti A, Meoded A, Bunge M, Fatemi A, Barrette P, Huisman TA, Salman MS. Novel diffusion tensor imaging findings in Krabbe disease. Eur J Paediatr Neurol. 2014;18(2):150–6.
145. Escolar ML, Poe MD, Smith JK, Gilmore JH, Kurtzberg J, Lin W, Styner M. Diffusion tensor imaging detects abnormalities in the corticospinal tracts of neonates with infantile Krabbe disease. AJNR Am J Neuroradiol. 2009;30(5):1017–21.
146. Guo AC, Petreall JR, Krutzberg J, Provenzale JM. Evaluation of white matter anisotropy in Krabbe disease with diffusion tensor MR imaging: initial experience. Radiology. 2001;218(3):809–15.
147. Zuccoli G, Narayanan S, Panigrahy A, Poe MD, Escolar ML. Midbrain morphology reflects extent of brain damage in Krabbe disease. Neuroradiology. 2015;57(7):739–45.
148. Loes DJ, Peters C, Krivit W. Globoid cell leukodystrophy: distinguishing early-onset from late-onset disease using a brain MR imaging scoring method. AJNR Am J Neuroradiol. 1999;20(2):316–23.

149. Livingston JH, Stivaros S, van der Knaap MS, Crow YJ. Recognizable phenotypes associated with intracranial calcification. Dev Med Child Neurol. 2013;55(1):46–57.
150. Livingston JH, Graziano C, Pysden K, Crow YJ, Mordekar SR, Moroni I, Uziel G. Intracranial calcification in early infantile Krabbe disease: nothing new under the sun. Dev Med Child Neurol. 2012;54(4):376–9.
151. Brockmann K, Dechent P, Wilken B, Rusch O, Frahm J, Hanefeld F. Proton MRS profile of cerebral metabolic abnormalities in Krabbe disease. Neurology. 2003;60(5):819–25.
152. Zarifi MK, Tzika AA, Astrakas LG, Poussaint TY, Anthony DC, Darras BT. Magnetic resonance spectroscopy and magnetic resonance imaging findings in Krabbe's disease. J Child Neurol. 2001;16:522–6.
153. van Rappard DF, Boelens JJ, Wolf NI. Metachromatic leukodystrophy: disease spectrum and approaches for treatment. Best Pract Res Clin Endocrinol Metab. 2015;29(2):261–73.
154. Gieselmann V. Metachromatic leukodystrophy: genetics, pathogenesis and therapeutic options. Acta Paediatr Suppl. 2008;97:15–21.
155. Groeschel S, Dali C, Clas P, Böhringer J, Duno M, Krarup C, Kehrer C, Wilke M, Krägeloh-Mann I. Cerebral gray and white matter changes and clinical course in metachromatic leukodystrophy. Neurology. 2012;79(16):1662–70.
156. Kim TS, Kim IO, Kim WS, Choi YS, Lee JY, Kim OW, Yeon KM, Kim KJ, Hwang YS. MR of childhood metachromatic leukodystrophy. AJNR Am J Neuroradiol. 1997;18(4):733–8.
157. Faerber EN, Melvin J, Smergel EM. MRI appearances of metachromatic leukodystrophy. Pediatr Radiol. 1999;29(9):669–72.
158. van der Voorn JP, Pouwels PJ, Kamphorst W, Powers JM, Lammens M, Barkhof F, van der Knaap MS. Histopathologic correlates of radial stripes on MR images in lysosomal storage disorders. AJNR Am J Neuroradiol. 2005;26(3):442–6.
159. Oguz KK, Anlar B, Senbil N, Cila A. Diffusion-weighted imaging findings in juvenile metachromatic leukodystrophy. Neuropediatrics. 2004;35(5):279–82.
160. Kruse B, Hanefeld F, Christen HJ, Bruhn H, Michaelis T, Hänicke W, Frahm J. Alterations of brain metabolites in metachromatic leukodystrophy as detected by localized proton magnetic resonance spectroscopy in vivo. J Neurol. 1993;241(2):68–74.
161. Sener RN. Metachromatic leukodystrophy. Diffusion MR imaging and proton MR spectroscopy. Acta Radiol. 2003;44(4):440–3.
162. Desnick RJ, Kaback MM. Advances in genetics: Tay-Sachs disease, Advances in genetics series, vol. 44. San Diego: Academic Press; 2001.
163. Maegawa GH, Stockley T, Tropak M, Banwell B, Blaser S, Kok F, Giugliani R, Mahuran D, Clarke JT. The natural history of juvenile or subacute GM2 gangliosidosis: 21 new cases and literature review of 134 previously reported. Pediatrics. 2006;118(5):e1550–62.
164. Aydin K, Bakir B, Tatli B, Terzibasioglu E, Ozmen M. Proton MR spectroscopy in three children with Tay-Sachs disease. Pediatr Radiol. 2005;35(11):1081–5.
165. Imamura A, Miyajima H, Ito R, Orii KO. Serial MR imaging and 1H-MR spectroscopy in monozygotic twins with Tay-Sachs disease. Neuropediatrics. 2008;39(5):259–63.
166. Migdalska-Richards A, Schapira AH. The relationship between glucocerebrosidase mutations and Parkinson disease. J Neurochem. 2016;139(Suppl 1):77–90.
167. Krishna SH, McKinney AM, Lucato LT. Congenital genetic inborn errors of metabolism presenting as an adult or persisting into adulthood: neuroimaging in the more common or recognizable disorders. Semin Ultrasound CT MR. 2014;35(2):160–91.
168. Abdel Razek AA, Abd El-Gaber N, Abdalla A, Fathy A, Azab A, Rahman AA. Apparent diffusion coefficient vale of the brain in patients with Gaucher's disease type II and type III. Neuroradiology. 2009;51(11):773–9.
169. Davies EH, Seunarine KK, Banks T, Clark CA, Vellodi A. Brain white matter abnormalities in paediatric Gaucher Type I and Type III using diffusion tensor imaging. J Inherit Metab Dis. 2011;34(2):549–53.
170. Mercimek-Mahmutoglu S, Gruber S, Rolfs A, Stadlbauer A, Woeber C, Kurnik P, Voigtlaender T, Moser E, Stoeckler-Ipsiroglu S. Neurological and brain MRS findings in patients with Gaucher disease type 1. Mol Genet Metab. 2007;91(4):390–5.
171. Yanjanin NM, Vélez JI, Gropman A, King K, Bianconi SE, Conley SK, Brewer CC, Solomon B, Pavan WJ, Arcos-Burgos M, Patterson MC, Porter FD. Linear clinical progression, independent of age of onset, in Niemann-Pick disease, type C. Am J Med Genet B Neuropsychiatr Genet. 2010;153B(1):132–40.
172. Huang JY, Peng SF, Yang CC, Yen KY, Tzen KY, Yen RF. Neuroimaging findings in a brain with Niemann-Pick type C disease. J Formos Med Assoc. 2011;110(8):537–42.
173. Walterfang M, Fahey M, Desmond P, Wood A, Seal ML, Steward C, Adamson C, Kokkinos C, Fietz M, Velakoulis D. White and gray matter alterations in adults with Niemann-Pick disease type C: a cross-sectional study. Neurology. 2010;75(1):49–56.
174. Lee R, Apkarian K, Jung ES, Yanjanin N, Yoshida S, Mori S, Park J, Gropman A, Baker EH, Porter FD. Corpus callosum diffusion tensor imaging and volume measures are associated with disease severity in pediatric Niemann-Pick disease type C1. Pediatr Neurol. 2014;51(5):669–74.e5.

175. Rieger D, Auerbach S, Robinson P, Gropman A. Neuroimaging of lipid storage disorders. Dev Disabil Res Rev. 2013;17(3):269–82.
176. Takanashi J, Hayashi M, Yuasa S, Satoh H, Terada H. Hypoyelination in I-cell disease; MRI, MR spectroscopy and neuropathological correlation. Brain and Development. 2012;34(9):780–3.
177. Altarescu G, Sun M, Moore DF, Smith JA, Wiggs EA, Solomon BI, Patronas NJ, Frei KP, Gupta S, Kaneski CR, Quarrell OW, Slaugenhaupt SA, Goldin E, Schiffmann R. The neurogenetics of mucolipidosis type IV. Neurology. 2002;59(3):306–13.
178. Frei KP, Patronas NJ, Crutchfield KE, Altarescu G, Schiffmann R. Mucolipidosis type IV: characteristic MRI findings. Neurology. 1998;51(2):565–9.
179. Geer JS, Skinner SA, Goldin E, Holden KR. Mucolipidosis type IV: a subtle pediatric neurodegenerative disorder. Pediatr Neurol. 2010;42(3):223–6.
180. Breningstall GN, Tubman DE. Magnetic resonance imaging in a patient with I-cell disease. Clin Neurol Neurosurg. 1994;96(2):161–3.
181. Wakabayashi K, Gustafson AM, Sidransky E, Goldin E. Mucolipidosis type IV: an update. Mol Genet Metab. 2011;104(3):206–13.
182. Schiffmann R, Mayfield J, Swift C, Nestrasil I. Quantitative neuroimaging in mucolipidosis type IV. Mol Genet Metab. 2014;111(2):147–51.
183. Bonavita S, Virta A, Jeffries N, Goldin E, Tedeschi G, Schiffmann R. Diffuse neuroaxonal involvement in mucolipidosis IV as assessed by proton magnetic resonance spectroscopic imaging. J Child Neurol. 2003;18:443–9.
184. Bonnefont JP, Djouadi F, Prip-Buus C, Gobin S, Munnich A, Bastin J. Carnitine palmitoyltransferases 1 and 2: biochemical, molecular and medical aspects. Genomics. 1994;24(1):195–7.
185. Gellera C, Verderio E, Floridia G, Finocchiaro G, Montermini L, Cavadini P, Zuffardi O, Taroni F. Assignment of the human carnitine palmitoyltransferase II gene (CPT1) to chromosome 1p32. Genomics. 1994;24(1):195–7.
186. Elpeleg ON, Hammerman C, Saada A, Shaag A, Golzand E, Hochner-Celnikier D, Berger I, Nadjari M. Antenatal presentation of carnitine palmitoyltransferase II deficiency. Am J Med Genet. 2001;102:183–7.
187. Isackson PJ, Bennett MJ, Lichter-Konecki U, Willis M, Nyhan WL, Sutton VR, Tein I, Vladutiu GD. CPT2 gene mutations resulting in lethal neonatal or severe infantile carnitine palmitoyltransferase II deficiency. Mol Genet Metab. 2008;94:422–7.
188. North KN, Hoppel CL, De Girolami U, Kozakewich HP, Korson MS. Lethal neonatal deficiency of carnitine palmitoyltransferase II associated with dysgenesis of the brain and kidneys. J Pediatr. 1995;127:414–20.
189. Pierce MR, Pridjian G, Morrison S, Pickoff AS. Fatal carnitine palmitoyltransferase II deficiency in a newborn: new phenotypic features. Clin Pediatr (Phila). 1999;38:13–20.
190. Ferreira CR, Silber MH, Chang T, Murnick JG, Kirmse B. Cerebral lipid accumulation detected by MRS in a child with carnitine palmitoyltransferase 2 deficiency: a case report and review of the literature on genetic etiologies of lipid peaks on MRS. JIMD Rep. 2016;28:69–74.
191. Bouchireb K, Teychene AM, Rigal O, de Lonlay P, Valayannopoulos V, Gaudelus J, Sellier N, Bonnefont JP, Brivet M, de Pontual L. Post-mortem MRI reveals CPT2 deficiency after sudden infant death. Eur J Pediatr. 2010;169(12):1561–3.
192. Seto T, Kono K, Morimoto K, Inoue Y, Shintaku H, Hattori H, Matsuoka O, Yamano T, Tanaka A. Brain magnetic resonance imaging in 23 patients with mucopolysaccharidoses and the effect of bone marrow transplantation. Ann Neurol. 2001;50(1):79–92.
193. Lee C, Dineen TE, Brack M, Kirsch JE, Runge VM. The mucopolysaccharidoses: characterization by cranial MR imaging. AJNR Am J Neuroradiol. 1993;14(6):1285–92.
194. Zafeiriou DI, Batzios SP. Brain and spinal MR imaging findings in mucopolysaccharidoses: a review. AJNR Am J Neuroradiol. 2013;34(1):5–13.
195. Rasalkar DD, Chu WCW, Hui J, Chu C-M, Paunipager BK, Li C-K. Pictorial review of mucopolysaccharidosis with emphasis on MRI features of brain and spine. Br J Radiol. 2011;84(1001):469–77. The British Institute of Radiology.
196. Calleja Gero ML, González Gutiérrez-Solana L, López Marín L, López Pino MA, Fournier Del Castillo C, Duat Rodríguez A. Neuroimaging findings in patient series with mucopolysaccharidosis. Neurologia. 2012;27(7):407–13.
197. Takahashi Y, Sukegawa K, Aoki M, Ito A, Suzuki K, Sakaguchi H, Watanabe M, Isogai K, Mizuno S, Hoshi H, Kuwata K, Tomatsu S, Kato S, Ito T, Kondo N, Orii T. Evaluation of accumulated mucopolysaccharides in the brain of patients with mucopolysaccharidoses by (1)H-magnetic resonance spectroscopy before and after bone marrow transplantation. Pediatr Res. 2001;49(3):349–55.
198. Clark JF, Cecil KM. Diagnostic methods and recommendations for the cerebral creatine deficiency syndromes. Pediatr Res. 2015;77(3):398–405.
199. Braissant O, Henry H. AGAT, GAMT and SLC6A8 distribution in the central nervous system, in relation to creatine deficiency syndromes: a review. J Inherit Metab Dis. 2008;31(2):230–9.
200. Braissant O, Henry H, Beard E, Uldry J. Creatine deficiency syndromes and the importance of creatine synthesis in the brain. Amino Acids. 2011;40:1315–24.
201. Cheillan D, Cognat S, Vandenberghe N, Des Portes V, Vianey-Saban C. Creatine deficiency syndromes. Rev Neurol (Paris). 2005;161:284–9.
202. Stence NV, Coughlin CR 2nd, Fenton LZ, Thomas JA. Distinctive pattern of restricted diffusion in

a neonate with molybdenum cofactor deficiency. Pediatr Radiol. 2013;43(7):882–5.
203. Higuchi R, Sugimoto T, Tamura A, Kioka N, Tsuno Y, Higa A, Yoshikawa N. Early features in neuroimaging of two siblings with molybdenum cofactor deficiency. Pediatrics. 2014;133(1):e267–71.
204. Vijayakumar K, Gunny R, Grunewald S, Carr L, Chong KW, DeVile C, Robinson R, McSweeney N, Prabhakar P. Clinical neuroimaging features and outcome in molybdenum cofactor deficiency. Pediatr Neurol. 2011;45(4):246–52.
205. Armstrong DD. Neuropathology of Rett syndrome. Ment Retard Dev Disabil Res Rev. 2002;8(2):72–6.
206. Carter JC, Lanham DC, Pham D, Bibat G, Naidu S, Kaufmann WE. Selective cerebral volume reduction in Rett syndrome: a multiple-approach MR imaging study. AJNR Am J Neuroradiol. 2008;29(3):436–41.
207. Dunn HG, Stoessl AJ, Ho HH, MacLeod PM, Poskitt KJ, Doudet DJ, Schulzer M, Blackstock D, Dobko T, Koop B, de Amorim GV. Rett syndrome: investigation of nine patients, including PET scan. Can J Neurol Sci. 2002;29(4):345–57.
208. Khong PL, Lam CW, Ooi CG, Ko CH, Wong VC. Magnetic resonance spectroscopy and analysis of MECP2 in Rett syndrome. Pediatr Neurol. 2002;26(3):205–9.
209. Gökcay A, Kitis O, Ekmekci O, Karasoy H, Sener RN. Proton MR spectroscopy in Rett syndrome. Comput Med Imaging Graph. 2002;26(4):271–5.
210. Smith DW, Lemli L, Opitz J. A newly recognized syndrome of multiple congenital anomalies. J Pediatr. 1964;64:210–7.
211. Irons M, Elias ER, Salen G, Batta AK, Frieden R, Chen TS, Salen G. Defective cholesterol biosynthesis in Smith-Lemli-Opitz syndrome. Lancet. 1993;341(8857):1414.
212. Trasimeni G, Di Biasi C, Iannilli M, Orlandi L, Boscherini B, Balducci R, Gualdi GF. MRI in Smith-Lemli-Opitz syndrome type I. Childs Nerv Syst. 1997;13(1):47–9.
213. Kelley RL, Roessler E, Hennekam RC, Feldman GL, Kosaki K, Jones MC, Palumbos JC, Muenke M. Holoprosencephaly in RSH/Smith-Lemli-Opitz syndrome: does abnormal cholesterol metabolism affect the function of Sonic Hedgehog? Am J Med Genet. 1996;66(4):478–84.
214. Lee RW, Conley SK, Gropman A, Porter FD, Baker EH. Brain magnetic resonance imaging findings in Smith-Lemili-Opitz syndrome. Am J Med Genet A. 2013;161(10):2407–19.
215. Lee RW, Yoshida S, Jung ES, Mori S, Baker EH, Porter FD. Corpus callosum measurements correlate with developmental delay in Smith-Lemli-Opitz syndrome. Pediatr Neurol. 2013;49(2):107–12.
216. Fitoz S, Atasoy C, Deda G, Erden I, Akyar S. Hippocampal malrotation with normal corpus callosum in a child with Opitz syndrome. Clin Imaging. 2003;27(2):75–6.
217. Caruso PA, Poussaint TY, Tzika AA, Zurakowski D, Astrakas LG, Elias ER, Bay C, Irons MB. MRI and 1H MRS findings in Smith-Lemli-Opitz syndrome. Neuroradiology. 2004;46(1):3–14.
218. Rodriguez D, Gauthier F, Bertini E, Bugiani M, Brenner M, N'guyen S, Goizet C, Gelot A, Surtees R, Pedespan JM, Hernandorena X, Troncoso M, Uziel G, Messing A, Ponsot G, Pham-Dinh D, Dautigny A, Boespflug-Tanguy O. Infantile Alexander disease: spectrum of GFAP mutations and genotype-phenotype correlation. Am J Hum Genet. 2001;69(5):1134–40.
219. van der Knaap MS, Naidu S, Breiter SN, Blaser S, Stroink H, Springer S, Begeer JC, van Coster R, Barth PG, Thomas NH, Valk J, Powers JM. Alexander disease: diagnosis with MR imaging. AJNR Am J Neuroradiol. 2001;22(3):541–52.
220. Gorospe JR, Naidu S, Johnson AB, Puri V, Raymond GV, Jenkins SD, Pedersen RC, Lewis D, Knowles P, Fernandez R, De Vivo D, van der Knaap MS, Messing A, Brenner M, Hoffman EP. Molecular findings in symptomatic and pre-symptomatic Alexander disease patients. Neurology. 2002;58(10):1494–500.
221. Johnson AB, Brenner M. Alexander's disease: clinical, pathologic, and genetic features. J Child Neurol. 2003;18(9):625–32.
222. Li R, Johnson AB, Salomons G, Goldman JE, Naidu S, Quinlan R, Cree B, Ruyle SZ, Banwell B, D'Hooghe M, Siebert JR, Rolf CM, Cox H, Reddy A, Gutiérrez-Solana LG, Collins A, Weller RO, Messing A, van der Knaap MS, Brenner M. Glial fibrillary acidic protein mutations in infantile, juvenile, and adult forms of Alexander disease. Ann Neurol. 2005;57(3):310–26.
223. Prust M, Wang J, Morizono H, Messing A, Brenner M, Gordon E, Hartka T, Sokohl A, Schiffmann R, Gordish-Dressman H, Albin R, Amartino H, Brockman K, Dinopoulos A, Dotti MT, Fain D, Fernandez R, Ferreira J, Fleming J, Gill D, Griebel M, Heilstedt H, Kaplan P, Lewis D, Nakagawa M, Pedersen R, Reddy A, Sawaishi Y, Schneider M, Sherr E, Takiyama Y, Wakabayashi K, Gorospe JR, Vanderver A. GFAP mutations, age at onset, and clinical subtypes in Alexander disease. Neurology. 2011;77(13):1287–94.
224. van der Knaap MS, Salomons GS, Li R, Franzoni E, Gutiérrez-Solana LG, Smit LM, Robinson R, Ferrie CD, Cree B, Reddy A, Thomas N, Banwell B, Barkhof F, Jakobs C, Johnson A, Messing A, Brenner M. Unusual variants of Alexander's disease. Ann Neurol. 2005;57(3):327–38.
225. Ni Q, Johns GS, Manepalli A, Martin DS, Geller TJ. Infantile Alexander's disease: serial neuroradiologic findings. J Child Neurol. 2002;17(6):463–6.
226. Mignot C, Desguerre I, Burglen L, Hertz-Pannier L, Renaldo F, Gadisseux JF, Gallet S, Pham-Dinh D, Boespflug-Tanguy O, Rodriguez D. Tumor-like enlargement of the optic chiasm in an infant

with Alexander disease. Brain and Development. 2009;31(3):244–7.
227. Van Poppel K, Broniscer A, Patay Z, Morris EB. Alexander disease: an important mimicker of focal brainstem glioma. Pediatr Blood Cancer. 2009;53(7):1355–6.
228. Biancheri R, Rossi A, Ceccherini I, Pezzella M, Prato G, Striano P, Minetti C. Magnetic resonance imaging "tigroid pattern" in Alexander disease. Neuropediatrics. 2013;44(3):174–6.
229. Imamura A, Orii KE, Mizuno S, Hoshi H, Kondo T. MR imaging and 1H-MR spectroscopy in a case of juvenile Alexander disease. Brain and Development. 2002;24(7):723–6.
230. Brockmann K, Dechent P, Meins M, Haupt M, Sperner J, Stephani U, Frahm J, Hanefeld F. Cerebral proton magnetic resonance spectroscopy in infantile Alexander disease. J Neurol. 2003;250(3):300–6.
231. Bassuk AG, Joshi A, Burton BK, Larsen MB, Burrowes DM, Stack C. Alexander disease with serial MRS and a new mutation in the glial fibrillary acidic protein gene. Neurology. 2003;61(7):1014–5.
232. van der Voorn JP, Pouwels PJ, Salomons GS, Barkhof F, van der Knaap MS. Unraveling pathology in juvenile Alexander disease: serial quantitative MR imaging and spectroscopy of white matter. Neuroradiology. 2009;51(10):669–75.
233. Nelson A, Kelley RE, Nguyen J, Palacios E, Neitzschman HR. MRS findings in a patient with juvenile-onset Alexander's leukodystrophy. J La State Med Soc. 2013;165(1):14–7.
234. Bhat MD, Bindu PS, Christopher R, Prasad C, Verma A. Novel imaging findings in two cases of biotinidase deficiency-a treatable metabolic disorder. Metab Brain Dis. 2015;30(5):1291–4.
235. Desai S, Ganesan K, Hegde A. Biotinidase deficiency: a reversible metabolic encephalopathy. Pediatr Radiol. 2008;38(8):848–56.
236. Burton BK, Roach ES, Wolf B, Weissbecker KA. Sudden death associated with biotinidase deficiency. Pediatrics. 1987;79:482–3.
237. Baykal T, Gokcay G, Gokdemir Y, Demir F, Seckin Y, Demirkol M, Jensen K, Wolf B. Asymptomatic adults and older siblings with biotinidase deficiency ascertained by family studies of index cases. J Inherit Metab Dis. 2005;28:903–12.
238. Wiznitzer M, Bangert BA. Biotinidase deficiency: clinical and MRI findings consistent with myelopathy. Pediatr Neurol. 2003;29(1):56–8.
239. Yang Y, Li C, Qi Z, Xiao J, Zhang Y, Yamaguchi S, Hasegawa Y, Tagami Y, Jiang Y, Xiong H, Zhang Y, Qin J, Wu XR. Spinal cord demyelination associated with biotinidase deficiency in 3 Chinese patients. J Child Neurol. 2007;22(2):156–60.
240. Mc Sweeney N, Grunewald S, Bhate S, Ganesan V, Chong WK, Hemingway C. Two unusual clinical and radiological presentations of biotinidase deficiency. Eur J Paediatr Neurol. 2010;14(6):535–8.
241. Cabasson S, Rivera S, Mesli S, Dulubac E. Brainstem and spinal cord lesions associated with skin changes and hearing loss: think of biotinidase deficiency. J Pediatr. 2015;166(3):771–1.e1.
242. Bottin L, Prud'hon S, Guey S, Giannesini C, Wolf B, Pindolia K, Stankoff B. Biotinidase deficiency mimicking neuromyelitis optica: initially exhibiting symptoms in adulthood. Mult Scler. 2015;21(12):1604–7.
243. Soares-Fernandes JP, Magalhães Z, Rocha JF, Barkovich AJ. Brain diffusion-weighted and diffusion tensor imaging findings in an infant with biotinidase deficiency. AJNR Am J Neuroradiol. 2009;30(9):E12.
244. Bunch M, Singh A. Peculiar neuroimaging and electrophysiological findings in a patient with biotinidase deficiency. Seizure. 2011;20(1):83–6.
245. Ginat-Israeli T, Hurvitz H, Klar A, Blinder G, Branski D, Amir N. Deteriorating neurological and neuroradiological course in treated biotinidase deficiency. Neuropediatrics. 1993;24(2):103–6.
246. Bousounis DP, Camfield PR, Wolf B. Reversal of brain atrophy with biotin treatment in biotinidase deficiency. Neuropediatrics. 1993;24(4):214–7.
247. Haagerup A, Andersen JB, Blichfeldt S, Christensen MF. Biotinidase deficiency: two cases of very early presentation. Dev Med Child Neurol. 1997;39(12):832–5.
248. Hoffman TL, Simon EM, Ficicioglu C. Biotinidase deficiency: the importance of adequate follow-up for an inconclusive newborn screening result. Eur J Pediatr. 2005;164(5):298–301.
249. Schürmann M, Engelbrecht V, Lohmeier K, Lenard HG, Wendel U, Gärtner J. Cerebral metabolic changes in biotinidase deficiency. J Inherit Metab Dis. 1997;20(6):755–60.

Index

J.S. Lewis, K.R. Keshari (eds.), *Imaging and Metabolism*, DOI 10.1007/978-3-319-61401-4

N

MIX
Papier aus verantwortungsvollen Quellen
Paper from responsible sources
FSC® C105338

If you have any concerns about our products,
you can contact us on
ProductSafety@springernature.com

In case Publisher is established outside the EU,
the EU authorized representative is:
Springer Nature Customer Service Center GmbH
Europaplatz 3, 69115 Heidelberg, Germany

Printed by Libri Plureos GmbH
in Hamburg, Germany